fMRI

Stephan Ulmer • Olav Jansen
Editors

fMRI

Basics and Clinical Applications

Third Edition

Springer

Editors
Stephan Ulmer
Department of Radiology
and Nuclear Medicine
Kantonsspital Winterthur
Winterthur, Switzerland

neurorad.ch
Zurich, Switzerland

Department of Radiology
and Neuroradiology
University Hospital Schleswig-Holstein
Kiel, Germany

Olav Jansen
Department of Radiology
and Neuroradiology
University Hospital Schleswig-Holstein
Kiel, Germany

ISBN 978-3-030-41876-2 ISBN 978-3-030-41874-8 (eBook)
https://doi.org/10.1007/978-3-030-41874-8

This Springer imprint is published by the registered company Springer Nature Switzerland AG
The registered company address is: Gewerbestrasse 11, 6330 Cham, Switzerland

Contents

Part I Basics

1 **Introduction** 3
Stephan Ulmer

2 **Neuroanatomy and Cortical Landmarks** 5
Stephan Ulmer

3 **The Electrophysiological Background of the fMRI Signal** 15
Christoph Kayser and Nikos K. Logothetis

4 **High-Field fMRI** 29
Elke R. Gizewski

5 **Resting-State fMRI: Preclinical Foundations** 47
Jonathan D. Power

6 **Spatial Resolution of fMRI Techniques** 65
Seong-Gi Kim, Tao Jin, and Mitsuhiro Fukuda

7 **Acquisition Aspects of Functional and Clinical Arterial Spin Labeling** 73
Dimo Ivanov and Yanina Kozovska

8 **fMRI Data Analysis Using SPM** 89
Guillaume Flandin and Marianne J. U. Novak

9 **Meta-Analyses in Basic and Clinical Neuroscience: State of the Art and Perspective** 117
Simon B. Eickhoff, Julius Kernbach, and Danilo Bzdok

Part II Clinical Applications

10 **Special Issues in fMRI Involving Children** 133
Lucie Hertz-Pannier and Marion Noulhiane

11 **Multimodal Brain Mapping in Patients with Early Brain Lesions** 149
Martin Staudt

12 Combining Transcranial Magnetic Stimulation with (f)MRI . . . 157
Gesa Hartwigsen, Tanja Kassuba, and Hartwig R. Siebner

13 Simultaneous EEG and fMRI Recordings (EEG–fMRI) 175
Friederike Moeller, Michael Siniatchkin, and Jean Gotman

14 Imaging Epileptic Seizures Using fMRI 193
David N. Vaughan and Graeme D. Jackson

15 The Functional Anatomy of Speech Processing: From Auditory Cortex to Speech Recognition and Speech Production 217
Gregory Hickok

16 Mapping of Recovery from Poststroke Aphasia: Comparison of PET and fMRI 225
Wolf-Dieter Heiss

17 Use of fMRI Language Lateralization for Quantitative Prediction of Naming and Verbal Memory Outcome in Left Temporal Lobe Epilepsy Surgery 241
Jeffrey R. Binder

18 Preoperative Blood Oxygen Level-Dependent (BOLD) Functional Magnetic Resonance Imaging (fMRI) of Motor and Somatosensory Function 265
Christoph Stippich and Anthony Tyndall

19 Resting State Functional MRI for Presurgical Planning 287
Joshua S. Shimony, Eric C. Leuthardt, Donna Dierker, Ki-Yun Park, Carl D. Hacker, and Abraham Z. Snyder

20 Functional Magnetic Resonance-Guided Resection of Intra-Axial Brain Tumors 303
Alexa Bodman and Walter Hall

21 Direct Cortical Stimulation and fMRI 311
H. Maximilian Mehdorn, Simone Goebel, and Arya Nabavi

22 Modeling Connectivity in Health and Disease: Examples from the Motor System 321
Simon B. Eickhoff and Christian Grefkes

23 Resting-State fMRI in Multiple Sclerosis 335
Maria A. Rocca, Ermelinda De Meo, and Massimo Filippi

24 The Perirhinal, Entorhinal, and Parahippocampal Cortices and Hippocampus: An Overview of Functional Anatomy and Protocol for Their Segmentation in MR Images 355
Sasa L. Kivisaari, Alphonse Probst, and Kirsten I. Taylor

25 Brain Network Functional Connectivity in Alzheimer's Disease and Frontotemporal Dementia 385
Juan Helen Zhou, Kwun Kei Ng, and Siwei Liu

26 fMRI in Parkinson's Disease 417
Hartwig R. Siebner, David Meder, and Damian M. Herz

27 Incidental Findings in Neuroimaging Research: Ethical Considerations 433
Stephan Ulmer, Thomas C. Booth, Guy Widdershoven, Olav Jansen, Gunther Fesl, Rüdiger von Kummer, and Stella Reiter-Theil

Index 441

Part I

Basics

1 Introduction

Stephan Ulmer

Thirty years ago, the very basic idea of fMRI has been introduced by Ogawa using T2*-weighted images to map changes in blood oxygenation. Since then the technique, paradigms, study designs, and analyzing software have evolved tremendously. Besides its application in basic brain research, it became a very powerful tool in daily clinical routine, especially in presurgical mapping. For the third time, his book focuses on these clinical applications starting from basics and the background, presenting current concepts and their application in a clinical setting.

Understanding brain function and localizing functional areas have ever since been the goal in neuroscience, and fMRI is a very powerful tool to approach this aim. Studies on healthy volunteers usually have a different approach and often a very complex study design, while clinical applications face other problems most commonly related to the limited compliance of the patients. Therefore, the application of fMRI in a clinical setting is a different challenge reflected in the study designs as well as in the analysis of algorithms of the data. Resting-state fMRI will open a new gate in clinical routine. As of now task-related fMRI, i.e., in motor tasks is more robust, but there always have been and will be modifications and improvements. fMRI using ASL might be a new approach. Also, we have learned that it's not a functional area but networks we're dealing with and functional connectivity is important.

Besides the classical definition of functional areas (such as motor- and language-related areas) that might have been shifted through a lesion or could be located in a distorted anatomy prior to neurosurgical resection, further clinical applications are mapping of recovery from stroke or trauma; cortical reorganization, if these areas were affected; and changes during the development of the brain or during the course of a disease. For psychiatric disorders fMRI offers new horizons in understanding the disease. fMRI also helps us to learn about Parkinson's disease and neurodegeneration such as Alzheimer's disease or frontotemporal dementia and changes associated with these diseases. There is also a gap between imaging and clinical findings in multiple sclerosis. Using fMRI, we can monitor functional adaptive or maladaptive reorganization that might help to develop therapeutic strategies. Understanding disorders such as epilepsy, we can now address what fMRI reveals about seizures directly from its onset in the interictal period, through to full clinical expression of the event and eventual termination, although there are technical challenges to do so.

Mapping children represents a twofold challenge. Normative data is not available, and com-

S. Ulmer (✉)
Department of Radiology and Nuclear Medicine, Kantonsspital Winterthur, Winterthur, Switzerland

neurorad.ch, Zurich, Switzerland

Department of Radiology and Neuroradiology, University Hospital Schleswig-Holstein, Kiel, Germany

S. Ulmer, O. Jansen (eds.), *fMRI*, https://doi.org/10.1007/978-3-030-41874-8_1

pliance is limited. In early childhood or in cognitively impaired children or just simply during brain development, cognitive tasks need to be modified individually, and that again causes problems in analyzing the data and interpreting the results.

Knowledge of basic neuroanatomy and understanding of the electrophysiological background of the fMRI signal, the physiology, and especially the possible pathophysiology of a disease that might affect the results are mandatory. Therefore, we need the results in healthy volunteers to understand the results in patients. In task-related fMRI, we need to monitor the patient in the scanner to guarantee that the results obtained will reflect activation caused by the stimulation, or why there is reduced or even missing activation. While the patient is still in the scanner, a repetition of the measurement can be performed; however, sometimes patients are not capable of performing the task. Here again resting-state fMRI might offer completely new options. A vascular stenosis or the steal effects of a brain tumor or an arteriovenous malformation (AVM) might corrupt the results. There are other sources of disturbance that might influence the results. For us interdisciplinary cooperation was and is the key.

Analyzing data is a science on its own. Fortunately, there is a variety of software solutions available free of charge for the most part. Task-synchronous or singular voluntary head motion during the experiment might corrupt the data to an extent that excludes a reliable interpretation of the data. Better than any available motion correction is avoidance of head movement altogether. As already stated, absence of an expected activation represents a real challenge and raises the question of the reliability of the method per se. Suppression of activation or task-related signal intensity decrease has also not been fully understood. Missing activation in a language task could mislead the neurosurgeon to resect a low-grade lesion close to the inferior frontal lobe and cause speech disturbance or memory loss after resection of a lesion close to the mesial temporal lobe, and therefore – depending on the close cooperation between the clinicians – healthy skepticism and combination with other modalities like direct cortical stimulation might be advisory. Comparison to other modalities of mapping brain functions will also be covered in detail. Again, resting-state fMRI will become more important in presurgical planning.

Prior to the introduction of echo planar imaging, temporal resolution was restricted. Spatial resolution requirements are much more important in individual cases than in a healthy control group, especially in the presurgical definition of the so-called eloquent areas. Higher field strengths might enable us to depict more signals but also more noise in the data as well.

With this book we try to answer some questions and give an overview on how fMRI can be applied for clinical purposes. It is a great honor for me to have this board of experts in the field involved in this project. I hope that you as a reader will enjoy this book as much as I have and that it will help you in your own daily work.

Neuroanatomy and Cortical Landmarks

2

Stephan Ulmer

2.1 Neuroanatomy and Cortical Landmarks of Functional Areas

Prior to any type of functional mapping, a profound knowledge of neuroanatomy is mandatory. Focusing on the clinical applications of fMRI, this chapter will present methods to identify characteristic anatomical landmarks and describe the course and shape of some gyri and sulci and how they can be recognized on MR imaging. As anatomy will be presented in neurofunctional systems, some redundancy is desired in order to course over cortical landmarks. If fMRI is not performed during clinical routine imaging, usually a 3D data set is acquired to overlay the results. Nowadays, fMRI is performed using echo planar imaging (EPI)(EPI) with anisotropic distortion, whereas 3D T1-weighted data sets, such as MPRAGE (magnetization-prepared rapid acquisition gradient echo) or SPGR (spoiled gradient-recalled acquisition in steady state) sequences, are usually isotropic. Normalization of the fMRI data may reduce this systemic error to some extent that is more pronounced at the very frontal aspect of the frontal lobe and the very posterior aspect of the occipital lobe. However, for individual data, normalization and overlaying fMRI results on anatomy remain crucial. No two brains, not even the two hemispheres within one subject, are identical at a macroscopic level, and anatomical templates represent only a compromise (Devlin and Poldrack 2007). Usage of templates like the Talairach space (based on the anatomy of one brain) or the MNI template (based on 305 brains) can cause registration error as well as additional variation and reduce accuracy; indeed, it does not warrant the shammed anatomical precision in the individual case.

2.1.1 Sensorimotor Cortex

2.1.1.1 Transverse Sections

There are various methods to identify the precentral gyrus (preCG; [3]), the central sulcus (CS) and the postcentral gyrus (postCG; [4]). From a craniocaudal point of view, the sensorimotor strip follows (from the apex to the Sylvian fissure [35b]) a medial-posterior-superior to lateral-anterior-inferior course. The precentral gyrus [3] fuses with the superior frontal gyrus (SFG; [1]) at the very upper convexity (Ebeling et al. 1986; Kido et al. 1980; Naidich et al. 1995; Ono et al. 1990). This can be well depicted on transverse sections (see Figs. 2.1 and 2.2). The precentral gyrus [3] is the most posterior part of the frontal lobe that extends inferiorly to the Sylvian fissure

S. Ulmer (✉)
Department of Radiology and Nuclear Medicine, Kantonsspital Winterthur, Winterthur, Switzerland

neurorad.ch, Zurich, Switzerland

Department of Radiology and Neuroradiology, University Hospital Schleswig-Holstein, Kiel, Germany

S. Ulmer, O. Jansen (eds.), *fMRI*, https://doi.org/10.1007/978-3-030-41874-8_2

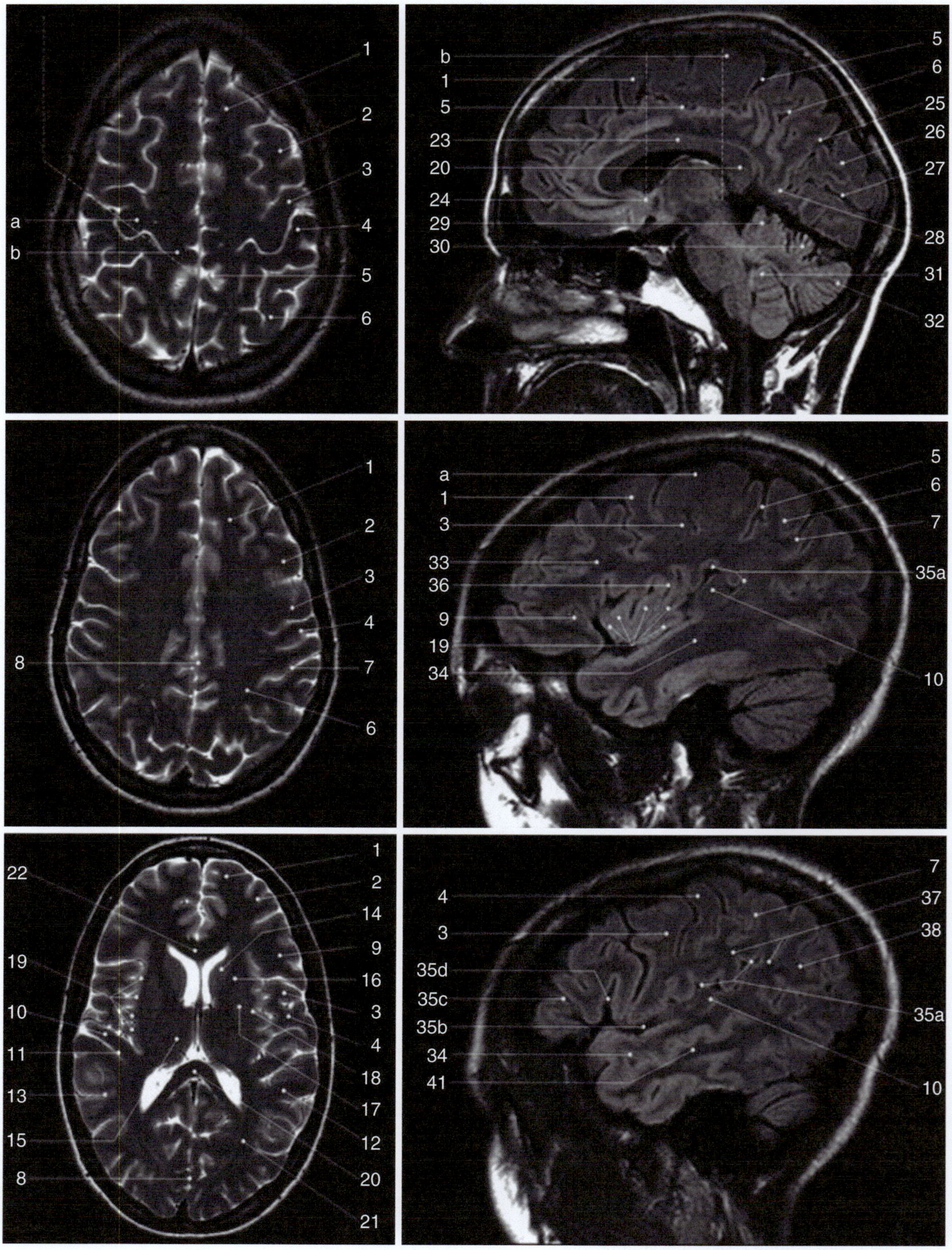

Fig. 2.1 Overview of the used sections. The numbers are explained within the text as well as in the other figure legends in detail

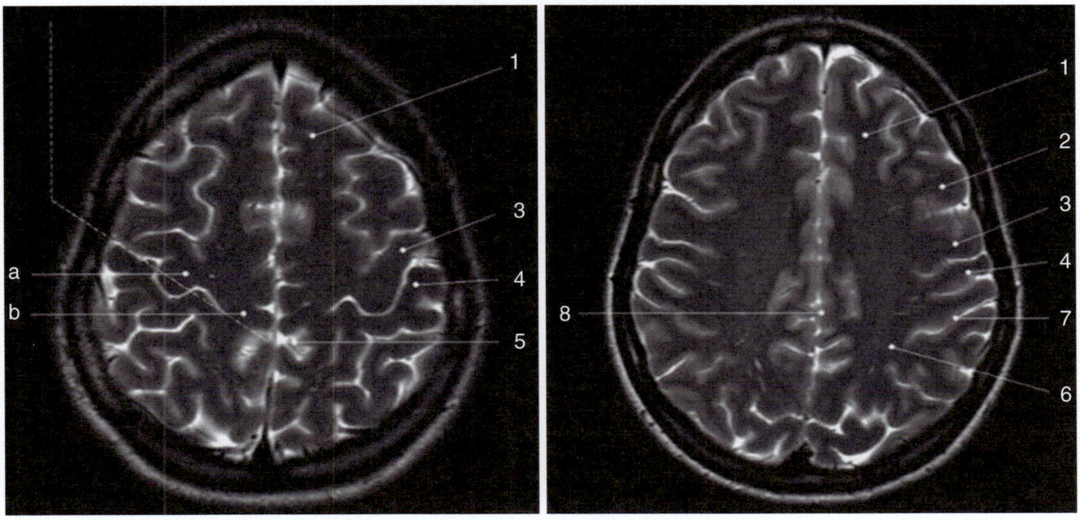

Fig. 2.2 Axial T2-weighted TSE MR images. *1* superior frontal gyrus; *2* medial frontal gyrus; *3* precentral gyrus; *4* postcentral gyrus; *5* "pars bracket," cingulated sulcus; *6* precuneus, parietal lobe; *7* intraparietal sulcus; *8* interhemispheric fissure; *a* hand knob; *b* paracentral lobule

[35b]. The precentral gyrus [3] is thicker than the postcentral gyrus [4] in anterior-posterior (ap) dimension (Naidich et al. 1995) as is the grey matter (Meyer et al. 1996). At the apex, the pre- [3] and postcentral gyri [4] form the paracentral lobule [b] as they fuse. Making a little detour to a lateral view (see Fig. 2.3), the cingulate sulcus [5] ascends at the medial interhemispheric surface dorsal to the paracentral lobule (pars marginalis) [b] and thus separates it from the precuneus [6]. This intersection can be appreciated on axial sections as the "bracket" sign (see Fig. 2.2; Naidich and Brightbill 1996) that borders the postcentral gyrus [4]. Somatotopographically, the apex harbours the cortical representation the lower extremity (Penfield and Rasmussen 1950). Following its course along the superficial convexity (from medial-posterior-superior to lateral-anterior-inferior), the cortical surface of the precentral gyrus increases at its posterior margin, building the omega-shaped motor hand knob ([a]; Yousry et al. 1995, 1997). Within this primary motor cortex (M1) of the hand, there is an additional somatotopic order of the individual digits (with interindividual overlap and variation). From medial to lateral, the hand

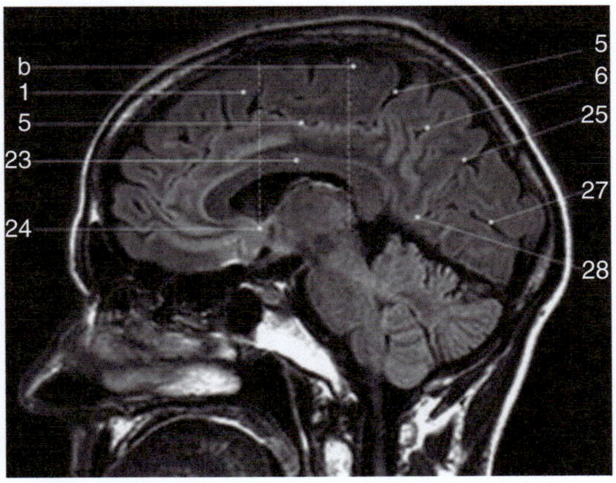

Fig. 2.3 Sagittal FLAIR image at the midline. *1* superior frontal gyrus; *5* "pars bracket," cingulate sulcus; *6* precuneus, parietal lobe; *23* body of the corpus callosum; *24* anterior commissure; *25* parietooccipital sulcus; *27* calcarine fissure; *b* paracentral lobule; *28* cuneal point

is organized beginning with digit 5 (D5) to the thumb representation (D1) being the most lateral (Dechent and Frahm 2003). The motor hand knob [a] is another typical landmark of the precentral gyrus [3]; however, as the CS and the postcentral gyrus [4] follow this course, there is also an omega-shaped structure in the postcentral gyrus (harbouring the somatosensory hand area). However, as described above, the ap-dimension of the postcentral gyrus [4] is smaller compared to the precentral gyrus [3], thus often enabling a differentiation. Somatotopographically, the cortical somatosensory representation follows the distribution of the precentral gyrus [3] (Penfield and Rasmussen 1950; Overduin and Servos 2004). Lateral to the SFG [1], the medial frontal gyrus [2] zigzags posteriorly and points towards the motor hand knob [a]. Beginning at this "junction" and lateral-inferior to this landmark, the ap-diameter of the preCG [3] decreases, but it increases again along the lower convexity. This has already been recognized by Eberstaller (1890). Using modern imaging techniques, the diameter had been measured, and the previous findings validated that the biggest diameter of the preCG [3] is found at the lower portion of the gyrus adjacent to the Sylvian fissure [35b] (Ono et al. 1990). This is the primary motor cortex (M1) of lip representation and tongue movements. In the axial sections, there is neither a typical shape or landmark of the gyrus nor measuring from the motor hand area or the ac (anterior commissure) that helps us to describe the location precisely. This can be solved on sagittal sections (see below).

Previously, the anatomy of the frontal lobe has been described partially. As the course of the medial frontal gyrus [2] can be followed nicely on axial sections, the lateral inferior aspect of the frontal lobe represents the inferior frontal gyrus. Anterior to the preCG [3], the prefrontal motor areas can be found. The inferior frontal gyrus borders and overhangs the insula [19] anteriorly. This part is the frontal operculum [9] harbouring the motor speech area of Broca (see below sagittal sections). The lateral ventricles with its anterior and posterior horn can easily be depicted on axial sections due to its typical form and typical signal caused by corticospinal fluid (CSF, see Figs. 2.1, 2.5 and 2.6). Their shape is formed through the head of the caudate nucleus [10] lateral to the anterior horn, the thalamus [11] lateral at its waist (III. ventricle) and posteriorly by the fibres of the antero-posteriorly running optic radiation [21] and left-right running fibres of the splenium [20] (see Figs. 2.5 and 2.6). Lateral to these structures, descending corticospinal fibres pass the internal capsule [16] and follow a certain somatotopic organization. The internal capsule is framed medial by the head of the caudate nucleus [10], the third ventricle and the thalamus [11] (at the posterior aspect of the third ventricle) and lateral by the globus pallidus [17]. From medial to lateral towards the insula [19], the globus pallidus, putamen and claustrum within the lentiform nucleus [17] can be differentiated. In the anterior limb and the genu of the internal capsule [16], corticospinal fibres from the tongue, lip and face descend, whereas in the posterior limb, fibres from the upper extremity, body and finally lower extremity are found.

2.1.1.2 Sagittal Sections

Previously sagittal sections have been described at the interhemispheric surface (see Fig. 2.3). The corpus callosum [20, 22, 23] represents the biggest connection between the two hemispheres. The frontal aspect is the genu [22], the medial part is the body [23], and the most rostral part is the splenium [20]. The corpus callosum encases the lateral ventricles. At the base, the anterior commissure (ac; [24]) can be identified as a roundish structure. Sometimes, the posterior commissure (pc) can also be defined, which represents a bundle of white fibres crossing the midline, at the dorsal aspect of the upper end of the cerebral aqueduct. Previously slice orientation of most fMRI studies had been performed according to this ac-pc line in order to have a reference system.

From the base to the apex, the corpus callosum is abutted by the callosal sulcus and the cingulate gyrus. The gyrus abutting the cingulate sulcus [5] is the medial part of the SFG [1]. In the region (at the medial cortical surface) framed by vertical lines perpendicular to the ac (Vac) or pc (Vpc; see Fig. 2.3), the supplementary motor area (SMA) is harboured in the cingulate gyrus and superior frontal gyrus. As described above, the cingulate sulcus [5] ascends at the medial interhemispheric surface (see Fig. 2.3) dorsal to the paracentral lobule ([b]; pars marginalis) and thus separates it from the precuneus [6]. This intersection can be can be nicely appreciated on axial sections as the "bracket" sign (see Fig. 2.2; Naidich and Brightbill 1996) that borders the postcentral gyrus [4]. The postcentral gyrus is already a part of the parietal lobe. The precuneus [6] is located dorsal to the postcentral sulcus. There is another important landmark that separates the parietal lobe from the occipital lobe (cuneus [26]), the parietooccipital sulcus [25]. It can be easy recognized in sagittal views (see Fig. 2.3), as the dorsal sulcus that follows an inferior-anterior to superior-posterior course, posterior to the ascending part of the cingulate sulcus [5]. It is advisable to follow one of these structures moving laterally through the brain in sagittal sections. Once the Sylvian fissure [35b] can be identified, anatomical landmarks are again easy to define.

In midsagittal sections (see Fig. 2.6), the motor hand knob [a] can again be recognized as a "hook" that rises out of the parenchyma and points dorsally. Further, laterally the sensorimotor cortex overhangs the insula [19]. The Sylvian fissure [35b] that separates the frontal lobe and the temporal lobe has an inferior-anterior to superior-posterior course. At its anterior margin, it ascends into the anterior horizontal ramus [35c] and more dorsally into the anterior ascending ramus [35d] of the frontal operculum [9] that also overhangs the anterior aspect of the insula [19]. The anterior horizontal ramus [35c] separates the pars orbitalis [40] from the pars triangularis [39], whereas the anterior ascending ramus [35d] separates the pars triangularis [39] from the pars opercularis [9] of the frontal operculum of the inferior frontal gyrus and thus forms an "M" (Naidich et al. 1995). The pars opercularis [9] of the frontal operculum of the inferior frontal lobe harbours Broca's area. At its posterior margin, the pars opercularis is delimited by the anterior subcentral sulcus. At the base of the sensorimotor strip, the precentral [3] and postcentral gyrus [4] fuse (Eberstaller 1890; Ono et al. 1990). This junction is delimited dorsally by the posterior subcentral sulcus. Movement of the lips or tongue induces an increase in BOLD signal at this portion (Fesl et al. 2003, own observations). The base of the sensorimotor area has, depending on anatomical variations, a "K" or an "N" shape that is built by the anterior subcentral sulcus and inferior precentral sulcus, the precentral gyrus, posterior subcentral sulcus, postcentral gyrus and postcentral sulcus that again borders the angular gyrus [38] (Eberstaller 1890; Ono et al. 1990, own observations; see Fig. 2.6). The posterior part of the Sylvian fissure separates—following its superior-posterior course—and ascends into the posterior ascending ramus [35a] flanked by the anterior and posterior aspect of the supramarginal gyrus [37] that has a horseshoe appearance.

2.1.2 The Insula

The insula [19] is covered by the superior temporal gyrus [34], the frontal operculum [9] and the base of the sensorimotor strip. Its anatomy is best depicted in sagittal sections (see Fig. 2.6).

2.1.2.1 Sagittal Sections

The insula [19] is separated by the CS [36] that runs from the superior-posterior towards the inferior-anterior located apex of the insula into an anterior lobule and a posterior lobule (see Fig. 2.6). The anterior lobule consists of three gyri (anterior, medial and posterior short insular gyri); the posterior lobule consists of two gyri, the anterior long insular gyrus and the posterior long insular gyrus separated by the postcentral gyrus (Naidich et al. 2004).

From a neurofunctional point of view, the insula has various functional areas. The anterior lobule was found to cause word-finding difficulties during electrical stimulation in epilepsy surgery (Ojemann and Whitaker 1978a, b) and to be responsible for speech planning (Wise et al. 1999; Price 2000). Speech apraxia is induced through lesions in the left precentral gyrus of the insula (Dronkers 1996; Nagao et al. 1999), whereas the right anterior lobule becomes activated during vocal repetition of nonlyrical tunes (Riecker et al. 2000). Stimulation of the right insula increases sympathetic tone, and stimulation of the left insula increases parasympathetic tone (Oppenheimer 1993), possibly playing a role in cardiac mortality in left insular stroke. Finally visual-vestibular interactions have been found (Brandt et al. 1998) to name a few systems.

2.1.2.2 Transverse Sections

The insular cortex [19] is delimited medially by the globus pallidus, putamen and claustrum (lentiform nucleus [17]) and separated by a small border of white matter (extreme capsule [18]). The gyri can be differentiated by counting each knob starting ventrally at the anterior peri-insular sulcus that abuts the pars opercularis [9] of the frontal operculum of the inferior frontal gyrus (see Figs. 2.4 and 2.5). Five knobs can be defined (anterior, medial and posterior short insular gyri and anterior and posterior long insular gyri).

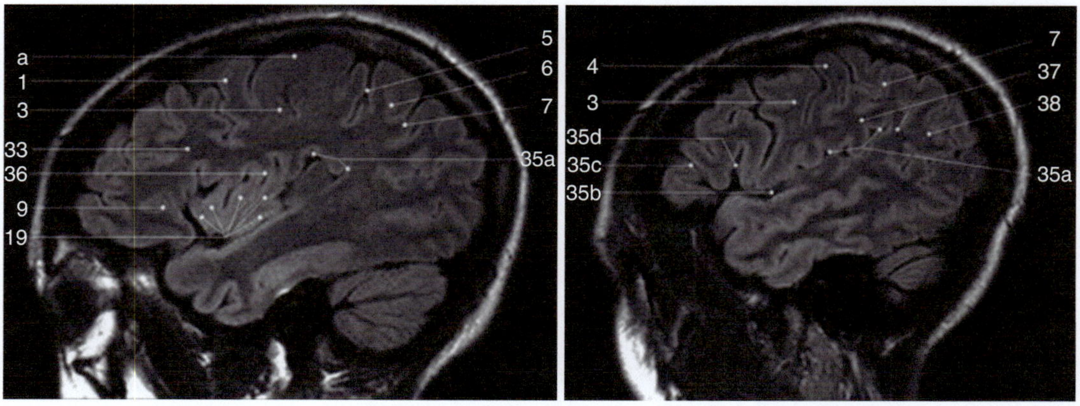

Fig. 2.4 Sagittal FLAIR images. *1* superior frontal gyrus; *3* precentral gyrus; *4* postcentral gyrus; *5* "pars bracket," cingulate sulcus; *6* precuneus, parietal lobe; *7* intraparietal sulcus; *9* pars opercularis, inferior frontal lobe, frontal operculum; *19* insula (anterior and posterior short insular gyri, anterior and posterior long insular gyri); *33* medial frontal gyrus; *35a* posterior ascending ramus of the Sylvian fissure; *35b* Sylvian fissure; *35c* anterior horizontal ramus of the Sylvian fissure; *35d* anterior ascending ramus of the Sylvian fissure; *36* central sulcus of the insula; *37* supramarginal gyrus; *38* angular gyrus; *a* hand knob

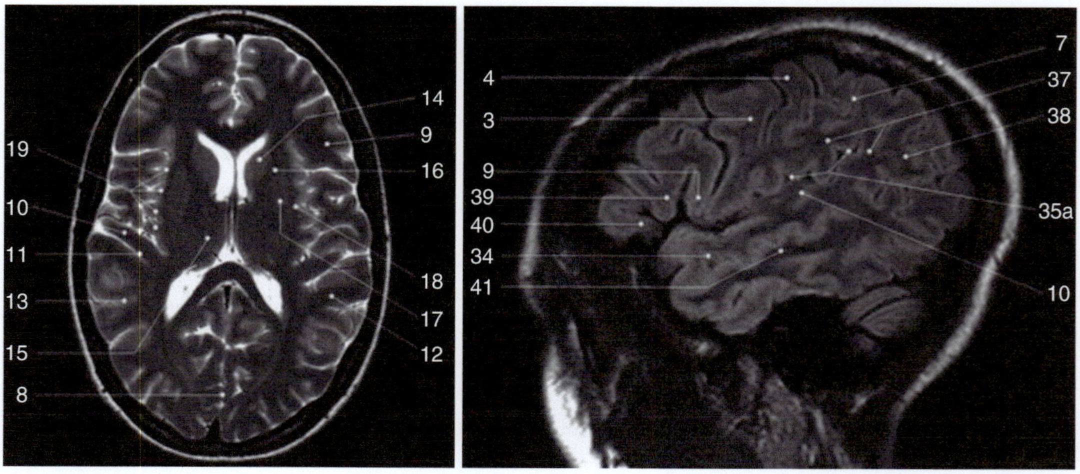

Fig. 2.5 Axial T2-weighted TSE MR and sagittal FLAIR images. *3* precentral gyrus; *4* postcentral gyrus; *7* intraparietal sulcus; *8* interhemispheric fissure; *9* pars opercularis, inferior frontal lobe, frontal operculum; *10* Heschl's gyrus; *11* Heschl's sulcus; *12* planum temporale; *13* superior temporal sulcus; *14* head of the caudate nucleus; *15* thalamus; *16* internal capsule; *17* globus pallidus, putamen, claustrum (lentiform nucleus); *18* extreme capsule; *19* insula (anterior and posterior short insular gyri, anterior and posterior long insular gyri); *34* superior temporal gyrus; *35a* posterior ascending ramus of the Sylvian fissure; *37* supramarginal gyrus; *38* angular gyrus; *39* pars triangularis, frontal operculum, inferior frontal gyrus; *40* pars orbitalis, frontal operculum, inferior frontal gyrus; *41* medial temporal gyrus

2.1.3 Speech-Associated Frontal Areas

2.1.3.1 Transverse Sections

In axial sections, the insula [19] can be found easily (see Figs. 2.5 and 2.6). From medial (ventricles) to lateral, the globus pallidus, putamen and claustrum, within the lentiform nucleus [17], can be differentiated followed by the extreme capsule [18] and the cortex of the insula [19]. The Sylvian fissure [35b] separates the insula [19] from the temporal lobe. As stated above, the insula—taking anatomic variations into account—has 4–5 knobs (anterior, medial and posterior short insular gyri divided by the CS, from the anterior and posterior long insular gyri). The insula [19] is covered by the superior temporal gyrus [34], the frontal operculum [9] and the base of the sensorimotor strip. After identifying the anterior short gyrus of the anterior lobule of the insular cortex, on a transverse view, the anterior border between the insula and inferior frontal lobe is the anterior peri-insular sulcus. It abuts the insula [19], on one hand, and the pars opercularis [9] of the frontal operculum of the inferior frontal gyrus, on the other. The pars opercularis [9] has a triangular shape in axial sections and covers the anterior part of the insula [19]. It can be followed into the anterior cranial fossa where it abuts the gyrus orbitalis that runs parallel to the gyrus rectus. The convolution anterior to the pars opercularis [9] on the lateral surface is the pars triangularis [39], separated by the anterior ascending ramus [35d] of the Sylvian fissure.

2.1.3.2 Sagittal Sections

Beginning at the lateral border of the brain (in sagittal views, see Figs. 2.4 and 2.5), there is the Sylvian fissure [35b] that runs anterior-inferior to posterior-superior. Previously, the posterior margins have been described (see above). The Sylvian fissure separates the temporal lobe from the frontal lobe. At its anterior margin, it ascends into the anterior horizontal ramus [35c] and more dorsally into the anterior ascending ramus [35d] of the frontal operculum [9] that also overhangs the anterior aspect of the insula [19]. The anterior horizontal ramus [35c] separates the pars orbitalis [40] from the pars triangularis [39], whereas the anterior ascending ramus [35d] separates the pars triangularis [39] from the pars opercularis [9] of the frontal operculum of the inferior frontal

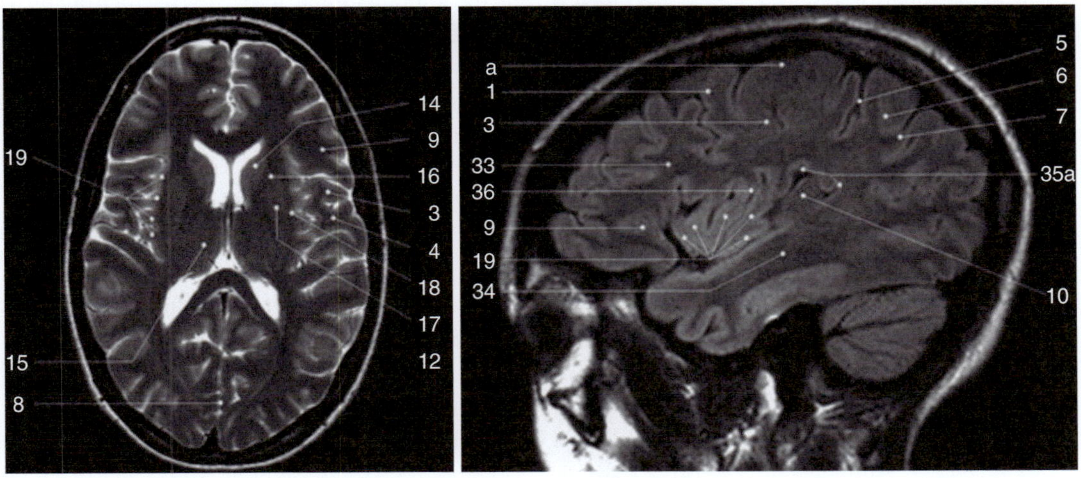

Fig. 2.6 Axial T2-weighted TSE MR and sagittal FLAIR images. *1* superior frontal gyrus; *3* precentral gyrus; *4* postcentral gyrus; *5* "pars bracket," cingulate sulcus; *6* precuneus, parietal lobe; *7* intraparietal sulcus; *8* interhemispheric fissure; *9* pars opercularis, inferior frontal lobe, frontal operculum; *10* Heschl's gyrus; *12* planum temporale; *14* head of the caudate nucleus; *15* thalamus; *16* internal capsule; *17* globus pallidus, putamen, claustrum (lentiform nucleus); *18* extreme capsule; *19* insula (anterior and posterior short insular gyri, anterior and posterior long insular gyri); *33* medial frontal gyrus; *34* superior temporal gyrus; *35a* posterior ascending ramus of the Sylvian fissure; *36* central sulcus of the insula

gyrus that forms an "M" (Naidich et al. 1995). The pars opercularis of the frontal operculum of the inferior frontal lobe harbours Broca's area. At its posterior margin, the pars opercularis is delimited by the anterior subcentral sulcus.

2.1.4 Auditory Cortex and Speech-Associated Temporoparietal Areas

2.1.4.1 Transverse Sections

From medial to lateral (see Figs. 2.5 and 2.6) towards the insula [19], the globus pallidus, putamen and claustrum within the lentiform nucleus [17] can be differentiated. Between the lentiform nucleus [17] and the cortex of the insula [19], the extreme capsule [18] is depicted as a small rim of white matter. The Sylvian fissure [35b] separates the insula [19] from the temporal lobe. This is an easy definable landmark on axial views. The insula—taking anatomic variations into account—has 4–5 knobs (anterior, medial and posterior short insular gyri divided by the CS [36], from the anterior and posterior long insular gyri). Posterior to the convolution that represents the section of the posterior long insular gyrus, a gyrus in the superior temporal lobe can be identified with a dorsomedial to anterior-lateral course, called the transverse temporal gyrus or Heschl's gyrus [10]. This is the primary auditory cortex (Mukamel et al. 2005; Devlin and Poldrack 2007). Number and size may vary (Penhune et al. 1996; Rademacher et al. 2001); however, this is another good landmark that is easy to define. Heschl's gyrus [10] might be interrupted by the sulcus intermedius of Beck. Two gyri on the right and only one on the left hemisphere can be found frequently (Shapleske et al. 1999). Heschl's sulcus [11], which borders Heschl's gyrus [10] posteriorly, is the anterior border of the planum temporale [12]. Although direct cortical stimulation intraoperatively may cause speech disturbances in this area (Sanai et al. 2008; Shapleske et al. 1999), the planum temporale [12] represents, more likely, the auditory association cortex. The planum temporale [12] extends on the superior surface of the temporal lobe and is delimited laterally by the superior temporal sulcus [13], posteriorly by the posterior ascending ramus and/or descending ramus of the Sylvian fissure and medially in the depth of the Sylvian fissure, which is less well defined (Shapleske et al. 1999). These borders are easier depicted in sagittal views; however, in transverse sections, remaining in the same plane in which Heschl's gyrus [10] can be found, the superior temporal sulcus [13] is the next biggest sulcus posterior to Heschl's sulcus [11]. Heschl's gyrus [10] bulges into the Sylvian fissure [35b]. The Sylvian fissure can therefore also be followed in ascending axial images. At the parietotemporal junction, sulci such as the Sylvian fissure or the superior temporal sulcus [13] ascend, whereas the sulcus intermedius primus descends. This hampers anatomical description in axial sections. Ascending in axial slice order, the superior temporal sulcus [13] diminishes. As Heschl's gyrus [10] bulges into the Sylvian fissure [35b], the Sylvian fissure can be followed on its course as posterior ascending ramus [35a] up to the level of the cella media of the lateral ventricles (in bicommissural orientation), as a big intersection posterior to Heschl's sulcus [11]. The posterior ascending ramus [35a] of the Sylvian fissure is imbedded in the supramarginal gyrus [37] which again is separated from the angular gyrus [38] by the sulcus intermedius primus. Descending in axial slice order, pre- and postcentral gyri can be identified as described above. The next sulcus dorsal to the postcentral sulcus is the intraparietal sulcus [7] which can be followed from the medial apical surface, laterally and dorsally in the parietal lobe [6]. Laterally, it ends above the sulcus intermedius primus and abuts the angular gyrus [38]. Size of the planum temporale [12] varies depending on sex, handedness and hemispherical dominance (Shapleske et al. 1999). Activation in functional imaging studies was found in verb generation tasks (Wise et al. 1991) and listening to tones, words and tone sequences (Binder et al. 1996, 1997, 2000).

2.1.4.2 Sagittal Sections

According to its dorsomedial to anterior-lateral course (see Fig. 2.6), the transverse temporal gyrus or Heschl's gyrus [10] abuts the base of the inferior sensorimotor strip (most likely the postcentral gyrus) at the lateral aspect and the posterior long gyrus of the insula [19] in more medially located sections. It is erected into the Sylvian fissure [35b]. Heschl's sulcus [11], which borders Heschl's gyrus [10] posteriorly, is the anterior border of the planum temporale [12]. The planum temporale [12] extends on the superior surface of the temporal lobe and is delimited laterally by the superior temporal sulcus [13], posteriorly by the posterior ascending ramus and/or descending ramus of the Sylvian fissure and medially in the depth of the Sylvian fissure, which is less well defined (Shapleske et al. 1999). The Sylvian fissure can be followed from the anterior ascending [35d] and horizontal rami [35c] in the frontal operculum [9] of the inferior frontal gyrus, dorsally to the ascending [35a] and descending rami at the temporoparietal junction. Medially it is flanked by the insula [19], laterally by the superior temporal gyrus [34] and inferior parts of the pre- and postcentral gyri. Parallel to the Sylvian fissure [35b], the superior temporal gyrus [34] also demonstrates an anterior-posterior course. The posterior ascending ramus [35a] of the Sylvian fissure is imbedded in the supramarginal gyrus [37] which has a horseshoe appearance. Posterior to the supramarginal gyrus [37], the superior-inferior running sulcus intermedius primus separates it from the angular gyrus [38]. The superior temporal sulcus [13] ascends at its posterior end and diminishes.

2.1.4.3 Coronal Sections

In coronal views, the Sylvian fissure separating the temporal lobe from the insula and the frontal lobe can easily be seen. Originating from the temporal lobe, Heschl's gyrus points towards the insula (not shown).

2.1.5 Visual Cortex

2.1.5.1 Sagittal Sections

At the medial surface of the occipital lobe, there is a sulcus that zigzags antero-posteriorly called the calcarine sulcus [27], along which the visual cortex is located. The calcarine sulcus [27] separates the superior lip from the inferior lip of the visual cortex.

References

Binder JR, Frost JA et al (1996) Function of the left planum temporale in auditory and linguistic processing. Brain 119:1239–1247

Binder JR, Frost JA et al (1997) Human brain language areas identified by functional imaging. J Neurosci 17:353–362

Binder JR, Frost JA et al (2000) Human temporal lobe activation by speech and nonspeech sounds. Cereb Cortex 10:512–528

Brandt T, Bartenstein P et al (1998) Reciprocal inhibitory visual-vestibular interactions: visual motion stimulation deactivates the parieto-insular vestibular cortex. Brain 121:1749–1758

Dechent P, Frahm J (2003) Functional somatotopy of finger representations in human primary motor cortex. Hum Brain Mapp 18:272–283

Devlin JT, Poldrack RA (2007) In praise of tedious anatomy. NeuroImage 37:1033–1041

Dronkers NF (1996) A new brain region for coordinating speech articulation. Nature 384:159–161

Ebeling U, Huber P et al (1986) Localization of the precentral gyrus in the computed tomogram and its clinical application. J Neurol 233(2):73–76

Eberstaller O (1890) Ein beitrag zur anatomie der oberfläche des grosshirns. Urban & Schwarzenberg, Wien/Leipzig

Fesl G, Moriggl B et al (2003) Inferior central sulcus: variations of anatomy and function on the example of the motor tongue area. NeuroImage 20(1):601–610

Kido DK, LeMay M et al (1980) Computed tomographic localization of the precentral gyrus. Radiology 135:373–377

Meyer JR, Roychowdhury S et al (1996) Location of the central sulcus via cortical thickness of the precentral and postcentral gyri on MR. AJNR Am J Neuroradiol 17(9):1699–1706

Mukamel R, Hagar G et al (2005) Coupling between neuronal firing, field potentials, and fMRI in human auditory cortex. Science 309:951–954

Nagao M, Takeda K et al (1999) Apraxia of speech associated with an infarct in the precentral gyrus of the insula. Neuroradiology 41:356–357

Naidich TP, Brightbill TC (1996) The pars marginalis: part I. A "bracket" sign for the central sulcus in axial plane CT and MRI. Int J Neuroradiol 2:3–19

Naidich TP, Valavanis AG et al (1995) Anatomic relationships along the low-middle convexity: part I – normal specimen and magnetic resonance imaging. Neurosurgery 36:517–532

Naidich TP, Kang E et al (2004) The insula: anatomic study and MR imaging display at 1.5 T. AJNR Am J Neuroradiol 25:222–232

Ojemann GA, Whitaker HA (1978a) The bilingual brain. Arch Neurol 35(7):409–412
Ojemann GA, Whitaker HA (1978b) Language localization and variability. Brain Lang 6(2):239–260
Ono M, Kubik S et al (eds) (1990) Atlas of the cerebral sulci. Georg Thieme, Stuttgart/New York
Oppenheimer S (1993) The anatomy and physiology of cortical mechanisms of cardiac control. Stroke 24:I3–I5
Overduin SA, Servos P (2004) Distributed digit somatotopy in primary somatosensory cortex. NeuroImage 23(2):462–472
Penfield W, Rasmussen T (1950) The cerebral cortex in man. Macmillan, New York
Penhune VB, Zatorre RJ et al (1996) Interhemispheric anatomical differences in human primary auditory cortex: probabilistic mapping and volume measurement from magnetic resonance scans. Cereb Cortex 6:661–672
Price CJ (2000) The anatomy of language: contributions from functional neuroimaging. J Anat 197:335–359
Rademacher J, Morosan P et al (2001) Probabilistic mapping and volume measurement of human auditory cortex. NeuroImage 13:669–683
Riecker A, Ackermann H et al (2000) Opposite hemispheric lateralization effects during speaking and singing at motor cortex, insula and cerebellum. Neuroreport 11:1997–2000
Sanai N, Mirzadeh Z et al (2008) Functional outcome after language mapping for glioma resection. N Engl J Med 358(1):18–27
Shapleske J, Rossell SL et al (1999) The planum temporale: a systematic review of its structural, functional and clinical significance. Brain Res Rev 29:26–49
Wise R, Chollet U et al (1991) Distribution of cortical neuronal networks involved in word comprehension and word retrieval. Brain 114:1803–1817
Wise RJ, Greene J et al (1999) Brain regions involved in articulation. Lancet 353:1057–1061
Yousry TA, Schmid UD et al (1995) Topography of the cortical motor hand area: prospective study with functional MR imaging and direct motor mapping at surgery. Radiology 195(1):23–29
Yousry TA, Schmid UD et al (1997) Localization of the motor hand area to a knob on the precentral gyrus. A new landmark. Brain 120(Pt 1):141–157

The Electrophysiological Background of the fMRI Signal

3

Christoph Kayser and Nikos K. Logothetis

3.1 Introduction

The ability to non-invasively study the architecture and function of the human brain constitutes one of the most exciting cornerstones for modern medicine, psychology and neuroscience. Current in vivo imaging techniques not only provide clinically essential information and allow new forms of treatment but also reveal insights into the mechanisms behind brain function and malfunction. This supremacy of modern imaging rests on its ability to study the structural properties of the nervous system simultaneously with the functional changes related to neuronal activity. As a result, imaging allows us to combine information about the spatial organization and connectivity of the nervous system with information about the underlying neuronal processes and provides the only means to link perception and cognition with the neural substrates in the human brain. Functional imaging techniques build on the interconnections of cerebral blood flow (CBF), the brain's energy demand and the neuronal activity (for reviews on this topic, see Heeger and Ress 2002; Logothetis 2002; Logothetis and Wandell 2004; Lauritzen 2005). Indeed, elaborate mechanisms exist to couple changes in CBF and blood oxygenation to the maintenance and restoration of ionic gradients and the synthesis, transport and reuptake of neurotransmitters. More than 125 years ago, Angelo Mosso had already realized that there must be a relation between energy demand and CBF when he observed increasing brain pulsations in a patient with a permanent skull defect performing a mental task (Mosso 1881). Similar observations on the coupling of blood flow to neuronal activity (from experiments on animals) led Roy and Sherrington to make the insightful statement that "… the chemical products of cerebral metabolism contained in the lymph that bathes the walls of the arterioles of the brain can cause variations of the calibre of the cerebral vessels: that is, in this reaction, the brain possesses an intrinsic mechanism by which its vascular supply can be varied locally in correspondence with local variations of functional activity" (Roy and Sherrington 1890).

Nowadays, there is little doubt about the usefulness of imaging to basic research and clinical diagnosis. In fact, with the wide availability of magnetic resonance imaging (MRI), functional imaging has become a self-sustaining branch of neuroscience research. Yet, and despite all this progress, it is still not clear how faithfully functional imaging replicates the patterns of neuronal activity underlying the changes in brain perfusion. Debating over the spatial and temporal precision

C. Kayser (✉)
Faculty of Biology, Department for Cognitive Neuroscience, Bielefeld University, Bielefeld, Germany
e-mail: christoph.kayser@uni-bielefeld.de

N. K. Logothetis
Department Physiology of Cognitive Processes, Max Planck Institute for Biological Cybernetics, Tübingen, Germany

S. Ulmer, O. Jansen (eds.), *fMRI*, https://doi.org/10.1007/978-3-030-41874-8_3

of the imaging signal, researchers have compared it to more direct measurements of electrical neuronal activity from electrophysiological approaches. This holds especially true for the blood-oxygenation level-dependent signal (BOLD-fMRI), which is probably the most widely used functional imaging technique (Ogawa et al. 1998). As direct measurements of neuronal activity can be obtained from mesoscopic recordings of electrical potentials on the scalp (EEG) as well as from spatially localized recordings using fine microelectrodes, they offer a wide variety of signals that characterize neuronal processes. Hence, before reviewing the neurophysiological basis of the functional imaging signal, it is worth considering the properties of the signals recorded using electrophysiological methods.

3.2 The Compound Neural Signal

Electrophysiological studies at the system level typically record extracellular signals, defined by the superposition of local currents. In contrast to the intracellular recordings that directly assess the membrane potential of individual neurons, extracellular signals can arise from a number of sources and are more difficult to interpret. Neurons are embedded in the extracellular medium, which acts as a volume conductor, allowing the passive spread of electrical signals across considerable spatial distances. For an extracellular recording point, the inflow of positively charged ions into the active sites of a neuron appears as a current sink (inward currents), while inactive membrane sites act as a source (outward currents) for the active regions. Given the resistive nature of the extracellular medium, these currents generate so-called extracellular field potentials (EFP) (Freeman 1975). The signal measured by an electrode placed at a neural site represents the mean EFP from the spatially weighted sum of sinks and sources along multiple cells at this particular site. In addition, by the superposition principle, the EFPs from multiple cells add up linearly throughout the volume conductor. Thus, for cells or cell compartments, with diametrically opposite orientations, currents of equal magnitude but opposite polarity will generate potentials that tend to cancel each other, while for well-aligned and elongated processes of neural elements, the currents add, resulting in a strongly oriented electric field. Despite these difficulties in interpreting the measured signals, EFP remains the most important tool for the systems neurophysiologist, as they convey a great deal of information about the underlying brain function.

If a small-tipped microelectrode is placed sufficiently close to the soma or axon of a neuron, then the measured EFP directly reports the spike (action potentials) of that neuron and possibly also of its immediate neighbours. The firing rates of such well-isolated neurons have been the critical measure for comparing neural activity with sensory processing or behaviour ever since the early development of microelectrodes (Adrian and Zotterman 1929). Indeed, measuring firing rates has been the mainstay of systems neuroscience for decades. Although a great deal has been learned from this measure of neuronal activity, the single-unit technique has the drawback of not providing information about subthreshold integrative processes or associational operations taking place at a given site. In addition, this recording technique suffers from a bias toward certain cell types and sizes (Towe and Harding 1970; Stone 1973). For large neurons, the active and passive regions are further apart, resulting in a substantially greater flow of membrane current and a larger extracellular spike than for a small cell. As a result, spikes generated by large neurons will remain above noise level over a greater distance from the cell than spikes from small neurons. It follows that typically measured spiking activity mostly represents the small population of large cells, which are the pyramidal cells in the neocortex. This bias is particularly pronounced in experiments with alert-behaving animals or humans, in which even slight movements of the subjects make it extremely difficult to record from smaller neurons for a sufficiently long time (Fried et al. 1997; Kreiman et al. 2000). As a result, most of the experiments using single-unit extracellular recordings report on the activity of large principal cells, which represent the output of the cortical area under study.

If the impedance of the microelectrode is sufficiently low or when no clear signal from individual neurons can be isolated, then the electrode can be used to monitor the totality of the action potentials in that region. Often, the multiunit activity (MUA) is characterized as compound electrical signal in a frequency range above 300–500 Hz. This signal has been shown to be site specific (Buchwald and Grover 1970) and to vary systematically with stimulus properties in the same way as the activity of single neurons (e.g. Kayser et al. (2007a)). There is good evidence that MUA activity reflects variations in the magnitude of extracellular spike potentials, with large-amplitude signal variations in the MUA reflecting large-amplitude extracellular potentials. Overall, the MUA seems to incorporate signals from a sphere with a radius of 150–300 mm, depending on the detailed electrode properties (Buchwald and Grover 1970; Legatt et al. 1980; Gray et al. 1989). Typically, such a region will contain thousands of neurons, suggesting that the MUA is especially sensitive to the synchronous firings of many cells, which is further enhanced by the principle of superposition mentioned above.

While the fast, high-frequency components of the aggregate field potentials mostly reflect the spiking activity of neighbouring neurons, the slower components of the EFP seem to reflect a different kind of activity. The so-called local field potential (LFP) is defined as the low-frequency component of the EFP and represents mostly slow events reflecting cooperative activity in neural populations. In contrast to the MUA, the magnitude of the LFP does not correlate with cell size but instead reflects the extent and geometry of local dendrites (Fromm and Bond 1964, 1967; Buchwald et al. 1966). A prominent geometric arrangement is formed by the pyramidal neurons with their apical dendrites running parallel to each other and perpendicular to the pial surface. They form a so-called open field arrangement, in which dendrites face in one direction and somata in another, producing strong dendrite-to-soma dipoles when they are activated by synchronous synaptic input. The spatial summation of the LFP has been suggested to reflect a weighted average of synchronized dendrosomatic components of the synaptic signals of a neural population within 0.5–3 mm of the electrode tip (Mitzdorf 1985, 1987; Juergens et al. 1999). The upper limits of the spatial extent of LFP summation were indirectly calculated by computing the phase coherence as a function of interelectrode distance in experiments with simultaneous multiple-electrode recordings (e.g. see Fig. 3.1). Combined intracellular and field potential recordings also suggest a synaptic/dendritic origin of the LFPs, representing locally averaged excitatory and inhibitory postsynaptic potentials, which are considerably slower than the spiking activity (Steriade and Amzica 1994; Steriade et al. 1998). In addition, the LFP can also include other types of slow activity unrelated to synaptic events, including voltage-dependent membrane oscillations (Juergens et al. 1999) and spike after potentials (Buzsaki et al. 1988).

In summary, three different signals can commonly be extracted from extracellular microelectrode recordings, each partially covering a different frequency regime of the acquired signal. Representing fast events, the MUA reflects

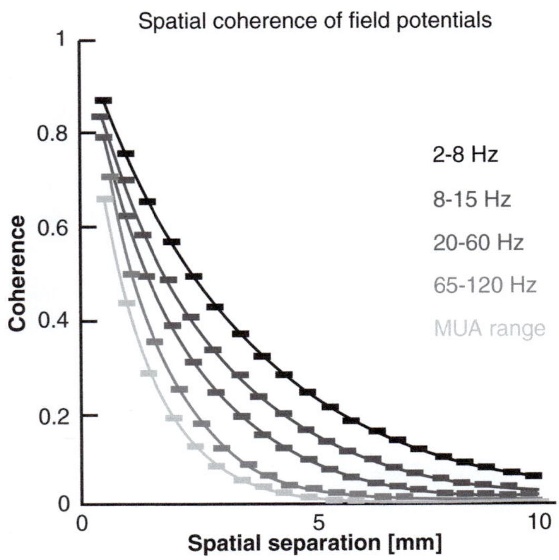

Fig. 3.1 Spatial coherence of the local field potential in primary visual cortex. Each graph displays the average coherence of the field potentials recorded from two electrodes as a function of the electrodes' spatial separation. Each *line* indicates a different frequency band

the averaged spiking activity of populations of neurons, with a bias for the larger, principal (projection) neurons. Covering the same frequency range, the single-unit activity reports mainly on the activity of the principal neurons that form the major output of a cortical area. In contrast and representing slower events, the LFP reflects slow waveforms such as synaptic potentials, afterpotentials and voltage-gated membrane oscillations that mostly reflect the input of a given cortical area as well as its local intracortical processing.

3.3 The Passive Electric Properties of the Brain

To better understand how the signal picked up by a microelectrode emerges from the underlying neuronal processes, especially with regard to the distinction of the different frequency regimes, it is important to know the basic electrical properties of brain tissue. The extracellular microenvironment consists of narrow gaps between cellular processes, probably not more than 200 Å wide on average. These spaces form a complex three-dimensional mosaic filled with extracellular fluid. Theoretical considerations suggest that currents and ions spread within this fluid but not through the cells (Robinson 1968). As a result, the resistance to electrical currents of this space depends on the detailed spatial layout of neuronal tissue, possibly resulting in an un-isotropic current flow that does not necessarily behave like that in a simple saline bath (Ranck 1963a, b; Mitzdorf 1985). Especially, from these considerations, it is unclear whether cortical tissue behaves like an ohmic resistor or whether signals of different frequencies experience frequency-dependent attenuation, that is, whether the tissue behaves like a capacitive filter.

A frequency-dependent behaviour was suggested by the fact that the activity of the slow wave measured by the EEG is largely independent of spiking responses, suggesting strong frequency-filtering properties of the tissue overlying the sources of the activity (Ajmone-Marsan 1965; Bedard et al. 2004, 2006). In addition, in extracellular unit recordings, the shape and amplitude of recorded spikes depend on the spatial position of the electrode relative to the neuron (Gold et al. 2006), while slow potentials show much less sensitivity to position and correlate over large spatial distances. Since the lower frequencies of the field potentials typically correlate over larger spatial distances than the higher frequencies of the same signal (Fig. 3.1), this can be interpreted as strong evidence for the cortical tissue to behave as a capacitive filter (Destexhe et al. 1999). Such a frequency-dependent impedance spectrum could selectively attenuate electric signals of some frequencies more than those of others, for example, high-frequency spiking events more than low-frequency potentials.

To clarify whether the brain's tissue behaves like an ohmic or a capacitive medium, we recently quantified the passive electrical spread of different signals in the brain in vivo. These measurements were conducted in the primary visual cortex, a typical model system for sensory processing, and on the scale of hundreds of micrometres to several millimetres, that is, the scale relevant to the typical functional imaging techniques such as fMRI-BOLD (Logothetis et al. 2007). At this scale, theoretical considerations suggest that the extracellular medium can be considered as largely homogenous and mostly isotropic (within the grey matter). Our results confirmed this and, more importantly, demonstrated that the cortical tissue does not behave like a capacitive filter but acts like an ohmic resistor, attenuating signals of different frequencies in the same manner.

In detail, we measured the voltage drop across two neighbouring electrodes induced by an injected current of predefined frequency (Fig. 3.2). Our measurements employed a four-point electrode system, allowing highly accurate and unperturbed measurements of resistance of cortical tissue in vivo. Over a wide range of current frequencies and for all tested spatial arrangements of the electrodes, the brain's grey matter tissue behaved like an isotropic and ohmic resistor. The white matter, in contrast, showed directional anisotropies, with lower resistance in one and higher resistance in the orthogonal direction. Yet, as for the grey matter, the white matter also behaved like an ohmic resistor. Altogether, our measurements clearly rejected the notion that the cortical tissue behaves like a frequency-dependent

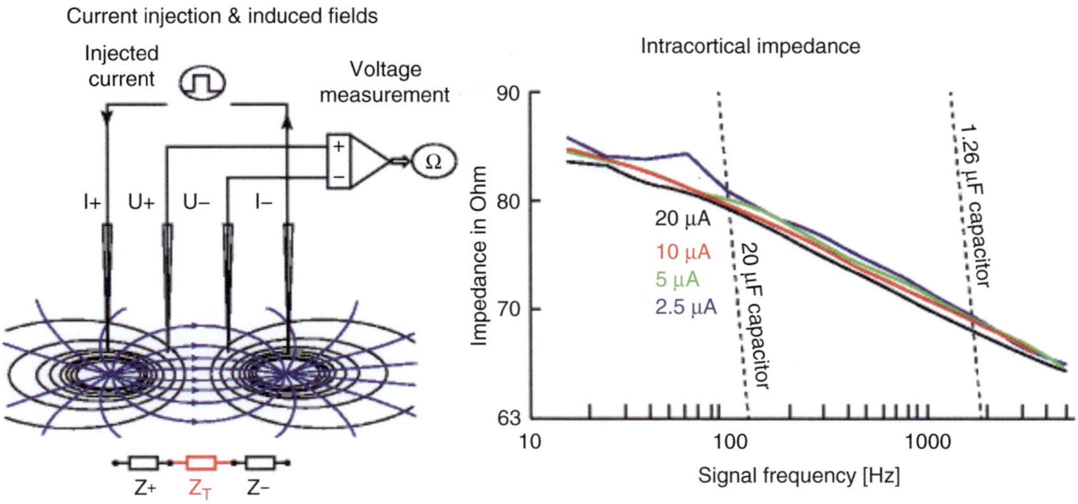

Fig. 3.2 Impedance spectrum of cortical tissue. The *left panel* displays the schematic representation of the impedance measurement. A current of a predefined frequency was injected (via electrodes I+ and I−), and the voltage difference was measured across electrodes U+ and U−. From this voltage difference, one can infer the cortical resistance (Z_T) as a function of current frequency, that is, the frequency-dependent impedance spectrum. The field *lines* indicate the current flow in a homogenous tissue. The *right panel* displays the measured impedance values for different current strengths in cortex (*solid lines*) and for electronic capacitances. Clearly, the impedance spectrum of the cortex is nearly flat compared to that of the capacitance, suggesting that the cortex does not behave like a frequency-dependent filter but rather like an ohmic resistor. For details, see Logothetis et al. (2007)

filter, at least on the spatial scale relevant to the typical functional imaging applications.

As a consequence of this finding, one has to conclude that some of the properties of the field potentials noted above, such as the different degree of spatial correlations in different frequency bands, are not the result of passive electrical spread in the tissue. In contrast, our findings suggest that the long-range correlations of the low-frequency signals, such as the theta or beta rhythms, result from properties of the generators of these signals, that is, from the spatial patterning of the connections mediating these oscillations, and hence might be a property that is also reflected in the functional imaging signal.

3.4 The Neural Correlate of the BOLD Signal

Given the distinction of the different signals that can be obtained from extracellular recordings, one can ask which signal best explains the activity patterns seen in functional imaging experiments. Or stated otherwise, which signal correlates best with the functional imaging signal? A growing body of work addresses this important question with two complementary approaches. An indirect approach asks whether both methodologies yield similar answers to a typical neuroscientific question, such as whether a certain region in the brain responds to a given stimulus. A direct approach, on the other hand, measures both signals at the same time to directly correlate the functional imaging activation with the different signals of neuronal activity.

A typical example for an indirect comparison was provided by Rees et al. who compared human fMRI measurements with electrophysiological data from single-unit recordings in monkeys (Rees et al. 2000). Both data sets were obtained from the motion-specific areas of the respective species and reflected how much the respective signal changed as a function of the stimulus' motion coherence. Comparing the slope of both signals, the authors concluded that the BOLD signal was directly proportional to the average firing rate, with a constant of proportionality of approximately nine spikes per second per percentage BOLD increase. Using the same strategy but focusing on the signal increase in primary visual cortex as a function of stimulus contrast, Heeger et al. confirmed such a linear relation of spiking activity and the BOLD signal, albeit with a smaller proportionality constant of 0.4 spikes per percentage BOLD increase (Heeger et al. 2000). While these results suggest a good correlation of the BOLD signal and firing rates in the same cortical region, they already indicate that the details of this relation, here the constant or proportionality, depend on detailed characteristics of each area.

While the above studies focused only on firing rates, another study on primary visual cortex extended this approach to a wider range of stimuli and physiological signals (Kayser et al. 2004). Studying the cat visual system, the BOLD signal was obtained from one group of animals, while MUA and field potential responses were recorded in a second group of animals. As a metric of comparison, the authors asked which of the different electrophysiological signals would yield similar relative responses to different stimuli as found in the BOLD signal. Stated otherwise, if stimulus A elicits a stronger BOLD response than stimulus B, which of the electrophysiological signal obeys the same relation across a large fraction of recording sites sampled in the same region of interest from which the BOLD signal is sampled (Fig. 3.3)? Overall, the MUA provided a worse match to the BOLD signal than did the LFP, although the latter showed strong frequency dependence. The best match between LFP and BOLD was obtained in the frequency range of 20–50 Hz, while slower oscillations generally showed a poor concordance with the imaging data. Noteworthy, this study also showed that the precise results of an indirect comparison can depend strongly on the specific stimuli employed: when the contrast involved grating stimuli, which elicit strong gamma band responses, a good match between the gamma band of the LFP and the BOLD was obtained. However, when the contrast involved only stimuli with less distinct activation patterns in the LFP, the correlation of LFP and BOLD also showed less frequency dependence.

While these studies only compared the average response strength of each signal, another extended the comparison to the temporal dimension and correlated the average time course obtained from fMRI with that obtained from neuronal responses (Mukamel et al. 2005). Using the human auditory cortex as a model system, these authors correlated the average fMRI responses obtained in a group of healthy subjects with intracortical recordings obtained from a group of epilepsy patients monitored for surgical treatment. While the BOLD signal again correlated well with the LFP, it showed an even stronger correlation with neuronal firing rates, contrasting the above result from visual cortex.

As these examples demonstrate, the results of an indirect comparison between the BOLD signal and neuronal responses may vary depending on the particular experimental paradigm and stimuli involved. In fact, an indirect comparison can only be conducted after the responses in the two measurements have each been highly averaged over trials. While such averaging will result in a robust estimate of the stimulus-related response, it will also remove the trial to trial variability of neuronal responses, the influence of the mental state and other brain state fluctuations that are not locked to the stimulus used to align the responses. As a result, one compares two "artificial" signals that do not necessarily resemble the pattern of neuronal activity seen during normal brain function. In addition, the temporal resolution of the imaging signal is often quite low, especially in human studies, resulting in a blurred signal which cannot be adequately compared to the fast changes of neuronal activity (see also below). An indirect comparison of functional imaging and neuronal activity can hence only speak about a certain, stimulus-driven aspect of the signals but does not generalize the complex interactions of feedforward and feedback processing that occur during normal conditions, where each activity pattern might be unique and non-repeatable.

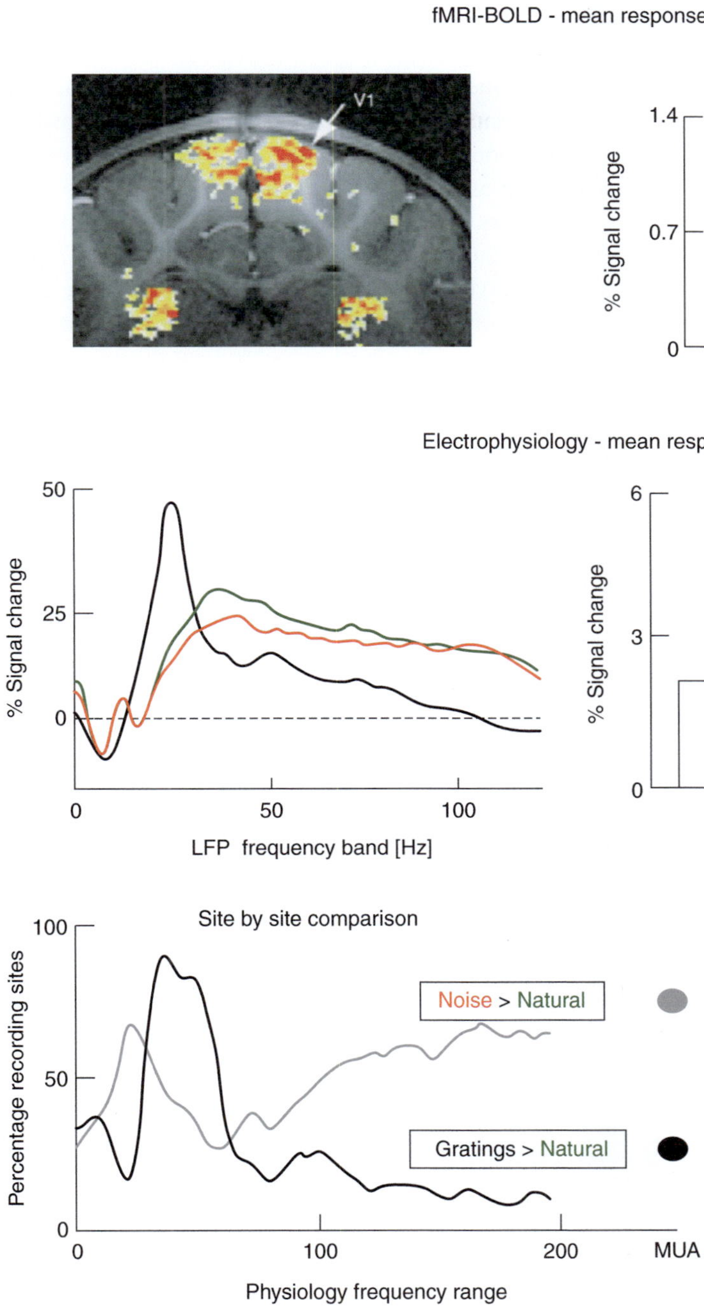

Fig. 3.3 Indirect comparison of BOLD and neurophysiological signals in cat primary visual cortex. The *upper panel* displays the average BOLD responses to the three kinds of stimuli used in this study, while the *middle panel* displays the average responses in the LFP and MUA. The *lower panel* displays the comparison between signals. This was done by counting the fraction of neurophysiological recording sites where the activity obeyed the same relations as found in the BOLD signal (noise > natural and gratings > natural). This comparison was performed separately for each LFP frequency band and MUA. For details, see Kayser et al. (2004)

To overcome the limitations of these indirect comparisons, our lab examined the relationship of the BOLD signal to neural activity directly by simultaneously acquiring electrophysiological and fMRI data from the same animals. To this end, we developed a 4.7 T vertical scanner environment specifically for combined neurophysiology and imaging experiments, including novel methods for interference compensation, microelectrodes and data denoising (Logothetis et al. 2001). Our measurements showed that the fMRI-BOLD response directly reflects a local increase in neural activity as assessed by the EFP signal. For the majority of recording sites, the BOLD signal was found to be a linear but not time-invariant function of LFPs, MUA and the firing rate of individual neurons (Fig. 3.4, upper panel). After stimulus presentation, a transient increase in power was typically observed across all LFP frequencies, followed by a lower level of activation that was maintained for the entire duration of stimulus presentation. The MUA, in contrast, often showed a more transient response, suggesting a lower correlation to the BOLD response. This hypothesis was confirmed using system identification techniques: while in general both LFPs and MUA served as good predictors for the BOLD, LFPs on average accounted for 7.6% more of the variance in the fMRI response than the MUA. This difference, albeit small, was statistically significant across experiments. In further experiments, we confirmed the same findings in alert animals, demonstrating that the correlation of BOLD and LFP holds good also during more complex, natural situations (Goense and Logothetis 2008). On the one hand, these findings confirm and extend the previous studies suggesting an anal-

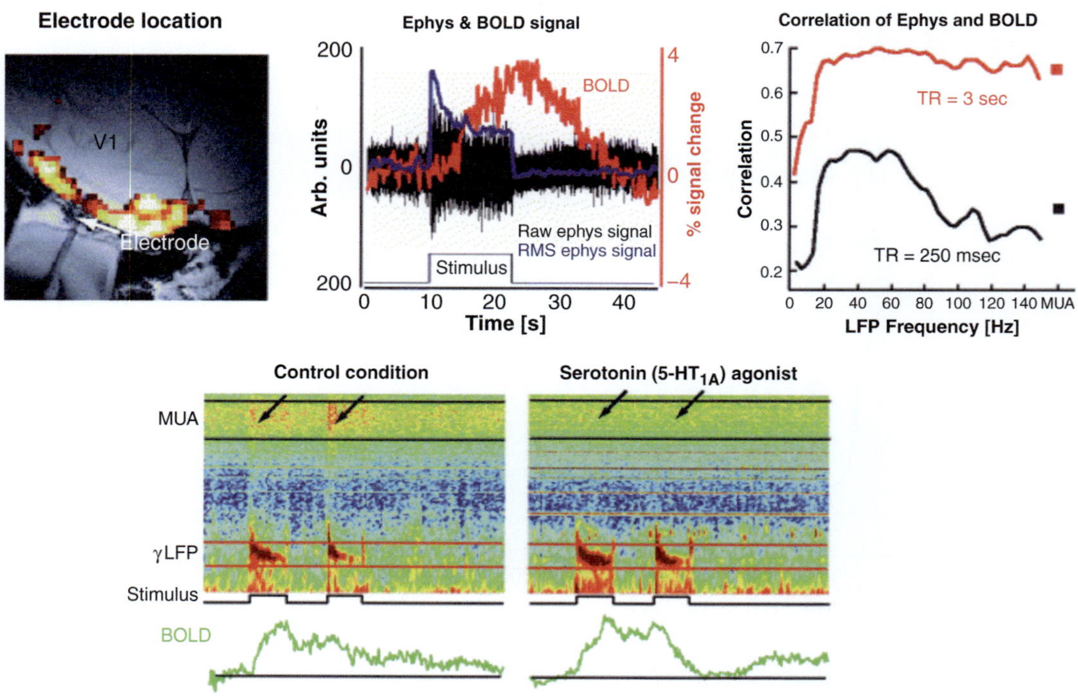

Fig. 3.4 Simultaneous measurement of BOLD and neurophysiological signals in the monkey primary visual cortex. In the *upper row*, the *left panel* displays the electrode location in V1, together with the functional response near the electrode (*red-yellow* colour code). The *middle panel* displays the simultaneously recorded BOLD and neuronal signals. The *right panel*, finally, displays the temporal correlation of both signals, once at high-temporal resolution (TR = 250 ms) and once using a smoothed, low-resolution signal (TR = 3 s). The *lower row* displays a dissociation of BOLD, MUA and LFP induced by the application of a serotonin agonist, which suppresses the firing of pyramidal neurons. During drug application, BOLD and LFP responses persist, while the MUA response ceases. For details, see Logothetis et al. (2001), Goense and Logothetis (2008) and Rauch et al. (2008)

ogy between spiking responses and the BOLD signal, while on the other hand, they reveal the strong contribution of field potentials to the BOLD signal, thereby suggesting that a direct translation of changes in the BOLD signal into changes in firing rates is misleading. Rather, we suggested on the basis of these observations that the BOLD signal reflects the input to a local region and its local processing, as reflected by the aggregate synaptic activity, more than its output, as reflected in the spiking activity of the principal cells.

A recent study in the cat visual cortex confirmed these findings by combining optical imaging to measure haemodynamic responses with simultaneous microelectrode recordings (Niessing et al. 2005). Along the lines of previous results, they found a frequency-dependent match between the imaging signal and LFPs. Especially, frequency bands below 10 Hz showed negative correlations with the imaging signal, that is, reduced field potential during increased blood flow response. Higher frequencies, especially between 50 and 90 Hz, showed good correlation with the imaging signal and, importantly, stronger correlations than observed for the MUA.

It is worth noting that the exact strength of the correlation between LFP, MUA and BOLD depends on the detailed properties of the paradigm and data acquisition. Especially, the different acquisition rates for functional imaging signals and neuronal responses can have profound influences, as can easily be demonstrated (Fig. 3.4, middle panel). Starting from a BOLD signal which was acquired using a temporal resolution of 250 ms, we subsequently decimated all signals to an effective temporal resolution of 3 s, the typical temporal resolution of human imaging studies. While the "fast" BOLD signal exhibits the well-established differential correlation of LFP and MUA with the BOLD, the "slow" signal shows an overall stronger correlation and less of a difference between LFP and MUA. Decreasing the temporal resolution effectively smoothens a signal and increases the coherence between LFP frequency bands hence the increased correlation. Not surprisingly, the correlation coefficients did not increase uniformly across frequency bands; the filtering particularly affected the high-frequency bands (>60 Hz), which are typically modulated on faster timescales. As a result, the smoothing unavoidably increases the correlation of MUA to the BOLD response as well. Such simple differences of the temporal resolution of the acquired signals can explain the different degree of correlations found in ours and in indirect human studies, since the latter heavily relied on temporally smoothed signals and subject-averaged signals (Mukamel et al. 2005). To conclude, care must be taken when interpreting correlations of haemodynamic and neuronal signals, as apparent conflicts can simply arise from methodological artefacts rather than true differences.

3.5 The Coupling of Synaptic Activity and CBF

A reason for the more gradual differences between LFP and MUA in their relation to the BOLD signal is that under many conditions, MUA and LFPs will vary together. In other words, in many stimulation conditions, the output of any processing station in subcortical and early cortical structures is likely to reflect the changes of the input, and the LFP-MUA relationship will be "tight," and both will be well correlated with BOLD. Yet, this scenario might be an "exception" when generating cognitive maps during complex tasks; as in such cases, the subject's "mental" state might be instantiated in diverse feedforward and feedback processes that do not necessarily increase the net output of cortical microcircuits. Hence, conditions might exist during which there is a dissociation of these signals, for example, a condition in which an increase in local input (LFP) results in a reduction in local output activity (MUA). Clearly, such situations could reveal important insights into the different processes underlying the different signals and their mutual relations. A powerful example of such a dissociation was provided by Mathiesen et al. (1998, 2000), Thomsen et al. (2004). These authors nicely exploited the synaptic organization of the cerebellar cortex, where electrical stimulation of the parallel fibres causes monosynaptic excitation of the Purkinje cells and disynaptic inhibition of the same neurons through the basket cells. This results in inhibition of the spiking activity in the Purkinje cells while at the same time increasing the synaptic input to these cells. Combining electrophysiological recordings with laser Doppler flowmetry to measure changes in CBF, Mathiesen et al. demonstrated a powerful dissociation of the spiking activity and the CBF. Both LFPs and CBF increased while spiking activity ceased, clearly demonstrating that increases in CBF or BOLD do not allow to make inferences about potential increases or decreases in the spiking activity of the stimulated region (Lauritzen and Gold 2003).

A similar dissociation of the imaging signal and neuronal firing rates could be seen in our studies (Logothetis et al. 2001). Often, the single- or multiunit activity showed strong response adaptation during the first few seconds, with a subsequent decay of the firing rates to baseline. In contrast to this, the BOLD signal and the LFP did persist above baseline throughout the stimulation period. As a result, during the sustained period of the stimulus, only the field potential can be associated with the imaging signal, but not the spiking activity. Importantly, there was no condition or observation period during which the opposite was observed. In addition to this naturally occurring dissociation, similar situations can be induced pharmacologically. For example, the application of a serotonin receptor agonist, which causes persistent hyperpolarization of pyramidal neurons, leads to a ceasing of the MUA responses (Fig. 3.4, lower panel). However, at the very same time, both the LFP and the BOLD signal still respond to visual stimulation, again demonstrating that the BOLD signal is not necessarily coupled to neuronal spiking responses (see Rauch et al. (2008) for further results along this line).

Is the CBF signal then linearly coupled to synaptic activity? While this indeed seems to hold good under some conditions, other conditions produce a nonlinear relation between afferent input and the haemodynamic response (Mathiesen et al. 1998; Norup Nielsen and Lauritzen 2001). Especially for very low or high levels of synaptic input, the CBF response can be decoupled from the input. For example, inducing deactivation of neuronal responses by either functional deactivation or application of TTX resulted in only a small reduction in baseline CBF (Gold and Lauritzen 2002). During such instances of neurovascular decoupling, the imaging data does not reflect all the changes in synaptic afferents, clearly highlighting the limited dynamic range of functional imaging. Such nonlinear relation between synaptic activity and CBF might, for example, arise from the unequal contribution of different receptors and channels to synaptic potentials and blood flow. For example, glutamatergic NMDA channels contribute to CBF but only little to the LFP (Hoffmeyer et al. 2007). As a result, blood flow responses might also exist in the absence of large changes in the LFP, providing strong evidence that it is not the extracellular current that causes increase in CBF but the intracellular signalling cascades related to neurotransmitter release, uptake and recycling. Indeed, while the haemodynamic response provides supplies of glucose and oxygen, it is not the processes that require the energy that call for an increase in CBF but rather the processes triggered in a feedforward manner by neurotransmitter-related signalling (Lauritzen 2005).

The notion that functional imaging measures the aggregate synaptic input to a local area also resolves a number of apparently conflicting results from imaging and electrophysiological experiments. Being sensitive to the synaptic input, functional imaging "sees" modulatory lateral and feedback projections, which might not be strong enough to induce significant changes in neuronal firing rates but nevertheless provides a larger proportion of the total synaptic input. For example, human imaging revealed influences of spatial attention in many visual areas, including primary visual cortex. At the same time, such attentional influences have been persistently difficult to demonstrate using single-neuron recordings or turned out to be much weaker than expected from human imaging (Luck et al. 1997; Kastner and Ungerleider 2000; Heeger and Ress 2002). Given that attentional influences are supposedly mediated by feedback projections from higher visual and frontoparietal regions, they might provide exactly this kind of input that is visible only using functional imaging. Along the same lines, it has been much easier to see cross-modal interactions, that is, influences of one sensory modality on another, using functional imaging than using electrophysiology (Calvert 2001; Kayser and Logothetis 2007). For example, functional imaging demonstrated that auditory cortex can be modulated and even activated by visual or somatosensory stimuli (Kayser et al. 2007b), while the same effects are only weakly present at the level of single-neuron firing rates. However, in full agreement with the above, visual modulation was well evident at the level of field potentials recorded in auditory cortex, again demonstrating a closer correspondence of the BOLD signal with field potentials than with firing rates (Kayser et al. 2008).

3.6 Conclusions

The haemodynamic responses characterized by functional imaging better reflect the aggregate synaptic activity and local processing that is characterized by the LFPs rather than providing information about the typical firing rates in the same region. This partly results from the mechanisms that drive increases in blood flow, which reside upstream from the axosomatic level and near the synaptic-dendritic level.

The collective findings of many studies provide good evidence for the notion that functional imaging reflects the input into a local region but not necessarily the output of the same. Under many normal conditions, the input and output of a local region will be related, and hence functional imaging will provide information about the typical neuronal firing rates in the same region. As a result of this sensitivity to synaptic input, functional imaging signals are more susceptible to modulatory feedback input, which often might provide only a minor contribution to the response strength of large principal neurons. However, for a priori and most experimental conditions, it is unclear what relationship to expect between in- and output, and hence feedforward- and feedback-related activations cannot be distinguished. As a result, it can sometimes be misleading, if not dangerous, to make direct inferences from imaging results about the underlying neuronal processes. Especially for applications with immediate consequences, such as clinical diagnostics and surgical planning, it seems prudent to establish well-defined paradigms in which the neural correlates of the imaging signal have been validated using combined electrophysiological and imaging approaches.

References

Adrian ED, Zotterman Y (1929) The impulses produced by sensory nerve endings, part 2. The response of a single end-organ. J Physiol 61:151–171

Ajmone-Marsan C (1965) Electrical activity of the brain: slow waves and neuronal activity. Isr J Med Sci 1:104–117

Bedard C, Kroger H et al (2004) Modeling extracellular field potentials and the frequency-filtering properties of extracellular space. Biophys J 86:1829–1842

Bedard C, Kroger H et al (2006) Model of low-pass filtering of local field potentials in brain tissue. Phys Rev E Stat Nonlinear Soft Matter Phys 73:051911

Buchwald JS, Grover FS (1970) Amplitudes of background fast activity characteristic of specific brain sites. J Neurophysiol 33:148–159

Buchwald JS, Halas ES et al (1966) Relationships of neuronal spike populations and EEG activity in chronic cats. Electroencephalogr Clin Neurophysiol 21:227–238

Buzsaki G, Bickford RG et al (1988) Nucleus basalis and thalamic control of neocortical activity in the freely moving rat. J Neurosci 8:4007–4026

Calvert GA (2001) Crossmodal processing in the human brain: insights from functional neuroimaging studies. Cereb Cortex 11:1110–1123

Destexhe A, Contreras D et al (1999) Spatiotemporal analysis of local field potentials and unit discharges in cat cerebral cortex during natural wake and sleep states. J Neurosci 19:4595–4608

Freeman W (1975) Mass action in the nervous system. Academic Press, New York

Fried I, MacDonald KA et al (1997) Single neuron activity in human hippocampus and amygdala during recognition of faces and objects. Neuron 18:753–765

Fromm GH, Bond HW (1964) Slow changes in the electrocorticogram and the activity of cortical neurons. Electroencephalogr Clin Neurophysiol 17:520–523

Fromm GH, Bond HW (1967) The relationship between neuron activity and cortical steady potentials. Electroencephalogr Clin Neurophysiol 22:159–166

Goense J, Logothetis N (2008) Neurophysiology of the BOLD fMRI signal in awake monkeys. Curr Biol 18:631–640

Gold L, Lauritzen M (2002) Neuronal deactivation explains decreased cerebellar blood flow in response to focal cerebral ischemia or suppressed neocortical function. Proc Natl Acad Sci U S A 99:7699–7704

Gold C, Henze DA et al (2006) On the origin of the extracellular action potential waveform: a modeling study. J Neurophysiol 95:3113–3128

Gray CM, Konig P et al (1989) Oscillatory responses in cat visual cortex exhibit inter-columnar synchronization which reflects global stimulus properties. Nature 338:334–337

Heeger DJ, Ress D (2002) What does fMRI tell us about neuronal activity? Nat Rev Neurosci 3:142–151

Heeger DJ, Huk AC et al (2000) Spikes versus BOLD: what does neuroimaging tell us about neuronal activity? Nat Neurosci 3:631–633

Hoffmeyer HW, Enager P et al (2007) Nonlinear neurovascular coupling in rat sensory cortex by activation of transcallosal fibers. J Cereb Blood Flow Metab 27:575–587

Juergens E, Guettler A et al (1999) Visual stimulation elicits locked and induced gamma oscillations in monkey intracortical- and EEG-potentials, but not in human EEG. Exp Brain Res 129:247–259

Kastner S, Ungerleider LG (2000) Mechanisms of visual attention in the human cortex. Annu Rev Neurosci 23:315–341

Kayser C, Logothetis NK (2007) Do early sensory cortices integrate cross-modal information? Brain Struct Funct 212:121–132

Kayser C, Kim M et al (2004) A comparison of hemodynamic and neural responses in cat visual cortex using complex stimuli. Cereb Cortex 14:881–891

Kayser C, Petkov CI et al (2007a) Tuning to sound frequency in auditory field potentials. J Neurophysiol 98:1806–1809

Kayser C, Petkov CI et al (2007b) Functional imaging reveals visual modulation of specific fields in auditory cortex. J Neurosci 27:1824–1835

Kayser C, Petkov CI et al (2008) Visual modulation of neurons in auditory cortex. Cereb Cortex 18:1560–1574. https://doi.org/10.1093/cercor/bhm187

Kreiman G, Koch C et al (2000) Category-specific visual responses of single neurons in the human medial temporal lobe. Nat Neurosci 3:946–953

Lauritzen M (2005) Reading vascular changes in brain imaging: is dendritic calcium the key? Nat Rev Neurosci 6:77–85

Lauritzen M, Gold L (2003) Brain function and neurophysiological correlates of signals used in functional neuroimaging. J Neurosci 23:3972–3980

Legatt AD, Arezzo J et al (1980) Averaged multiple unit activity as an estimate of phasic changes in local neuronal activity: effects of volume-conducted potentials. J Neurosci Methods 2:203–217

Logothetis NK (2002) The neural basis of the blood-oxygen-level-dependent functional magnetic resonance imaging signal. Philos Trans R Soc Lond Ser B Biol Sci 357:1003–1037

Logothetis NK, Wandell BA (2004) Interpreting the BOLD signal. Annu Rev Physiol 66:735–769

Logothetis NK, Pauls J et al (2001) Neurophysiological investigation of the basis of the fMRI signal. Nature 412:150–157

Logothetis NK, Kayser C et al (2007) In vivo measurement of cortical impedance spectrum in monkeys: implications for signal propagation. Neuron 55:809–823

Luck SJ, Chelazzi L et al (1997) Neural mechanisms of spatial selective attention in areas V1, V2, and V4 of macaque visual cortex. J Neurophysiol 77:24–42

Mathiesen C, Caesar K et al (1998) Modification of activity-dependent increases of cerebral blood flow by excitatory synaptic activity and spikes in rat cerebellar cortex. J Physiol 512(Pt 2):555–566

Mathiesen C, Caesar K et al (2000) Temporal coupling between neuronal activity and blood flow in rat cerebellar cortex as indicated by field potential analysis. J Physiol 523(Pt 1):235–246

Mitzdorf U (1985) Current source-density method and application in cat cerebral cortex: investigation of evoked potentials and EEG phenomena. Physiol Rev 65:37–100

Mitzdorf U (1987) Properties of the evoked potential generators: current source-density analysis of visually evoked potentials in the cat cortex. Int J Neurosci 33:33–59

Mosso A (1881) Ueber den Kreislauf des Blutes im Menschlichen Gehirn. von Veit, Leipzig

Mukamel R, Gelbard H et al (2005) Coupling between neuronal firing, field potentials, and FMRI in human auditory cortex. Science 309:951–954

Niessing J, Ebisch B et al (2005) Hemodynamic signals correlate tightly with synchronized gamma oscillations. Science 309:948–951

Norup Nielsen A, Lauritzen M (2001) Coupling and uncoupling of activity-dependent increases of neuronal activity and blood flow in rat somatosensory cortex. J Physiol 533:773–785

Ogawa S, Menon RS et al (1998) On the characteristics of functional magnetic resonance imaging of the brain. Annu Rev Biophys Biomol Struct 27:447–474

Ranck JB (1963a) Analysis of specific impedance or rabbit cerebral cortex. Exp Neurol 7:153–174

Ranck JB (1963b) Specific impedance of rabbit cerebral cortex. Exp Neurol 7:144–152

Rauch A, Rainer G et al (2008) The effect of a serotonin induced dissociation between spiking and perisynaptic activity on BOLD functional MRI. Proc Natl Acad Sci 108:6759–6764

Rees G, Friston K et al (2000) A direct quantitative relationship between the functional properties of human and macaque V5. Nat Neurosci 3:716–723

Robinson DA (1968) The electrical properties of metal microelectrodes. Proc IEEE 56:1065–1071

Roy CS, Sherrington CS (1890) On the regulation of the blood supply of the brain. J Physiol 11:85–108

Steriade M, Amzica F (1994) Dynamic coupling among neocortical neurons during evoked and spontaneous spike-wave seizure activity. J Neurophysiol 72:2051–2069

Steriade M, Amzica F et al (1998) Spike-wave complexes and fast components of cortically generated seizures. II Extra- and intracellular patterns. J Neurophysiol 80:1456–1479

Stone J (1973) Sampling properties of microelectrodes assessed in the cat's retina. J Neurophysiol 36:1071–1079

Thomsen K, Offenhauser N et al (2004) Principal neuron spiking: neither necessary nor sufficient for cerebral blood flow in rat cerebellum. J Physiol 560:181–189

Towe AL, Harding GW (1970) Extracellular microelectrode sampling bias. Exp Neurol 29:366–381

High-Field fMRI

4

Elke R. Gizewski

4.1 Introduction

In recent years, functional magnetic resonance imaging (fMRI) has become a widely used approach for neuroscience. However, this method has the potential to be improved with regard to both spatial and temporal resolution. The blood-oxygenation level-dependent (BOLD) contrast represents signal changes in T2- or T2*-weighted images. These sequences are presumed to be well suited to high magnetic field strength, as fMRI sequences benefit from higher signal-to-noise ratio (SNR) and higher signal in BOLD contrast images (Vaughan et al. 2001). However, their sensitivity to susceptibility also causes problems, e.g. in-plane dephasing and signal dropouts near tissue-air boundaries.

To achieve greater insights into brain function, ultra-high-field fMRI has been applied in some studies to attain higher spatial resolutions (Duong et al. 2003; Pfeuffer et al. 2002a). These studies focused on high-resolution images which can be acquired rapidly and with good temporal and special resolution. Additionally, the signal increase advantage in high-field MRI has been studied (Pfeuffer et al. 2002b). Nearly all of these early studies, therefore, accepted restrictions in the field of view and the number of slices for 7-T imaging and avoided areas near tissue-air boundaries. For broader application including pre-surgical fMRI and for analysing cognitive functions, however, a more extended coverage of the brain is needed to reveal network activation involving multiple areas. This chapter will give insights into the pros and cons of high- and ultra-high-field fMRI and into ongoing developments to overcome the restrictions referred to and improve the benefits.

4.2 Benefits and Limitations of High- and Ultra-High-Field MRI

The introduction of ultra-high-field MRI systems has brought MRI technology closer to the physical limitations, and greater development effort is required to achieve appropriate sequences and images. 3-T MRI systems are high-field systems maintaining a relatively high-comfort level for the user similar to 1.5-T MRI systems (Alvarez-Linera 2008; Norris 2003). Theoretically, the SNR at high-field MRI should, according to the Boltzmann equation, show a linear increase with increasing magnetic field strength. But, the interactions of the magnetic field and other influencing factors, e.g. relaxation times, radio frequency (RF) pulses and coils performance during image acquisition, are very complex. One important factor is the change in RF pulses in higher magnetic field strengths. Changing the field strength

E. R. Gizewski (✉)
Department for Radiology, University Clinic for Neuroradiology, Medical University Innsbruck, Innsbruck, Austria
e-mail: elke.gizewski@i-med.ac.at

S. Ulmer, O. Jansen (eds.), *fMRI*, https://doi.org/10.1007/978-3-030-41874-8_4

from 1.5 to 3 T results in a fourfold increase in the required energy, resulting in an increase in specific absorption rate (SAR) (Ladd 2007). The increase in SAR leads to limitations in image acquisition, as the absorption of energy in the tissue cannot be allowed to exceed certain thresholds. Therefore, restrictions in the number of slices and achieving homogenous excitation of the nuclei increase with higher field strength.

Current 3-T scanners have been significantly improved since their introduction, especially with regard to coil developments and sequence techniques; therefore, today the advantages, such as faster acquisition time and/or higher resolution, are greater than the disadvantages, such as higher costs and in some cases instability in running the systems (Scheef et al. 2007). For higher field strength, e.g. 7 T, the developments have also improved in the recent time but are still in the process of improvement.

Another important point is the magnet design. Especially at 7-T whole-body systems, the magnet is very long compared to a typical 1.5-T magnet. The bore is 60 cm as for a long time at common 1.5 T but due to the length gives a narrow impression (Fig. 4.1). Therefore, anxiety is again a problem for imaging. However, newer studies could demonstrate that the acceptance of 7-T imaging procedures in subjects and patients was acceptable (Theysohn et al. 2008). A final important point is the contraindication of every metal implant at 7 T. Even non-ferromagnetic material can be influenced due to induced electrical currents. When located in the centre of imaging, such material, e.g. a surgical calotte fixation, would lead to disturbing artefacts.

Some recent studies addressed the possible side effects of ultra-high-field MRI as increasing spread of high-field and ultra-high-field scanners has encouraged new discussion of the safety aspects of MRI. Studies on possible cognitive effects of MRI examinations could not reveal any significant influence of high field strength and the application of HF impulses during and after normal scanning procedures (Schlamann et al. 2010a). However, one study showed that immediately after MRI exposure, the cortical silent period during transcranial magnetic stimulation was highly significantly prolonged in normal subjects (Schlamann et al. 2010b). Interestingly this was found for 1.5 and 7 T with no significant difference or dependency on the field strength.

4.3 Special Aspects of High-Field fMRI

BOLD contrast images are normally acquired using a gradient echo-planar technique (EPI). Optimal sequence design has to take into account echo times and sampling period; the variation in sensitivity between tissues with different baseline T2∗, the effects of physiological noise and non-exponential signal decay are relevant influencing factors (Gowland and Bowtell 2007). In high-field fMRI, the optimal TE is shorter than at 1.5 T. The shortening of T2∗ is proportional to the magnetic field (Okada et al. 2005). The TE used in optimized 3-T fMRI imaging is between 30 and 35 ms (Preibisch et al. 2008). The optimum TE for 7 T has been reported to be around 25 ms in focused fMRI in the occipital cortex (Yacoub et al. 2001).

As mentioned above, the SNR should increase with the magnetic field strength. Some studies have revealed a BOLD signal increase up to fivefold in 7-T fMRI compared to 1.5-T BOLD signals. Studies focusing on an increase in resolution and small field of view (Pfeuffer et al. 2002c) could reveal a higher signal increase at 7 T than studies with whole-brain coverage (Gizewski et al. 2007). This variability can be explained taking into account the above-mentioned factors influencing the SNR. Additionally, the impact of these factors increases with higher field strength, resulting in a greater variability of BOLD signal between different measurements and subjects at 7 T compared to 1.5 T. The relatively wide range of relative BOLD signal changes compared to 1.5 T and even 3 T may also be explained by the difficulty in achieving a uniform static magnetic field shim and a uniform RF excitation field at 7 T. The fMRI experiments at 7 T are therefore more dependent on field inhomogeneities, and these have to be taken into account during image analysis.

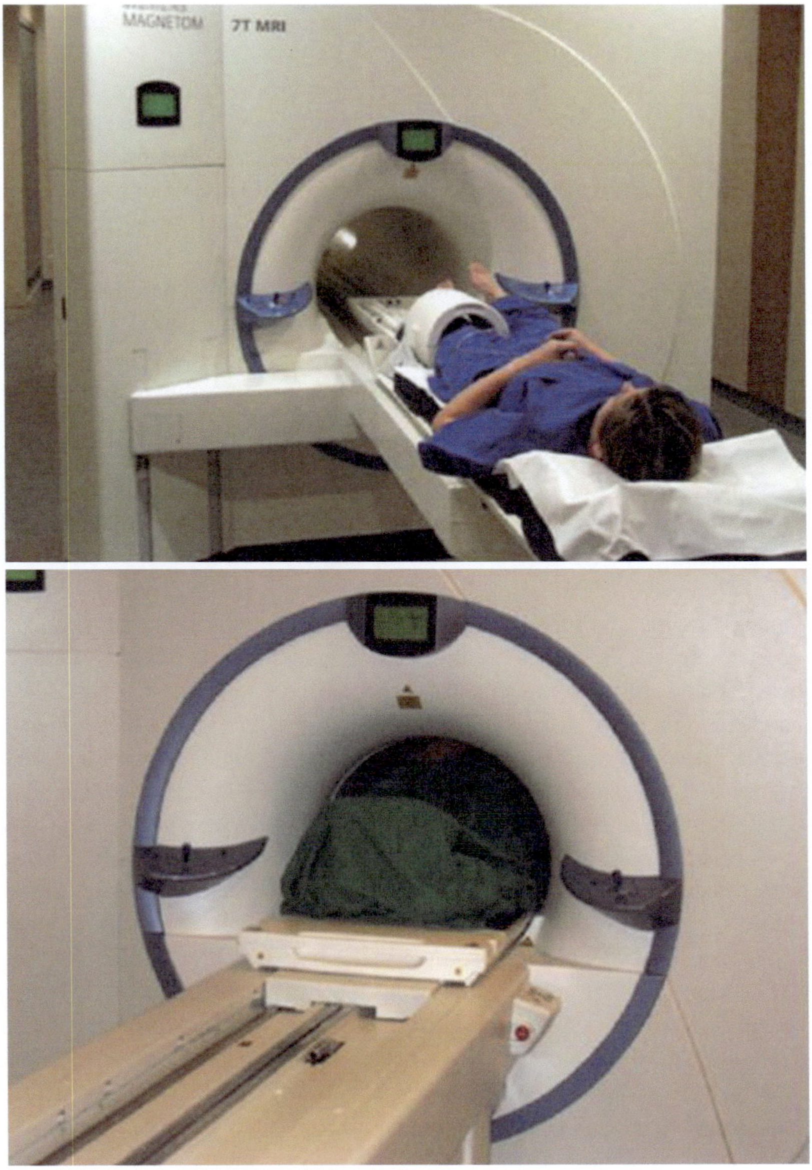

Fig. 4.1 7-T MR scanner with a bore of 60 cm and a length of 3.50 m. The MR is surrounded by 425 tonnes of steel. The *upper figure* shows a person before positioned feet first into the scanner. The *lower figure* shows a person head first in the scanner with the head in the isocentre, the feet covered with a sheet. The scanner used here is located at the Erwin L. Hahn Institut, Essen, Germany

The BOLD effect at higher field strength increases less in vessels larger than the voxel size and is thus more pronounced in vessels smaller than the voxel size. By using smaller voxels at higher field strength compared to 1.5 T, the BOLD signal can become more specific and reliable (Shimada et al. 2008; Zou et al. 2005). Therefore, the signal changes should be more closely linked to the cortical activity. With the increasing signal and enhanced stability of the BOLD signal at higher field strength, the repetition of events can be reduced. At ultra-high fields, even single events can give reliable BOLD signal as discussed in more detail below (Sect. 4.5).

Recent studies have addressed further aspects of SNR and BOLD signal improvement: Newton et al. (2012) evaluated the potential benefits of higher fields for detecting and analysing functional connectivity. The authors measured the influence of spatial resolution (from 1-mm up to 3-mm slice thickness) during a motor task at 7 T on estimates of functional connectivity through decreased partial volume averaging. They could show that resting-state correlations within the sensorimotor system increase as voxel dimensions decreased from 3 × 3 × 2 to 1 × 1 × 2 mm. These results suggest that the true representation of sensorimotor network is more focal than could be resolved with larger voxels. The authors conclude that the described increase may be due to decreased partial volume averaging and that functional connectivity within the primary seed region might be heterogeneous on the scale of single voxels.

A main problem at high field strength is the achievement of good response functions even in areas suffering from in-plane dephasing and signal dropouts near tissue-air boundaries. A further central problem is the increasing chemical shift, proportional to the magnetic field strength. All these limitations lead to errors when reading the echo. Therefore, the optimization of scanning parameters and coil construction is of much greater importance than in routine 1.5-T scanners. Today, many improvements are achieved and lead to increased use of 7 T for fMRI studies as discussed below. The following paragraphs will give some examples of these developments in ultra-high-field BOLD and structural imaging.

The shimming, especially at 7 T, should be performed manually by the user. Although the standard shimming algorithm may be used, multiple repetitions should be performed with close verification of the result before starting the EPI sequence. At higher field strengths, a per slice shimming may be necessary to account for increased B0 distortions. Additionally, the phase correction parameters can be calculated slice by slice using three non-phase-encoded navigator echoes before the EPI readout (Heid 1997). Excellent B0 homogeneity has been demonstrated recently in the human brain at 7 Tesla with the dynamic multi-coil technique (DYNAMITE) for magnetic field shimming (Juchem et al. 2011). Recently, this groups also report the benefits of DYNAMITE shimming for multi-slice EPI and T2∗ mapping (Juchem et al. 2015). Furthermore, high-degree and high-order B0 shimming was on gradient-echo EPI at 7 T with improvement especially for cortical regions (Kim et al. 2017). But also specially designed coils have been developed to overcome those limitations, e.g. multichannel-phased array transmit coils with homogenous excitation across the visual cortex (Sengupta et al. 2016).

Nevertheless, there are increased susceptibility artefacts at 3 and 7 T compared to 1.5 T. Significant improvement can be reached by using more advanced head coils than circularly polarized (CP) coils. Multichannel coils allow application of parallel acquisition techniques (Mirrashed et al. 2004). Multiple channels provide further increases in SNR and, coupled with parallel imaging, reduce artefacts, e.g. due to susceptibility differences near tissue-air boundaries as is known from experience at 1.5 T. It has been demonstrated that the use of parallel imaging at 3 T results in an increase of BOLD signal depending on the employed parallel imaging method and its implementation (Preibisch et al. 2008). At 7 T, the coil equipment has to be newly developed, as the 7-T MRI systems require combined transmit and receive (t/r) coils. The first t/r coils were CP designs which did not enable parallel imaging techniques, but multichannel designs with up to 32 receiver channels are now available. Some groups also design their own coils in respect to higher resolution using more than 32 channels. As multichannel t/r coils for 7 T are now available more easily, nearly all experimental groups switched from CP to multichannel coils.

A further disadvantage at high field could be a restriction in the number of slices due to SAR restrictions and inhomogeneous resolution over the brain (Wiggins et al. 2005). Therefore, the coils and sequences have to be chosen depending on the paradigms to be applied. Again, parallel imaging can be useful for reducing the RF load on the tissue and enabling more slices. It was shown that at 3 T, a reduction factor of 2 in parallel imaging can be used with only little penalty with regard to sensitivity (Preibisch et al. 2008).

Some problems in image distortion can be solved using spin-echo instead of gradient-echo EPI sequences, but they are, so far, not routinely used. The blood contribution that dominates Hahn spin-echo (HSE)-based BOLD contrast at low magnetic fields and degrades specificity is highly attenuated at high fields because the apparent T2 of venous blood in an HSE experiment decreases quadratically with increasing magnetic field. In contrast, the HSE BOLD contrast increases supralinearly with the magnetic field strength. Yacoub et al. report the results of detailed quantitative evaluations of HSE BOLD signal changes for functional imaging in the human visual cortex at 4 and 7 T (Yacoub et al. 2003). They used the increased SNR of higher field strengths and surface coils to avoid partial volume effects. Furthermore, they could show that high-resolution acquisitions lead to a CNR increase with voxel sizes <1 mm^3. It was concluded that the high-field HSE fMRI signals originated largely from the capillaries and that the magnitude of the signal changes associated with brain function reached sufficiently high levels at 7 T to make it a useful approach for mapping on the millimetre to submillimetre spatial scale.

Recently, balanced-steady-state free precession (b-SSFP) fMRI was developed utilizing the passband of the b-SSFP off-resonance response to measure MR signal changes elicited by changes in tissue oxygenation during increases in neuronal activity. This sequence allows distortion-free full-brain coverage with only two acquisitions and is a candidate for improved fMRI also at 7 T. Malekian et al. (2018) used a non-balanced SSFP at 7 T with the conclusion that this sequence with suitable modifications can be regarded as a robust SSFP-based method for high spatial specificity fMRI techniques. Furthermore, a 3D-GRASE with variable flip angles was tested at 7 T fMRI (Kemper et al. 2016). The authors could show that variable flip angle refocusing schemes increase usability of 3D-GRASE for high-resolution f MRI as it results in a reduction of blurring and increase in spatial coverage. A further approach to overcome the distortion problem was the use of a T2-preparation module to induce BOLD contrast, followed by a single-shot 3D fast gradient-echo readout with short TE (Hua et al. 2014).

The problem that thermal and physiological noise dominates the SNR of the fMRI time course at high spatial resolutions at high field strengths can be a prominent issue if a high-resolution matrix and a thin slice thickness are used. The problem is acquiring data at lower resolution, which is then dominated by physiological noise. A solution would be to acquire data at high resolution and smooth the data back to the desired lower resolution. In such cases, the physiological noise can limit some benefits of high-field acquisition, since increases in image SNR produce only small increases in time course SNR if the 1.5-T resolution is used (Triantafyllou et al. 2006). But, some problems even at 3 T remain; low-frequency periodic fluctuations were found to have increased as well as the time-dependent increase in noise, especially in long EPI sessions (Shimada et al. 2008).

The Nyquist ghost also increases at higher field strength and is an important factor in BOLD imaging at 7 T. There are strategies to improve the traditional Nyquist ghost correction approach in EPI at high fields. One group describes schemes based on the reversal of the EPI readout gradient polarity for every other volume throughout an fMRI acquisition train as one improvement. The authors concluded that at high B0 fields, substantial gains in Nyquist ghost correction of echo-planar time series are possible by this alternating method (van der Zwaag et al. 2009).

The gradient-echo EPI sequences are mostly used for fMRI, especially for clinical applications. Therefore, the optimization of EPI sequences and reduction in artefacts are of great importance. Multichannel coils are basically an array of surface coils with higher signal in the periphery than in the centre. At higher field strength, the signal even in the centre of multichannel coils is higher compared to 1.5 T. Results obtained at 3 T using a combination of multichannel coil and parallel imaging showed that BOLD sensitivity improved by 11% in all brain regions, with larger gains in areas typically affected by strong susceptibility artefacts. The use of parallel imaging markedly reduces image distortion, and hence, the method has found widespread application in functional brain imaging (Poser et al. 2006). Recently, a new technique for 2D gradient-recalled gradient-echo EPI termed "variable slice thickness" (VAST) was introduced, which reduces signal losses caused by through-slice susceptibility artefacts, while keeping the volume TR manageable (Brunheim et al. 2017).

A further interesting approach for BOLD imaging might be the three-dimensional segmented echo-planar imaging (3D-EPI). Single-shot EPI at 7 T often suffers from significant geometric distortions partly due to low bandwidth in the phase-encoded direction and amplified physiological noise. The 3D sequence could further improve high-resolution fMRI as it provides an increased SNR at similar temporal resolution to traditional multi-slice 2D-EPI readouts, in total, leading to increased volume coverage and decreased geometric distortions. The study of van der Zwaag et al. (2012) could reveal that during fMRI experiments at 7 T with a motor task, the 3D-EPI outperforms the 2D-EPI in terms of temporal SNR and sensitivity to detect activated brain regions. Similar results were reported in a further study using a 3D PRESTO sequence (Barry and Strother 2011).

In summary, an extended optimization of sequences and new coil developments, especially new transmit-receive coils, was done in the recent years with increasing evidence of optimized fMRI at ultra-high-field MRI. Furthermore, new aspects of multimodal imaging in functional MRI are more and more coming up. One example is the combination of neurochemical and BOLD MRI at 7 T. There are some reports about small concentration changes in lactate, glutamate, aspartate and glucose in the human cortex during prolonged stimuli. However, a correlation to BOLD-fMRI signals was unclear. Bednarik et al. (2015) could show that MRS at 7 T is sensitive to analyse such small signal changes and that BOLD-fMRI signals were positively correlated with glutamate and lactate concentration changes. As at 3 T and also at ultra-high-field MRI, the combination of DTI and fMRI is more and more used. For example, the functional specificity of the cortico-subcortical loops depending on varying levels of cognitive hierarchy as well as their structural connectivity was addressed using high-resolution fMRI and DTI (Jeon et al. 2014).

4.3.1 7 T and Beyond

The main driving force for the trend to higher and higher field strengths is the gain in intrinsic SNR, which is expected to grow at least linearly with field strength. However, as mentioned above, with increasing static field restrictions have to overcome, the homogeneity of the RF fields declines; the longitudinal relaxation time T1 increases, while T2 and T2∗ decrease; construction of RF coils for high frequencies becomes more and more important. An excellent overview of the development and comparison of 3 T, 7 T and 9.4 T is given by the paper of Pohmann et al. (2016). Their experiments could show that in standard experimental conditions, SNR increased supralinearly with field strength. But also, to take full advantage of this gain, the deteriorating B1 homogeneity and the decreasing T2 (∗) have to be overcome. Therefore, recent papers have described solutions for these challenges, for example, the higher-degree whole-brain B0 shimming at 9.4 T (Chang et al. 2018). They emphasized the necessity of calibrating the shim system and concluded that better B_0 homogeneity drastically reduces signal dropout and distortions for echo-planar imaging and significantly improves the linewidths of MR spectroscopy imaging. Similar to 7 T (as described above), a possible solution for fMRI is the use of SSFP imaging. First results have been presented for high-resolution mapping of neural activation in the visual brain areas at 9.4 T (Scheffler and Ehses 2016).

However, due to the mentioned increasing challenges at higher field strength, further studies and developments have to be done since we fully can take advantage of the high SNR increase at higher fields.

4.4 Ultra-High-Field fMRI: Recent Neurocognitive Studies

Early experiments have, besides motor paradigms, addressed retinotopic maps at 7 T. An identification of visual areas in the occipitoparietal cortex was found (Hoffmann et al. 2009). It was demonstrated that the mean coherence increased with magnetic field strength and with voxel size. At 7 T, the occipital cortex could be sampled with high sensitivity in a single short session at high resolution. Therefore, retinotopic mapping at 7 T opens the possibility of detailed understanding of the cortical visual field representations and of their plasticity in visual system pathologies. A further study analysed the use of spin-echo BOLD with 1.8-mm resolution at 3- and 7-T imaging for retinotopic mapping in comparison to gradient sequences (Olman et al. 2010). As mentioned above, some early studies could demonstrate the use of spin-echo sequences for fMRI. Olman et al. could now show that GE BOLD and at 7-T SE BOLD had no systematic differences in either the area or the boundary locations for V1, V2 and V3. Therefore, the feasibility of high-resolution spin-echo BOLD experiments with good sensitivity throughout multiple visual areas was demonstrated. However, the highest resolution at ultra-high-field fMRI is restricted due to biological point-spread of the haemodynamic signal. The extent of this spread is described to be determined by the local vascular distribution and by the spatial specificity of blood flow regulation. Apart from this, there is influence from the measurement parameters. A recent study introduced a laminar surface-based analysis method and studied the relationship between spatial localization and activation strength as a function of laminar depth by acquiring an isotropic, single-shot EPI at 7 T (Polimeni et al. 2010). The BOLD signal was sampled exclusively from the superficial, middle or deep cortical laminae. This group could show that avoiding surface laminae improved spatial localization. They conclude that optimal spatial resolution in functional imaging of the cortex can be achieved using anatomically informed spatial sampling to avoid large pial vessels.

Apart from analyses of direct motor tasks as described in the clinical application discussion below, the sensorimotor network has recently been the focus on 7-T fMRI studies. Hale et al. used resting-state fMRI at 3 and 7 T to assess connectivity in the sensorimotor network and default mode network at different spatial smoothing levels (Hale and Brookes 2010). The authors found higher temporal correlation coefficients for both sensorimotor network and default mode network at 7 T compared to 3 T for all smoothing levels. The maximum physiological noise contribution was higher at 7 T. However, no significant difference in the spatial correlation of maps following physiological correction was found. Whole-brain high-resolution (down to 1-mm isotropic voxels) resting-state fMRI at 7 T using parallel imaging technology could be performed without restrictions in temporal resolution or brain coverage (De Martino and Esposito 2011). Since those first reports, further resting-state fMRI experiments have been published. For example, the higher resolution was used to characterize resting-state fMRI signal time course properties and evaluate different seed placements within and around haemorrhagic traumatic axonal injury lesions (Lee et al. 2018).

Up to now, some studies have and further studies will have to also address cognitive functions involving more challenging brain areas. One study evaluated BOLD responses due to visual sexual stimuli at 7 T (Walter et al. 2008). This study could demonstrate that fMRI at high fields provides an ideal tool to investigate functional anatomy of subcortical structures. Furthermore, due to an increased SNR, functional scans of short duration can be acquired at high resolution. Coming back to experiments involving areas with high sensitivity to susceptibility artefacts, first results revealed acceptable image quality using an 8-channel head coil at 7 T compared to 3 T (Fig. 4.2). Additionally, in these results, the hippocampal activation during a memory-encoding task improved from 3 to 7 T (Theysohn et al. 2013). However, the dropout of volunteers due to image inhomogeneities was higher at 7 T.

Using the above-mentioned improvements in BOLD imaging at 7 T, further studies were published addressing subregional network architecture. The medial temporal lobe substructures with its integral role in memory functions have been analysed using 7 T resting-state fMRI (Shah et al. 2018). They found a moderate structural and strong functional inter-hemispheric symmetry. Furthermore, several bilateral hippocampal

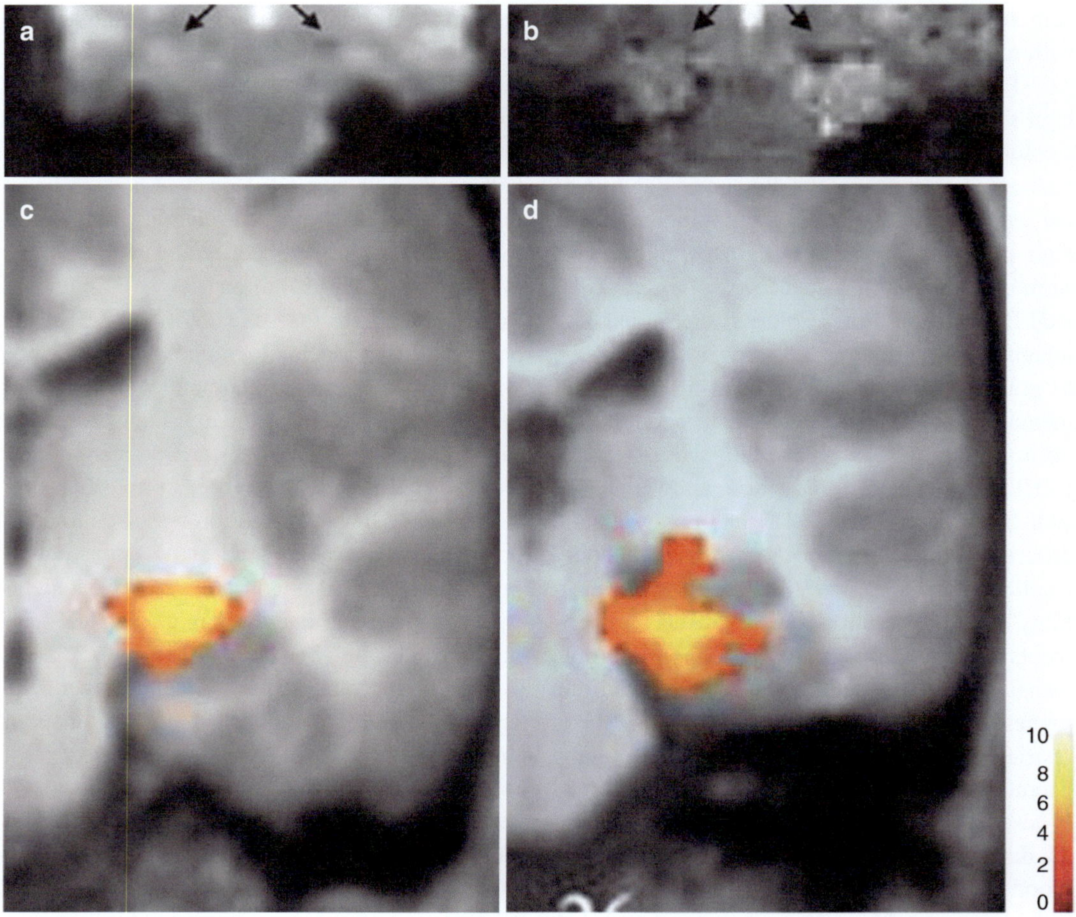

Fig. 4.2 EPI images with its sensitivity for susceptibility artefacts are compared at 3 T (**a**) and 7 T (**b**) imaging. Parallel acquisition techniques for reduction of these artefacts were used at both scanners (matrix 92 × 92 m^2 in this case at both scanners with 8-channel head coil). (**c** and **d**) The images show that the improvement of 7-T imaging techniques leads to acceptable image quality, allowing fMRI studies of the hippocampal region

subregions (CA1, dentate gyrus and subiculum) could be identified as functional network hubs. Another mapping was done using intraneural microstimulation of single mechanoreceptive afferent units in the median nerve in humans (Sanchez Panchuelo et al. 2016). With this method an opportunity is given to bridge the gap between first-order mechanoreceptive afferent input codes and their spatial, dynamic and perceptual representations in the human cortex. Another structure with small size and connection to other small regions, the bed nucleus of the stria terminalis was another target to use fMRI at 7 T (Torrisi et al. 2015). This region is implicated in the pathophysiology of anxiety and addiction disorders but easily addressed by conventional methods. This group used seed-based resting-state functional connectivity to map the bed nucleus resting-state network. They could demonstrate the in vivo reproduction of many human bed nucleus connections previously described in animal research.

4.5 Ultra-High-Field fMRI and Possible Clinical Applications

3-T fMRI is increasingly used in clinical and experimental studies in most countries. In addition to developments in coil technology, 3-T MRI provides an excellent solution for higher resolution and/or signal changes with an acceptable increase in susceptibility artefacts (Alvarez-Linera 2008).

3-T fMRI has been used in a variety of experiments so far. The initial dip in the motor and visual areas was examined simultaneously using a visually guided finger-tapping paradigm (Yacoub and Hu 2001). Other experiments could show that fMRI measurements quantifying the strength of activity and centres of mass in response to tasks offer sensitive measurements of change over repeated imaging sessions. Therefore, fMRI at high field strength can be used for serial investigations of individual participants using simple motor and cognitive tasks in a simple block design (Goodyear and Douglas 2008). These results are very promising in respect to advanced clinical use of high-field fMRI. At 1.5 T, one main problem is the restriction in obtaining individual activation maps due to lack of sensitivity and specificity. This can be overcome with the more stable haemodynamic response function and higher BOLD signal at 3 T and even more at higher field strength, e.g. 7 T.

Within the recent years, the number of fMRI studies using 3-T scanners has much grown as those scanners become more and more available. Besides experimental studies like evaluation of gender differences, encoding and recognition of pseudowords (Banks et al. 2012) or differences in humour (Kohn et al. 2011), clinical studies also revealed improvement of activation at 3 T compared to 1.5 T (Blatow et al. 2011). Figure 4.3 gives a typical clinical example of the use of 3-T (f)MRI in tumour patients. In the everyday setting, such significant activation during a finger-tapping task can be achieved robustly in a short block design and a scanner-associated post-processing with overlay on structural 3D T1 image after contrast application (MPRAGE). Recently, the mapping of substructures was published not only for visual and auditory cortex but also for human finger somatotopy ((Martuzzi et al. 2014). Cortical representations of fingers are of particular interest, and therefore these results have impact to clinical imaging.

The first 7-T studies were performed to demonstrate the feasibility of BOLD fMRI using EPI and to characterize the BOLD response in humans at 7 T using visual stimulation. These results indicate that fMRI can be reliably performed at 7 T and that at this field strength, both the sensitivity and spatial specificity of the BOLD response are increased. These studies suggest that ultra-high-field MR systems are advantageous for functional mapping in humans (Yacoub et al. 2001).

Decreasing the voxel size at high field strength and simultaneously obtaining high temporal resolution are major challenges and are mainly limited by gradient performance. Pfeuffer et al. used an optimized surface coil set-up for zoomed functional imaging in the visual cortex (Pfeuffer et al. 2002c). With a single-shot acquisition at submillimetre resolution (500 × 500 mm^2) in the human brain and a high temporal resolution of 125 ms, activation of single-trial BOLD responses was obtained. Therefore, the possibilities of event-related functional imaging in the human brain were expanded. One recent study in relation to brain-computer-interface (BCI) technology research used a real-time fMRI at 7 T to evaluate the potential benefit of this method for BCI interactions (Andersson et al. 2010).

For clinical use, the activation in eloquent areas such as the sensorimotor areas and coverage of larger brain volumes are of great importance. One study at 7 T revealed activation in all sensorimotor motor areas at 7 T: SI, MI, SII, SMA, thalamus and contralateral cerebellar areas involved in sensorimotor processing (Gizewski et al. 2007). Even when using a t/r CP coil, the signal change was a factor of 2–5 higher at 7 T than at 1.5 T. At 7 T, susceptibility artefacts were present especially in the basal brain structures, but a well-fitted response curve could be detected in all sensorimotor areas at 7 T, even in areas suffering from susceptibility such as the cerebellum (Fig. 4.4). In contrast to the results at 1.5 T, thalamic activation was found in all subjects and revealed an excellent response function. Even single-block analyses at 7 T revealed similar or even higher response strength than multi-block measurements at 1.5 T. These results indicate that fMRI can be robustly performed at 7 T, covering the whole brain using a t/r CP head coil with

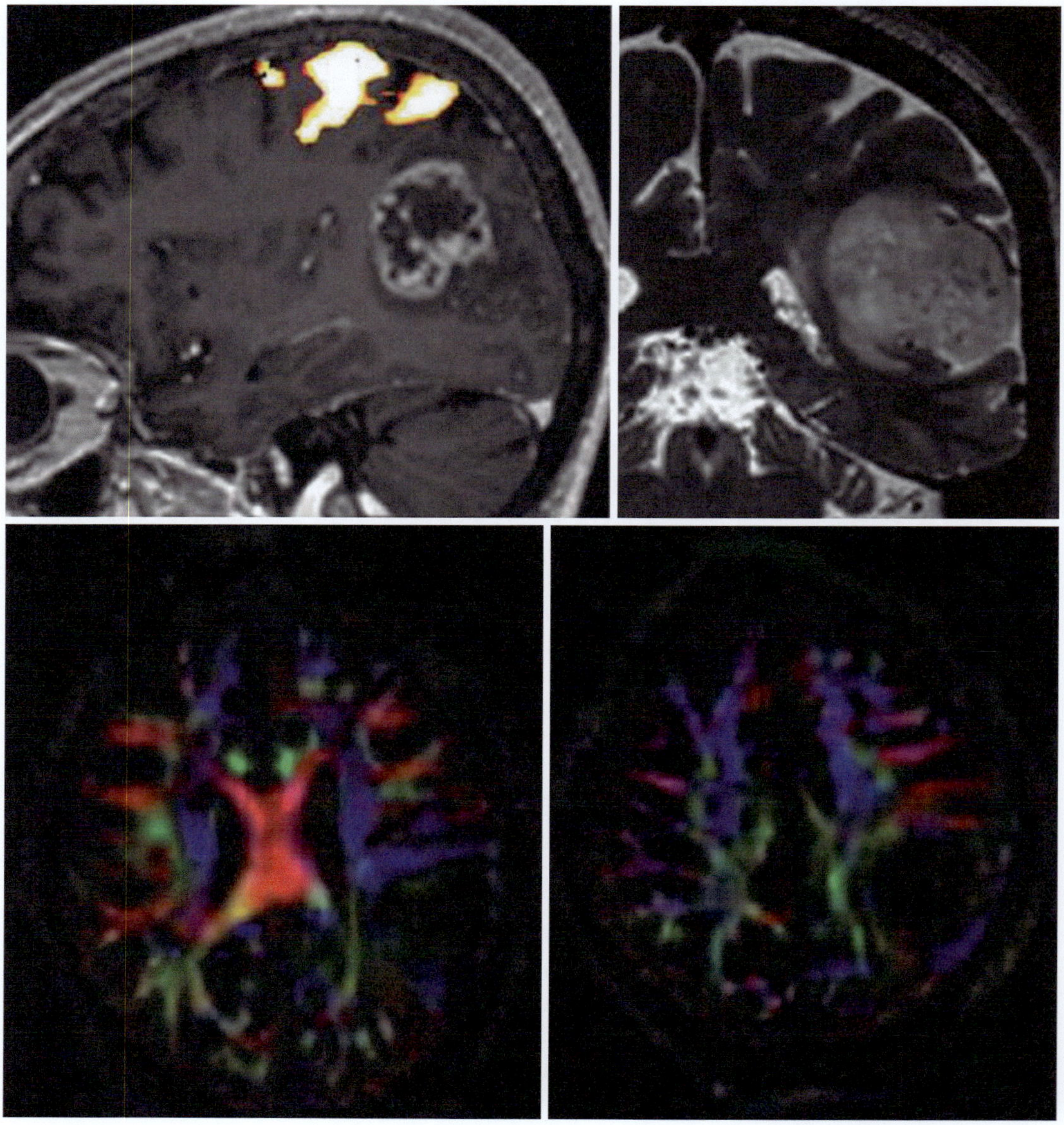

Fig. 4.3 Clinical application of 3 T: significant activation during a finger-tapping task performed by a patient with a brain tumour near the central area in a short block design. Results are presented after scanner-associated post-processing with overlay on structural 3D T1 image after contrast application (MPRAGE). In the same session, normally T2-weighted 3D images and a DTI are added to the fMRI task

higher signal and increased stability of the haemodynamic response curve. The excellent response functions and signal change elevations shown in this study using a well-established, simple sensorimotor paradigm indicate that even in susceptibility problematic brain regions, ultra-high-field fMRI is possible. A further study used a 16-channel head coil at 7 T to measure the topographic representation of the digits in human somatosensory cortex at 1-mm isotropic resolution in individual subjects (Sanchez-Panchuelo and Schluppeck 2010). This study using a tactile stimulation of each finger could show an orderly map of the digits on the postcentral gyrus. Those activations were robust and could be made in individual subjects, leading to a wide use of this method in clinical and experimental settings. These results are very interesting

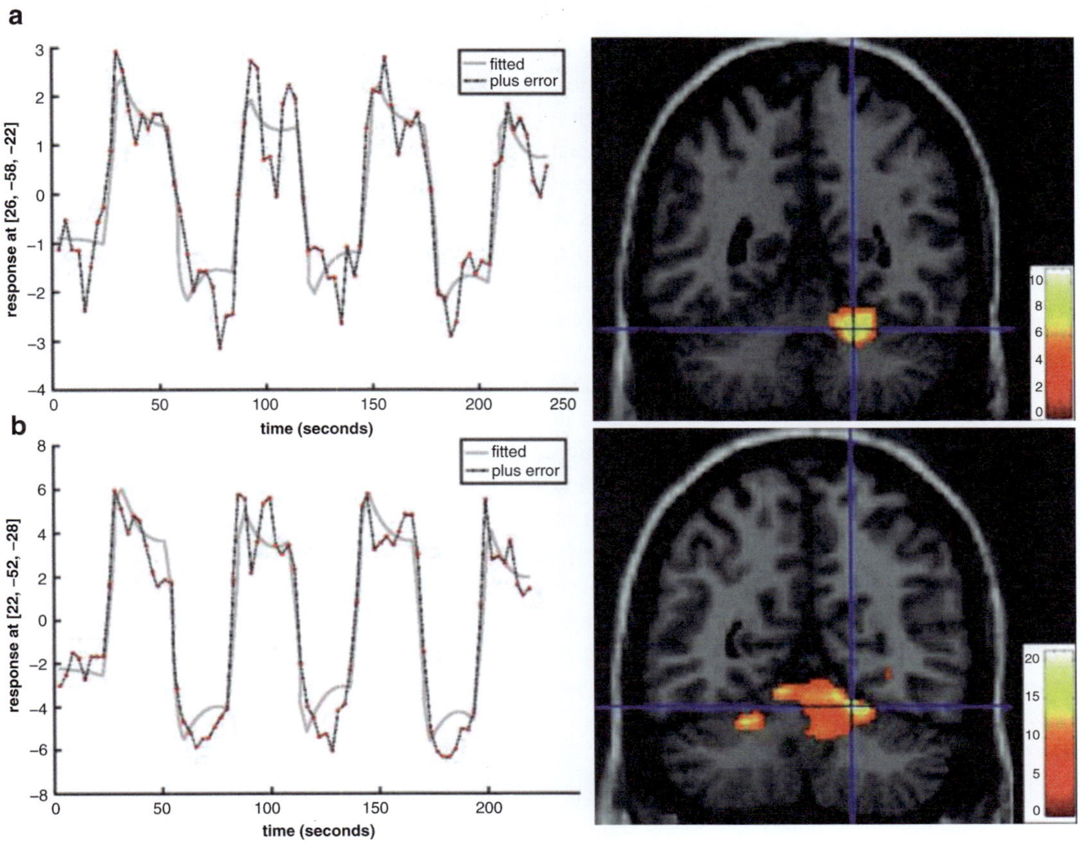

Fig. 4.4 (**a**) Plot of fitted response function at the main cluster in the cerebellar sensorimotor areas at 1.5 T (representative subject). Statistical parametric maps of activation within all subjects performing the finger-tapping task compared with rest period at 1.5 T. Task-related increase in MR signal is superimposed on coronal section of a 3D T1-weighted standard brain. Statistically corrected threshold is $p < 0.05$. Results show main activation in the cerebellum. (**b**) Plot of fitted response function at the main cluster in the cerebellar sensorimotor areas at 7 T (representative subject). Statistical parametric maps of activation within all subjects performing the finger-tapping task compared with rest period at 7 T. Statistically corrected threshold is $p < 0.005$. Results show main activation in the cerebellum

in relation to a similar study performed at 3 T (Olman et al. 2012). This group found strong evidence of BOLD selectivity in the hemisphere contralateral to the cued digit; however, they found no evidence for an orderly spatial topography. One can discuss the differences in respect to slight differing settings but also in respect to the influence of higher field strength.

As mentioned above the signal increase in ultra-high-field fMRI depends on many factors, not only on the magnetic field strength. Some studies have revealed a signal increase of up to fivefold using imaging parameters focused on increased spatial resolution and small field of view (Pfeuffer et al. 2002a, b). The sensitivity is somewhat constrained by the SNR characteristics if a CP head coil is used in conjunction with standard voxel sizes from 1.5 T. It has been shown that a reduction in voxel size leads to an improvement in time series SNR through a decrease in physiological noise (Triantafyllou et al. 2005). The relatively small BOLD changes in certain brain areas in the CP study might be explained by this effect, but the use of larger voxels allows whole-brain coverage.

It is likely that future studies will not strive for exceptional resolution in one area of the brain but be targeted at analysing complex networks.

Especially cognitive functions but also clinical applications require more slices and coverage of extended brain areas. Furthermore, some interesting structures such as the hippocampal region can, as in the cerebellum, suffer from signal dropouts near tissue-air boundaries. The recent developments in coil technique and sequences as well as post-processing have much improved the use of ultra-high field even in the mentioned problematic areas. Some examples were described in the cognitive section above. Figure 4.5 shows a further example with possible use not only in experimental settings but also in clinical applications: a representative activation of the dentate nucleus during a finger-tapping task. With such technique, even examination of activation of the dentate nucleus in a verb-generation task in normal volunteers was possible using the increase in signal-to-noise ratio (Thürling et al. 2011). For image processing, a newly developed region of interest-driven normalization method of the dentate nuclei was applied. This experiment suggests that the human dentate nucleus can be subdivided into a rostral and more dorsal motor domain and a ventrocaudal non-motor domain. Such findings represent the benefit of high-field fMRI with its higher SNR and possibility to reveal deep brain structures more reliable.

Further interesting structures with the need of higher resolution also in clinical applications are the brainstem and deep brain nuclei. This region also suffers from signal dropouts near tissue-air boundaries and pulsation artefacts, for example, due to the basilar artery (Fig. 4.6). For anatomical and fibre tracking methods (DTI), the sequences have been optimized resulting in depiction of substructures within the brainstem (Deistung et al. 2013, Gizewski et al. 2014). The anatomy of the human brainstem in vivo was mainly achieved by acquiring and generating images with multiple contrasts: T2/PD-weighted images,

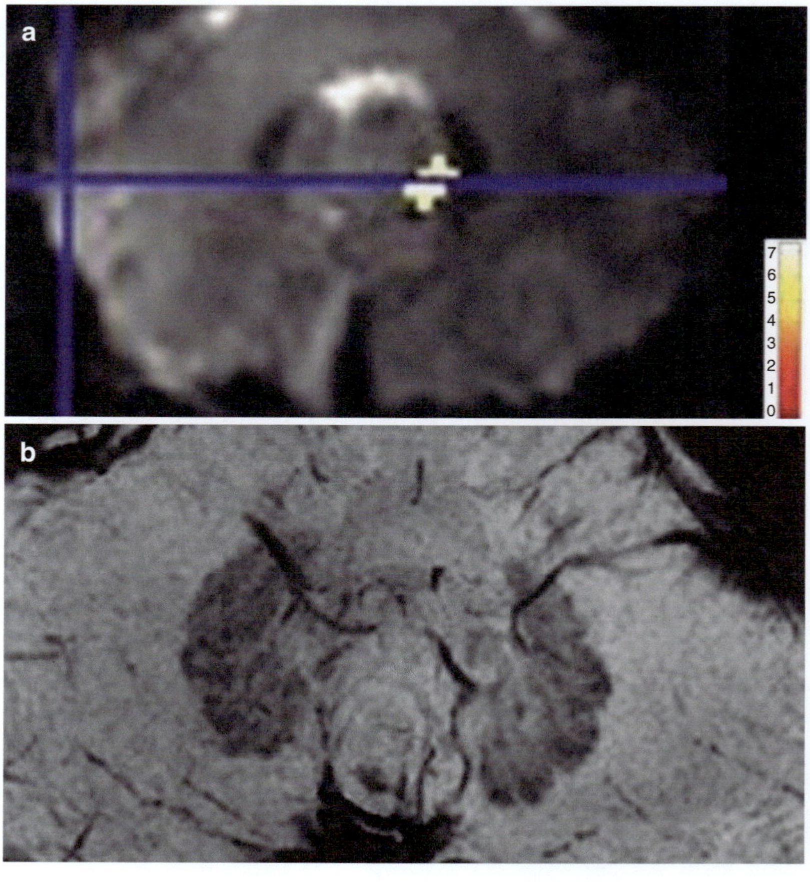

Fig. 4.5 Statistical parametric maps of activation of a single subject performing finger-tapping task compared with rest period at 7 T superimposed on EPI transverse orientation (**a**) and the high-resolution SWI imaging of dentate nucleus at 7 T (**b**). Statistically corrected threshold is $p < 0.001$

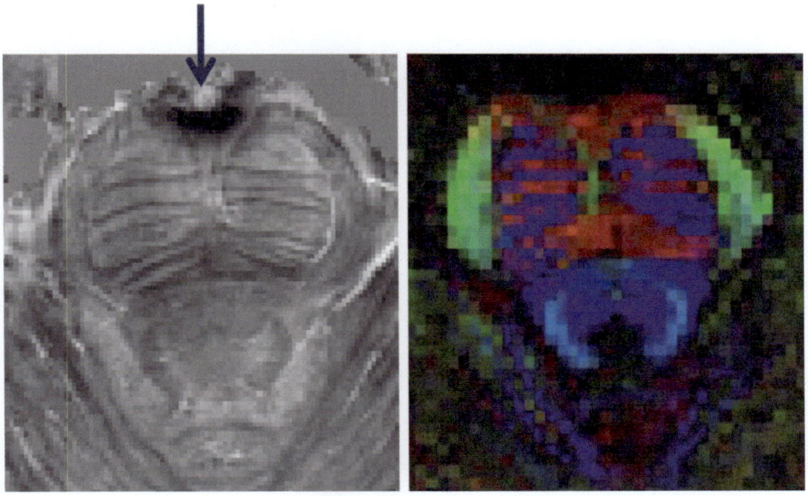

Fig. 4.6 SWI with pulsation artefact due to basilar artery, however, excellent resolution in DTI. Measurements in cooperation with Dr. Sina Straub, DKFZ, Heidelberg, Germany

quantitative maps of longitudinal relaxation rate (R1∗ maps), magnetic susceptibility maps (SWI with quantitative mapping) and DTI. For fMRI further challenges have to be solved in this region. The haemodynamic response function (HRF) may vary substantially in subcortical structures, and adoption in designing and interpretation of fMRI studies of these regions are needed. Lewis et al. (2018) studied the temporal properties and non-linearities of the HRF across the human subcortical visual system (superior colliculus, lateral geniculate nucleus of the thalamus, primary visual cortex). They concluded that subcortical visual structures exhibit fast and nonlinear haemodynamic responses and that these dynamics enable detection of fast BOLD signals even within small deep brain structures when imaging at 7 T. The high-resolution structural images of the brainstem with delineation of brainstem nuclei were further used to identify seed regions in resting-state fMRI (Bianciardi et al. 2016). Here, the connectomes of 11 brainstem nuclei of the ascending arousal, motor and autonomic systems from 12 controls could be presented.

A further substructure of the brainstem, which can be clearly visualized at 7 T, is the periaqueductal grey, a key region in autonomic function. Some 3 T studies have shown involvement of this region in some autonomic functions, e.g. pain processing. However, to identify these subregions was still impossible. Faull et al. (2015) then showed deactivation in the lateral and dorsomedial columns of the PAG corresponding with short breath holds and cortical activations demonstrating the involvement of these subregions of PAG in the network of conscious respiratory control for the first time in humans.

Basal ganglia circuits are important in neurological disorders such as Parkinson's disease (PD) and target in advanced therapies such as deep brain stimulation (DBS). Knowledge about the connectivity of the human basal ganglia and thalamus has evolved over recent years but still suffers from restricted resolution and sensitivity in in vivo imaging. One group presented an imaging and computational protocol to overcome this problems (Lenglet et al. 2012). High-resolution structural and functional images were acquired with 7 T and revealed detailed structural and connectivity representations of the human basal ganglia and thalamus. These data provides more information on basal ganglia circuitry and has impact for pre-surgical planning in individual human subjects. This optimized fMRI for basal ganglia using a reduction of echo time and spatial resolution was used by de Hollander et al. (2017). They also revealed that an fMRI protocol at 3 T with identical resolution to the 7 T showed no robust BOLD sensitivity in any of the BG nuclei. Therefore, this application is a well-confirmed benefit of ultra-high-field fMRI in clinical applications.

In respect to more direct clinical application, first experiments with a speech paradigm could

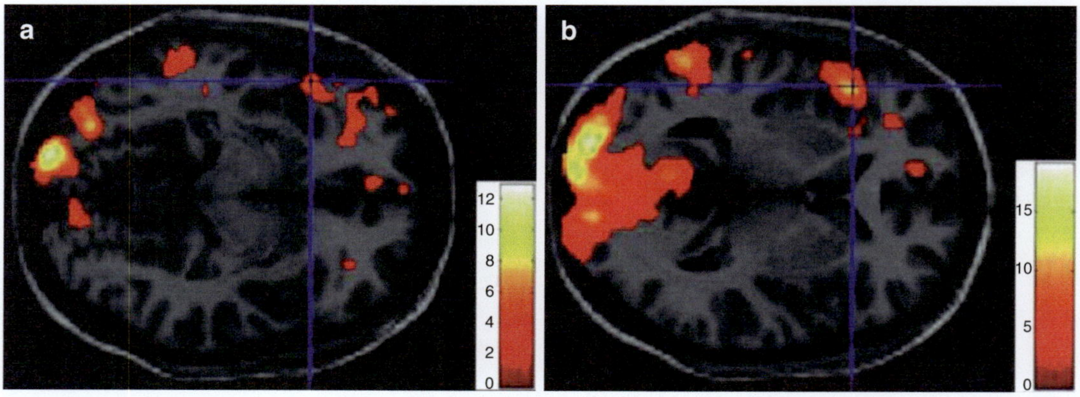

Fig. 4.7 Statistical parametric maps of activation within all subjects performing the verb-generation task compared with rest period at 1.5 T (**a**) and 7 T (**b**) superimposed on a standard brain in transverse orientation. Statistically corrected threshold is $p < 0.005$. Activated areas of Broca and Wernicke regions are shown at both field strengths but with more extended clusters and higher signal change at 7 T

reveal the advantages of 7-T fMRI combined with an 8-channel head coil and a parallel acquisition technique (Fig. 4.7). Even using the parallel acquisition technique, an increase in BOLD signal could be obtained, and a more extended activation and detection of lateralization could be found. Furthermore, the application of parallel imaging led to a significant reduction of artefacts (Fig. 4.2). Therefore, a reliable co-registration of high-resolution structural images with the EPI images could be performed. Figure 4.8 shows a patient with a cavernoma scanned pre-surgically at 1.5 T (a) and 7 T (b). The speech paradigm was a verb-generation task in both measurements in a block design. The activation maps are superimposed on susceptibility-weighted images (SWI) at 1.5 and 7 T. In addition to the higher BOLD signal and the more extended activation at 7 T, the higher spatial resolution of the structural images confers further benefit for surgical planning. One recent study could demonstrate the clinical benefit of 7-T fMRI. The primary motor hand area was analysed at 3 and 7 T in 17 patients (Beisteiner and Robinson 2011). However, as in former studies, 7-T data suffered from significant increase of artefacts (ghosting, head motion).

With the higher resolution and further optimized sequences, spinal cord structures come to the focus of interest. Recently, a group reported their findings of resting-state functional connectivity in the human spinal cord in a cohort of healthy volunteers. They observed robust functional connectivity between left and right ventral motor horns and between left and right dorsal sensory horns (Barry et al. 2016).

Besides fundamental experimental interests, e.g. for cognitive studies, clinical indications of 7-T fMRI can be imagined. Pre-surgical fMRI in patients with brain tumours could benefit from either higher resolution or faster imaging. Even patients impaired with respect to motor function are for the most part able to perform a short-finger movement sufficient for a single-block examination.

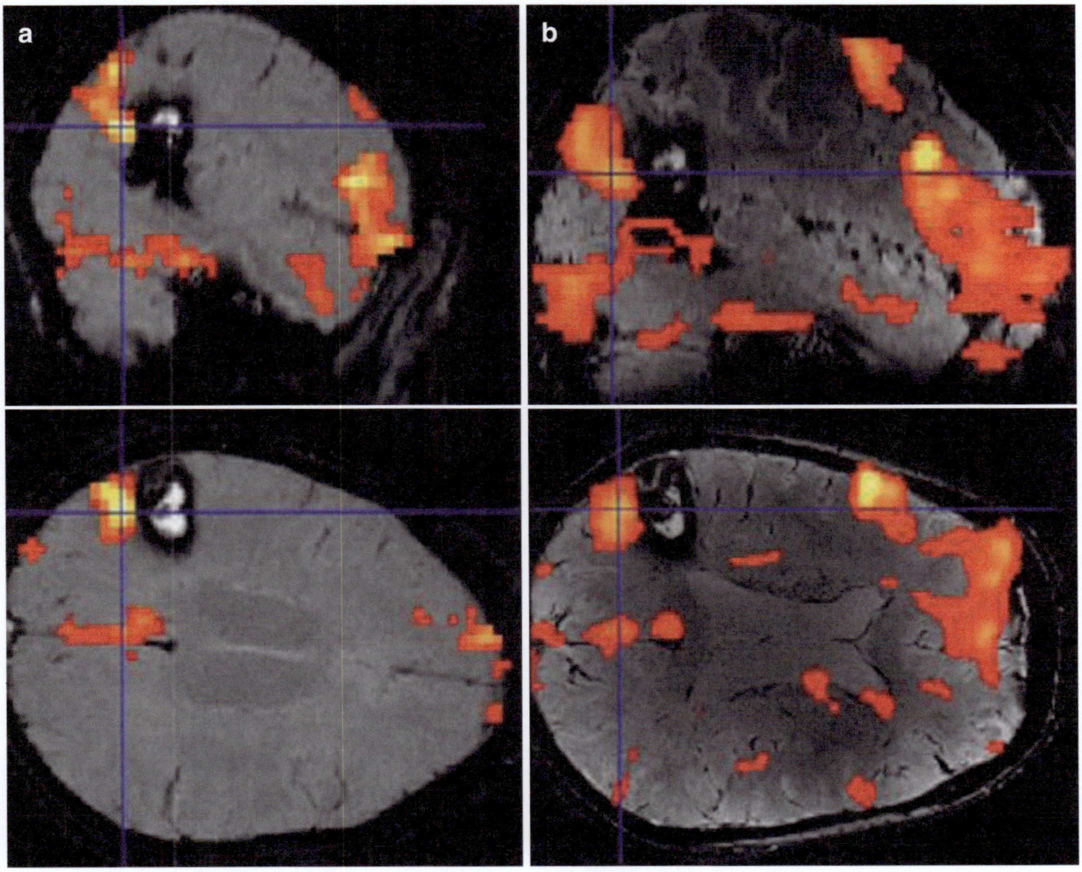

Fig. 4.8 Statistical parametric maps of activation within one patient performing the verb-generation task compared with rest period at 1.5 T (**a**) and 7 T (**b**) superimposed on SWI images. Statistically corrected threshold is $p < 0.005$. Activated areas of Broca and Wernicke regions are shown at both field strengths but with more extended clusters and higher signal change at 7 T. Furthermore, the structural images have a higher in-plane resolution at 7 T with enhanced tumour-brain differentiation and superior depiction of the inner structure of the cavernoma

References

Alvarez-Linera J (2008) 3 T MRI: advances in brain imaging. Eur J Radiol 67(3):415–426

Andersson P, Ramsey NF et al (2010) BCI control using 4 direction spatial visual attention and real-time fMRI at 7 T. Conf Proc IEEE Eng Med Biol Soc 2010:4221–4225

Banks SJ, Jones-Gotman M et al (2012) Sex differences in the medial temporal lobe during encoding and recognition of pseudowords and abstract designs. NeuroImage 59(2):1888–1895

Barry RL, Strother SC (2011) Data-driven optimization and evaluation of 2D EPI and 3D PRESTO for BOLD fMRI at 7 Tesla: I. Focal coverage. NeuroImage 55(3):1034–1043

Barry RL, Rogers BP, Conrad BN, Smith SA, Gore JC (2016) Reproducibility of resting state spinal cord networks in healthy volunteers at 7 Tesla. NeuroImage 133:31–40

Bednařík P, Tkáč I, Giove F, DiNuzzo M, Deelchand DK, Emir UE, Eberly LE, Mangia S (2015 Mar 31) Neurochemical and BOLD responses during neuronal activation measured in the human visual cortex at 7 Tesla. J Cereb Blood Flow Metab 35(4):601–610

Beisteiner R, Robinson S (2011) Clinical fMRI: evidence for a 7T benefit over 3T. NeuroImage 57(3):1015–1021

Bianciardi M, Toschi N, Eichner C, Polimeni JR, Setsompop K, Brown EN, Hämäläinen MS, Rosen BR, Wald LL (2016 Jun) In vivo functional connectome of human brainstem nuclei of the ascending arousal, autonomic, and motor systems by high spatial resolution 7-Tesla fMRI. MAGMA 29(3):451–462

Blatow M, Reinhardt J et al (2011) Clinical functional MRI of sensorimotor cortex using passive motor and sensory stimulation at 3 Tesla. J Magn Reson Imaging 34(2):429–437

Brunheim S, Johst S, Pfaffenrot V, Maderwald S, Quick HH, Poser BA (2017 Dec) Variable slice thickness (VAST) EPI for the reduction of susceptibility artifacts in whole-brain GE-EPI at 7 Tesla. MAGMA 30(6):591–607

Chang P, Nassirpour S, Henning A (2018 Jan) Modeling real shim fields for very high degree (and order) B0 shimming of the human brain at 9.4 T. Magn Reson Med 79(1):529–540

de Hollander G, Keuken MC, van der Zwaag W, Forstmann BU, Trampel R (2017 Jun) Comparing functional MRI protocols for small, iron-rich basal ganglia nuclei such as the subthalamic nucleus at 7 T and 3 T. Hum Brain Mapp 38(6):3226–3248

De Martino F, Esposito F (2011) Whole brain high-resolution functional imaging at ultra high magnetic fields: an application to the analysis of resting state networks. NeuroImage 57(3):1031–1044

Deistung A, Schäfer A, Schweser F, Biedermann U, Güllmar D, Trampel R, Turner R, Reichenbach JR (2013) High-resolution MR imaging of the human brainstem in vivo at 7 Tesla. Front Hum Neurosci 7:710

Duong TQ, Yacoub E et al (2003) Microvascular BOLD contribution at 4 and 7 T in the human brain: gradient-echo and spin-echo fMRI with suppression of blood effects. Magn Reson Med 49(6):1019–1027

Faull OK, Jenkinson M, Clare S, Pattinson KT (2015 Jun) Functional subdivision of the human periaqueductal grey in respiratory control using 7 Tesla fMRI. NeuroImage 113:356–364

Gizewski ER, de Greiff A et al (2007) FMRI at 7 T: whole-brain coverage and signal advantages even infratentorially? NeuroImage 37(3):761–768

Gizewski ER, Maderwald S, Linn J, Dassinger B, Bochmann K, Forsting M, Ladd ME (2014 Mar) High-resolution anatomy of the human brain stem using 7-T MRI: improved detection of inner structures and nerves? Neuroradiology 56(3):177–186

Goodyear BG, Douglas EA (2008) Minimum detectable change in motor and prefrontal cortex activity over repeated sessions using 3 T functional MRI and a block design. J Magn Reson Imaging 28(5):1055–1060

Gowland PA, Bowtell R (2007) Theoretical optimization of multi-echo fMRI data acquisition. Phys Med Biol 52(7):1801–1813

Hale JR, Brookes MJ (2010) Comparison of functional connectivity in default mode and sensorimotor networks at 3 and 7 T. MAGMA 23(5–6):339–349

Heid O (1997) Robust EPI phase correction. In: Proceedings of the ISMRM, Vancouver, 1997

Hoffmann MB, Stadler J et al (2009) Retinotopic mapping of the human visual cortex at a magnetic field strength of 7 T. Clin Neurophysiol 120(1):108–116

Hua J, Qin Q, van Zijl PC, Pekar JJ, Jones CK (2014 Dec) Whole-brain three-dimensional T2-weighted BOLD functional magnetic resonance imaging at 7 Tesla. Magn Reson Med 72(6):1530–1540

Jeon HA, Anwander A, Friederici AD (2014 Jul 9) Functional network mirrored in the prefrontal cortex, caudate nucleus, and thalamus: high-resolution functional imaging and structural connectivity. J Neurosci 34(28):9202–9212

Juchem C, Nixon TW, McIntyre S, Boer VO, Rothman DL, de Graaf RA (2011 Oct) Dynamic multi-coil shimming of the human brain at 7 T. J Magn Reson 212(2):280–288

Juchem C, Umesh Rudrapatna S, Nixon TW, de Graaf RA (2015 Jan 15) Dynamic multi-coil technique (DYNAMITE) shimming for echo-planar imaging of the human brain at 7 Tesla. NeuroImage 105:462–472

Kemper VG, De Martino F, Yacoub E, Goebel R (2016 Sep) Variable flip angle 3D-GRASE for high resolution fMRI at 7 Tesla. Magn Reson Med 76(3):897–904

Kim T, Lee Y, Zhao T, Hetherington HP, Pan JW (2017 Nov) Gradient-echo EPI using a high-degree shim insert coil at 7 T: implications for BOLD fMRI. Magn Reson Med 78(5):1734–1745

Kohn N, Kellermann T et al (2011) Gender differences in the neural correlates of humor processing: implications for different processing modes. Neuropsychologia 49(5):888–897

Ladd ME (2007) High-field-strength magnetic resonance: potential and limits. Top Magn Reson Imaging 18(2):139–152

Lee S, Polimeni JR, Price CM, Edlow BL, McNab JA (2018 Jun) Characterizing signals within lesions and mapping brain network connectivity after traumatic axonal injury: a 7 Tesla resting-state FMRI study. Brain Connect 8(5):288–298

Lenglet C, Abosch A, Yacoub E, De Martino F, Sapiro G, Harel N (2012) Comprehensive in vivo mapping of the human basal ganglia and thalamic connectome in individuals using 7T MRI. PLoS One 7(1):e29153

Lewis LD, Setsompop K, Rosen BR, Polimeni JR (2018 Jun 20) Stimulus-dependent hemodynamic response timing across the human subcortical-cortical visual pathway identified through high spatiotemporal resolution 7T fMRI. NeuroImage 181:279–291

Malekian V, Nasiraei-Moghaddam A, Khajehim M (2018 Jul) A robust SSFP technique for fMRI at ultra-high field strengths. Magn Reson Imaging 50:17–25

Martuzzi R, van der Zwaag W, Farthouat J, Gruetter R, Blanke O (2014 Jan) Human finger somatotopy in areas 3b, 1, and 2: a 7T fMRI study using a natural stimulus. Hum Brain Mapp 35(1):213–226

Mirrashed F, Sharp JC et al (2004) High-resolution imaging at 3 T and 7 T with multiring local volume coils. MAGMA 16(4):167–173

Newton AT, Rogers BP et al (2012) Improving measurement of functional connectivity through decreasing partial volume effects at 7 T. NeuroImage 59(3):2511–2517

Norris DG (2003) High field human imaging. J Magn Reson Imaging 18(5):519–529

Okada T, Yamada H et al (2005) Magnetic field strength increase yields significantly greater contrast-to-noise ratio increase: measured using BOLD contrast in the primary visual area. Acad Radiol 12(2):142–147

Olman CA, Van de Moortele PF et al (2010) Retinotopic mapping with spin echo BOLD at 7 T. Magn Reson Imaging 28(9):1258–1269

Olman CA, Pickett KA et al (2012) Selective BOLD responses to individual finger movement measured with fMRI at 3 T. Hum Brain Mapp 33(7): 1594–1606

Pfeuffer J, Adriany G et al (2002a) Perfusion-based high-resolution functional imaging in the human brain at 7 Tesla. Magn Reson Med 47(5):903–911

Pfeuffer J, Van de Moortele PF et al (2002b) Correction of physiologically induced global off-resonance effects in dynamic echo-planar and spiral functional imaging. Magn Reson Med 47(2):344–353

Pfeuffer J, Van de Moortele PF et al (2002c) Zoomed functional imaging in the human brain at 7 Tesla with simultaneous high spatial and high temporal resolution. NeuroImage 17(1):272–282

Pohmann R, Speck O, Scheffler K (2016 Feb) Signal-to-noise ratio and MR tissue parameters in human brain imaging at 3, 7, and 9.4 Tesla using current receive coil arrays. Magn Reson Med 75(2):801–809

Polimeni JR, Fischl B et al (2010) Laminar analysis of 7 T BOLD using an imposed spatial activation pattern in human V1. NeuroImage 52(4):1334–1346

Poser BA, Versluis MJ et al (2006) BOLD contrast sensitivity enhancement and artifact reduction with multiecho EPI: parallel-acquired inhomogeneity-desensitized fMRI. Magn Reson Med 55(6):1227–1235

Preibisch C, Wallenhorst T et al (2008) Comparison of parallel acquisition techniques generalized autocalibrating partially parallel acquisitions (GRAPPA) and modified sensitivity encoding (mSENSE) in functional MRI (fMRI) at 3 T. J Magn Reson Imaging 27(3):590–598

Sanchez Panchuelo RM, Ackerley R, Glover PM, Bowtell RW, Wessberg J, Francis ST, McGlone F (2016) Mapping quantal touch using 7 Tesla functional magnetic resonance imaging and single-unit intraneural microstimulation. Elife 5. pii: e12812

Sanchez-Panchuelo RM, Schluppeck D (2010) Mapping human somatosensory cortex in individual subjects with 7T functional MRI. J Neurophysiol 103(5):2544–2556. https://doi.org/10.1152/jn.01017.2009

Scheef L, Landsberg MW et al (2007) Methodological aspects of functional neuroimaging at high field strength: a critical review. Rofo 179(9):925–931

Scheffler K, Ehses P (2016 Jul) High-resolution mapping of neuronal activation with balanced SSFP at 9.4 Tesla. Magn Reson Med 76(1):163–171

Schlamann M, Voigt MA et al (2010a) Exposure to high-field MRI does not affect cognitive function. J Magn Reson Imaging 31(5):1061–1066

Schlamann M, Yoon MS et al (2010b) Short term effects of magnetic resonance imaging on excitability of the motor cortex at 1.5 T and 7 T. Acad Radiol 17(3):277–281

Sengupta S, Roebroeck A, Kemper VG, Poser BA, Zimmermann J, Goebel R, Adriany G (2016) A specialized multi-transmit head coil for high resolution fMRI of the human visual cortex at 7T. PLoS One.11(12):e0165418

Shah P, Bassett DS, Wisse LEM, Detre JA, Stein JM, Yushkevich PA, Shinohara RT, Pluta JB, Valenciano E, Daffner M, Wolk DA, Elliott MA, Litt B, Davis KA, Das SR (2018 Feb) Mapping the structural and functional network architecture of the medial temporal lobe using 7T MRI. Hum Brain Mapp 39(2):851–865

Shimada Y, Kochiyama T et al (2008) System stability of a 3 T-MRI during continuous EPI scan. Nippon Hoshasen Gijutsu Gakkai Zasshi 64(12):1504–1512

Theysohn JM, Maderwald S et al (2008) Subjective acceptance of 7 Tesla MRI for human imaging. MAGMA 21(1–2):63–72

Theysohn N, Qin S, Maderwald S, Poser BA, Theysohn JM, Ladd ME, Norris DG, Gizewski ER, Fernandez G, Tendolkar I (2013 Oct) Memory-related hippocampal activity can be measured robustly using FMRI at 7 Tesla. J Neuroimaging 23(4):445–451

Thürling M, Küper M et al (2011) Activation of the dentate nucleus in a verb generation task: a 7 T MRI study. NeuroImage 57(3):1184–1191

Torrisi S, O'Connell K, Davis A, Reynolds R, Balderston N, Fudge JL, Grillon C, Ernst M (2015 Oct) Resting state connectivity of the bed nucleus of the stria terminalis at ultra-high field. Hum Brain Mapp 36(10):4076–4088

Triantafyllou C, Hoge RD et al (2005) Comparison of physiological noise at 1.5 T, 3 T and 7 T and optimization of fMRI acquisition parameters. NeuroImage 26(1):243–250

Triantafyllou C, Hoge RD et al (2006) Effect of spatial smoothing on physiological noise in high-resolution fMRI. NeuroImage 32(2):551–557

van der Zwaag W, Marques JP et al (2009) Minimization of Nyquist ghosting for echo-planar imaging at ultra-high fields based on a "negative readout gradient" strategy. J Magn Reson Imaging 30(5):1171–1178

van der Zwaag W, Marques JP et al (2012) Temporal SNR characteristics in segmented 3D-EPI at 7 T. Magn Reson Med 67(2):344–352

Vaughan JT, Garwood M et al (2001) 7 T vs. 4 T: RF power, homogeneity, and signal-to-noise comparison in head images. Magn Reson Med 46(1):24–30

Walter M, Stadler J et al (2008) High resolution fMRI of subcortical regions during visual erotic stimulation at 7 T. MAGMA 21(1–2):103–111

Wiggins GC, Potthast A et al (2005) Eight-channel phased array coil and detunable TEM volume coil for 7 T brain imaging. Magn Reson Med 54(1): 235–240

Yacoub E, Hu X (2001) Detection of the early decrease in fMRI signal in the motor area. Magn Reson Med 45(2):184–190

Yacoub E, Shmuel A et al (2001) Imaging brain function in humans at 7 Tesla. Magn Reson Med 45(4): 588–594

Yacoub E, Duong TQ et al (2003) Spin-echo fMRI in humans using high spatial resolutions and high magnetic fields. Magn Reson Med 49(4):655–664

Zou KH, Greve DN et al (2005) Reproducibility of functional MR imaging: preliminary results of prospective multi-institutional study performed by biomedical informatics research network. Radiology 237(3):781–789

5 Resting-State fMRI: Preclinical Foundations

Jonathan D. Power

5.1 Introduction

The purpose of this chapter is to orient readers, especially clinicians, to a relatively new and rapidly expanding approach to using functional magnetic resonance imaging (fMRI) called resting-state fMRI. The approach is called resting state because subjects simply lie quietly in a scanner for a period of time and do nothing but stare ahead while fMRI data are collected. Somewhat surprisingly, this simple scan can reveal much about the brain's organization. Other names for the technique are functional connectivity MRI or intrinsic fMRI; in this chapter the term RSFC will denote resting-state functional connectivity. A chapter on this topic is new to this edition, and the addition reflects the hope that RSFC scans will deliver clinically relevant information on individual persons in the near future.

A basic literacy in RSFC techniques is important to clinicians because RSFC scans are shifting from purely scientific instruments to increasingly a preclinical and even clinical tool. In the mid-2000s, only a few dozen RSFC papers were published each year, exclusively in neuroscience journals. By contrast, in 2017, conservatively, about two thousand papers used RSFC techniques judging by PubMed search. It is now common to open an issue of *Brain* or *The American Journal of Psychiatry* and to find RSFC studies. The approach of this chapter is not to review clinical findings but rather to show the kinds of data that are obtained in RSFC analyses and the kinds of findings that have caused excitement in scientific and clinical communities. In this way the reader develops a sense of what is important in RSFC analyses and the possible applications and developments that are on the horizon.

5.2 Conceptual Overview

The study of resting-state fMRI data represents a paradigm shift in functional neuroimaging. The first 20 years of fMRI studies, beginning in the early 1990s, were largely concerned with tasks, such as tasks of visual perception or language generation. Clinical studies tended to emphasize tasks that seemed relevant to symptomatology, such as having depressed versus nondepressed participants judge angry versus neutral (i.e., valenced) facial expressions. The analysis of task fMRI data entailed finding signal changes that were time-locked to the experimental paradigm. In block designs (e.g., where participants viewed alternating checkerboards for 20 s then rested for 20 s), one sought differential signals during stimulus periods versus rest periods. In event-related designs (e.g., where subjects made living/nonliving judgments on a series of words), one could

J. D. Power (✉)
Department of Psychiatry, Weill Cornell Medical College, Sackler Institute for Developmental Psychobiology, New York, NY, USA
e-mail: jdp9009@nyp.org

S. Ulmer, O. Jansen (eds.), *fMRI*, https://doi.org/10.1007/978-3-030-41874-8_5

model signal changes to different categories of stimuli and even temporal interactions between successive stimuli. By averaging many presentations of stimuli, noise could be suppressed and relevant signals extracted. The kinds of conclusions these data supported were often of the form "brain location X shows increased/decreased signal during period A versus period B" (e.g., signal increase in primary visual cortex during checkerboard presentation periods compared to rest periods) or "signal patterns at brain location Y discriminate condition A versus condition B" (e.g., medial parietal signals discriminating remembered versus forgotten stimuli). The overarching point is that the task provided both the rationale for the contrast of interest (where/how/why a stimulus/demand was processed) and the ability to identify the signal of interest (via the task-timing structure).

RSFC data necessitate a different approach. In the first place, the task-free format means investigators are not specifying a process or manipulation. This lack of constraint can be viewed as an asset, for a wide variety of populations can be studied that would normally not comply with a task (e.g., young children, subjects with low IQ, etc.). It can also be viewed as a weakness, for little to nothing about the signals under study is specified (an early criticism of RSFC was that it studied people as they made grocery lists). Additionally, since there is no task timing to isolate signals of interest, it is not (usually) possible to study time-locked signal changes as in task fMRI. In fact, the dominant approach to RSFC analysis is to examine patterns of signal covariance in the data. Covariance-based approaches to the data cause two challenges: (i) huge numbers of outcome measures can be generated (N signals can yield ~N^2 pairwise correlations) creating many opportunities for false-positive findings, and (ii) without task timing, it is difficult to separate "signal" from "noise" in a scan.

The first RSFC study was published in 1995 and it contained provocative findings (detailed below). The fact that over the next decade only a handful of major studies were published using the technique is a telling index of the strength of reservations about RSFC held by many knowledgeable persons in the field (i.e., few were willing to risk paying for fMRI scans of noise while people constructed grocery lists). Many of those reservations were, in retrospect, well-grounded and prescient, and much of this chapter will address those and other concerns about the technique. However, as the chapter should also show, despite the limitations and challenges of RSFC studies, new and important information about brain organization has been gathered from these scans and is being put to use to better understand human anatomy, behavior, and illness.

5.3 Basic Facts about Resting-State fMRI Scans

For the last 15 years, the large majority of RSFC scans collected has been from subjects resting in an fMRI scanner for about 5 min (Van Dijk et al. 2010). Subjects are typically not given much instruction besides to lie quietly and to hold still. They may see a white, gray, or black screen, with or without a crosshair to focus on, and sometimes subjects are asked to close their eyes. The eyes-closed versus eyes-open choice turns out to have mattered more than initially appreciated, because many subjects with eyes closed fall asleep without investigators being aware of it (and patterns of neural activity differ across these states) (Tagliazucchi and Laufs 2014). Accompanying measures are sometimes recorded to monitor physiologic processes that can impact fMRI scans, most often pulse oximetry (for heart rate) and elastic abdominal belt traces (for respiratory patterns) and, less frequently, eye tracking data, galvanic skin responses, electrocardiograms, electroencephalograms, and expired gas measures (e.g., end-tidal pCO_2).

Prior to the simultaneous multi-slice sequences that have gained popularity in the last 5 years, most RSFC scans used single-slice echo planar imaging with volumes acquired every 2–4 s and voxels (the 3D pixels that comprise MRI images) of 2–4 mm per side. With the multi-slice accelerations, sub-second sampling intervals have become common, and voxels are often around 2 mm or smaller per side. Additionally, the length of scans has increased. Whereas 5 min was long viewed as adequate (with dissenters), for advanced analyses, it has become clear that substantial gains in reliability are made throughout the first 60–90 min of scanning (Laumann et al. 2015). It is now common to see scans of 10 or 15 min or more in studies.

RSFC data, due to its task-free nature, is amenable to aggregation across protocols and sites. Several large repositories of data exist, and tens of thousands of scans are publicly available to any interested party. Initial efforts, such as ABIDE, gathered dozens to hundreds of ~5-min scans from multiple sites. More recent notable resources include the Human Connectome Project, a 1200-subject study which includes an hour of RSFC data per subject (as well as genetic, behavioral, and multimodal imaging data) (Marcus et al. 2013); the MyConnectome project, which includes 14 h of RSFC scans on a single individual over a year with a variety of diary, blood draw, and behavioral data (Poldrack et al. 2015); and the Midnight Scan Club, which for 10 subjects includes 5 h of RSFC data, 6 h of task data, and behavioral and structural imaging data (Gordon et al. 2017). Large federally funded extensions of the Human Connectome Project are ongoing for developmental, aging, and clinical populations in the United States, and similar projects exist in the European Union and in China.

5.4 Basic Properties of RSFC Scans: The Bad News

As stated above, one of the challenges of RSFC analyses is that neurally caused "signal" is hard to separate from "noise" since there is no experimental manipulation (Murphy et al. 2013). The importance of signal denoising in RSFC is easily appreciated by looking at a few individual scans. Figure 5.1 shows two scans from a cohort analyzed in (Power et al. 2017a) following a pictorial format described in (Power 2017). The rainbow of colors at the top show head position over time

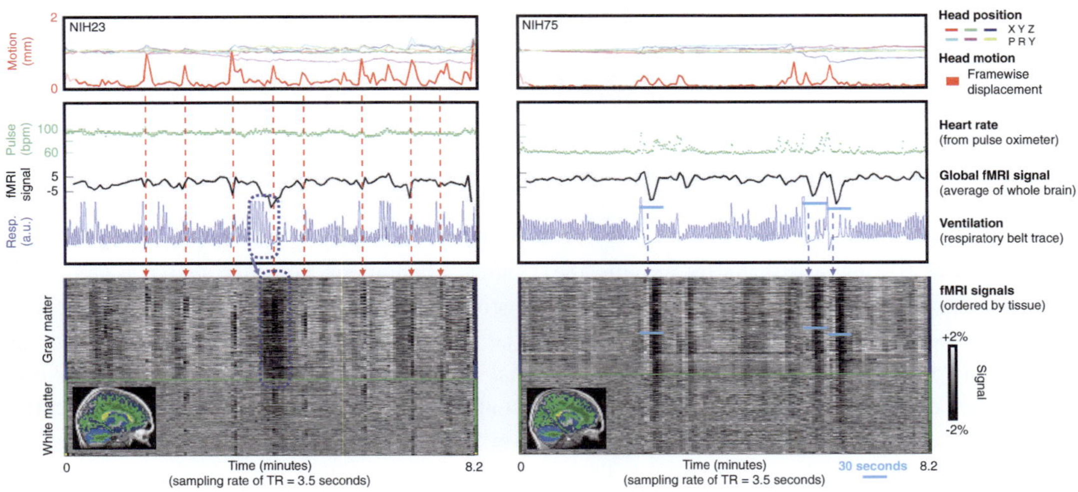

Fig. 5.1 Seeing fMRI timeseries. Data from two subjects are shown. At top, head position and head motion traces. In the middle, heart rate derived from pulse oximetery in green, a respiratory belt trace in blue, and the whole-brain fMRI signal in black. At bottom, using tissue compartments shown in the inset image, all voxel signals in the gray and white matter and ventricles are shown, organized by tissue compartment (see colored bars at sides and corresponding colors in the inset images). The bright green line separates gray from white matter signals. Red arrows indicate periods of motion, during and immediately after which spatially specific signal abnormalities are seen in the heatmaps of fMRI signals. Blue arrows denote several deep breaths followed by pauses in breathing, patterns which reflect sighs or yawns. The fMRI data show brief increases and then prolonged signal decreases lasting approximately 30 s following these respiratory changes. In the scan at left, a dotted box encloses a period of deepened breathing and subsequent accompanying signal decrease in fMRI signals

(X, Y, and Z for head position and pitch, roll, and yaw for head angle); the thick red line shows head motion (the derivative of position). The gray scale heatmap at the bottom shows all voxel signals in the scan, with time on the x-axis and tissue compartments ordering the y-axis: gray matter signals are above the bright green horizontal line, and white matter signals are below the line. Typically signals in the white matter are interpreted as artifacts. In the left scan, motion is time-locked to widespread and large signal changes throughout the brain (red arrows). This is motion artifact. The blue trace in the middle panel shows the respiratory rhythms of the subject measured by an elastic abdominal belt. In the right scan, at several points, there are large increases in the abdominal belt trace followed by pauses, reflecting deep breaths such as sighs or yawns. In the 30 s subsequent to these breaths, large signal decreases (vertical black bands) are seen throughout the gray matter and in the white matter (blue arrows). These are respiratory signals, a kind of impulse response function to deep breaths. In the left scan, there is also a period midway through the scan where many deep breaths occurred, and about a minute of decreased fMRI signals follows this period (dotted blue boxes). There are other influences on RSFC signals, but these motion and respiratory signals are sufficient to make the point that very large signal changes in RSFC data are often due to unwanted factors during the scan.

Head motion causes artifacts by moving the head position relative to scanner hardware (especially the receive coils) and also by disrupting the proton spin histories that underpin the physics of tissue excitation and signal readout. These motion artifacts tend to be spatially specific, impacting different portions of a volume differently depending on when and how the head moved (Power et al. 2017b). The net effect of motion in terms of signal covariance (which is what matters most in RSFC analyses) is to drive up correlations between signals of nearby voxels and to drive correlations between signals of distant voxels toward zero or negative values (Power et al. 2012; Satterthwaite et al. 2012; Van Dijk et al. 2012).

Respiratory signals, unlike motion artifact, are blood oxygen-level-dependent (BOLD) signals, the same signals caused by neural activity and studied in fMRI studies. BOLD signals are strongly influenced by levels of deoxyhemoglobin in the blood (among a few factors). Recall that the mechanism of BOLD contrast is neural signals causing locally excessive blood flow causing increased blood oxygenation causing changes in blood magnetic properties that are well-captured by sequences designed to detect these changes (i.e., BOLD-weighted sequences). For respiratory patterns, in a similar fashion to neurally induced BOLD changes, hypoventilation causes hypercapnia which potently increases cerebral blood flow which causes enriched oxygenation and BOLD-weighted signal increases. Hyperventilation produces complementary changes. Because respiratory signals are shared across all gray matter, they tend to drive up correlations between signals throughout the brain, regardless of how distant the signals are (Power et al. 2018).

Respiration and head motion are related, as are the artifacts they produce (Power 2017; Power et al. 2018). Breathing produces head motion, both in the sense of ongoing, cyclic, small respirations of normal breathing and in sense of large intermittent breaths that produce larger transient motions such as those shown in Fig. 5.1. Thus, when a dataset exhibits motion, one can expect both overall increases in covariance due to respiratory phenomena and also distance-dependent increases in covariance due to motion artifacts (i.e., increased covariance between proximal signal pairs relative to distal signal pairs) (Power et al. 2015). The balance of frank motion artifact versus respiratory phenomena determines the relative contributions of these two motion-associated patterns in the data. The importance of these details will be clear shortly.

There are other kinds of artifacts in fMRI scans (Murphy et al. 2013), but enough have been illustrated that the reader understands they must be taken seriously, for they can obviously impact signal covariance. The chief problems in RSFC related to artifacts are (i) not all artifacts are known or well-characterized; (ii) artifacts like motion and respiration, which are well-characterized, are difficult to selectively remove from scans; and (iii) variables of interest, like age or diagnosis, correlate with head motion and thus with the prevalence of major artifacts and their associated signal properties. These considerations underscore the importance of signal denoising, which is discussed later. But prior to that, to balance the bad news in this section, the next section lays out why RSFC scans are so interesting.

5.5 Basic Properties of RSFC Scans: The Good News

The field of RSFC was born out of the observation that if one mapped out the parts of the brain where BOLD signal changed during finger tapping (here, bluntly called the finger motor system) and if one then examined the spontaneous fMRI signals among regions of the finger motor system, one would find that these signals were selectively and highly correlated while the subject lay at rest not moving their fingers (Biswal et al. 1995). These correlations were strongest at low frequencies with periods of 10–100 s, much slower than the typical evoked BOLD responses studied in task fMRI. Such findings were soon extended to the auditory system and the visual system (Lowe et al. 1998; Cordes et al. 2000). In each of these cases, task fMRI was used to map out functionally related brain regions, and then RSFC correlations were found to be selectively high among these sets of regions. Such findings led to the general hypothesis that covariance in fMRI signals in the absence of explicit tasks could index the functional relatedness of the tissue giving rise to those signals. In other words, functional connectivity MRI could serve as a "functional pseudo-tracer." It is worth emphasizing that RSFC does not directly measure neural connectivity or even neural activity—it measures temporal coherence in blood magnetic properties. In optimal circumstances, with successful denoising, RSFC isolates indirect consequences of neural processes, via the BOLD signal, and allows one to study the spatial and temporal patterns of these shared processes. Other chapters in this volume provide greater detail on the mechanisms linking neural activity to fMRI signals.

RSFC findings can be expressed in several ways. The most basic way is to obtain signals at two regions of interest (ROIs), which can be single voxels or collections of voxels, and then to compare these signals with one another via correlation coefficients. Figure 5.2a shows a made-up illustration of a 2-ROI comparison. When more than two ROIs are involved, it is convenient to represent the correlations as a matrix, where the entry at row I and column J shows the correlation of the signals at ROIs I and J. Figure 5.2b shows a schematized illustration of this approach with a set of made-up ROIs. In the case of Pearson correlations, the matrix is symmetric about the diagonal (because the correlation of signals I and J is equal to the correlation of signals J and I). In this matrix, the correlation between the tan and blue nodes is high, and they are both part of a cluster of ROIs with correlated signals (within the dotted blue box), whereas the red and pink ROIs have a low correlation and are part of separate clusters (the orange and green boxes, respectively). When sets of ROIs are considered together, they are sometimes pictorially represented by "spring embedding" plots, where the ROIs (also called nodes) are positioned in space by the strength of their "connections," here meaning the RSFC correlations. The ball and stick diagram in Fig. 5.2 is a made-up and partial but appropriate spring embedded layout of the matrix, showing how such diagrams help to understand large and complex sets of relationships such as correlation matrices. In this case only very strong correlations and a handful of nodes are shown.

Another version of the correlation matrix is to correlate the signal from an ROI (the "seed") with the signals at every voxel in the brain. This generates a 3D volume of the brain populated by correlation coefficients, called a "seed map." A common way of displaying the seed map is to show a high-resolution anatomical scan (or a brain surface) and overlay it with a heatmap of where the seed map exceeds some statistical threshold. In terms of a correlation matrix, the seed map is akin to using all voxels as ROIs and

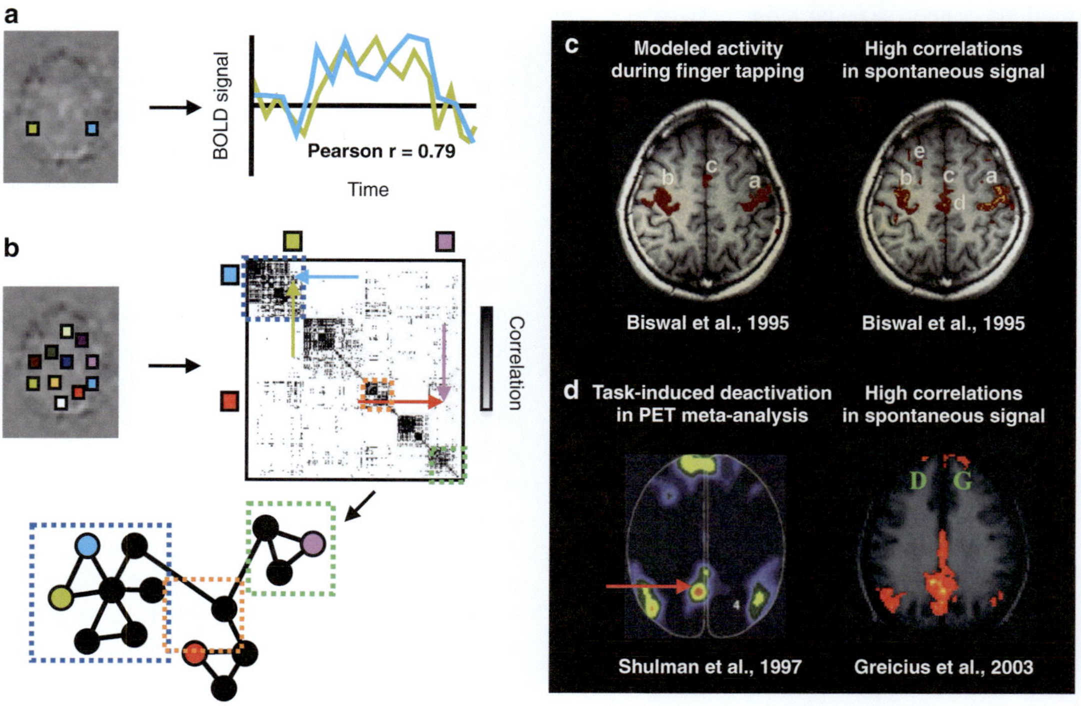

Fig. 5.2 Presenting RSFC data. (**a**) Pairwise correlation coefficients: two colored boxes denote regions of interest (ROIs), and made-up RSFC signals are shown for the ROIs along with a made-up correlation coefficient. (**b**) Correlation matrices: several colored ROIs are shown, and a matrix of correlations is shown (reflecting many more nodes than are shown at left; this is a real RSFC matrix from 264 ROIs), with locations of the entries for two pairs of ROIs shown by the arrows. A made-up ball-and-stick spring embedded diagram shows a layout consistent with the clustering structure of the matrix—the blue and tan ROIs (with high correlation) are in the same cluster (dotted blue box), whereas the pink and red ROIs (with low correlation) belong to different clusters (the orange and green boxes, respectively). (**c**) Seed maps: at left, a statistical map of where BOLD signals change during a finger-tapping task. At right, an RSFC seed map produced from an ROI defined by the finger tapping task. (**d**) Seed map: at left, a statistical map of where metabolic activity decreased during a variety of goal-oriented tasks. At right, an RSFC seed map produced from the posterior cingulate (where the red arrow points in the left map). Note the correspondence in (**c**) and (**d**) of functionally defined sets of regions and RSFC signal correlation patterns

designating ROI J as the seed (for a seed of a single voxel), with row J containing the seed map. ROIs (here, voxels) with correlation coefficients over a threshold are displayed anatomically on a brain surface or brain volume.

An important pair of statistical maps is shown in Fig. 5.2c. The first map shows where finger tapping changed BOLD signal, outlining the finger motor system. The second map is an RSFC seed map produced from an ROI defined from the finger-tapping task. The correspondence is not complete, but it is compelling: task-defined functionally related regions display correlated spontaneous fMRI signals. This map was the first published RSFC finding (Biswal et al. 1995). Figure 5.2d shows another landmark pair of statistical maps. At left is a map from a meta-analysis of positron emission tomography (PET) studies, showing where metabolic activity *decreased* during task performance. This is the first map of what is now called the default mode network, so called because metabolic activity in these regions is higher at rest than during task performance (for most tasks) (Shulman et al. 1997). At right is an RSFC seed map produced from the posterior midline region of the default mode network (Greicius et al. 2003). Again, a compelling correspondence is seen between task-defined functionally related regions and the patterns of correlation in RSFC signals.

The first decade of RSFC studies were mainly concerned with producing such maps for a variety of task-defined systems and with demonstrating that such maps were neither trivial byproducts of structured noise in scans nor due to conscious or suggested neural activity. Maps were initially produced for the motor, auditory, and visual systems, then for the default mode network, and then for various attention and control networks (Oakes et al. 2005; Dosenbach et al. 2007; Seeley et al. 2007). By the late 2000s, several groups were attempting not just to replicate known systems but to mine RSFC data for its natural clustering structure—to see how many groups of correlated signals existed and their anatomical organization across the brain (Smith et al. 2009; Yeo et al. 2011; Power et al. 2011). Results of two such studies are shown at the top of Fig. 5.3. In these studies, all voxels given a particular color strongly display a major signal, and each voxel is colored in a "winner-take-all" fashion such that it belongs to one and only one cluster. This approach is an oversimplification of the data, since the neural populations captured in a voxel certainly represent more than one signal at a time, but it is a useful beginning step to understanding the signal patterns. Readers may think of these analyses as mapping out continents on a globe. In each study, visual signals cluster together, and default mode signals cluster together, reflecting the correlated signals found in the seed maps mentioned above. But many other distributed patterns of RSFC correlation also exist, indicating that the cortex, subcortical nuclei, and cerebellum are organized into a set of large-scale and often distributed RSFC patterns. The patterns in these two studies are not identical, but they are similar in many respects and have been replicated many times since.

The studies discussed above were group studies, where correlation patterns were averaged across large numbers (dozens to hundreds) of subjects. More recent efforts have been directed toward producing such maps in individual persons. One of the first attempts to firmly establish a single person's RSFC patterns was via the MyConnectome scans, shown in the bottom left of Fig. 5.3 (Laumann et al. 2015). There is an obvious overall similarity between the individual and a group average, but there are also several differences, and, importantly, these differences are reliable and are not "noise" or "artifacts." Note the smooth contours of clusters in the group map compared to the more jagged, bulbous pattern of the individual or the existence of a little dot of yellow in the individual medial prefrontal region. These details are real—they are recapitulated in task activation patterns and are found in split portions of the RSFC data—but they are not apparent in a group due to averaging. In other words, there are idiosyncrasies of an individual that are averaged away in the group. At bottom middle and the right side are data from eight individuals of the Midnight Scan Club, first with their average RSFC clustering structure and then with each individual's structure (Gordon et al. 2017). These individual structures all look recognizably like a group average, but all contain idiosyncrasies as well. The significance of the individual structures is not yet clear—it is unknown whether the amount of cortex prominently displaying a certain kind of signal (here, a color) has any kind of behavioral significance, if it matters whether one has a yellow dot or a black dot or no dot amidst the red swathe of medial prefrontal cortex, whether some people lack certain signal distinctions altogether, and so on. Investigations of these topics are underway.

These developments have several implications for clinical efforts to utilize RSFC scans. (i) The clinician treats the individual, not the cohort, and it is thus welcome news that reliable RSFC estimates can be obtained in single subjects. However, the caveat is that presently between 60 and 90 min are needed to obtain highly reliable estimates, which is not practical for most clinical purposes. That number may (or may not) drop in the future with technical advances. (ii) The individual variability in RSFC organization is substantial, at least in the first few dozen individuals who have been analyzed extensively and published. This variability has deep implications for neuroimaging and for clinical efforts to therapeutically target brain regions, for example, by transcranial magnetic stimulation (TMS). First, a given stereotaxic coordinate may not identify the

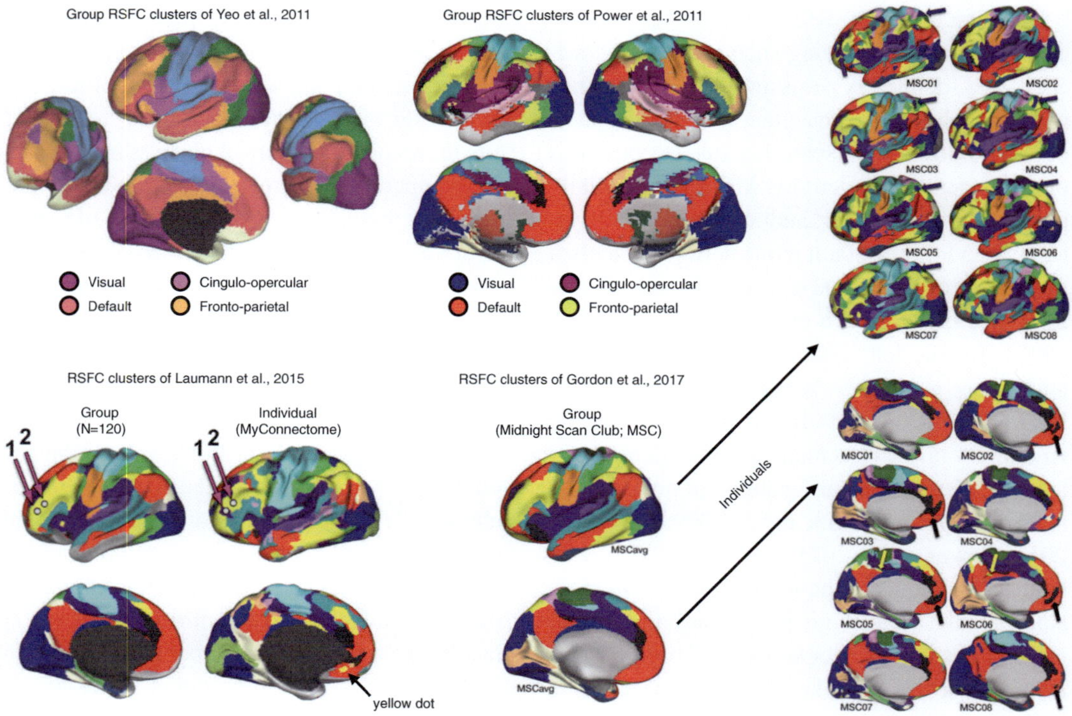

Fig. 5.3 Clustering structure of RSFC scans. At top, two group average clustering structures of RSFC data are shown. Each color on a surface reflects a predominant signal, and often signals are found at multiple locations of the cortex. At bottom left, the first well-characterized individual clustering structure, published from the MyConnectome database. At right and bottom middle of the figure are 8 individual clustering structures and their group average. There are clear similarities across individuals of clustering structures and also reliable idiosyncrasies of the individual structures

same functional part of the brain across subjects. This was always assumed to be the case, but the RSFC clustering patterns—and their recapitulation in task fMRI activation patterns—bring this fact into stark relief. Second, it is possible that individuals may differ in a qualitative sense in some aspects of brain organization—that is, it may be not only that a border of an RSFC map is shifted a few millimeters but that some people may have medial prefrontal yellow or black dots and some people may not or that some people may not have entire signal distinctions that others have. The combination of these two observations leads to a certain basic skepticism about using spatial systems to approach brains, for example, the nearly universal use of spatial landmarks to register neuroimaging scans (which essentially stretch or warp scans to all conform to one another or a target brain) or the nearly universal use of stereotaxic coordinates or external landmark systems to target TMS protocols. The underlying limitation is always the same: sampling a stereotaxic signal, or stimulating a stereotaxic coordinate, may on average target a certain neural population or process, but there is enough individual variability that much inaccuracy is likely entering studies and protocols, degrading the ability to measure or produce desired results. The silver lining to these observations is that the existence of reliable RSFC patterns in individuals suggests that it may be possible to identify, in an individually tailored fashion, desired functional parts of the brain and to use tailored approaches for image registration and therapeutic purposes.

The progress outlined above should demonstrate why both scientists and clinicians are excited about RSFC scans—the data are relatively easy to acquire and can be used to map, in very broad strokes, the functional topography of an individual brain. Other notable areas of investigation are to use RSFC signals to try to delineate functional areas of individual brains (akin to Brodmann maps), to link the cluster-level cortical patterning of RSFC to expression gradients of biochemical molecules and gene expression patterns, and to find RSFC correlates of disease. We will expand on clinical findings below, but next the topic of signal denoising will be discussed in greater detail.

5.6 Basic Properties of RSFC Scans: Links between Artifacts and Variables of Interest

This section deals with one of the most challenging aspects of RSFC scans: the fact that variables of interest often correlate with the prevalence of artifacts in the signals (Siegel et al. 2016). The problem is that if artifacts are only partially removed during scan denoising, one runs a risk of identifying an artifact as an effect of interest.

Nowhere has this challenge been more evident than in the study of development. In the mid-2000s, several groups began to scan children and adolescents, hoping to derive a trajectory of RSFC maturation into young adulthood. Each of these groups reported a clear and striking cross-sectional finding: at young ages the RSFC organization was predominantly local with few strong long-distance correlations, but over adolescence and into adulthood, the local correlations were weaker, and the longer-distance correlations were stronger (Kelly et al. 2009; Fair et al. 2009; Supekar et al. 2009). In other words, there was a distance-dependent developmental trajectory. Recall that motion artifact causes distance-dependent changes in RSFC covariance (a fact that was unknown at the time of the developmental studies) (Power et al. 2012; Satterthwaite et al. 2012; Van Dijk et al. 2012). Unfortunately, children have high levels of head motion, adolescents have intermediate levels, and young adults have the lowest levels of head motion (Fig. 5.4). In retrospect, the developmental RSFC findings mentioned above were mostly if not entirely attributable to inadequately removed motion

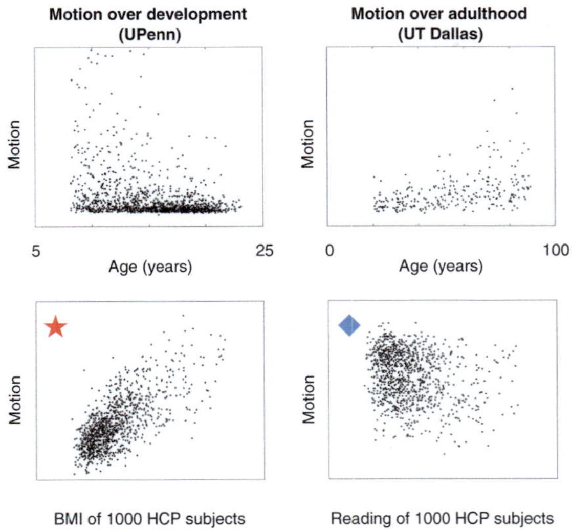

Correlation of behavioral/physiological measures with motion in 1000 Human Connectome Project subjects

Measure	First 500	Next 500
★ Body Mass Index (BMI)	0.66	0.69
Weight	0.52	0.55
Systolic blood pressure	0.23	0.18
Diastolic blood pressure	0.18	0.22
Fluid intelligence (Raven's matrices)	-0.17	-0.24
◆ Reading (English)	-0.23	-0.23
Vocabulary (pictures)	-0.19	-0.19
Years of education	-0.17	-0.23
Dimensional Change Card Sorting	-0.18	-0.15
Manual dexterity (pegboard)	-0.18	-0.14
Spatial orientation (Penn Line)	-0.17	-0.21

Fig. 5.4 Links between motion and variables of interest. At top left, scatter plots in two representative datasets showing motion decreasing over school-age development, and then increasing in later adulthood, establishing a U-shaped motion curve across the lifespan. At right, a table showing correlations of behavioral, physiological, and cognitive measures with subject motion, first in the first 500 subjects of the Human Connectome Project, and then in the next 500 subjects. At bottom left, two scatter plots show the basis of two of the correlations in the table (marked with symbols), plotting data from all 1000 subjects

artifacts. Subsequent developmental studies in the same age range with stricter quality control procedures have found RSFC developmental effects to be much attenuated although of a similar character as the initial findings, and it is not clear that these remaining effects are not actually attributable to still-unremoved motion artifact (Satterthwaite et al. 2013).

Artifacts indexed by motion also create challenges for studying aging because older adults move more than younger adults, illustrated in an aging cohort in Fig. 5.4. In general, simply due to motion, one would expect for old populations to display stronger short-distance RSFC correlations and weaker long-distance correlations than young adults. Tellingly, an initial RSFC finding in aging studies was one of "disconnection" of brain regions that are far away but within the same cluster (e.g., disconnection of the posterior cingulate from the medial prefrontal cortex, both parts of the default mode network) (Andrews-Hanna et al. 2007). This is unfortunately also the kind of effect one would expect from under-removed motion artifact. Studies with stricter quality control for motion find attenuated results in aging, much like the developmental story (Van Dijk et al. 2012). An additional challenge in aging is that as the brain ages it shrinks, sulci widen, and cerebrospinal fluid (CSF) fills the opened gaps, causing voxels to sample increasing amounts of CSF with age. CSF has very different signal properties than the gray matter. Thus, multiple kinds of signal properties correlate with subject age.

Motion is a problem even in studies of young adults. In large cohorts of young adults, when subjects are stratified by motion, distance-dependent changes in covariance are evident in every cohort that has been examined, demonstrating that motion artifacts are present in the data (e.g., (Power et al. 2017b; Yan et al. 2013; Burgess et al. 2016)). In the Human Connectome Project scans of neurotypical adults, several behavioral and physiological variables correlate with motion, some of which are shown in Fig. 5.4 (Siegel et al. 2016). These correlations were initially reported for the first 500 subjects of the HCP dataset, and they replicate in the next 500 subjects. Body mass index and weight are particularly strongly correlated with head motion, likely due to links between body habitus and how respiration causes head movement. There are also weaker but significant and replicable correlations of motion with cognitive measures such as reading ability and manual dexterity. It should be no surprise then that RSFC correlates of behavioral and physiological variables have been found, but the question is whether these correlates are due to motion and the artifacts it indexes or due to neural underpinnings of the variables of interest (or both). Naturally, the answer to that question hinges on scan denoising, and the next section surveys this topic.

5.7 Basic Properties of RSFC Scans: Signal Denoising

The single most important question, usually, when interpreting RSFC findings, is whether signal denoising was adequate. It should be clear from the discussion above that artifacts can have major influences on RSFC covariance and that artifacts correlate with variables of interest. It is thus essential to either remove signal artifacts or somehow equate groups when searching for "neural" correlates of variables of interest.

The field of RSFC denoising is too broad and too rapidly evolving to survey in a chapter. This text will instead outline a few high-level organizing principles and then will survey the performance of a small number of common denoising approaches. Readers who wish to gain expertise in RSFC signal denoising are referred to an entire special issue of *NeuroImage* on the topic (volume 154, the July 2017 issue, e.g., (Bulte and Wartolowska 2017; Ciric et al. 2017; Zaitsev et al. 2017; Liu 2017)).

There are two basic approaches to signal denoising. One approach is to record external variables and then use certain assumptions or rules to model the impact of those variables on signals and then to remove that predicted variance from scans. The other approach is to take signals from scans and use them in an internal, data-driven way to identify and remove noise from the same scans. Model-driven approaches tend to try to measure motion or physiological parameters like respiration, heart rate, or pupil size and to predict the signal variance that should be associated with these variables. Examples of this approach are "RETROICOR" (for instantaneous cardiac and respiratory effects (Glover et al. 2000)), "RVTcor" (for delayed respiratory effects (Birn et al. 2008)), or the use of head position estimates as nuisance regressors (Friston et al. 1996). These models are attractive for having clear predictions and relationships, but they unfortunately fail to capture much of the variance they ought to model (Power et al. 2017a). This fact has been made clear both for motion and respiratory phenomena in recent studies, and these approaches will not be considered further in this chapter. Data-driven approaches fall into two major categories: those approaches that take signals from only nuisance compartments (i.e., places aside from the gray matter, like the ventricles, cranium, or white matter) and those approaches that take signals mainly or only from the gray matter. Examples of the former approaches include removing average white matter or average ventricle signals from a scan, whereas examples of the latter approach include removing average cortical signals from the scan. Data-driven approaches are attractive for having few presumptions about the data, but they range widely in what they accomplish, as will be discussed below.

There are three common ways that data-driven denoising treats signals from a compartment (whether a nuisance or gray matter compartment): average signals, principal component analysis (PCA) of signals, and independent component analysis (ICA) of signals. Average signals are easy enough to understand, but PCA and ICA deserve some explanation. PCA simplifies large sets of signals into a much smaller set of summary signals in descending order of explanatory power. The first principal component is typically the average signal or something very close to it, because this signal usually explains the most variance in the data. The second signal explains the next most variance, etc. A common use of PCA would be, for example, to take thousands of white matter signals and condense them into a small number of signals (e.g., 3 or 5) that would be regressed out of gray matter time series (this approach falls in the "CompCor" family of techniques in the RSFC literature (Behzadi et al. 2007)). Like PCA, ICA also simplifies large sets of signals into small sets of summary signals. However, in ICA, the signals are not identified via explanatory power alone but are instead identified by maximizing some kind of dissimilarity in where the signals come from. Signals can be dissimilar in either time or space, but spatial ICA is by far the most common approach used in denoising. So, in other words, spatial ICA is designed to find spatially specific groupings of signals. A common use of ICA for denoising would be to decompose all gray matter signals into spatial ICA components and then to label component signals as "signal" or "noise" depending on their spatial patterning or their temporal characteristics or other properties. Techniques like "FIX-ICA" and "ICA-AROMA" are in this category of techniques (Salimi-Khorshidi et al. 2014; Pruim et al. 2015).

By considering the characteristics of the artifacts discussed so far, one can anticipate the kind of denoising that would be needed to remove the artifact. Motion artifacts are spatially specific and time-limited, and thus methods targeted in space or time are best suited to removing motion artifacts. ICA is well-suited to find spatially specific patterns, and other spatially tailored approaches could also identify such signals (e.g., using the white matter proximal to a gray matter voxel to derive its nuisance signals (Jo et al. 2010)). In contrast, average cortical signals cannot contain the variety of spatially specific changes produced by motion because those specific changes often cancel one another out. Another approach to motion artifacts, since motion is time-limited in its effects, would be to remove from analysis the time points affected by motion and perhaps those just after motion, an approach called censoring or scrubbing (Power et al. 2012). Respiratory signals are slow, global signals. Such signals are well-identified by average gray or average white matter signals or by PCA of those compartments (Power et al. 2018). Spatial ICA is poorly suited to identifying global signals because they are not spatially specific. In summary, each denoising technique has particular properties that become strengths and weaknesses in the context of different kinds of artifacts. No single denoising technique identifies all kinds of artifact, and combinations of techniques are needed to properly denoise RSFC data (Ciric et al. 2017).

One useful way to understand RSFC denoising is to look at gray plots like those in Fig. 5.1 before and after denoising. An example of a scan before and after FIX ICA is shown in Fig. 5.5. In this denoising procedure, a large number of spatial ICA components are identified in the gray matter and are then classified as signal to be retained or discarded. What is obvious is that several vertical black bands representing respiratory effects persist through denoising (pink arrows). Less obvious is that many motion artifacts and the head-position-dependent horizontal strand-like patterns in the undenoised data are removed. Both of these properties matter. In general, spatial ICA does an excellent job at removing spatially specific motion artifacts, but it does very little for global respiratory artifacts. In contrast, removing average gray matter signals eliminates respiratory artifacts (and other global signals) but has almost no impact on spatially specific motion artifacts.

The overarching message of this section is that multiple techniques are needed to target the multiple kinds of artifacts present in fMRI data.

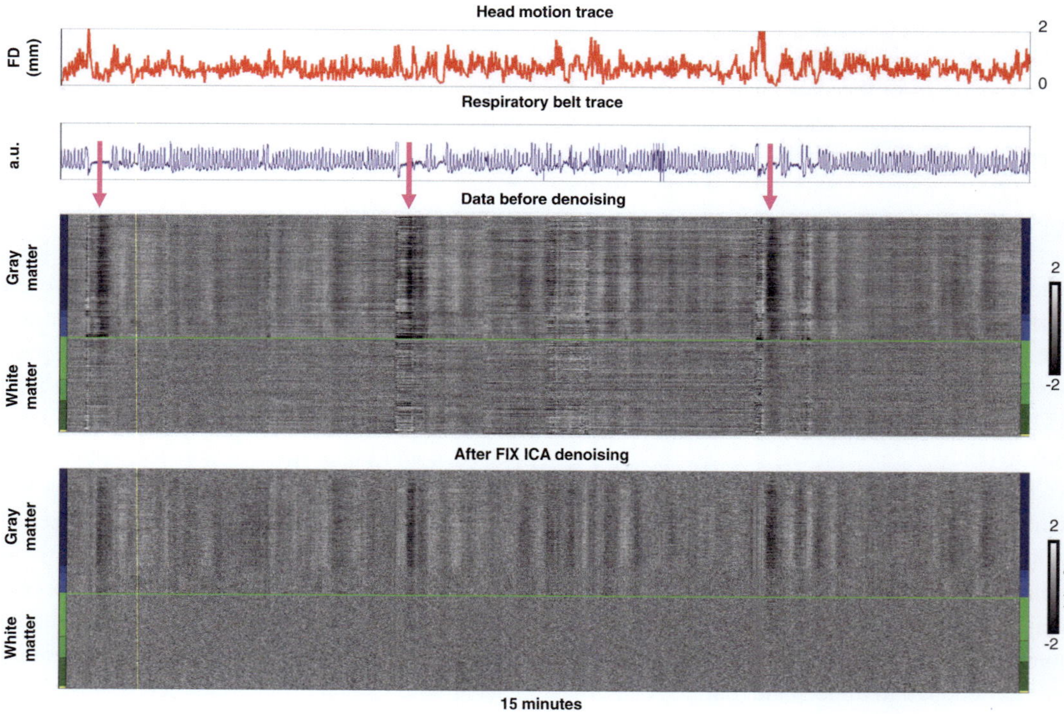

Fig. 5.5 An example of global respiratory artifacts persisting through denoising. These data are from a single 15-min fMRI scan from the Human Connectome Project (HCP156637). At top in red, head motion is shown via a Framewise Displacement (FD) trace. Below, a respiratory belt trace shows when deep breaths and shallow breathing occurred. The grayscale heatmaps show thousands of signals from the gray matter (above the green lines) and white matter (below the green lines). Signals present in both compartments are considered artifacts. The pink arrows note several instances of deep breaths followed by periods of shallow breathing or apnea, which produce large decreases in fMRI signals throughout the brain (black vertical bands). These global respiratory artifacts are not removed by the FIX-ICA denoising procedure. The color bars at the sides of the gray-scale plots denote cortical (dark blue), subcortical (medium blue) and cerebellar (bright blue) signals, superficial (bright green), deeper (darker green), and deepest (dark green) white matter signals, and ventricle signals (yellow)

The details of these techniques may seem arcane, but they are vital to the interpretation of RSFC studies. Progress in using RSFC studies to understand individual differences in healthy subjects and diagnostic and prognostic patterns in patients is dependent on effective denoising. Readers with an interest in RSFC are strongly encouraged to consult the reviews on the topic mentioned above.

5.8 Clinical Uses of RSFC Data

This chapter concludes by discussing some of the nascent clinical uses of RSFC. In general, RSFC scans are not yet used by psychiatrists and neurologists, though there is an expectation that RSFC will eventually come into use in these fields. Neurosurgeons and radiologists can use RSFC to map functional boundaries of individual brains, and an example of use in surgical planning is shown below. Rather than trying to survey the field, a few interesting and preliminary clinical uses of RSFC are presented in some detail.

One use of RSFC is to map tumor extent. A dominant influence on BOLD signals across the brain is respiration, which depends on intact homeostatic mechanisms linking vasomotor responses in local vasculature to the pCO_2 and pO_2 levels detected in arterial blood. In an intact brain, if a seed ROI is taken of the whole brain (yielding the global signal), a seed map tends to highlight all gray matter, which is where respiratory effects are most prominent. If vasomotor coupling to blood gas concentration is disrupted, as is the case in and around some tumors, RSFC signals within and around the tumor will no longer reflect the global signals found at all other portions of the brain. RSFC seed maps can then be used to help map out the extent of pathology. Figure 5.6 shows an example of this use of RSFC scans. A T1-weighted scan with intravenous contrast shows ring-shaped enhancement around a glioblastoma, and a FLAIR sequence shows peritumoral hyperintensity reflecting edema where the blood-brain barrier and vasomotor responses are likely compromised (Chow et al. 2016). If seed ROIs are created of the enhancing region and of the entire contralateral hemisphere (which will practically yield the global signal of healthy tissue), then highly disparate seed maps are found in RSFC data. The important finding is that the global "control" seed map has a "hole" where the tumor and peritumoral tissue are found. Using localized biopsies, this disruption of vascular function around the tumor has been verified to be related to local tumor burden, and RSFC may thus serve as a measure of infiltration (Bowden et al. 2018). Furthermore, the infiltration pattern detected by RSFC differs across categories of tumors (i.e., by IDH1 mutation status), which may help explain why some tumors have high rates of recurrence after treatment (Englander et al. 2018). Note that in this example, the data and techniques are RSFC, but the interpretation has to do with hemodynamics and not neural processing.

Other uses of RSFC in the neurosurgical and neurological domains include using RSFC to map eloquent cortex during surgical planning, using RSFC to track the consequences of epilepsy surgery (e.g., after resection or callosotomy), using RSFC to track poststroke recovery, and using RSFC to track plasticity due to constraint-induced movement therapy (e.g., casting a good arm to force a patient to use a weak arm).

In the psychiatric domain, there is hope of finding endophenotypes of mental illness via RSFC. The present diagnostic system is organized around the *Diagnostic Statistical Manual of Mental Disorders, Fifth Edition* (DSM-V), which creates diagnostic categories via sets of criteria. The criteria are not biological measures (e.g., a pressure, a concentration, a genotype) but are rather symptoms described by the patient or behaviors observed by a clinician or others. Progress in treatment is typically captured by questionnaires and/or detailed personal interviews. While no one would question the value of clinical assessments or the validity of many of the diagnostic criteria sets, they are necessarily subjective, time-intensive avenues to diagnosis, and they are based on behavior and self-report and thus only indirectly on neurobiology. Further, within a given diagnosis, there is often little information to identify optimal medical therapies

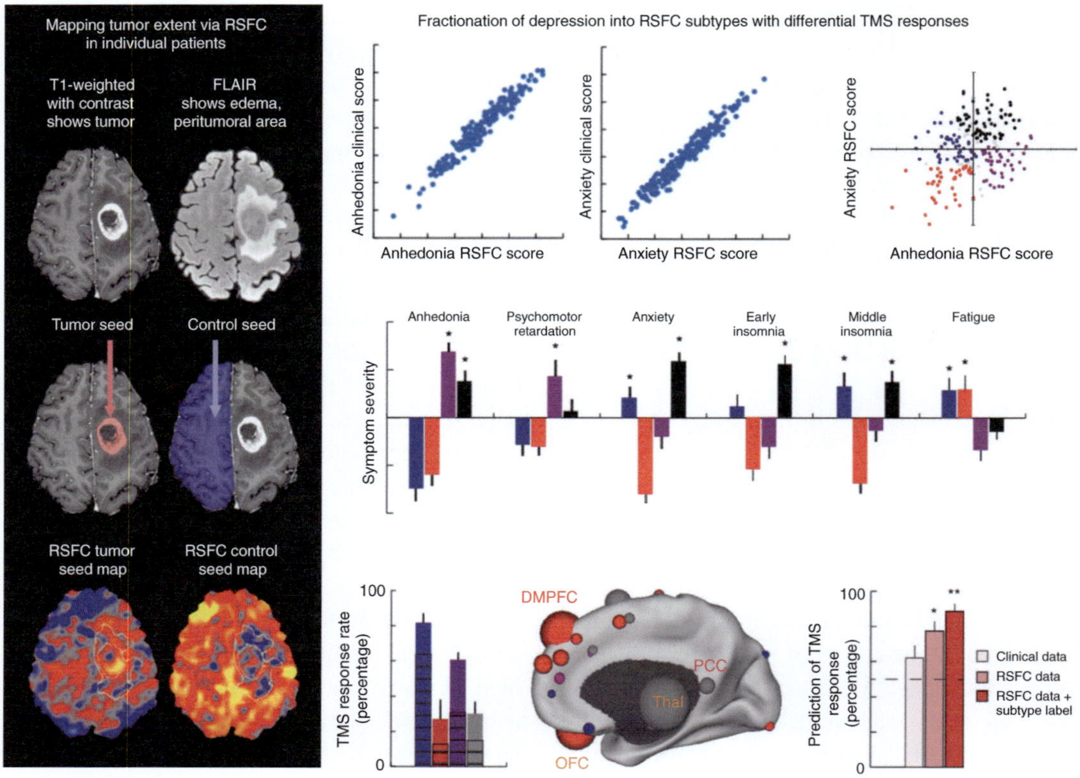

Fig. 5.6 Clinical uses of RSFC. At left, scans from a single subject are shown. The T1-weighted image shows a contrast-enhancing tumor, and the FLAIR image shows peri-tumoral edema. The middle panels show ROIs of the tumor and unaffected control tissue in the contralateral hemisphere, and the bottom panels show RSFC seed maps of these seeds. In RSFC seed maps, the tumor seed maps the area of enhancement, whereas the control seed maps everything but the tumor and peritumoral area. At right, results from the largest RSFC study of depression to date. Clinical assessments yielded symptom scores, which were then used to identify two large-scale patterns in RSFC data related to anhedonic and anxiety symptom severity. Clustering along these two dimensions yielded four clusters, which contained differential symptom profiles. Response to TMS differed among these subtypes, with the best response in the blue and pink clusters. The surfaces show locations of the ROIs with signals most predictive of RSFC subtypes. Notably, clinical scores were less predictive of TMS response than the RSFC patterns

(e.g., lithium versus valproic acid versus atypical antipsychotics in patients with bipolar disorder) other than the side effect and pharmacokinetic profiles of the medications. It would be a great aid to psychiatry to define brain imaging signatures with diagnostic and prognostic implications.

For these reasons, there has been excitement over a recent, large-scale RSFC study of depressed patients (Drysdale et al. 2017). While this study has not yet been replicated, it was well-conducted and gathered the largest cohort of depressed patients yet studied via RSFC by combining data from several independent sites. Some of the findings are shown in Fig. 5.6. The analysis was as follows. First, large numbers (many hundreds) of patients contributed RSFC data, a set of several hundred ROIs was used, and about 30,000 pairwise correlations were calculated in each subject after denoising. Then, among depressed patients, scores on a standard questionnaire about depression (the Hamilton Depression Rating Scale (HAM-D)) were correlated with the RSFC measures to identify RSFC patterns (patterns referring to sets of correlations) that scaled systematically with symptom patterns. Broadly, this analysis yielded two RSFC patterns: one pattern that scaled with anhedonic symptoms and one pattern that scaled with anxiety symptoms (top row of Fig. 5.6). When patient RSFC data were plotted in terms of these two patterns, four clusters were identified, which were labeled depression subtypes (top row of Fig. 5.6, far right, in colors). These subtypes, which were defined based on RSFC patterns, contained different profiles of symptoms on the HAM-D, shown in the middle row of Fig. 5.6, as one would expect since symptoms were used to define the initial two RSFC patterns. Importantly, TMS conducted on depressed patients was variably effective depending on the RSFC subtype of depression: subtypes 1 and 3 (blue and pink colors) responded at much higher rates than did subtypes 2 and 4 (bottom left). And interestingly, response to TMS was better predicted by RSFC measures than by clinical measures (bottom right). The results of this study should be viewed as preliminary, and they need to be replicated, but they are suggestive of an eventual role of RSFC in psychiatric practice.

There are numerous other clinical findings worth discussing that could not be included in a single chapter. Such omissions are made in part due to space constraints, but it must also be mentioned that for most clinical conditions there are presently numerous conflicting or at least inconsistent clinical RSFC studies. In part, these inconsistencies may reflect diagnostic heterogeneity or a lack of power. But surely the inconsistencies are in part due to the wide variety of denoising strategies used across the field, which have widely variable efficacy in removing various artifacts. For the typical reader of this chapter, it is not practical to develop the expertise needed to critically appraise RSFC studies with purported clinical or behavioral relevance, and a "wait and see" perspective on the emerging RSFC literature would be prudent. By the time the next edition of this volume emerges, many more clinical studies will have emerged, which should help clarify which findings are most durable and attention-worthy.

5.9 Conclusions

RSFC has evolved from a scientific curiosity in the mid-1990s to a widely used scientific tool in the mid-2010s, and it is beginning to make inroads into clinical practice as the year 2020 approaches. The kinds of findings surveyed here should excite curiosity about the technique and what it may reveal about the human brain. Over the last decade, it has become possible to derive large-scale maps of cortical, subcortical, and cerebellar brain organization in individual persons. Just as all human faces have the same parts (e.g., nose, eyes, etc.) but are individually distinct, the overall RSFC structure across individuals appears similar but with reliable distinctions in each individual. Ongoing research is trying to link individual RSFC properties to individual differences in behavior and cognition. In terms of clinical studies, nearly the entire literature is cross-sectional, involving correlates between RSFC measures and clinical scores. There are some preliminary demonstrations of how RSFC might be clinically useful, such as the uses shown above, but the literature is young, and much work remains to be done to affirm and refine the role of RSFC in clinical practice.

Acknowledgments The author thanks Julie Penzner, Meredith Pittman, and Thomas Pearce for their comments on the manuscript. J.D.P. is supported by a gift from the Mortimer D. Sackler, MD, family.

Conflict of Interest: The author declares no conflicts of interest.

References

Andrews-Hanna JR, Snyder AZ, Vincent JL, Lustig C, Head D, Raichle ME et al (2007) Disruption of large-scale brain systems in advanced aging. Neuron 56(5):924–935

Behzadi Y, Restom K, Liau J, Liu TT (2007) A component based noise correction method (CompCor) for BOLD and perfusion based fMRI. NeuroImage 37(1):90–101

Birn RM, Smith MA, Jones TB, Bandettini PA (2008) The respiration response function: the temporal dynamics of fMRI signal fluctuations related to changes in respiration. NeuroImage 40(2):644–654

Biswal B, Yetkin FZ, Haughton VM, Hyde JS (1995) Functional connectivity in the motor cortex of resting human brain using echo-planar MRI. Magn Reson Med 34(4):537–541

Bowden SG, Gill BJA, Englander ZK, Horenstein CI, Zanazzi G, Chang PD et al (2018) Local glioma cells are associated with vascular dysregulation. AJNR Am J Neuroradiol 39(3):507–514

Bulte D, Wartolowska K (2017) Monitoring cardiac and respiratory physiology during FMRI. NeuroImage 154:81–91

Burgess GC, Kandala S, Nolan D, Laumann TO, Power JD, Adeyemo B et al (2016) Evaluation of denoising strategies to address motion-correlated artifacts in resting-state functional magnetic resonance imaging data from the human Connectome Project. Brain Connect 6(9):669–680

Chow DS, Horenstein CI, Canoll P, Lignelli A, Hillman EM, Filippi CG et al (2016) Glioblastoma induces vascular dysregulation in nonenhancing peritumoral regions in humans. AJR Am J Roentgenol 206(5):1073–1081

Ciric R, Wolf DH, Power JD, Roalf DR, Baum GL, Ruparel K et al (2017) Benchmarking of participant-level confound regression strategies for the control of motion artifact in studies of functional connectivity. NeuroImage 154:174–187

Cordes D, Haughton VM, Arfanakis K, Wendt GJ, Turski PA, Moritz CH et al (2000) Mapping functionally related regions of brain with functional connectivity MR imaging. AJNR Am J Neuroradiol 21(9):1636–1644

Dosenbach NU, Fair DA, Miezin FM, Cohen AL, Wenger KK, Dosenbach RA et al (2007) Distinct brain networks for adaptive and stable task control in humans. Proc Natl Acad Sci U S A 104(26):11073–11078

Drysdale AT, Grosenick L, Downar J, Dunlop K, Mansouri F, Meng Y et al (2017) Resting-state connectivity biomarkers define neurophysiological subtypes of depression. Nat Med 23(1):28–38

Englander ZK, Horenstein CI, Bowden SG, Chow DS, Otten ML, Lignelli A et al (2018) Extent of BOLD vascular dysregulation is greater in diffuse gliomas without isocitrate dehydrogenase 1 R132H mutation. Radiology 287(3):965–972

Fair DA, Cohen AL, Power JD, Dosenbach NU, Church JA, Miezin FM et al (2009) Functional brain networks develop from a "local to distributed" organization. PLoS Comput Biol 5(5):e1000381

Friston KJ, Williams S, Howard R, Frackowiak RS, Turner R (1996) Movement-related effects in fMRI time-series. Magn Reson Med 35(3):346–355

Glover GH, Li TQ, Ress D (2000) Image-based method for retrospective correction of physiological motion effects in fMRI: RETROICOR. Magn Reson Med 44(1):162–167

Gordon EM, Laumann TO, Gilmore AW, Newbold DJ, Greene DJ, Berg JJ et al (2017) Precision functional mapping of individual human brains. Neuron 95(4):791–807. e7

Greicius MD, Krasnow B, Reiss AL, Menon V (2003) Functional connectivity in the resting brain: a network analysis of the default mode hypothesis. Proc Natl Acad Sci U S A 100(1):253–258

Jo HJ, Saad ZS, Simmons WK, Milbury LA, Cox RW (2010) Mapping sources of correlation in resting state FMRI, with artifact detection and removal. NeuroImage 52(2):571–582

Kelly AM, Di Martino A, Uddin LQ, Shehzad Z, Gee DG, Reiss PT et al (2009) Development of anterior cingulate functional connectivity from late childhood to early adulthood. Cereb Cortex 19(3):640–657

Laumann TO, Gordon EM, Adeyemo B, Snyder AZ, Joo SJ, Chen MY et al (2015) Functional System and Areal Organization of a Highly Sampled Individual Human Brain. Neuron 87(3):657–670

Liu TT (2017) Reprint of 'noise contributions to the fMRI signal: an overview'. NeuroImage 154:4–14

Lowe MJ, Mock BJ, Sorenson JA (1998) Functional connectivity in single and multislice echoplanar imaging using resting-state fluctuations. NeuroImage 7(2):119–132

Marcus DS, Harms MP, Snyder AZ, Jenkinson M, Wilson JA, Glasser MF et al (2013) Human Connectome Project informatics: quality control, database services, and data visualization. NeuroImage 80:202–219

Murphy K, Birn RM, Bandettini PA (2013) Resting-state fMRI confounds and cleanup. NeuroImage 80:349–359

Oakes TR, Johnstone T, Ores Walsh KS, Greischar LL, Alexander AL, Fox AS et al (2005) Comparison of fMRI motion correction software tools. NeuroImage 28(3):529–543

Poldrack RA, Laumann TO, Koyejo O, Gregory B, Hover A, Chen MY et al (2015) Long-term neural and physiological phenotyping of a single human. Nat Commun 6:8885

Power JD (2017) A simple but useful way to assess fMRI scan qualities. NeuroImage 154:150–158

Power JD, Cohen AL, Nelson SM, Wig GS, Barnes KA, Church JA et al (2011) Functional network organization of the human brain. Neuron 72(4):665–678

Power JD, Barnes KA, Snyder AZ, Schlaggar BL, Petersen SE (2012) Spurious but systematic correlations in functional connectivity MRI networks arise from subject motion. NeuroImage 59(3):2142–2154

Power JD, Schlaggar BL, Petersen SE (2015) Recent progress and outstanding issues in motion correction in resting state fMRI. NeuroImage 105:536–551

Power JD, Plitt M, Laumann TO, Martin A (2017a) Sources and implications of whole-brain fMRI signals in humans. NeuroImage 146:609–625

Power JD, Plitt M, Kundu P, Bandettini PA, Martin A (2017b) Temporal interpolation alters motion in fMRI scans: magnitudes and consequences for artifact detection. PLoS One 12(9):e0182939

Power JD, Plitt M, Gotts SJ, Kundu P, Voon V, Bandettini PA et al (2018) Ridding fMRI data of motion-related influences: removal of signals with distinct spatial and physical bases in multiecho data. Proc Natl Acad Sci U S A 115(9):E2105–E2E14

Pruim RH, Mennes M, van Rooij D, Llera A, Buitelaar JK, Beckmann CF (2015) ICA-AROMA: a robust ICA-based strategy for removing motion artifacts from fMRI data. NeuroImage 112:267–277

Salimi-Khorshidi G, Douaud G, Beckmann CF, Glasser MF, Griffanti L, Smith SM (2014) Automatic denoising of functional MRI data: combining independent component analysis and hierarchical fusion of classifiers. NeuroImage 90:449–468

Satterthwaite TD, Wolf DH, Loughead J, Ruparel K, Elliott MA, Hakonarson H et al (2012) Impact of in-scanner head motion on multiple measures of functional connectivity: relevance for studies of neurodevelopment in youth. NeuroImage 60(1):623–632

Satterthwaite TD, Wolf DH, Ruparel K, Erus G, Elliott MA, Eickhoff SB et al (2013) Heterogeneous impact of motion on fundamental patterns of developmental changes in functional connectivity during youth. NeuroImage 83:45–57

Seeley WW, Menon V, Schatzberg AF, Keller J, Glover GH, Kenna H et al (2007) Dissociable intrinsic connectivity networks for salience processing and executive control. J Neurosci 27(9):2349–2356

Shulman GL, Fiez JA, Corbetta M, Buckner RL, Miezin FM, Raichle ME et al (1997) Common blood flow changes across visual tasks: II. Decreases in cerebral cortex. J Cogn Neurosci 9(5):648–663

Siegel JS, Mitra A, Laumann TO, Seitzman BA, Raichle M, Corbetta M et al (2016) Data quality influences observed links between functional connectivity and behavior. Cereb Cortex 27(9):4492–4502

Smith SM, Fox PT, Miller KL, Glahn DC, Fox PM, Mackay CE et al (2009) Correspondence of the brain's functional architecture during activation and rest. Proc Natl Acad Sci U S A 106(31):13040–13045

Supekar K, Musen M, Menon V (2009) Development of large-scale functional brain networks in children. PLoS Biol 7(7):e1000157

Tagliazucchi E, Laufs H (2014) Decoding wakefulness levels from typical fMRI resting-state data reveals reliable drifts between wakefulness and sleep. Neuron 82(3):695–708

Van Dijk KR, Hedden T, Venkataraman A, Evans KC, Lazar SW, Buckner RL (2010) Intrinsic functional connectivity as a tool for human connectomics: theory, properties, and optimization. J Neurophysiol 103(1):297–321

Van Dijk KR, Sabuncu MR, Buckner RL (2012) The influence of head motion on intrinsic functional connectivity MRI. NeuroImage 59(1):431–438

Yan CG, Cheung B, Kelly C, Colcombe S, Craddock RC, Di Martino A et al (2013) A comprehensive assessment of regional variation in the impact of head micromovements on functional connectomics. NeuroImage 76:183–201

Yeo BT, Krienen FM, Sepulcre J, Sabuncu MR, Lashkari D, Hollinshead M et al (2011) The organization of the human cerebral cortex estimated by intrinsic functional connectivity. J Neurophysiol 106(3):1125–1165

Zaitsev M, Akin B, LeVan P, Knowles BR (2017) Prospective motion correction in functional MRI. NeuroImage 154:33–42

Spatial Resolution of fMRI Techniques

6

Seong-Gi Kim, Tao Jin, and Mitsuhiro Fukuda

6.1 Introduction

Following its introduction over three decades ago, functional magnetic resonance imaging (fMRI) based on the blood oxygenation-level-dependent (BOLD) contrast (Ogawa et al. 1990) has become the tool of choice for visualizing neural activity in the human brain. The conventional BOLD approach has been extensively used for pinpointing functional foci of vision, motor, language, and memory in normal and clinical patients. Intraoperative localization of functional foci will greatly improve surgical planning for epilepsy and tumor dissection and, potentially, for deep brain stimulation. Therefore, it is critical to understand the spatial resolution of fMRI relative to the actual neural active site (see review articles (Kim and Ogawa 2002; Kim and Ugurbil 2003)).

In order to reliably determine the functional foci, high signal-to-noise ratio (SNR), which can be achieved using optimized imaging techniques, is critical. However, high SNR of fMRI techniques is not sufficient for high-resolution functional mapping if the signals that are being imaged do not have a high *specificity* to the local neural activity. Therefore, it is important to understand the signal source of BOLD fMRI and its fundamental limit of spatial resolution. Increased neural activity induces an increase in tissue metabolic demands. Thus, imaging the metabolic change (e.g., 2-fluorodeoxyglucose positron emission tomography) will yield high spatial specificity as metabolism will occur at the tissue at the site of the neuronal activity and not in the vasculature. Changes in neural activity and metabolism could directly or indirectly modulate the hemodynamic responses, including the cerebral blood flow (CBF), the cerebral blood volume (CBV), and the venous oxygenation levels. It has been well established that the magnitude of CBF change is well correlated with that of metabolic change. Thus, CBF mapping can pinpoint the most active spot of neural activity even if the exact spatial extent of the CBF response is controversial ((Malonek and Grinvald 1996) vs. (Duong et al. 2001)). The most commonly used BOLD technique is sensitive to paramagnetic deoxyhemoglobin (dHb), which is located at the capillaries and the venous draining vascular system (Ogawa et al. 1993),

S.-G. Kim (✉)
Center for Neuroscience Imaging Research, Institute for Basic Science,
Suwon, South Korea

Department of Radiology, University of Pittsburgh, Pittsburgh, PA, USA

Department of Biomedical Engineering, Sungkyunkwan University,
Suwon, South Korea
e-mail: kimsg@pitt.edu; seonggikim@skku.edu

T. Jin · M. Fukuda
Department of Radiology, University of Pittsburgh, Pittsburgh, PA, USA
e-mail: taj6@pitt.edu; mif5@pitt.edu

S. Ulmer, O. Jansen (eds.), *fMRI*, https://doi.org/10.1007/978-3-030-41874-8_6

reducing spatial specificity of the gradient-echo BOLD signal. Often in fMRI studies, higher-resolution BOLD images appear localized to large venous vessels because of larger contributions of venous signals due to the reduced volume fraction of tissue.

To understand the spatial resolution of hemodynamic responses, functional changes of different vascular origins should be carefully considered. In this chapter, we will discuss the intrinsic limitations and the improvements of spatial resolution.

6.2 Vascular Structure and Hemodynamic Response

As all fMRI signals originate from changes in hemodynamics, it is important to examine vascular structure. Detailed human brain vasculature was studied anatomically by Duvernoy et al. (1981). In short, vessels can be classified into pial and parenchymal vessels. Superficial pial arterial and venous vessels are numerous; arterial vessels with ~40–280 μm diameter have lesser branches than venous vessels with a ~130–380 μm diameter. These vessels can run a few centimeters and even longer. At the surface of the cortex, pial vessels connect to penetrating arteries and emerging veins at a right angle.

Parenchymal vessels can be divided into arteries, veins, and capillary network. Capillaries with ~5 μm average diameter and ~100 μm length are most abundant at the middle of the cortex (Pawlik et al. 1981). Intracortical arteries and veins can be further classified into their cortical depths (Duvernoy et al. 1981): group 1 and 2 vessels (with 10–20 μm diameter for arterial vessels and 20–30 μm for venous vessels) reach the upper cortical layers (layers 2–3), group 3 (with 15–30 μm for arterial vessels and 45 μm for venous vessels) the middle of the cortex (layers 3–5), group 4 (with 30–40 μm for arterial vessels and 65 μm for venous vessels) the lower cortical region (layer 6), and group 5 (with 30–75 μm for arterial vessels and 80–125 μm for venous vessels) the white matter. The number of intracortical arteries is ~4 times the number of intracortical veins (Duvernoy et al. 1981).

The intrinsic limit of spatial specificity of hemodynamic-based fMRI can be dependent on how finely CBF and CBV are regulated. Blood in each intracortical artery will supply a certain tissue volume, which is referred to as "the volume of arterial unit"; the volume of arterial unit is a volume with 0.33–0.5 mm diameter around a vessel for groups 2–3 and 0.5–2 mm for group 5 (Duvernoy et al. 1981). If an individual intracortical artery can be independently regulated, spatial resolution can be 0.33–0.5 mm if arterial vessels or capillary changes are detected. Our fMRI studies suggest that intrinsic CBF and CBV changes are reasonably specific to submillimeter functional domains (Duong et al. 2001; Zhao et al. 2005), which are in the order of 0.5–0.7 mm diameter in cats. If the regulation point exists at precapillary arterioles or capillaries, then spatial resolution is even better. Recent papers indicate that precapillary arterioles indeed dilate during stimulation via astrocyte-capillary signaling (Zonta et al. 2003; Mulligan and MacVicar 2004; Metea and Newman 2006; Schummers et al. 2008; Petzold and Murthy 2011). In fact, the capillary network responds precisely in regions of neural activity in rat olfactory bulb, suggesting that spatial resolution of ~100 μm is achievable (Chaigneau et al. 2003).

When an imaging technique is sensitive to changes in intracortical veins, its spatial resolution is determined by the volume of tissue draining to each vein, which is considered to be "the volume of venous unit." The volume of venous units is a volume with 0.75–1 mm diameter around a vessel for groups 3–4 vessels and 1–4 mm diameter for group 5 (Duvernoy et al. 1981). Thus, spatial resolution cannot be better than 0.75 mm even if one single intracortical artery regulates precisely and downstream vessels respond. Intracortical venous vascular structures can be visualized with MRI. Figure 6.1 shows venographic images of cat brain, which were obtained using the BOLD contrast at 9.4 T. Venous vessels appear as dark lines or dots because venous blood has short T_2^* relative to tissue and arterial blood. Furthermore, blood

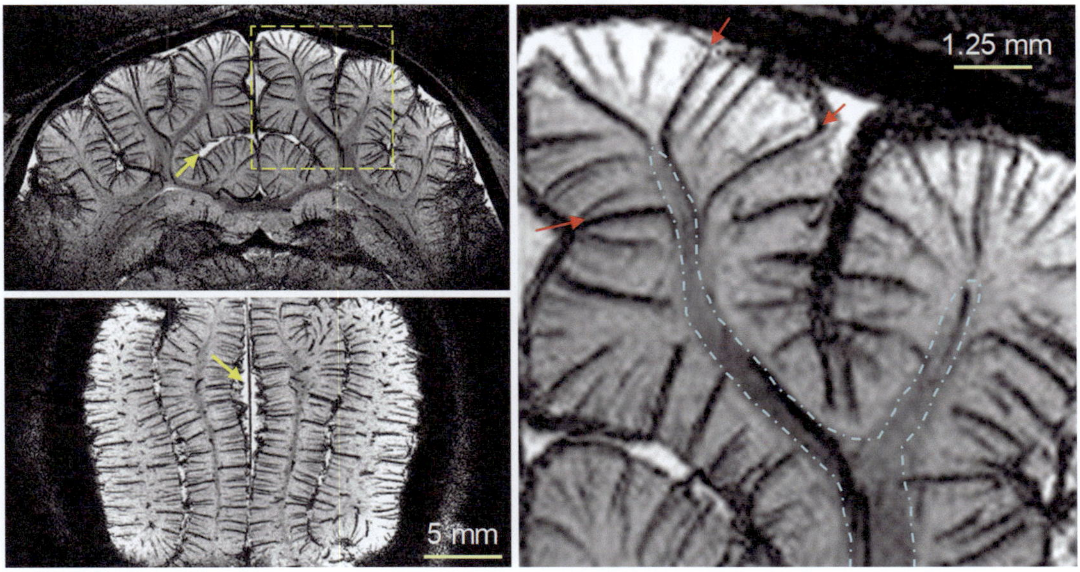

Fig. 6.1 Visualization of venous vessels in a cat brain. A 3-D T_2^*-weighted MR image was obtained at 9.4 T with 78 μm isotropic resolution and field of view of 2 × 2 × 4 cm³. A gradient-echo time of 20 ms was used to maximize the contrast between venous vessels and tissue. Data acquisition and processing methods were reported elsewhere (Park et al. 2008). 1.25-mm-thick slabs were selected, and minimum intensity projection was performed to enhance the contrast of venous vessels. As a surface coil was used, the ventral section in the coronal slice (*top left*) had poor signal-to-noise ratio (SNR), and thus, vessels could not be detected in that region. White matter areas (*contours in right*) can be distinguished from the gray matter. *Dotted yellow box* in the coronal image was expanded 4 times into the right. *Yellow arrows* cerebrospinal fluid (CSF) areas; *red arrows* venous vessels draining from the white matter, which are "group 5." *Scale bar*, 5 mm for *left* and 1.25 mm for *right*

susceptibility effect extends to tissue, enlarging apparent venous vessel size. Clearly, in groups 3–5, intracortical veins can be easily visualized, and group 3 is the most numerous. Typical distance between intercortical veins is ~0.5–1 mm (Fig. 6.1).

6.3 Spatial Resolution of BOLD fMRI

Since blood travels from capillaries to intracortical veins, and finally pial veins, a change in dHb concentration in blood can also occur far away from the actual gray matter region with increased neural activity, reducing effective spatial resolution. However, there is considerably more dilution of dHb change farther downstream from the neuronally active region due to larger blood contribution from inactive regions. This dilution issue is also closely related to strength and spatial extent of neural activity. When the area of activation is small, this deoxygenated blood is diluted with blood from inactivated regions, effectively reducing the oxygenation level change. Thus BOLD fMRI is capable of differentiating small functional modules such as single whisker barrels (Yang et al. 1996). However, when the area of activation is large, blood drained from active regions can travel far away without much dilution.

Conventional BOLD response is related to a change in dHb contents within a voxel, thus directly correlated with (baseline dHb content) times (oxygenation change). Since a pixel with draining veins has high baseline dHb content, the BOLD response is particularly sensitive to large draining veins. Thus, spatial resolution of conventional BOLD signal can be much worse than that determined by the volume of venous unit. It is a reasonable assumption that conventional BOLD-based *high-resolution* fMRI may mostly detect the functionally less-specific large-vessel signals. To precisely localize functional foci, it is desirable to remove or minimize large-vessel contributions.

In order to understand which size of venous vessels can be detected by BOLD fMRI, we review the source of BOLD fMRI signals. Detailed biophysical models and explanations can be found in others (Ogawa et al. 1993; Weisskoff et al. 1994; Kim and Ugurbil 2003). The BOLD contrast induced by dHb arises from both intravascular (IV) and extravascular (EV) components. Since exchange of water between these two compartments (typical lifetime of the water in capillaries >500 ms) is relatively slow when compared with the imaging time (echo time < 100 ms), MRI signals from these can be treated as separate pools.

The IV component is considered to be uniform within vessels because water rapidly exchanges between red blood cells (RBC) with paramagnetic dHb and plasma (average water residence time in RBCs = ~5 ms) and travels through space by exchange and diffusion. Thus, "dynamic" time averaging occurs over the many different fields induced by dHb. All water molecules inside the vessel will experience similar dynamic averaging, resulting in reduction of blood water T_2 in the venous pool. At high magnetic fields, venous blood T_2 can be shorter than tissue T_2 because R_2 ($=1/T_2$) of venous blood is quadratically dependent on magnetic field (Thulborn et al. 1982). Thus, at a higher magnetic field, IV contribution can be reduced by setting echo time much longer than blood T_2 (or T_2*) (Lee et al. 1999; Jin et al. 2006). Alternatively, the IV signal can be reduced by applying bipolar gradients (as employed in diffusion-weighted images), which, with a b value of >30 s/mm^2, are expected to leave only the microvascular/extravascular contribution (Le Bihan et al. 1986).

The EV BOLD phenomenon has two biophysical sources (Ogawa et al. 1993; Weisskoff et al. 1994): one is due to intra-voxel dephasing of the magnetization in the presence of susceptibility-induced gradients, and the other is due to diffusion across the steep, susceptibility-induced gradients around small vessels (capillaries and venules). The first component induces high-percentage signal changes around large venous vessels, regardless of magnetic field strength. Since field gradient decreases by $(r/a)^2$ where r is the distance from vessel to the region of interest and a is the vessel radius, the dephasing effect around a larger vessel is more spatially widespread. However, the dephasing effect of the static field can be refocused by the 180° radiofrequency (RF) pulse. Therefore, the EV contribution of large vessels can be reduced by using the spin-echo technique (which is similar to T_2-weighting in diagnostic imaging). The second component induces small signal changes in areas around capillaries and small venules. The reason is that tissue water around capillaries and small venules will be "dynamically" averaged over the many different fields during TE, similar to the IV component. This effect is larger at a higher magnetic field due to an increased susceptibility gradient within the water diffusion distance during TE. The dynamic diffusion-induced signals can be detected by either GE or SE approach. It is conceivable that the T_2-based BOLD technique is better localized to neuronal active region than T_2*-based BOLD if the IV component of large vessels is removed (Zhao et al. 2004, 2006). However, the sensitivity of spin-echo techniques is less than gradient-echo BOLD signal.

To examine the spatial resolution of GE and SE BOLD fMRI, we used cortical layers as a model because layer 4 has the highest metabolic and CBF responses during neural activity as well as the highest synapse density and cytochrome oxidase activity (Woolsey et al. 1996). If the fMRI technique is highly specific to metabolic response and/or neural activity, the middle of the cortex should have the highest signal change. Figure 6.2 shows GE and SE BOLD fMRI maps of one isoflurane-anesthetized cat obtained during visual stimulation at 9.4 T (Zhao et al. 2006). To view the cortical cross section within a plane resolution of 156 × 156 μm^2, a 2-mm-thick imaging slice was selected perpendicular to the cortical surface. In both GE and SE BOLD maps,

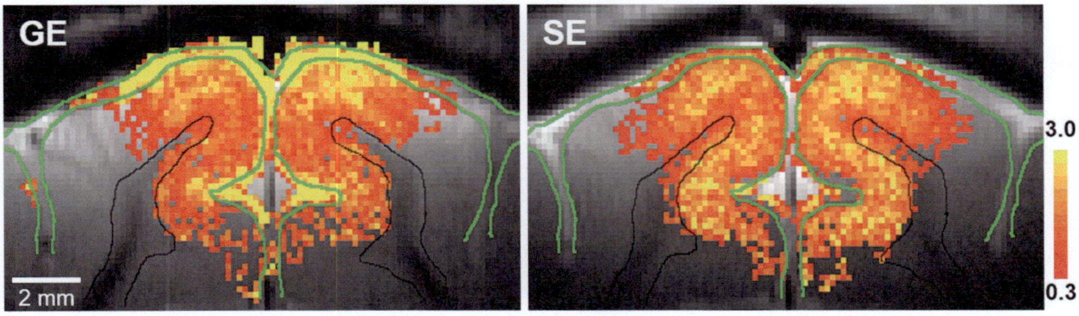

Fig. 6.2 High-resolution GE (*left*) and SE BOLD (*right*) fMRI maps of cat brain during visual stimulation overlaid on anatomical EPI images (Zhao et al. 2006). Coronal 2-mm-thick images with 156 × 156 μm² in-plane resolution were acquired using the four shot EPI technique at 9.4 T with gradient-echo time of 20 ms and spin-echo time of 40 ms. To determine statistically significant pixels, Student's *t* test was performed on a pixel-by-pixel basis with a t-value threshold of 2.0. Then, percentage signal changes were calculated for statistically active pixels. *Green contours* CSF area, *black contours* white matter, *scale bar* 2 mm, *color scale bar* 0.3–3%

signal intensities increased during visual stimulation, indicating an increase in venous oxygenation. In conventional GE BOLD fMRI (Fig. 6.2), the highest-percentage signal changes (yellow pixels) were seen in the CSF space (within the green contours), where pial veins are located. This large-vessel contribution to BOLD signals is reduced using the SE technique (Fig. 6.2) because the dephasing around large vessels refocuses. This result is consistent with high-field SE BOLD observations (Lee et al. 1999; Yacoub et al. 2003; Zhao et al. 2004).

SE BOLD fMRI is an excellent alternative approach if high spatial resolution is required and high magnetic field (such as 7 T) is available (Moon et al. 2007; Yacoub et al. 2008). Otherwise, conventional GE BOLD fMRI should be used with post-processing approaches to remove or minimize large-vessel contributions. Location of large pial venous vessels can be determined from venographic images obtained with high-resolution T_2*-weighted MR techniques (see Fig. 6.1) or from anatomical structures such as sulci and CSF. Large venous vessel areas tend to induce large BOLD percent change (see also Fig. 6.2) (Kim et al. 1994), delayed response (Lee et al. 1995), significant phase change (Menon 2002), and large baseline fluctuations (Kim et al. 1994). Although these criteria are subjective, they are effective in detecting and reducing large-vessel contamination.

6.4 Perfusion-Based fMRI Approaches

Alternative to the BOLD approach, CBF-weighted techniques which are sensitive mainly to parenchyma should be considered for mapping functional foci. CBF-weighted functional images can be obtained using MR by employing arterial blood water as an endogenous flow tracer. Arterial spin labeling (ASL) can be achieved by RF pulse(s). Then, labeled spins move into capillaries in the imaging slice and exchange with tissue water spins. To obtain only perfusion-related images, two images are acquired, one with ASL and the other without labeling. The difference between the two images is directly related to CBF, and relative CBF changes due to physiological perturbations can be measured. Most of the labeled water molecules extract into tissue, and the remaining labeled water lose most of their labeling by the time they reach the draining veins due to its relatively short half-life (i.e., T_1 of blood). Thus, CBF-weighted MRI signals predominantly originate from tissue/capillary as well as arterial vessels (Ye et al. 1997; Lee et al. 2002; Kim and Kim 2005). Sensitivity of perfusion-weighted signals increases with magnetic field strength due to an increase in arterial blood T_1. ASL techniques include continuous ASL (Detre et al. 1992), flow-sensitive alternating inversion recovery (FAIR) (Kim 1995;

Kwong et al. 1995), and various other techniques (Edelman et al. 1994; Wong et al. 1998).

Perfusion-based MR techniques have been used for fMRI studies. The spatial specificity of CBF-based fMRI is superior compared to GE BOLD techniques (Duong et al. 2001). Figure 6.3 shows BOLD and CBF functional maps during finger movements obtained at 4 T (Kim et al. 1997). The FAIR technique was used with inversion time of 1.4 s; the BOLD map was obtained from non-slice-selective inversion recovery images, while the CBF map was from subtraction of non-slice-selective from slice-selective inversion recovery images. Generally, activation areas are consistent between the maps measured by both techniques. However, pixel-wise comparison shows discrepancy between the two maps. Large signal changes in BOLD are located at draining veins indicated by arrows in the middle slice, while no signal change was observed in CBF. Tissue areas with high-percent CBF changes have low BOLD signal changes. This indicates that the CBF approach is more specific to tissue than GE BOLD fMRI. To further confirm human fMRI results, BOLD and CBF fMRI were also compared in the cat's layer model. Figure 6.4 shows GE BOLD and CBF fMRI maps obtained during visual stimulation at 9.4 T (Jin and Kim 2008). CBF data were obtained using the FAIR technique with inversion time of 1.25 s, while gradient -echo BOLD data were obtained with TE of 20 ms. The highest GE BOLD signal changes occur at the surface of the cortex, while the highest CBF changes occur at the middle of the cortex.

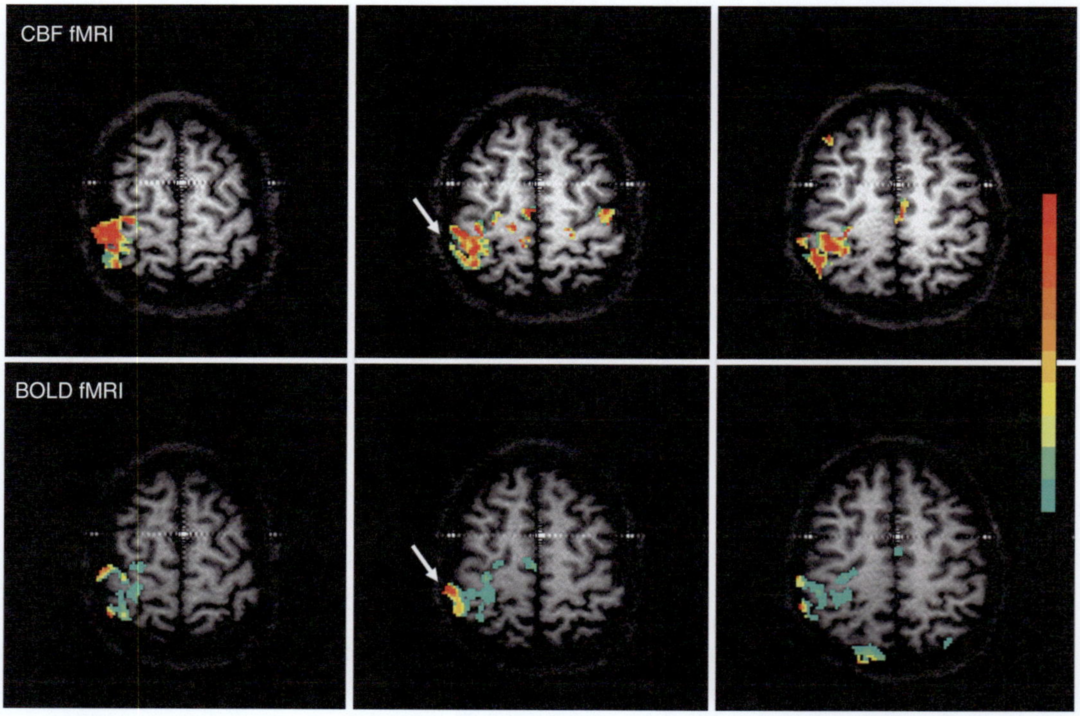

Fig. 6.3 BOLD and CBF functional maps of left-hand finger opposition, overlaid on T_1-weighted EPI (Kim et al. 1997). The flow-sensitive alternating inversion recovery (FAIR) technique was used to acquire BOLD (*bottom*) and CBF (*top*) contrast simultaneously at 4.0 T. BOLD maps were obtained from non-slice-selective inversion recovery (IR) images, while CBF maps were calculated from differences between slice-selective and non-slice-selective IR images. A cross-correlation value of 0.3 was used for threshold. For BOLD images, each color increment represents a 1% increment starting from the bottom 1%, while for CBF images, each color increment represents a 10% increment starting from the bottom 10%. The oblique arrow at the middle slice, indicating the right (contralateral) central sulcus, shows no activation in the CBF map, but large signal increase in the BOLD map, suggesting BOLD is sensitive to large draining veins

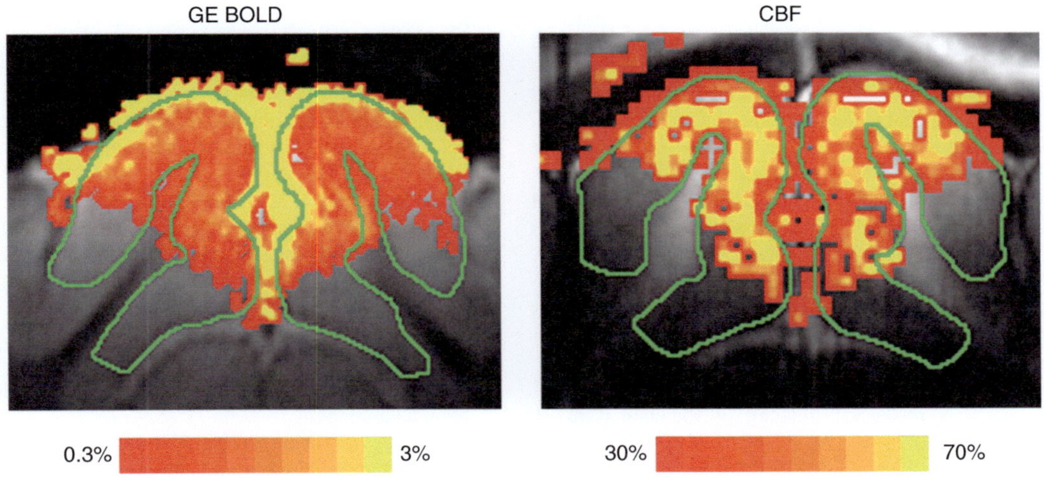

Fig. 6.4 BOLD and CBF fMRI maps of cat brain during visual stimulation overlaid on anatomical EPI images (Jin and Kim 2008). Coronal 2-mm-thick images with $312 \times 312\ \mu m^2$ in-plane resolution were acquired at 9.4 T; BOLD fMRI (*left*) was obtained with TE of 20 ms, while CBF (*right*) was detected with the FAIR technique with inversion time of 1.25 s. Maps were obtained by thresholding with a P value <0.05 and number of contiguous active pixels ≥3. The gray matter areas are outlined by *green contours*. The highest BOLD signal changes are observed at the surface of the cortex, while the highest CBF changes occur at the middle of the cortex. *Color bar* 0.3–3.0% for BOLD and 30–70% for CBF

This again demonstrates that perfusion-based fMRI technique is superior to GE BOLD for pinpointing functional foci precisely.

Proper CBF contrast is achieved only when enough time is allowed for the labeled arterial water to travel into the region of interest and exchange with tissue water. This makes it difficult to detect changes in CBF with a temporal resolution greater than T_1 of arterial blood water. Acquisition of a pair of images can further reduce temporal resolution and consequently SNR. Thus, it is difficult to obtain whole-brain fMRI rapidly. However, baseline CBF value can be obtained, in addition to quantitative functional response. An additional advantage is less sensitivity to baseline signal drifts because slow non-activation-related signal changes can be removed by the pairwise subtraction (Kim 1995), and it is more stable to low-frequency stimulation compared to BOLD. Therefore, perfusion-based fMRI techniques are preferable for repetitive measurements over a long time period such as weeks and months, allowing investigations of functional reorganization and development. In clinical applications of fMRI where precise mapping is required around abnormal regions, the CBF-based fMRI technique is most appropriate because parenchymal signals are dominant.

Acknowledgments This work was supported in part by IBS-R15-D1. The authors thank their colleagues in the neuroimaging laboratory at the University of Pittsburgh for providing the figures and for helpful discussion.

References

Chaigneau E, Oheim M et al (2003) Two-photon imaging of capillary blood flow in olfactory bulb glomeruli. Proc Natl Acad Sci U S A 100(22):13081–13086

Detre JA, Leigh JS et al (1992) Perfusion imaging. Magn Reson Med 23:37–45

Duong TQ, Kim D-S et al (2001) Localized cerebral blood flow response at submillimeter columnar resolution. Proc Natl Acad Sci U S A 98:10904–10909

Duvernoy HM, Delon S et al (1981) Cortical blood vessels of the human brain. Brain Res Bull 7(5):519–579

Edelman RR, Siewert B et al (1994) Qualitative mapping of cerebral blood flow and functional localization with echo-planar MR imaging and signal targeting with alternating radio frequency. Radiology 192:513–520

Jin T, Kim SG (2008) Cortical layer-dependent dynamic blood oxygenation, cerebral blood flow and cerebral blood volume responses during visual stimulation. NeuroImage 43(1):1–9

Jin T, Wang P et al (2006) Source of nonlinearity in echo-time-dependent BOLD fMRI. Magn Reson Med 55:1281–1290

Kim S-G (1995) Quantification of relative cerebral blood flow change by flow-sensitive alternating inversion recovery (FAIR) technique: application to functional mapping. Magn Reson Med 34:293–301

Kim T, Kim S-G (2005) Quantification of cerebral arterial blood volume and cerebral blood flow using MRI with modulation of tissue and vessel (MOTIVE) signals. Magn Reson Med 54:333–342

Kim S-G, Ogawa S (2002) Insights into new techniques for high resolution functional MRI. Curr Opin Neurobiol 12:607–615

Kim S-G, Ugurbil K (2003) High-resolution functional magnetic resonance imaging of the animal brain. Methods 30:28–41

Kim SG, Hendrich K et al (1994) Potential pitfalls of functional MRI using conventional gradient-recalled echo techniques. NMR Biomed 7(1–2):69–74

Kim S-G, Tsekos NV et al (1997) Multi-slice perfusion-based functional MRI using the FAIR technique: comparison of CBF and BOLD effects. NMR Biomed 10:191–196

Kwong KK, Chesler DA et al (1995) MR perfusion studies with T1-weighted echo planar imaging. Magn Reson Med 34:878–887

Le Bihan D, Breton E et al (1986) MR imaging of intravoxel incoherent motions: application to diffusion and perfusion in neurologic disorders. Radiology 161:401–407

Lee AT, Glover GH et al (1995) Discrimination of large venous vessels in time-course spiral blood-oxygen-level-dependent magnetic resonance functional neuroimaging. Magn Reson Med 33:745–754

Lee S-P, Silva AC et al (1999) Diffusion-weighted spin-echo fMRI at 9.4 T: microvascular/tissue contribution to BOLD signal change. Magn Reson Med 42:919–928

Lee S-P, Silva AC et al (2002) Comparison of diffusion-weighted high-resolution CBF and spin-echo BOLD fMRI at 9.4 T. Magn Reson Med 47:736–741

Malonek D, Grinvald A (1996) Interactions between electrical activity and cortical microcirculation revealed by imaging spectroscopy: implication for functional brain mapping. Science 272:551–554

Menon RS (2002) Postacquisition suppression of large-vessel BOLD signals in high-resolution fMRI. Magn Reson Med 47:1–9

Metea M, Newman E (2006) Glial cells dilate and constrict blood vessels: a mechanism of neurovascular coupling. J Neurosci 26:2862–2870

Moon CH, Fukuda M et al (2007) Neural interpretation of blood oxygenation level-dependent fMRI maps at submillimeter columnar resolution. J Neurosci 27:6892–6902

Mulligan S, MacVicar B (2004) Calcium transients in astrocyte endfeet cause cerebrovascular constrictions. Nature 431:195–199

Ogawa S, Lee T-M et al (1990) Oxygenation-sensitive contrast in magnetic resonance image of rodent brain at high magnetic fields. Magn Reson Med 14:68–78

Ogawa S, Menon RS et al (1993) Functional brain mapping by blood oxygenation level-dependent contrast magnetic resonance imaging. A comparison of signal characteristics with a biophysical model. Biophys J 64(3):803–812

Park SH, Masamoto K et al (2008) Imaging brain vasculature with BOLD microscopy: MR detection limits determined by in vivo two-photon microscopy. Magn Reson Med 59:855–865

Pawlik G, Rackl A et al (1981) Quantitative capillary topography and blood flow in the cerebral cortex of cats: an in vivo microscopic study. Brain Res 208:35–58

Petzold GC, Murthy VN (2011) Role of astrocytes in neurovascular coupling. Neuron 71:782–797

Schummers J, Yu H et al (2008) Tuned responses of astrocytes and their influence on hemodynamic signals in the visual cortex. Science 320:1638–1643

Thulborn KR, Waterton JC et al (1982) Oxygenation dependence of the transverse relaxation time of water protons in whole blood at high field. Biochim Biophys Acta 714:265–270

Weisskoff RM, Zuo CS et al (1994) Microscopic susceptibility variation and transverse relaxation: theory and experiment. Magn Reson Med 31:601–610

Wong E, Buxton R et al (1998) Quantitative imaging of perfusion using a single subtraction (QUIPSS anf QUIPSS II). Magn Reson Med 39:702–708

Woolsey TA, Rovainen CM et al (1996) Neuronal units linked to microvascular modules in cerebral cortex: response elements for imaging the brain. Cereb Cortex 6:647–660

Yacoub E, Duong TQ et al (2003) Spin-echo fMRI in humans using high spatial resolutions and high magnetic fields. Magn Reson Med 49:655–664

Yacoub E, Harel N et al (2008) High-field fMRI unveils orientation columns in humans. Proc Natl Acad Sci U S A 105:10607–10612

Yang X, Hyder F et al (1996) Activation of single whisker barrel in rat brain localized by functional magnetic resonance imaging. Proc Natl Acad Sci U S A 93:475–478

Ye FQ, Mattay VS et al (1997) Correction for vascular artifacts in cerebral blood flow values by using arterial spin tagging techniques. Magn Reson Med 37:226–235

Zhao F, Wang P et al (2004) Cortical depth-dependent gradient-echo and spin-echo BOLD fMRI at 9.4 T. Magn Reson Med 51:518–524

Zhao F, Wang P et al (2005) Spatial specificity of cerebral blood volume-weighted fMRI responses at columnar resolution. NeuroImage 27:416–424

Zhao F, Wang P et al (2006) Cortical layer-dependent BOLD and CBV responses measured by spin-echo and gradient-echo fMRI: insights into hemodynamic regulation. NeuroImage 30:1149–1160

Zonta M, Angulo MC et al (2003) Neuron-to-astrocyte signaling is central to the dynamic control of brain microcirculation. Nat Neurosci 6:43–50

7 Acquisition Aspects of Functional and Clinical Arterial Spin Labeling

Dimo Ivanov and Yanina Kozovska

7.1 Introduction

Tissue perfusion is a fundamental physiological variable that refers to the delivery of blood to capillary beds. Perfusion is important because it determines the rate of delivery of oxygen and nutrients (glucose, etc.) to the tissue and the rate of clearance of waste products. Disorders of perfusion such as stroke account for much of the medical morbidity, and blood flow (perfusion) alterations also commonly accompany other pathophysiological changes such as cancer, epilepsy, and neurodegenerative diseases. Tissue perfusion is quantified by the amount of blood delivered to the tissue per unit time, for a unit volume or mass of tissue (e.g., ml of blood/min/100 g of tissue).

A number of blood flow-related parameters can be measured using a range of magnetic resonance imaging (MRI) methodologies. Noninvasive quantitative measurements of tissue perfusion can be obtained using arterial spin labeling (ASL) (Detre et al. 1992; Williams et al. 1992). In the ASL approach, arterial blood water is used as an endogenous diffusible tracer. The tracer is created by inverting the magnetization of the blood in the arteries with radiofrequency (RF) pulses (see Sect. 7.2), before it flows into the target tissue. After the "labeled" blood flows into the tissue, the resulting magnetization is reduced, and images collected downstream from the labeling location appear slightly darker. By subtracting the labeled images from control images, acquired without inverting the blood's magnetization, the amount of blood that entered the tissue since the beginning of the labeling can be calculated. A time series of interleaved labeled and control image pairs is usually acquired, enabling dynamic perfusion measurements. Simple pair-wise subtraction can be employed provided functional studies are not performed. The majority of ASL applications have been in the brain due to its high perfusion rates, spatially consolidated blood supply, the lack of major motion issues, and the tight coupling between regional cerebral blood flow (CBF) and neural activity (Raichle 1998). The lifetime of the endogenous label is governed by the longitudinal relaxation time (T_1) of blood, which is on the order of 1–2 s (Zhang et al. 2013). ASL implementation parameters are largely influenced by the fact that this lifetime is similar to the arterial transit time (ATT), i.e., the transport time from the labeling position to the tissue. The time between the image acquisition and the end of the labeling is called post-labeling delay (PLD). A fundamental trade-off is that a short PLD does not allow for complete delivery of the labeled blood water to the tissue, whereas a long PLD results in

D. Ivanov (✉)
Department of Cognitive Neuroscience, Faculty of Psychology and Neuroscience, Maastricht Brain Imaging Centre (M-BIC), Maastricht University, Maastricht, The Netherlands
e-mail: dimo.ivanov@maastrichtuniversity.nl

Y. Kozovska
Department of Vascular Surgery, Kerckhoff-Klinik, Bad Nauheim, Germany

S. Ulmer, O. Jansen (eds.), *fMRI*, https://doi.org/10.1007/978-3-030-41874-8_7

strong T_1 decay and therefore reduced signal-to-noise ratio (SNR). The ATT varies regionally and allows defining vascular and watershed territories (Hendrikse et al. 2008) or collateral flow sources (Petersen et al. 2010; Bokkers et al. 2009). In addition, ATT differs between healthy and pathological tissue as well as among individuals.

The noninvasive nature of ASL and its ability to dynamically and quantitatively measure CBF make it an attractive approach for both neuroscience research and clinical applications (Detre et al. 1998; Detre and Wang 2002). ASL has been applied to study cerebrovascular disease (Detre and Wang 2002; Donahue et al. 2012), to identify abnormal neurovascular coupling mechanisms (Blicher et al. 2012; Donahue et al. 2010) and flow territory asymmetry (Hendrikse et al. 2005; Donahue et al. 2014). The capability of ASL to concurrently measure functional changes of CBF and BOLD signal has proven to be useful for investigating the brain's physiology in health and disease (Bulte et al. 2012; Buxton et al. 2014). Surround subtraction approaches should be employed in functional studies to minimize cross talk between the CBF and BOLD signal during activations (Lu et al. 2006; Liu et al. 2002). In these techniques, consecutive control images are either averaged or interpolated to the time of the label image that is acquired in between, with the intent of maintaining a similar blood oxygenation level of the resulting combined control image and the label image. Baseline CBF has been used to study longitudinal intra-subject changes due to, for example, learning, experience, and plasticity and also to examine inter-subject differences in baseline brain physiology in healthy subjects and patients (Detre and Wang 2002; Krieger et al. 2014). In functional experiments, ASL generally has higher time course stability than BOLD fMRI for long duration block designs (Aguirre et al. 2002) and, owing to its quantitative and noninvasive contrast mechanism, is ideally suited for evaluating longitudinal changes. Functional ASL changes have been shown to be less variable across healthy subjects and better localized to the site of neural activation than the BOLD signal and quantitatively more directly related to neuronal activity (Duong et al. 2001; Tjandra et al. 2005; Cavusoglu et al. 2012; Havlicek et al. 2015).

Nevertheless, compared to BOLD fMRI, CBF measurements using ASL present some drawbacks (Alsop et al. 2015), such as lower SNR of the perfusion-weighted signal due to the low microvascular density (~1–2% of the local tissue volume). ASL has a reduced temporal resolution compared to BOLD fMRI, because of the need to acquire pairs of label and control images. Also a PLD is necessary to allow the labeled blood to reach the imaging slab. T_1 decay of the labeled blood and increased power deposition limit ASL's brain coverage in comparison to BOLD imaging. To overcome these drawbacks, different ASL approaches have been proposed. It is important to stress that despite these limitations, accurate CBF estimates can be obtained with ASL when it is implemented properly. An overview of how to tackle these drawbacks, together with protocol recommendations, is given in (Alsop et al. 2015), while in this chapter we will focus mainly on the strategies to improve the SNR and temporal resolution of ASL in neuroimaging. The implications of the different ASL parameter choices on the BOLD functional sensitivity will also be discussed below.

The aforementioned ASL limitations have also largely determined the design of the functional perfusion experiments performed. Due to the low temporal resolution, it is advised to acquire only the brain areas of interest to avoid unnecessary increases in the repetition time (TR). The ASL TRs of at least 2.5 s are also the reason why block design experiments with block durations of at least 20 s are typically employed. Furthermore, paradigms that elicit large functional responses such as visual, motor, or pharmacological stimuli are predominantly used with ASL. One of the main benefits for ASL is that the magnitude of the CBF modulations for such stimuli is an order of magnitude larger than the corresponding BOLD responses, increasing the ease of detection. It is likely that this relation holds true for a broad range of stimuli, but experimental evidence on this is still lacking. A useful notion to remember about the functional ASL time course is that the envelope (the control's signal intensity) represents the BOLD signal, whereas the magnitude of the difference between control and label is proportional to the CBF. Therefore, during functional activation, both the control signal intensity and the difference between the control and label signal increase.

ASL has a low SNR, which can be increased by means of a low spatial resolution (typically 2–4 mm voxels) and signal averaging across multiple repetitions. ASL's limited perfusion temporal SNR (tSNR) leads to low CBF functional sensitivity that rarely allows high spatial resolutions and inflicts longer scanning durations in fMRI studies. The perfusion tSNR is determined by the control image tSNR, labeling bolus length (amount of labeled blood), PLD, and the degree of background suppression (see Sect. 7.3). Other imaging parameters, such as the voxel size, partial Fourier factor, or the RF coil employed, influence the perfusion tSNR only indirectly through the control tSNR. The relationship between perfusion tSNR and control tSNR is complex as decreases in control tSNR also lead to reduction in perfusion tSNR, but the two become decoupled when background suppression is applied. Background suppression diminishes the static tissue signal and to a smaller extent the control tSNR. In contrast, perfusion tSNR is increased when background suppression is applied due to the reduction of physiological noise in the ASL time series. The control tSNR is influenced by a large number of factors including echo time (TE), voxel size, RF receive array, use of parallel imaging, and magnetic field strength. Some of these parameters also directly impact the perfusion tSNR like the field strength and TE. Other factors only modulate the perfusion tSNR through the control tSNR, like the receive array and voxel size. The TE is mainly determined by the readout (acquisition) approach employed. The readout options are reviewed in Sect. 7.4 and range from the commonly used 2D single-shot EPI, through 2D single-shot spiral, to 3D segmented spin-echo (SE) approaches. Newer readout techniques include 2D simultaneous multi-slice (SMS) EPI techniques (Feinberg et al. 2013; Kim et al. 2013; Ivanov et al. 2017a) and 2D turboFLASH (TFL)) (Zuo et al. 2013; Wang et al. 2015). The 3D SE approaches with their increased SNR and optimal combination with background suppression have become commonly used (Vidorreta et al. 2013). The PLD is mostly determined by the research question and physiological constraints and therefore offers a relatively limited opportunity to influence the ASL (t)SNR. The amount of labeled blood is determined by the bolus length and depends on the labeling technique employed. Pulsed, continuous, pseudo-continuous, and velocity-selective approaches (see Sect. 7.2) have been proposed.

7.2 Labeling Approaches

Several techniques have been proposed for achieving arterial blood labeling. The first is called continuous ASL (CASL), and in it the arterial blood is continuously and selectively labeled as it passes through a labeling plane (Detre et al. 1992; Williams et al. 1992). Pulsed ASL (PASL) was introduced shortly thereafter, and it uses a short RF pulse or a train of pulses to instantaneously invert the magnetization of blood and tissue. In PASL, the pulses can be applied either below the brain (Kim 1995; Wong et al. 2006) or to the entire brain with subsequent inversion of the imaging slices to produce a magnetization difference between blood and brain water (Detre et al. 1994). Pseudo-continuous ASL (pCASL) is a hybrid approach that mimics CASL using many short pulses to provide better sensitivity and compatibility with modern clinical scanner hardware (Alsop and Detre 1998; Edelman and Chen 1998). Velocity-selective arterial spin labeling (VSASL) has been explored as a means of eliminating the dependence on arterial transit time (Aslan et al. 2010; Dai et al. 2012).

Pulsed and (pseudo-)continuous ASL labeling methods differ fundamentally not only in the spatial extent but also in the duration of the labeling (Fig. 7.1). In CASL and pCASL, the labeling occurs over a longer period, typically 1–3 s, and the process is known as flow-driven adiabatic inversion. The labeling is performed using one long RF pulse and a constant gradient in CASL,

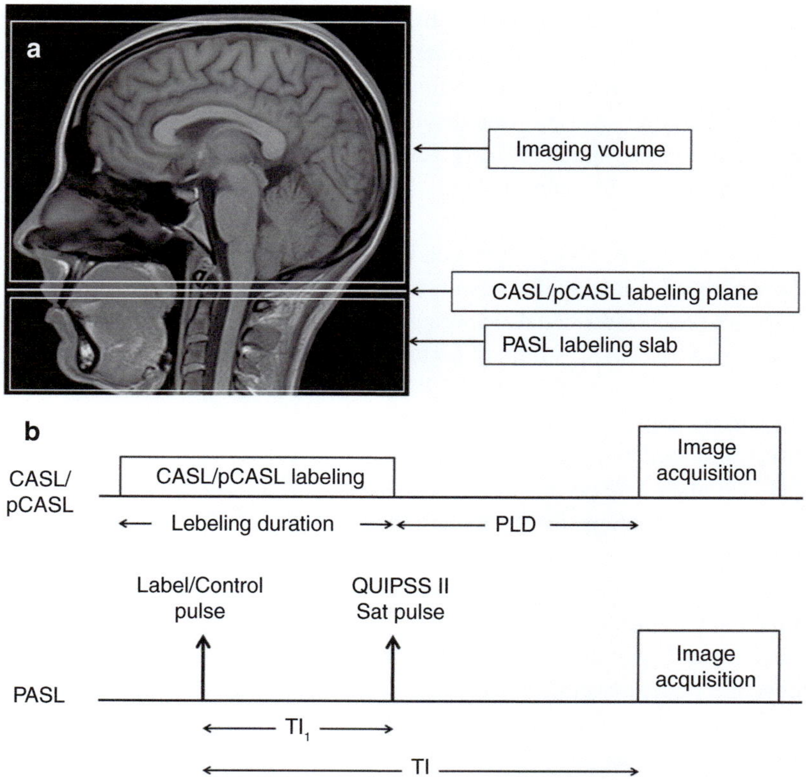

Fig. 7.1 (**a**) Schematic diagram of imaging and labeling regions for CASL/pCASL and PASL. In CASL/pCASL, labeling occurs as blood flows through a single labeling plane, while in PASL, a slab of tissue, including arterial blood, is labeled. (**b**) Timing diagram for CASL/pCASL and PASL. For QUIPSS (quantitative imaging of perfusion using single subtraction) II PASL, TI_1 is the bolus duration and is analogous to the labeling duration in CASL/pCASL. TI is the time between the inversion pulse and image acquisition in PASL. The PLD in CASL/pCASL is equal to the quantity ($TI-TI_1$) in QUIPSS II PASL

whereas in pCASL more than a 1000 slice-selective RF pulses are applied at a rate of approximately one per millisecond along with a train of gradient pulses. CASL produces significant saturation of brain tissue through magnetization transfer effects, biasing the perfusion estimates. CASL pulse sequence modifications that have been introduced to reduce this bias lead to decreased labeling efficiency and therefore lower SNR. An approach that largely eliminates magnetization transfer effects in CASL involves the application of separate labeling coils (Trampel et al. 2002). However, such hardware is incompatible with most MR scanners, which prevented the widespread use of this approach. In pCASL, larger gradients are present during the RF pulses, decreasing magnetization transfer effects and increasing the labeling efficiency on standard scanner hardware, which make pCASL preferred over CASL. The ASL's SNR increases with the labeling duration. However, longer label durations lengthen the TR and thereby reduce the temporal resolution and the number of averages obtainable per unit time. Long labeling durations also increase the ASL signal dependence on the tissues' T_1 but may help preserve signal when the arterial transit time is unexpectedly long. The optimal labeling duration in pCASL is determined by the T_1 of arterial blood, as the SNR gains diminish with label durations much longer than the arterial blood's T_1. An important issue for pCASL is the positioning of the labeling plane. In the ideal case, the labeling plane should be located in a region where the relevant feeding arteries are relatively straight and perpendicular to the labeling plane. This is often accomplished using an angiogram since one, adequate for this purpose, can be obtained in less than a minute. Inefficient labeling leads to image artifacts and can occur when the labeling RF pulses have insufficient amplitude or are applied at a location different from the labeling plane.

In PASL, a single RF pulse or a short (10–50 ms) train of pulses inverts a slab of tissue, including the feeding arteries, proximal to the area of interest. Many PASL labeling approaches, and associated acronyms, have been introduced to realize this inversion, but overall, their performance is fairly similar. One important difference between them is in the labeling of blood that flows into the region of interest from the distal side. When whole-brain coverage is specified, then this region is outside the head, and this distinction becomes irrelevant. For smaller imaging slabs, vessels entering from above the slab (mostly veins) may produce ASL signals, and their contribution should be considered when comparing perfusion values across ASL techniques. For flow-sensitive alternating inversion recovery (FAIR) (Kim 1995) and its variants, inflow from above will cause a positive ASL signal. For EPISTAR (echo planar imaging and signal targeting with alternating RF) (Edelman and Chen 1998), inflow from above will result in a negative signal, and for PICORE (proximal inversion with a control for off-resonance effects) (Wong et al. 1997) and PULSAR (pulsed star labeling of arterial regions) (Golay et al. 2005), inflow from above produces no ASL signal. In PASL, several techniques have been devised to minimize potential artifacts. For efficient inversion (inversion efficiency greater than 95%), adiabatic RF pulses (Frank et al. 1997; Yongbi et al. 1998) are preferred due to their robustness against transmit RF field inhomogeneities. Moreover, the total RF power during the label and control conditions is matched to minimize magnetization transfer effects, which can bias the perfusion estimates (Zhang et al. 1995). The inversion profile of the slab-selective inversion pulse is also optimized to avoid overlap with the imaging volume (Frank et al. 1997; Yongbi et al. 1998). Finally, saturation of the imaging volume just before and/or after the labeling pulses is applied to minimize any residual label/control differences and as an initial step in the background suppression process described in Sect. 7.3.

The primary advantages of PASL relative to (p)CASL are low RF power deposition, shorter achievable TR, and that the inversion efficiency is high and consistent. Nevertheless, PASL's perfusion (t)SNR is fundamentally lower than that of pCASL, because of the shorter labeled bolus. In PASL, the bolus size is limited by the spatial coverage of the RF transmit coil, while in pCASL the bolus' temporal width is controlled by the duration of the labeling. The optimal thickness of the labeling slab in PASL is not simply "as large as possible" since several factors limit its dimensions. First, for FAIR, the width of the transition zone between inverted and uninverted blood at the edge of the labeled bolus is proportional to the thickness of the imaging slab. For all other PASL labeling methods, the width of this transition zone is proportional to the thickness of the labeling slab. For a large slab thickness, the transition zone becomes bigger, requiring a greater gap between the labeling and imaging slabs, which in turn increases arterial transit times and requires longer delays for the labeled blood to travel from the labeling location to the tissue. Therefore, increasing the PASL labeling slab thickness beyond a certain value does not lead to higher ASL SNR. Second, the RF transmit coil is limited in size, and the transmit RF field falls off with distance from its center. For accurate CBF quantification, the labeled bolus should consist of completely inverted blood, and to ensure this, the labeling slab needs to be limited to the region of relative homogeneity of the transmit RF field. Finally, if the labeling bolus extends beyond the homogeneous transmit RF region, any partially inverted blood will take additional time to clear from the labeling slab, requiring a longer TR before the next labeling pulse and thus lowering the temporal efficiency. Empirically, a 15–20 cm labeling slab thickness is a good compromise between these factors for most RF coils, but the bolus' exact temporal width will remain unknown. It should be noted that the width of the bolus will also vary among individuals. It is possible to control the labeling bolus width by means of the QUIPSS II (quantitative imaging of perfusion using single subtraction II) modification (Wong et al. 1998), in which a slab-selective saturation pulse that matches the labeling slab is used to remove the tail end of the labeled bolus (see Fig. 7.1b). This adaptation is necessary for quantification of CBF using PASL at a single delay time.

In both CASL and PASL, the label is applied to arterial blood that is proximal to the tissue of interest (Fig. 7.1a). This necessarily produces a transit delay, a delay required for the labeled blood to travel from the labeling location to the tissue. In order to minimize the influence of this transit time on the CBF estimation, a PLD is inserted into the pulse sequence to allow for the delivery of the label prior to image acquisition (Fig. 7.1b). In healthy human brains with normal flow, ATT can vary between 500 and 1900 ms depending on the labeling location and the tissue location in the brain, so a PLD equal to the longest ATT is sufficient to allow for complete delivery of the label. However, in the presence of vascular disease and in the deep white matter, the ATT can be longer than 2000 ms and therefore significantly longer than T_1 of blood. Thus, the use of a PLD that is longer than the ATT would result in very low SNR due to T_1 decay of the label. It should be mentioned that the ATT for pCASL is generally longer than for PASL, because the labeling in pCASL happens further upstream. The shorter ATT and bolus length in PASL allows higher temporal resolution, which is valuable in fMRI studies. The choice of PLD is a compromise, such that perfusion SNR is acceptable and that in the large majority of cases the ASL signal will accurately reflect CBF. However, low perfusion-weighted signal may reflect some combination of low CBF and unusually long ATT, and not solely low CBF. In many cases, long ATT can be identified by the presence of intraluminal signal in the same vascular distribution due to label remaining in the arteries. VSASL (Wong et al. 2006) was introduced specifically to address the transit delay problem. In VSASL, the labeling pulse is velocity-selective, and not spatially selective. The overall concept is based on the fact that arterial blood is decelerating, while tissue water and venous blood are not. This difference permits selective arterial labeling even within the imaging region, which minimizes the transit delay. Unfortunately, the current VSASL implementations have lower SNR than pCASL, which prevents their widespread adoption. It is worth mentioning that apart from the minimum achievable TR, the choice of labeling approach has little effect on the BOLD functional sensitivity.

7.3 Background Suppression

The perfusion signal is typically only ~1–2% of the equilibrium tissue signal. In order to provide adequate ASL SNR, low spatial resolution and signal averaging are typically employed. Using low spatial resolutions, the fluctuations in the signal are dominated not by thermal noise but come largely from physiological sources such as cardiac, respiratory, and subject motion. These fluctuations are proportional to the signal intensity in the raw images and can easily mask the modulation due to perfusion itself. Therefore, if it is possible to decrease the static tissue signal intensity without a proportional reduction in the perfusion signal, the perfusion tSNR can be improved substantially. A decrease of the signal intensity unmodulated by labeling can be accomplished using a combination of spatially selective saturation and inversion pulses applied after the labeling pulses. This process is known as background suppression (Dixon et al. 1991; Ye et al. 2000; Garcia et al. 2005). It is important to realize that while the longitudinal magnetization always decays with T_1 toward its equilibrium value, the *perfusion-weighted signal* decays with T_1 toward *zero*. The perfusion signal is not affected by a global inversion when it is applied to both the label and control conditions.

For CASL and pCASL, the background suppression inversion pulses should cover the area that is distal to the labeling plane, including the imaging area, while in PASL the background suppression inversion pulse should cover the labeling slab itself and the imaging volume. This ensures that labeled blood is fully inverted with each background suppression inversion pulse, regardless of whether it has flowed into the imaging region yet or not. There is a trade-off in the number of inversion pulses used for background suppression. The larger the number of inversion pulses, the more accurately static tissue can be suppressed over a wide range of tissue T_1 values. The trade-off is that each inversion pulse slightly reduces the measured ASL signal as well. The efficiency of the inversion pulses is high but not perfect and is typically ~95%, so each inversion pulse reduces the ASL signal by ~5%. Two inversion pulses can be employed for moderate tissue signal suppression, and four inversion pulses result in background suppression higher than 95% as demonstrated in Fig. 7.2. It is important to note that background suppression increases the RF power deposition, but unless the SAR limits are exceeded, it does not reduce the ASL temporal resolution.

Background suppression results in minimal static tissue magnetization at a selected point in time. Even though background suppression can be combined with any readout approach, its effectiveness differs across approaches. Background suppression is most effective for techniques where there is only one RF excitation following each label. This includes single-slice 2D imaging, single-shot 3D imaging, or 3D imaging segmented across TR periods (Vidorreta et al. 2013). For sequential multi-slice readouts, where each slice is acquired at a different time point, the effectiveness of background suppression varies between slices. For segmented 3D imaging, background suppression is especially important, as inconsistency between segments can result in ghosting artifacts that are large compared to the ASL signal if the static tissue signal is not suppressed.

Apart from increasing the perfusion tSNR and CBF sensitivity, background suppression also decreases the BOLD detection sensitivity as the latter depends on the background tissue signal. Fortunately, the decrease in BOLD sensitivity is significantly smaller than the decrease in tissue signal at least for 2D EPI readouts (Ghariq et al. 2014). Nevertheless, this sensitivity decrease has often hindered researchers interested in concurrent CBF and BOLD data to employ background suppression in their acquisitions. The background suppression influence on the BOLD sensitivity for 3D spin-echo readouts is difficult to separate from the effect of the readout, but also their lower static tissue signal leads to lower BOLD sensitivity.

7.4 Imaging Readouts

A wide range of readouts can be and has been used for ASL acquisitions. Each of the readouts has advantages and disadvantages, which favor its utilization for a specific application. Most generally, readouts are either single-shot or segmented. In single-shot approaches, an MR image is acquired very rapidly, i.e., within 100 ms. In segmented techniques, the image acquisition is slower—from several hundred milliseconds to minutes. The short acquisition time of single-shot readouts allows high temporal resolution and

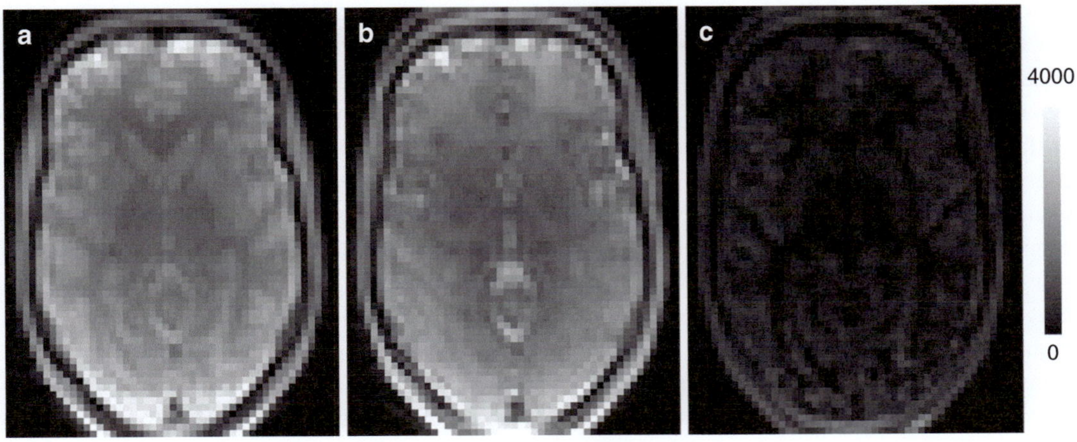

Fig. 7.2 (**a**) An axial slice through a 3D GRASE volume obtained without background suppression. (**b**) The corresponding slice from a 3D GRASE control volume acquired with 2 background suppression pulses scaled by a factor of 10 showing a different tissue contrast and moderate signal suppression. (**c**) The corresponding slice from a 3D GRASE control volume acquired with 4 background suppression pulses scaled by a factor of 10 demonstrating more than 95% brain tissue suppression

freezes out motion and physiological fluctuations that can corrupt segmented MR images. This makes single-shot approaches preferred for fMRI studies. The disadvantage of single-shot compared to segmented readouts is the increased number of artifacts such as signal dropout, image distortions, and blurring. Another distinction between imaging approaches is whether they are 2D or 3D. In 3D techniques, data from the whole imaging volume is collected every time, whereas in 2D readouts the volume is split into multiple 2D slices. Conventionally, the 2D slices are sequentially acquired. The 2D SMS approach enables the simultaneous acquisition of multiple 2D slices, increasing the temporal efficiency of the readout. The most commonly used readout trajectories in 2D are rectilinear for segmented approaches and EPI and spiral for single-shot techniques. In 3D, these trajectories are simply repeated, so stacks of EPIs or spirals are usually employed. It is worth mentioning that due to timing constraints most single-shot readouts are 2D and most 3D readouts are segmented. However, 2D segmented (such as TFL) and 3D single-shot readouts are also used. Parallel imaging allows shortening the readout duration through data undersampling, increasing the temporal efficiency and reducing image artifacts due to main magnetic field inhomogeneities. The disadvantage of parallel imaging is that it decreases SNR, which is why segmentation is often used in ASL when the readout duration needs to be shortened, instead. Nevertheless, segmentation severely penalizes the temporal efficiency and can lead to artifacts, which is why it should be used with caution. Another distinction between acquisition techniques is whether or not they utilize spin echoes. Those that use spin echoes are called spin-echo (SE) approaches and those that do not – gradient echo (GRE) techniques. GRE techniques are more time-efficient but suffer more from artifacts caused by main magnetic field inhomogeneities compared to SE techniques. Finally, 2D single-shot readouts can be repeated several times with different TEs, leading to multi-echo methods.

For clinical CBF mapping, 3D SE readouts, such as 3D turbo spin echo (TSE), stack of spirals (SoS), and 3D gradient and spin echo (GRASE), have been recommended due to their optimal combination with background suppression and relative insensitivity to main magnetic field inhomogeneities (Alsop et al. 2015). The high RF power deposition of 3D SE techniques makes them impractical at fields above 3 T, where GRE approaches are preferred. An example would be 2D SMS TFL (Wang et al. 2015). For functional CBF mapping at any field strength, high temporal resolution is key, and therefore in this case single-shot methods are favored. 2D GRE EPI and 2D GRE spirals are popular ASL fMRI techniques also due to the possibility to concurrently acquire CBF and BOLD data, especially in their multi-echo versions. The recent growth of SMS EPI approaches has not missed the ASL domain. This is due to their increased efficiency and better combination with background suppression than conventional 2D readouts. Finally, 3D EPI (Poser et al. 2010) may gain popularity in the future due to its very low power deposition, homogeneous PLD and SNR across slices, high temporal efficiency, and compatibility with background suppression.

3D SE readouts provide nearly optimal SNR for measurement of the ASL magnetization by striking a balance between the susceptibility insensitivity of pure SE methods and the temporal efficiency of EPI or spiral acquisitions. The main weakness of 3D SE approaches is that with long spin-echo trains T_2-related signal modulation across echoes can result in through-plane blurring. In case partial brain coverage or thicker slices for whole-brain coverage are not acceptable, the number of spin echoes per TR needs to be reduced using either parallel imaging or segmentation. Typically, the segmented option was chosen because until recently no 3D SE techniques with efficient (low SNR loss) parallel imaging acceleration were available. Segmented approaches require data consistency between excitations, so background suppression is essential to prevent motion-related artifacts from dominating the ASL signal. To achieve the most accurate "control-label difference," the label and control conditions for a given shot are acquired sequentially in time, i.e., the label/control modulation is the inner-most loop of the acquisition.

The motion insensitivity of the 3D SoS acquisition is improved through the natural oversampling at the center of k-space. However, 3D SoS is also susceptible to in-plane blurring due to off-resonance offsets. In contrast, 3D GRASE typically does not oversample k-space, and resonance offsets result in in-plane distortion rather than blurring. The main disadvantage of segmented 3D SE approaches is the poor temporal resolution, where the respective techniques with parallel imaging acceleration (undersampling) in one (Vidorreta et al. 2017), two (Ivanov et al. 2017b; Boland et al. 2016), and three dimensions (Chang et al. 2017) prove valuable. With modern receive coil arrays, the more spatial dimensions the acceleration is spread over, the smaller the SNR penalty accompanying parallel imaging will be. Currently, reconstructions using 1D undersampling in 3D SoS or 1D/2D undersampling for 3D GRASE can be performed online at the scanner, while the reconstruction in the remaining cases needs to be done offline. This favors the utilization of those with immediate reconstruction especially for clinical and functional CBF imaging. One example utilizing 3D GRASE with 2D acceleration and CAIPIRINHA can be seen in Fig. 7.3.

TFL-based readouts exhibit reduced sensitivity to T_2* effects, similar to the SE approaches. Nevertheless, the reduced resonance offset (and importantly BOLD) sensitivity does not come from refocusing as in SE techniques, but from the use of a very short TE. The high phase-encoding bandwidth, along with the segmented readout,

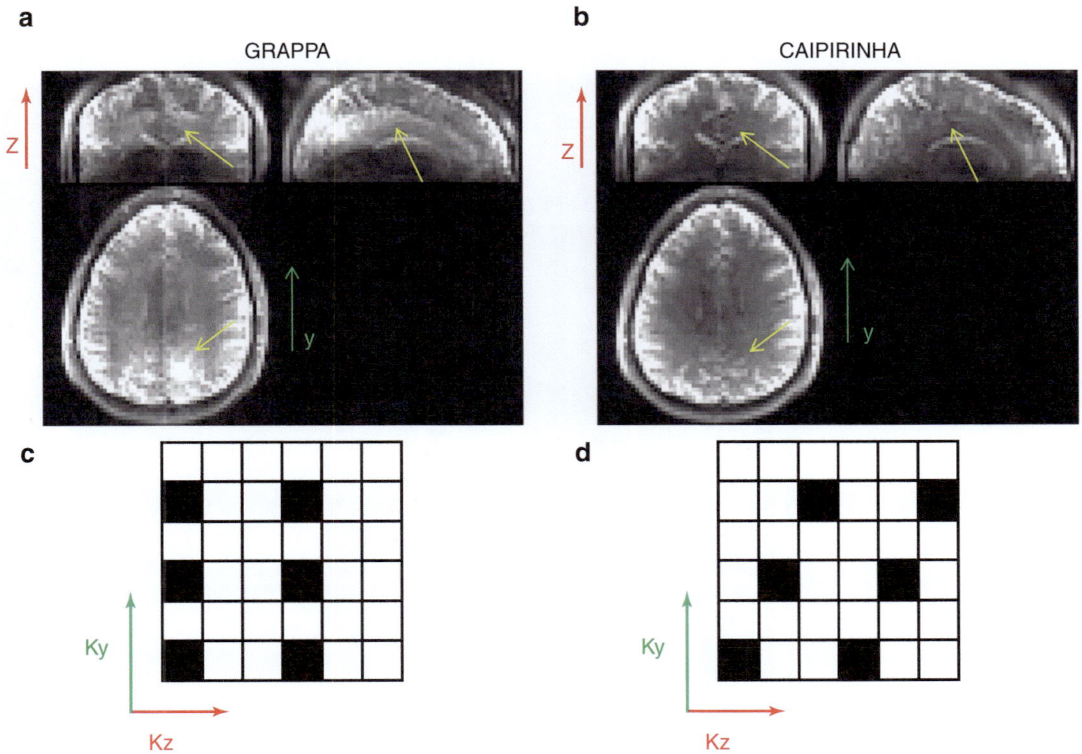

Fig. 7.3 Example single-shot 3D GRASE images (scaled identically) acquired with 2 × 3 acceleration and the corresponding 2D sampling units. The yellow arrows indicate the locations where residual alias can be seen in the images reconstructed with GRAPPA in **a**, but not in **b**. The CAIPIRINHA images are free from these artifacts, despite the high total acceleration factor employed. The red and green arrows show the phase-encoding (y) and partition-encoding (z) directions. The sampling unit corresponding to GRAPPA is depicted in **c**, whereas that used in CAIPIRINHA (with a z-shift of 1) in **d**

ensures the absence of geometrical distortions and dropouts in areas affected by susceptibility gradients. The main disadvantages of TFL readouts are the decreased temporal efficiency and increased physiological noise compared to EPI. SMS and background suppression have been proposed to tackle these TFL weaknesses, respectively. 3D SoS also employs a short TE, whereas the echo times in 3D GRASE are comparable to the ones used in EPI. This makes 3D GRASE the ASL readout approach with highest BOLD sensitivity after GRE EPI. The key difference to EPI comes from the fact that SE BOLD, as obtained using 3D GRASE, is much weaker than the GRE BOLD measured with EPI.

2D EPI is well-suited for high temporal resolution, simultaneous functional CBF, and BOLD mapping, especially in the low spatial resolution regime. The simultaneous multi-slice 2D EPI significantly increases the brain coverage with only a slight SNR penalty (Ivanov et al. 2017a). 3D EPI readouts (Poser et al. 2010) also allow simultaneous CBF and BOLD measurements (Gai et al. 2011). 3D EPI can be combined with background suppression and has been successfully implemented at 7 T (Hall et al. 2010; Ivanov et al. 2016) because of their low-power deposition. 3D EPI sensitivity is higher than that of 2D EPI in the thermal-noise-dominated regime of high spatial resolutions (Fig. 7.4), but they are comparable in the physiological-noise-dominated regime (Poser et al. 2010; Huber et al. 2018). The advantage of 3D EPI over 2D EPI for ASL lies in the improved temporal efficiency, since in the former a longer readout (and a larger brain coverage) with optimal PLD is possible. CBF sensitivity improvements without loss of temporal resolution and small BOLD sensitivity reduction may be obtained by the utilization of background suppression in 3D EPI such as in 3D EPI combined with the double-acquisition background-suppressed (DABS) FAIR (Wesolowski et al. 2009).

For studies focusing solely on perfusion, acquisition at shorter TE is beneficial as it increases the perfusion-weighted signal and suppresses the susceptibility contamination of CBF values (St Lawrence and Wang 2005). Readouts that intrinsically allow this include 2D spiral and

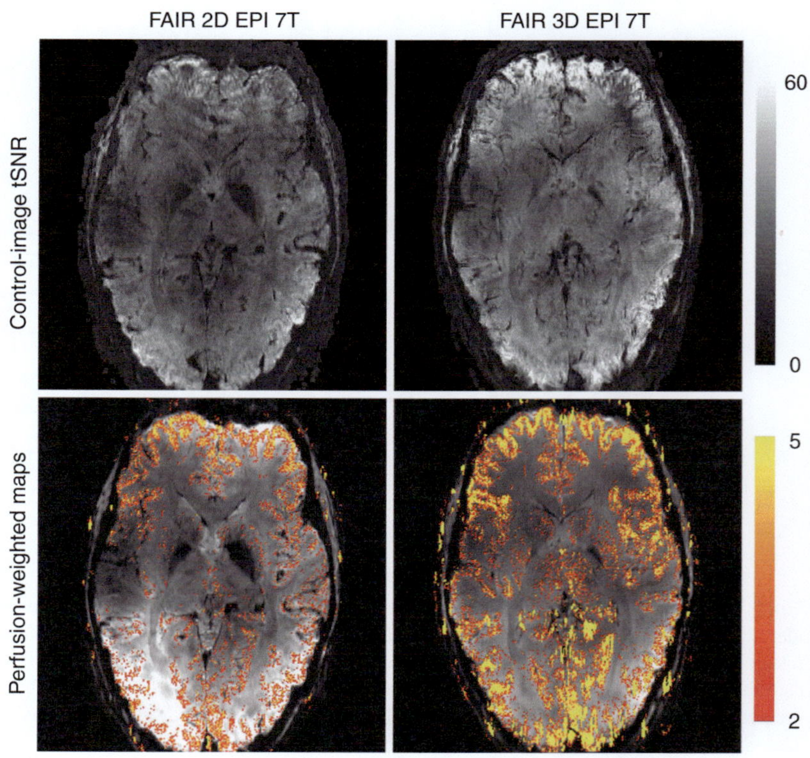

Fig. 7.4 Identically scaled control tSNR and perfusion-weighted maps from FAIR 2D EPI (left) and FAIR 3D EPI (right) acquired using the same scanning time

2D TFL. They prove particularly helpful for high-resolution and white matter CBF imaging, where the longer minimum TE of EPI presents a major drawback. The application of parallel imaging and/or partial Fourier allows keeping the TE and readout duration in EPI short. If a study is interested in measuring BOLD in addition to CBF, EPI will still be a viable option, especially compared to TFL as the latter cannot simultaneously acquire CBF and GRE BOLD images without further ado. Dual-echo spiral and EPI readouts offer the largest flexibility when it comes to concurrent measurements of perfusion and BOLD. In the case of a single-echo approach, a compromise between CBF and BOLD sensitivities typically needs to be made. Dual-echo is beneficial when the second TE is close to the optimal TE for BOLD imaging at the employed field strength, while the first TE is as short as possible.

When comparing the CBF and BOLD sensitivity of different readouts, it is important to keep in mind that different aspects might contribute to the particular CBF and BOLD sensitivities. For instance, background suppression increases the CBF sensitivity and reduces BOLD sensitivity. Longer TE raises BOLD sensitivity and decreases CBF sensitivity. SE readouts boost the CBF sensitivity and diminish the BOLD sensitivity. Readouts that combine several of the features increasing CBF sensitivity like 3D SE SoS will outperform 2D GRE EPI in that aspect, but the latter will be superior in terms of BOLD sensitivity. Due to these conflicting requirements for the BOLD and CBF sensitivities, the combination of a background-suppressed single-shot 3D GRASE readout for the CBF and 2D EPI for BOLD imaging has been proposed (Fernandez-Seara et al. 2016). The disadvantage of this approach is the reduced temporal resolution as the TR needs to accommodate both readouts.

7.5 High Magnetic Fields

Performing ASL at ultrahigh field (UHF; i.e., 7 T and higher) offers several advantages (Ivanov et al. 2017a; Gardener et al. 2009). The image SNR increases with field strength (Norris 2003; Pohmann et al. 2016), which, for instance, improves perfusion measurements in the white matter (Gardener and Jezzard 2015). In addition, the increased T_1 values at higher fields (Rooney et al. 2007; Wright et al. 2008) reduce the label decay during the PLD and image acquisition, resulting in higher perfusion SNR. These advantages allow increasing the brain coverage and/or using longer PLD to avoid vascular artifacts due to incomplete transfer of the labeled blood to the local tissue. The advantages of UHF for BOLD imaging, demonstrated in numerous studies (e.g., (Uludag et al. 2009; van der Zwaag et al. 2009; Donahue et al. 2011), and references therein), render simultaneous CBF and BOLD imaging using ASL at UHF particularly attractive.

Despite the aforementioned gains, UHF ASL has not found widespread use in humans due to significant technical challenges. First, the spatial homogeneity and efficiency of the labeling are significantly degraded at UHF due to main magnetic field inhomogeneities and transmit RF field inhomogeneities (Teeuwisse et al. 2010; Luh et al. 2013). Second, SAR constraints not only make SE approaches impractical but also limit the utilization of pCASL and background suppression. As a consequence, to remain within SAR limits, many UHF ASL implementations employed poor temporal resolutions that are not compatible with the requirements of adequately sampling the fMRI hemodynamic response (Zuo et al. 2013; Luh et al. 2013; Ghariq et al. 2012; Bause et al. 2016; Zimmer et al. 2016). For example, the increased power deposition at 7 T leads to doubling of the minimum achievable TR of pCASL at 3 T, even with low flip-angle readouts (Zuo et al. 2013; Wang et al. 2015). Third, resolution loss along the phase-encoding direction and blurring in EPI can be observed for readout lengths typically used at lower fields due to the faster T_2* decay at UHF (Farzaneh et al. 1990; de Zwart et al. 2006). Parallel imaging addresses some of these issues by shortening the EPI readout and reducing the effective echo spacing. Since parallel imaging involves data undersampling, it also leads to decreases in image SNR and to a smaller extent tSNR (de Zwart et al.

2006), especially in the center of the brain, where the g-factor penalty is largest.

A recent study by Ivanov and colleagues demonstrated that a 7 T PASL EPI technique using optimized TR FOCI inversion pulses and dielectric pads outperformed 3 T ASL EPI for all resolutions and labeling schemes investigated, when parallel imaging was used (Ivanov et al. 2017c). In contrast, without parallel imaging, 3 T ASL superseded 7 T PASL in terms of perfusion tSNR, because of the reduced labeling efficiency and increased physiological noise at UHF. These results indicate that the image SNR increase (when parallel imaging is used) rather than the longer T_1s at 7 T plays the decisive role for the advantages of 7 T ASL with respect to 3 T ASL. It is worth mentioning that the application of dielectric pads and optimized TR FOCI inversion pulses significantly improved the labeling efficiency at 7 T compared to the case without them. Overall, the optimized 7 T PASL approach offered higher CBF and BOLD sensitivity than the examined 3 T techniques. In particular, the cross-field functional ASL comparison of Ivanov et al. entailed 8.5-min visual stimulation experiments performed at each of the following in-plane resolutions: 1.5, 2.0, 2.5, and 3.0 mm. The stimulation protocol consisted of an initial rest period (gray screen) of 30 s and 8 blocks each presenting 25-s 8 Hz-flickering-checkboard hemifield stimulation followed by 35-s rest. The results from the activated hemisphere presented in Fig. 7.5 demonstrate the substantially smaller sensitivity of CBF vs. BOLD at both field strengths. Further, a reduction of the significantly activated CBF cortical area with increasing resolution due to SNR decrease can be seen at both fields. Finally, the significantly activated areas for both CBF and BOLD were larger at 7 T than at 3 T for all resolutions underscoring the improved functional sensitivity at higher field (Fig. 7.5).

The improved image SNR at 7 T compared to 1.5 and 3 T can also be utilized to image the

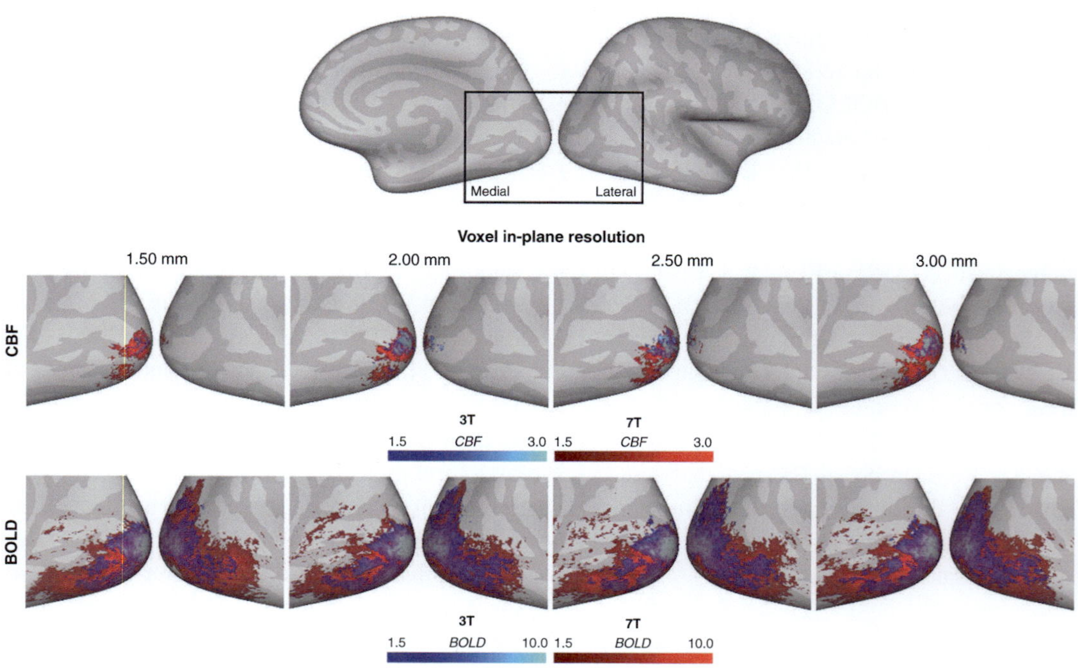

Fig. 7.5 CBF and BOLD activations. Significant CBF and BOLD activation for the different in-plane resolutions: results from 3 T FAIR are overlaid on the 7 T FAIR ones to facilitate across-field-strength comparison. The top row shows the CBF activation and the bottom row the BOLD activation. The Z-values are color-coded from dark to light blue for 3 T FAIR and from dark to light red for 7 T FAIR. A different maximum value was chosen for CBF and BOLD (i.e., 3.0 and 10.0, respectively) to better suit their specific dynamic ranges

human brain at higher spatial resolution. Pfeuffer and colleagues demonstrated at 7 T in humans that functional CBF mapping has superior spatial specificity than the typically employed GRE BOLD signal (Pfeuffer et al. 2002). Only a few studies have shown CBF maps with in-plane resolution below 1.5 mm (Zuo et al. 2013; Pfeuffer et al. 2002; Duong et al. 2002). It is worth noting that these studies utilized diverse readout approaches—SE EPI, GRE EPI, and TFL—but were all performed at 7 T, indicating its capability for high-resolution CBF imaging.

7.6 Summary

As low SNR has been the main issue in ASL, many of the approaches devised and described above aim to boost the perfusion sensitivity. Background suppression and short TE are parameters that will ensure higher CBF sensitivity irrespective of the readout approach chosen. Unfortunately, exactly they also cause a decreased BOLD sensitivity. Therefore, multi-echo EPI or spiral readouts offer a good compromise between CBF and BOLD sensitivity when their concurrent measurement is required. The labeling approach (duration) and PLD also have a major influence on the ASL's SNR. Longer labeled bolus increases ASL's SNR, while longer PLD decreases it. Often a compromise for their combined duration needs to be made to avoid unnecessary increase in TR and thereby decrease of temporal resolution. This is just an example of the recurring situation where the researcher needs to trade SNR for temporal resolution and/or artifact reduction. Another aforementioned case of this trade-off is segmentation in 3D SE acquisitions. Recently, advanced parallel imaging strategies that enable substantial acquisition acceleration with minor SNR penalties, irrespective of the readout, have been proposed, and these will become more widely used in the future. Both clinical and functional ASL will largely benefit from these technologies as they allow rapid, accurate, and reliable measurements of perfusion. Finally, ultrahigh magnetic fields will realize their full potential for CBF sensitivity increases, once the remaining challenges related to power deposition and field inhomogeneities are tackled by developments in hardware and parallel transmission technologies.

Acknowledgments The authors would like to thank Kamil Uludag, Benedikt Poser, Laurentius Huber, Anna Gardumi, Sriranga Kashyap, Roy Haast, Josef Pfeuffer, Denizhan Kurban and Jordi Kleinloog for their help and support with ASL developments and/or proofreading this work.

References

Aguirre GK, Detre JA, Zarahn E, Alsop DC (2002) Experimental design and the relative sensitivity of BOLD and perfusion fMRI. NeuroImage 15(3):488–500. https://doi.org/10.1006/nimg.2001.0990

Alsop DC, Detre JA (1998) Multisection cerebral blood flow MR imaging with continuous arterial spin labeling. Radiology 208(2):410–416. https://doi.org/10.1148/radiology.208.2.9680569

Alsop DC, Detre JA, Golay X, Gunther M, Hendrikse J, Hernandez-Garcia L et al (2015) Recommended implementation of arterial spin-labeled perfusion MRI for clinical applications: a consensus of the ISMRM perfusion study group and the European consortium for ASL in dementia. Magn Reson Med 73(1):102–116. https://doi.org/10.1002/mrm.25197

Aslan S, Xu F, Wang PL, Uh J, Yezhuvath US, van Osch M et al (2010) Estimation of labeling efficiency in pseudocontinuous arterial spin labeling. Magn Reson Med 63(3):765–771. https://doi.org/10.1002/mrm.22245

Bause J, Ehses P, Mirkes C, Shajan G, Scheffler K, Pohmann R (2016) Quantitative and functional pulsed arterial spin labeling in the human brain at 9.4 T. Magn Reson Med 75(3):1054–1063. https://doi.org/10.1002/mrm.25671

Blicher JU, Stagg CJ, O'Shea J, Ostergaard L, MacIntosh BJ, Johansen-Berg H et al (2012) Visualization of altered neurovascular coupling in chronic stroke patients using multimodal functional MRI. J Cereb Blood Flow Metab 32(11):2044–2054. https://doi.org/10.1038/jcbfm.2012.105

Bokkers RP, van der Worp HB, Mali WP, Hendrikse J (2009) Noninvasive MR imaging of cerebral perfusion in patients with a carotid artery stenosis. Neurology 73(11):869–875. https://doi.org/10.1212/WNL.0b013e3181b7840c

Boland M, Stirnberg R, Stöcker T (2016) CAIPIRINHA-accelerated 3D GRASE ASL for brain perfusion imaging: A comparison with segmented and GRAPPA-accelerated acquisitions. Proceedings of the 33rd Annual meeting of the ESMRMB2016. p. 63

Bulte DP, Kelly M, Germuska M, Xie J, Chappell MA, Okell TW et al (2012) Quantitative measurement of cerebral physiology using respiratory-calibrated

MRI. NeuroImage 60(1):582–591. https://doi.org/10.1016/j.neuroimage.2011.12.017

Buxton RB, Griffeth VE, Simon AB, Moradi F, Shmuel A (2014) Variability of the coupling of blood flow and oxygen metabolism responses in the brain: a problem for interpreting BOLD studies but potentially a new window on the underlying neural activity. Front Neurosci 8:139. https://doi.org/10.3389/fnins.2014.00139

Cavusoglu M, Bartels A, Yesilyurt B, Uludag K (2012) Retinotopic maps and hemodynamic delays in the human visual cortex measured using arterial spin labeling. NeuroImage 59(4):4044–4054. https://doi.org/10.1016/j.neuroimage.2011.10.056

Chang YV, Vidorreta M, Wang Z, Detre JA (2017) 3D-accelerated, stack-of-spirals acquisitions and reconstruction of arterial spin labeling MRI. Magn Reson Med 78(4):1405–1419. https://doi.org/10.1002/mrm.26549

Dai W, Robson PM, Shankaranarayanan A, Alsop DC (2012) Reduced resolution transit delay prescan for quantitative continuous arterial spin labeling perfusion imaging. Magn Reson Med 67(5):1252–1265. https://doi.org/10.1002/mrm.23103

de Zwart JA, van Gelderen P, Golay X, Ikonomidou VN, Duyn JH (2006) Accelerated parallel imaging for functional imaging of the human brain. NMR Biomed 19(3):342–351. https://doi.org/10.1002/nbm.1043

Detre JA, Wang J (2002) Technical aspects and utility of fMRI using BOLD and ASL. Clin Neurophysiol 113(5):621–634

Detre JA, Leigh JS, Williams DS, Koretsky AP (1992) Perfusion imaging. Magn Reson Med 23(1):37–45

Detre JA, Zhang W, Roberts DA, Silva AC, Williams DS, Grandis DJ et al (1994) Tissue specific perfusion imaging using arterial spin labeling. NMR Biomed 7(1–2):75–82

Detre JA, Alsop DC, Vives LR, Maccotta L, Teener JW, Raps EC (1998) Noninvasive MRI evaluation of cerebral blood flow in cerebrovascular disease. Neurology 50(3):633–641

Dixon WT, Sardashti M, Castillo M, Stomp GP (1991) Multiple inversion recovery reduces static tissue signal in angiograms. Magn Reson Med 18(2):257–268

Donahue MJ, Near J, Blicher JU, Jezzard P (2010) Baseline GABA concentration and fMRI response. NeuroImage 53(2):392–398. https://doi.org/10.1016/j.neuroimage.2010.07.017

Donahue MJ, Hoogduin H, van Zijl PC, Jezzard P, Luijten PR, Hendrikse J (2011) Blood oxygenation level-dependent (BOLD) total and extravascular signal changes and DeltaR2∗ in human visual cortex at 1.5, 3.0 and 7.0 T. NMR Biomed 24(1):25–34. https://doi.org/10.1002/nbm.1552

Donahue MJ, Strother MK, Hendrikse J (2012) Novel MRI approaches for assessing cerebral hemodynamics in ischemic cerebrovascular disease. Stroke 43(3):903–915. https://doi.org/10.1161/STROKEAHA.111.635995

Donahue MJ, Hussey E, Rane S, Wilson T, van Osch M, Hartkamp N et al (2014) Vessel-encoded arterial spin labeling (VE-ASL) reveals elevated flow territory asymmetry in older adults with substandard verbal memory performance. J Magn Reson Imaging 39(2):377–386. https://doi.org/10.1002/jmri.24150

Duong TQ, Kim DS, Ugurbil K, Kim SG (2001) Localized cerebral blood flow response at submillimeter columnar resolution. Proc Natl Acad Sci U S A 98(19):10904–10909. https://doi.org/10.1073/pnas.191101098

Duong TQ, Yacoub E, Adriany G, Hu X, Ugurbil K, Vaughan JT et al (2002) High-resolution, spin-echo BOLD, and CBF fMRI at 4 and 7 T. Magn Reson Med 48(4):589–593

Edelman RR, Chen Q (1998) EPISTAR MRI: multislice mapping of cerebral blood flow. Magn Reson Med 40(6):800–805

Farzaneh F, Riederer SJ, Pelc NJ (1990) Analysis of T2 limitations and off-resonance effects on spatial resolution and artifacts in echo-planar imaging. Magn Reson Med 14(1):123–139

Feinberg DA, Beckett A, Chen L (2013) Arterial spin labeling with simultaneous multi-slice echo planar imaging. Magn Reson Med 70(6):1500–1506. https://doi.org/10.1002/mrm.24994

Fernandez-Seara MA, Rodgers ZB, Englund EK, Wehrli FW (2016) Calibrated bold fMRI with an optimized ASL-BOLD dual-acquisition sequence. NeuroImage 142:474–482. https://doi.org/10.1016/j.neuroimage.2016.08.007

Frank LR, Wong EC, Buxton RB (1997) Slice profile effects in adiabatic inversion: application to multislice perfusion imaging. Magn Reson Med 38(4):558–564

Gai ND, Talagala SL, Butman JA (2011) Whole-brain cerebral blood flow mapping using 3D echo planar imaging and pulsed arterial tagging. J Magn Reson Imaging 33(2):287–295. https://doi.org/10.1002/jmri.22437

Garcia DM, Duhamel G, Alsop DC (2005) Efficiency of inversion pulses for background suppressed arterial spin labeling. Magn Reson Med 54(2):366–372. https://doi.org/10.1002/mrm.20556

Gardener AG, Jezzard P (2015) Investigating white matter perfusion using optimal sampling strategy arterial spin labeling at 7 Tesla. Magn Reson Med 73(6):2243–2248. https://doi.org/10.1002/mrm.25333

Gardener AG, Gowland PA, Francis ST (2009) Implementation of quantitative perfusion imaging using pulsed arterial spin labeling at ultra-high field. Magn Reson Med 61(4):874–882. https://doi.org/10.1002/mrm.21796

Ghariq E, Teeuwisse WM, Webb AG, van Osch MJ (2012) Feasibility of pseudocontinuous arterial spin labeling at 7 T with whole-brain coverage. MAGMA 25(2):83–93. https://doi.org/10.1007/s10334-011-0297-0

Ghariq E, Chappell MA, Schmid S, Teeuwisse WM, van Osch MJ (2014) Effects of background suppression on the sensitivity of dual-echo arterial spin labeling MRI for BOLD and CBF signal changes.

NeuroImage 103:316–322. https://doi.org/10.1016/j.neuroimage.2014.09.051

Golay X, Petersen ET, Hui F (2005) Pulsed star labeling of arterial regions (PULSAR): a robust regional perfusion technique for high field imaging. Magn Reson Med 53(1):15–21. https://doi.org/10.1002/mrm.20338

Hall EL, Gowland P, Francis ST (eds) (2010) 3D-EPI ASL at ultra high field. Joint annual meeting ISMRM-ESMRMB. ISMRM, Stockholm, Sweden

Havlicek M, Roebroeck A, Friston K, Gardumi A, Ivanov D, Uludag K (2015) Physiologically informed dynamic causal modeling of fMRI data. NeuroImage 122:355–372. https://doi.org/10.1016/j.neuroimage.2015.07.078

Hendrikse J, van der Zwan A, Ramos LM, van Osch MJ, Golay X, Tulleken CA et al (2005) Altered flow territories after extracranial-intracranial bypass surgery. Neurosurgery 57(3):486–494; discussion-94

Hendrikse J, Petersen ET, van Laar PJ, Golay X (2008) Cerebral border zones between distal end branches of intracranial arteries: MR imaging. Radiology 246(2):572–580. https://doi.org/10.1148/radiol.2461062100

Huber L, Ivanov D, Handwerker DA, Marrett S, Guidi M, Uludag K et al (2018) Techniques for blood volume fMRI with VASO: from low-resolution mapping towards sub-millimeter layer-dependent applications. NeuroImage 164:131–143. https://doi.org/10.1016/j.neuroimage.2016.11.039

Ivanov D, Poser BA, Kashyap S, Gardumi A, Huber L, Uludag K (2016) Sub-millimeter human brain perfusion maps using arterial spin labelling at 3 and 7 T. ISMRM Workshop on Ultra High Field MRI2016. p. 14

Ivanov D, Poser BA, Huber L, Pfeuffer J, Uludag K (2017a) Optimization of simultaneous multislice EPI for concurrent functional perfusion and BOLD signal measurements at 7T. Magn Reson Med 78(1):121–129. https://doi.org/10.1002/mrm.26351

Ivanov D, Pfeuffer J, Gardumi A, Uludag K, Poser BA (2017b) 2D CAIPIRINHA improves accelerated 3D GRASE ASL. Proceedings of the 25th Annual Meeting of the ISMRM2017. p. 3630

Ivanov D, Gardumi A, Haast RAM, Pfeuffer J, Poser BA, Uludag K (2017c) Comparison of 3T and 7T ASL techniques for concurrent functional perfusion and BOLD studies. NeuroImage 156:363–376. https://doi.org/10.1016/j.neuroimage.2017.05.038

Kim SG (1995) Quantification of relative cerebral blood flow change by flow-sensitive alternating inversion recovery (FAIR) technique: application to functional mapping. Magn Reson Med 34(3):293–301

Kim T, Shin W, Zhao T, Beall EB, Lowe MJ, Bae KT (2013) Whole brain perfusion measurements using arterial spin labeling with multiband acquisition. Magn Reson Med 70(6):1653–1661. https://doi.org/10.1002/mrm.24880

Krieger SN, Gauthier CJ, Ivanov D, Huber L, Roggenhofer E, Sehm B et al (2014) Regional reproducibility of calibrated BOLD functional MRI: implications for the study of cognition and plasticity. NeuroImage 101:8–20. https://doi.org/10.1016/j.neuroimage.2014.06.072

Liu TT, Wong EC, Frank LR, Buxton RB (2002) Analysis and design of perfusion-based event-related fMRI experiments. NeuroImage 16(1):269–282. https://doi.org/10.1006/nimg.2001.1038

Lu H, Donahue MJ, van Zijl PC (2006) Detrimental effects of BOLD signal in arterial spin labeling fMRI at high field strength. Magn Reson Med 56(3):546–552. https://doi.org/10.1002/mrm.20976

Luh WM, Talagala SL, Li TQ, Bandettini PA (2013) Pseudo-continuous arterial spin labeling at 7 T for human brain: estimation and correction for off-resonance effects using a Prescan. Magn Reson Med 69(2):402–410. https://doi.org/10.1002/mrm.24266

Norris DG (2003) High field human imaging. J Magn Reson Imaging 18(5):519–529. https://doi.org/10.1002/jmri.10390

Petersen ET, Mouridsen K, Golay X, all named co-authors of the Qt-rs (2010) The QUASAR reproducibility study, part II: results from a multi-center arterial spin labeling test-retest study. NeuroImage 49(1):104–113. https://doi.org/10.1016/j.neuroimage.2009.07.068

Pfeuffer J, Adriany G, Shmuel A, Yacoub E, Van De Moortele PF, Hu X et al (2002) Perfusion-based high-resolution functional imaging in the human brain at 7 Tesla. Magn Reson Med 47(5):903–911. https://doi.org/10.1002/mrm.10154

Pohmann R, Speck O, Scheffler K (2016) Signal-to-noise ratio and MR tissue parameters in human brain imaging at 3, 7, and 9.4 Tesla using current receive coil arrays. Magn Reson Med 75(2):801–809. https://doi.org/10.1002/mrm.25677

Poser BA, Koopmans PJ, Witzel T, Wald LL, Barth M (2010) Three dimensional echo-planar imaging at 7 Tesla. NeuroImage 51(1):261–266

Raichle ME (1998) Behind the scenes of functional brain imaging: a historical and physiological perspective. Proc Natl Acad Sci U S A 95(3):765–772

Rooney WD, Johnson G, Li X, Cohen ER, Kim SG, Ugurbil K et al (2007) Magnetic field and tissue dependencies of human brain longitudinal 1H2O relaxation in vivo. Magn Reson Med 57(2):308–318. https://doi.org/10.1002/mrm.21122

St Lawrence KS, Wang J (2005) Effects of the apparent transverse relaxation time on cerebral blood flow measurements obtained by arterial spin labeling. Magn Reson Med 53(2):425–433. https://doi.org/10.1002/mrm.20364

Teeuwisse WM, Webb AG, van Osch MJR (2010) Arterial spin labeling at ultra-high field: all that glitters is not gold. Int J Imag Syst Tech 20(1):62–70. https://doi.org/10.1002/ima.20218

Tjandra T, Brooks JC, Figueiredo P, Wise R, Matthews PM, Tracey I (2005) Quantitative assessment of the reproducibility of functional activation measured with BOLD and MR perfusion imaging: implications for clinical trial design. NeuroImage 27(2):393–401. https://doi.org/10.1016/j.neuroimage.2005.04.021

Trampel R, Mildner T, Goerke U, Schaefer A, Driesel W, Norris DG (2002) Continuous arterial spin labeling using a local magnetic field gradient coil. Magn Reson Med 48(3):543–546. https://doi.org/10.1002/mrm.10228

Uludag K, Muller-Bierl B, Ugurbil K (2009) An integrative model for neuronal activity-induced signal changes for gradient and spin echo functional imaging. NeuroImage 48(1):150–165. https://doi.org/10.1016/j.neuroimage.2009.05.051

van der Zwaag W, Francis S, Head K, Peters A, Gowland P, Morris P et al (2009) fMRI at 1.5, 3 and 7 T: characterising BOLD signal changes. NeuroImage 47(4):1425–1434. https://doi.org/10.1016/j.neuroimage.2009.05.015

Vidorreta M, Wang Z, Rodriguez I, Pastor MA, Detre JA, Fernandez-Seara MA (2013) Comparison of 2D and 3D single-shot ASL perfusion fMRI sequences. NeuroImage 66:662–671. https://doi.org/10.1016/j.neuroimage.2012.10.087

Vidorreta M, Wang Z, Chang YV, Wolk DA, Fernandez-Seara MA, Detre JA (2017) Whole-brain background-suppressed pCASL MRI with 1D-accelerated 3D RARE stack-of-spirals readout. PLoS One 12(8):e0183762. https://doi.org/10.1371/journal.pone.0183762

Wang Y, Moeller S, Li X, Vu AT, Krasileva K, Ugurbil K et al (2015) Simultaneous multi-slice Turbo-FLASH imaging with CAIPIRINHA for whole brain distortion-free pseudo-continuous arterial spin labeling at 3 and 7T. NeuroImage 113:279–288. https://doi.org/10.1016/j.neuroimage.2015.03.060

Wesolowski R, Gowland P, Francis ST (2009) Double acquisition background suppressed (DABS) FAIR at 3 T and 7 T: advantages for simultaneous BOLD and CBF acquisition. Proceedings of the 17th Annual Meeting of the ISMRM2009. p. 1526

Williams DS, Detre JA, Leigh JS, Koretsky AP (1992) Magnetic resonance imaging of perfusion using spin inversion of arterial water. Proc Natl Acad Sci U S A 89(1):212–216

Wong EC, Buxton RB, Frank LR (1997) Implementation of quantitative perfusion imaging techniques for functional brain mapping using pulsed arterial spin labeling. NMR Biomed 10(4–5):237–249

Wong EC, Buxton RB, Frank LR (1998) Quantitative imaging of perfusion using a single subtraction (QUIPSS and QUIPSS II). Magn Reson Med 39(5):702–708

Wong EC, Cronin M, Wu WC, Inglis B, Frank LR, Liu TT (2006) Velocity-selective arterial spin labeling. Magn Reson Med 55(6):1334–1341. https://doi.org/10.1002/mrm.20906

Wright PJ, Mougin OE, Totman JJ, Peters AM, Brookes MJ, Coxon R et al (2008) Water proton T1 measurements in brain tissue at 7, 3, and 1.5 T using IR-EPI, IR-TSE, and MPRAGE: results and optimization. MAGMA 21(1–2):121–130. https://doi.org/10.1007/s10334-008-0104-8

Ye FQ, Frank JA, Weinberger DR, McLaughlin AC (2000) Noise reduction in 3D perfusion imaging by attenuating the static signal in arterial spin tagging (ASSIST). Magn Reson Med 44(1):92–100

Yongbi MN, Branch CA, Helpern JA (1998) Perfusion imaging using FOCI RF pulses. Magn Reson Med 40(6):938–943

Zhang W, Silva AC, Williams DS, Koretsky AP (1995) NMR measurement of perfusion using arterial spin labeling without saturation of macromolecular spins. Magn Reson Med 33(3):370–376

Zhang X, Petersen ET, Ghariq E, De Vis JB, Webb AG, Teeuwisse WM et al (2013) In vivo blood T(1) measurements at 1.5 T, 3 T, and 7 T. Magn Reson Med 70(4):1082–1086. https://doi.org/10.1002/mrm.24550

Zimmer F, O'Brien K, Bollmann S, Pfeuffer J, Heberlein K, Barth M (2016) Pulsed arterial spin labelling at ultra-high field with a B 1 (+) -optimised adiabatic labelling pulse. MAGMA 29(3):463–473. https://doi.org/10.1007/s10334-016-0555-2

Zuo Z, Wang R, Zhuo Y, Xue R, St Lawrence KS, Wang DJ (2013) Turbo-FLASH based arterial spin labeled perfusion MRI at 7 T. PLoS One 8(6):e66612. https://doi.org/10.1371/journal.pone.0066612

fMRI Data Analysis Using SPM

8

Guillaume Flandin and Marianne J. U. Novak

Abbreviations

DCM	Dynamic causal model
EPI	Echo planar imaging
FFX	Fixed-effects analysis
fMRI	Functional magnetic resonance imaging
FPR	False-positive rate
FWE	Family-wise error
FWHM	Full width at half maximum
GLM	General linear model
HRF	Haemodynamic response function
MIP	Maximum intensity projection
PET	Positron emission tomography
RFT	Random field theory
RFX	Random-effects analysis
SPM	Statistical parametric map(ping)
SVC	Small volume correction
TR	Time to repeat
VBM	Voxel-based morphometry

G. Flandin (✉)
Wellcome Centre for Human NeuroImaging, UCL Queen Square Institute of Neurology, London, UK
e-mail: g.flandin@ucl.ac.uk

M. J. U. Novak
Department of Neurology, Royal Free Hospital, London, UK
e-mail: marianne.novak@nhs.net

8.1 Introduction

Statistical parametric mapping (SPM) is an established statistical data analysis framework through which regionally specific effects in structural and functional neuroimaging data can be characterised. SPM is also the name of a free and open source academic software package through which this framework (amongst other things) can be implemented. In this chapter, we will give an overview of the underlying concepts of the SPM framework and will illustrate this by describing how to analyse a typical block-design functional MRI (fMRI) data set using the SPM software. An exhaustive description of SPM would be beyond the scope of this introductory chapter; for more information, we refer interested readers to *Statistical Parametric Mapping: The Analysis of Functional Brain Images* (Friston et al. 2007).

The aim of the SPM software[1] is to communicate and disseminate neuroimaging data analysis methods to the scientific community. It is developed by the SPM co-authors, who are associated with the Wellcome Centre for Human Neuroimaging, including the Functional Imaging Laboratory, UCL Queen Square Institute of Neurology. For those interested, a history of SPM can be found in a special issue of the NeuroImage journal, produced to mark 20 years of fMRI (Ashburner 2011). In brief, SPM was created by Karl Friston in approximately 1991 to carry out statistical analysis of positron

[1] https://www.fil.ion.ucl.ac.uk/spm/.

S. Ulmer, O. Jansen (eds.), *fMRI*, https://doi.org/10.1007/978-3-030-41874-8_8

emission tomography (PET) data. Since then, the SPM project has evolved to support newer imaging modalities such as functional magnetic resonance imaging (fMRI), EEG and MEG (M/EEG) and to incorporate constant developments and improvements of existing methods. The current released version of SPM is SPM12.

The SPM framework is summarised in Fig. 8.1 (Flandin and Friston 2008). The analysis pipeline starts with a raw imaging data sequence at the top left corner of the figure and ends with a statistical parametric map (also abbreviated to SPM) showing the significance of regional effects in the bottom right corner. The SPM framework can be partitioned into three key components, all of which will be described in this chapter:

- Preprocessing, or spatially transforming data: images are spatially aligned to each other to correct for the effect of subject movement during scanning (realignment/motion correction), then spatially normalised into a standard space and smoothed.
- Modelling the preprocessed data: parametric statistical models are applied at each voxel (a *vo*lume *el*ement, the three-dimensional extension of a pixel in 2D) of the data, using a general linear model (GLM) to describe the data in terms of experimental effects, confounding effects and residual variability.
- Statistical inference on the modelled data: classical statistical inference is used to test hypotheses that are expressed in terms of

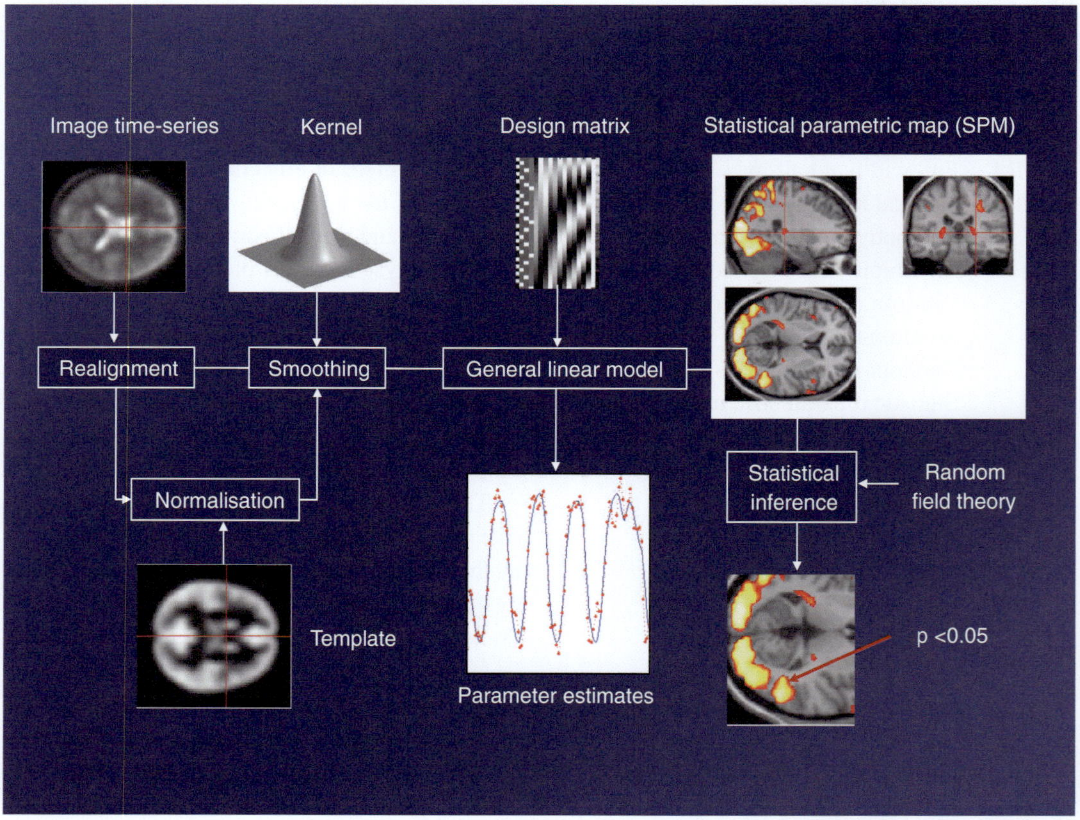

Fig. 8.1 Flowchart of the SPM processing pipeline, starting with raw imaging data and ending with a statistical parametric map (*SPM*). The raw images are motion-corrected, then subject to non-linear warping so that they match a template that conforms to a standard anatomical space. After smoothing, the general linear model is employed to estimate the parameters of a model encoded by a design matrix containing all possible predictors of the data. These parameters are then used to derive univariate test statistics at every voxel; these constitute the SPM. Finally, statistical inference is performed by assigning *p* values to unexpected features of the SPM, such as high peaks or large clusters, through the use of the random field theory

GLM parameters. This results in an image in which the voxel values are statistics: this is a statistical parametric map (SPM). For such classical inferences, a multiple comparisons problem arises from the application of mass-univariate tests to images with many voxels. This is solved through the use of random field theory (RFT), resulting in inference based on corrected *p* values.

In this chapter, we will illustrate the concepts underpinning SPM through the analysis of an actual fMRI data set. The data set we will use was the first ever fMRI data set collected and analysed at the Functional Imaging Laboratory (by Geraint Rees, under the direction of Karl Friston) and is locally known as the Mother of All Experiments. The data set can be downloaded from the SPM website,[2] allowing readers to reproduce the analysis pipeline that we will describe on their own computers. (For more detailed step-by-step instructions to this analysis, we refer readers to the SPM manual.[3]) The purpose of the experiment was to explore equipment and techniques in the early days of fMRI. The experiment consisted of a single session in a single subject; the subject was presented with alternating blocks of rest and auditory stimulation, starting with a rest block. The auditory stimulation consisted of binaurally, bi-syllabic words presented at a rate of 60 words/min. Ninety-six whole brain echo planar imaging (EPI) scans were acquired on a modified 2 T Siemens MAGNETOM Vision System, with a repetition time (TR) of 7 s. Each block lasted for six scans, and there were 16 blocks in total, each lasting for 42 s. Each scan consisted of 64 contiguous slices ($64 \times 64 \times 64$, $3 \times 3 \times 3$ mm^3 voxels). A structural scan was also acquired prior to the experiment ($256 \times 256 \times 54$, $1 \times 1 \times 3$ mm^3 voxels).

Acquisition techniques have tremendously improved since this data set was acquired—a TR of 7 s seems very slow in comparison with today's standards—but the analysis pipeline is identical to that of more recent data sets and fits nicely with the purpose of illustration in this chapter. While analysing this block, or epoch, designed experiment, we will point out the few steps that differ in the analysis of event-related data sets.

After an overview of the SPM software, we will describe in the next sections the three key components of an SPM analysis, namely, (1) spatial transformations, (2) modelling and (3) statistical inference.

8.2 SPM Software Overview

8.2.1 Requirements

The SPM software is written in MATLAB[4] (The MathWorks, Inc.), a high-level technical computing language and interactive environment. SPM is distributed under the terms of the GNU General Public Licence. The software consists of a library of MATLAB M-files and a small number of C-files (which perform some of the most computationally intensive operations) and will run on any platform supported by MATLAB: 64-bit Microsoft Windows, Apple macOS and Linux. This means that a prospective SPM user must first install commercially available software MATLAB. More specifically, SPM12 requires either MATLAB version 7.4 (R2007a) or any more recent version (up to 9.6 (R2019a) at time of writing). Only core MATLAB software is required; no extra MATLAB toolboxes are needed.

A standalone version of SPM12, compiled using the MATLAB Compiler, is also available from the SPM development team upon request. This allows the use of all of the SPM functions without the need for a MATLAB licence (although this comes at the expense of being able to modify the software).

8.2.2 Installation

The installation of SPM simply consists of unpacking a ZIP archive from the SPM website on the user computer and then adding the root SPM directory to the MATLAB path. If needed,

[2] https://www.fil.ion.ucl.ac.uk/spm/data/auditory/.

[3] https://www.fil.ion.ucl.ac.uk/spm/doc/manual.pdf.

[4] https://www.mathworks.com/.

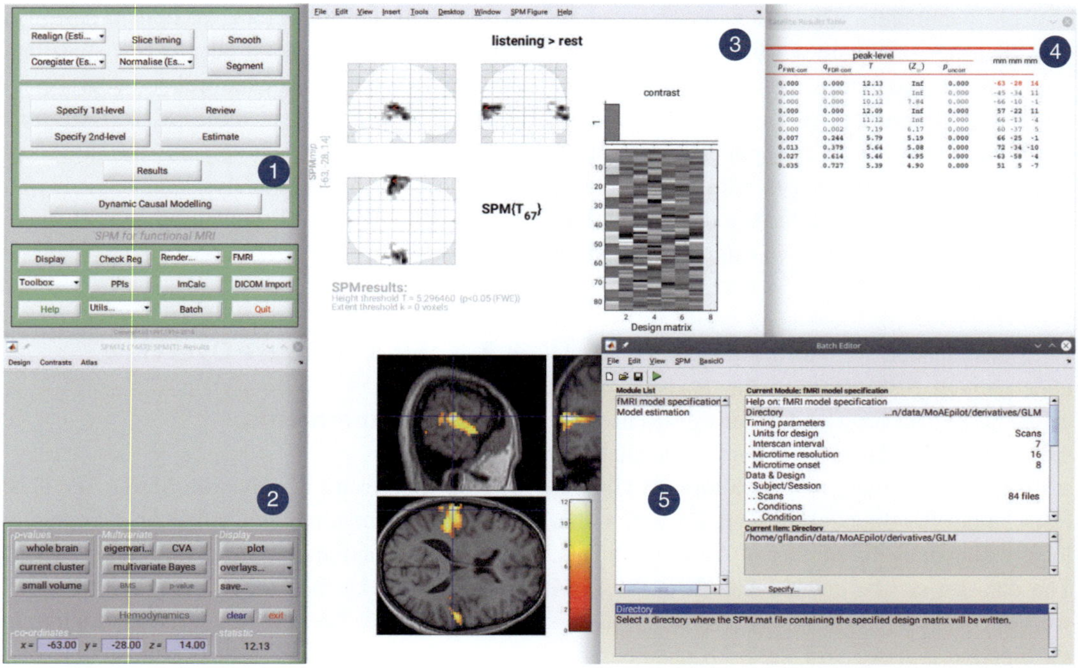

Fig. 8.2 Interface of the SPM12 software for the fMRI modality: (*1*) Menu window, (*2*) Interactive window, (*3*) Graphics window, (*4*) Satellite Results window and (*5*) Batch editor interface

more details on the installation can be found on the SPM wiki on Wikibooks.[5]

SPM updates (which include bug fixes and improvements to the software) take place regularly (approximately every 6 months) and are advertised on the SPM mailing list.[6] SPM is a constantly evolving software package, and we therefore recommend that users either subscribe to the mailing list or check the SPM website so that they can benefit from ongoing developments. Updates can be easily installed by unpacking the update ZIP archive on top of the existing installation so that newer files overwrite existing ones. We would, however, advise users not to install updates mid-analysis (unless a specific update is needed), to ensure consistency within an analysis.

8.2.3 Interface

To start up SPM, simply type *spm* in the MATLAB command line and choose the modality in which you wish to use SPM in the new window that opens. A shortcut is to directly type *spm fmri*. The SPM interface consists of three main windows, as shown in Fig. 8.2. The Menu window (1) contains entry points to the various functions contained in SPM. The Interactive window (2) is used either when SPM functions require additional information from the user or when an additional function-specific interface is available. The Graphics window (3) is the window in which results and figures are shown. Additional windows can appear, such as the Satellite Graphics window (4), in which extra results can be displayed, or the Batch Editor window (5). SPM can run in batch mode (in which several SPM functions can be set up to run consecutively through a single analysis pipeline), and the Batch Editor window is the dedicated interface for this. The window can be accessed through the 'Batch' button in the Menu window.

The Menu window is subdivided into three sections, which reflect the key components of an SPM analysis: spatial preprocessing, modelling and inference.

[5]https://en.wikibooks.org/wiki/SPM/.

[6]https://www.fil.ion.ucl.ac.uk/spm/support/.

8.2.4 File Formats

In general, the first step when using SPM is to convert the raw data into a format that the software can read. Most MRI scanners produce image data that conform to the DICOM (Digital Imaging and Communications in Medicine) standard.[7] The DICOM format is very flexible and powerful, but this comes at the expense of simplicity. As a consequence, the neuroimaging community agreed in 2004 to use a simpler image data format, the NIfTI (Neuroimaging Informatics Technology Initiative)[8] format, to facilitate interoperability between fMRI data analysis software.

A NIfTI image file can consist either of two files, with the extensions *.hdr* and *.img*, or a single file, with the extension *.nii*. The two versions can be used in SPM interchangeably (note that you can also come across a compressed version of these files with a *.gz* extension; it is recommended to uncompress such files before use in SPM). The *header* (*.hdr*) file contains meta-information about the data, such as the voxel size, the number of voxels in each direction and the data type used to store values. The *image* (*.img*) file contains the raw 3D array of voxel values. A file with the *.nii* extension contains all of this information in one file. A key piece of information stored in the header is the *voxel-to-world mapping*: this is a spatial transformation that maps from the stored data coordinates (voxel column *i*, row *j*, slice *k*) into a real-world position (*x*, *y*, *z mm*) in space. The real-world position can be in either a standardised space such as Talairach and Tournoux space or Montreal Neurological Institute (MNI) space or a subject-specific space based on scanner coordinates.

FMRI data can be considered as 4D data—a time series of 3D data—and can therefore be stored as a single file in the NIfTI format where the first three dimensions are in space and the fourth is in time. It is sometimes more convenient to use a set of 3D files instead of a single 4D file in SPM12; we are going to use a 4D file here.

DICOM image data can be converted into NIfTI files in SPM using the 'DICOM Import' button in the Menu window. This is usually a straightforward process. If needed, however, NIfTI data obtained from other file converters (such as dicm2nii[9] or dcm2niix[10]) can also be used in SPM; the output NIfTI images are interoperable between software packages.

The auditory data set used in this chapter has already been converted from the DICOM format. We have one 4D NIfTI functional file, namely *sub-01_task-auditory_bold.nii*, and one NIfTI structural file, namely *sub-01_T1w.nii*, organised according to the Brain Imaging Data Structure (BIDS) (Gorgolewski et al. 2016), a community-led standard format for organizing and describing neuroimaging experiments datasets.

Images can be displayed in SPM using the 'Display' and 'Check Reg' buttons from the Menu window. The first function displays a single image and some information from its header, while the second displays up to 15 images at the same time. This can be used to check the accuracy of alignment, for example.

8.3 Spatial Transformations

A number of preprocessing steps must be applied to the fMRI data to transform them into a form suitable for statistical analysis. Most of these steps correspond to some form of image registration, and Fig. 8.3 illustrates a typical preprocessing pipeline. There is no universal pipeline to use in all circumstances—options depend on the data themselves and the aim of the analysis—but the one presented here is fairly standard.

The first preprocessing step is to apply a motion correction algorithm to the fMRI data (this is the *realignment function*). This may eventually include some form of distortion correction.

[7]https://dicomstandard.org/.

[8]https://nifti.nimh.nih.gov/.

[9]https://www.mathworks.com/matlabcentral/fileexchange/42997.

[10]https://www.nitrc.org/plugins/mwiki/index.php/dcm2nii:MainPage.

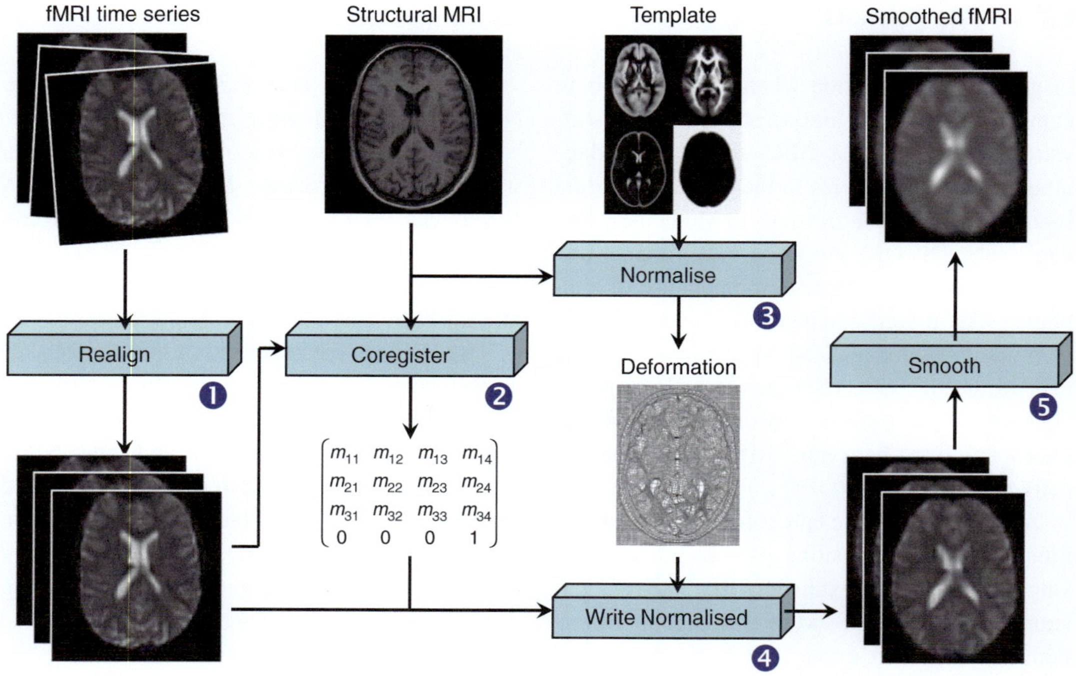

Fig. 8.3 Flowchart of a standard pipeline to preprocess fMRI data. After realignment (*1*) to correct for movement, structural and functional images are coregistered (*2*) then normalised (*3*, *4*) to conform to a standard anatomical space (e.g. MNI space) before being spatially smoothed using a Gaussian kernel (*5*)

A structural MRI of the same subject is often acquired and should be brought into alignment with the fMRI data in a second step (*coregister function*). The warps needed to spatially normalise the structural image into some standard space should then be estimated (*normalise function*) and applied to the motion-corrected functional images to normalise them into the same standard space (*write normalise function*). The final step will typically be to smooth the functional data spatially by applying a Gaussian kernel to them (*smooth function*).

The type of spatial *transformations* that should be applied to data depends on whether the data to be transformed all come from the same subject (*within-subject* transformations) or from multiple different subjects (*between-subject* transformations). The choice of *objective function* (the criterion to assess the quality of the registration) used to estimate the deformation also depends on the modality of data in question. Realignment is a *within-subject, within-modality* registration, while coregistration is a *within-subject, between-modality* registration. Normalisation is a *between-subject* registration. Within-subject registration will generally involve a *rigid body* transformation, while a between-subject registration will need estimation of affine or non-linear warps; this is because a more complex transformation is required to warp together the anatomically variable brains of different subjects than to warp together different images of the same brain. A criterion to compare two images of the same modality can be the sum of squares of the differences of the two images, while the comparison between two images of different modalities will involve more advanced criteria. An *optimisation algorithm* is then used in the registration step to maximise (or minimise) the objective function. Once the parameters have been estimated, the target image can be transformed to match the source image by resampling the data using an *interpolation* scheme. This step is referred to as *reslicing* when dealing with rigid transformations.

8.3.1 Data Preparation

Before preprocessing an fMRI data set, the first images acquired in a session should be discarded. This is because much of the very large signal change that they contain is due to the time it takes for magnetisation to reach equilibrium. This can be easily seen by looking at the first few images at the beginning of the time series using the display function. Some scanners might handle these '*dummy scans*' automatically by acquiring a few scans before the real start of the acquisition, but this should be checked. In our example data set organised according to BIDS, the first 12 scans have already been discarded, leaving us with 84 scans. This is more than necessary here but it preserves the simplicity of the experimental design as it corresponds to one complete cycle of auditory stimulation and rest.

It is good practice to manually reorient the images next so that they roughly match the normalised space that SPM uses (MNI space). This will help the convergence of the registration algorithms used in preprocessing; the algorithms use a local optimisation procedure and can fail if the initial images are not in rough alignment. In practice, the origin (*0, 0, 0* mm) should be within 5 cm of the anterior commissure (a white matter track which connects the two hemispheres across the midline), and the orientation of the images should be within about 20° of the SPM template. To check the orientation of images, display one image of the time series using the 'Display' button and manually adjust their orientation using the translation (right, forward, up) and rotation (pitch, roll, yaw) parameters in the bottom left panel until the prerequisites are met. To actually apply the transformation to the data, you need to press the 'Set Origin' button followed by the 'Reorient' button and select all the images to reorient. With the auditory data set, the structural image is already correctly orientated, but the functional scans should be translated by about [*0, −31, −36*] mm. See Fig. 8.4 for a screenshot of the 'Display' interface illustrating how to change the origin of a series of images.

8.3.2 Realignment

As described above, the first preprocessing step is to realign the data to correct for the effects of subject movement during the scanning session. Despite restraints on head movement, cooperative subjects still show displacements of up to several millimetres, and these can have a large impact on the significance of the ensuing inference; in the unfortunate situation where a subject's movements are correlated with the experimental task, spurious activations can be observed if no correction was performed prior to statistical analysis. Alternatively, movements correlated with responses to an experimental task can inflate unwanted variance components in the voxel time series and reduce statistical power.

The objective of realignment is to determine the rigid body transformation that best maps the series of functional image volumes into a common space. A rigid body transformation can be parameterised by six parameters in 3D: three translations and three rotations. The realignment process involves the estimation of the six parameters that minimise the mean squared difference between each successive scan and a reference scan (usually the first or the average of all scans in the time series) (Friston et al. 1995).

Unfortunately, even after realignment, there may still be some motion-related artefacts remaining in the functional data (Friston et al. 1996b); this is mainly because the linear, rigid body realignment transformation cannot capture non-linear effects. These non-linear effects can be the consequence of subject movement between slice acquisition, interpolation artefacts, magnetic field inhomogeneities or spin-excitation history effects. One solution is to use the movement parameter estimates as covariates of no interest during the modelling of the data. This will effectively remove any signal that is correlated with functions of the movement parameters but can still be problematic if the movement effects are correlated with the experimental design. An alternative option is to use the 'Realign and Unwarp' function (Andersson et al. 2001). The assumption in this function is that the residual movement variance can be largely explained

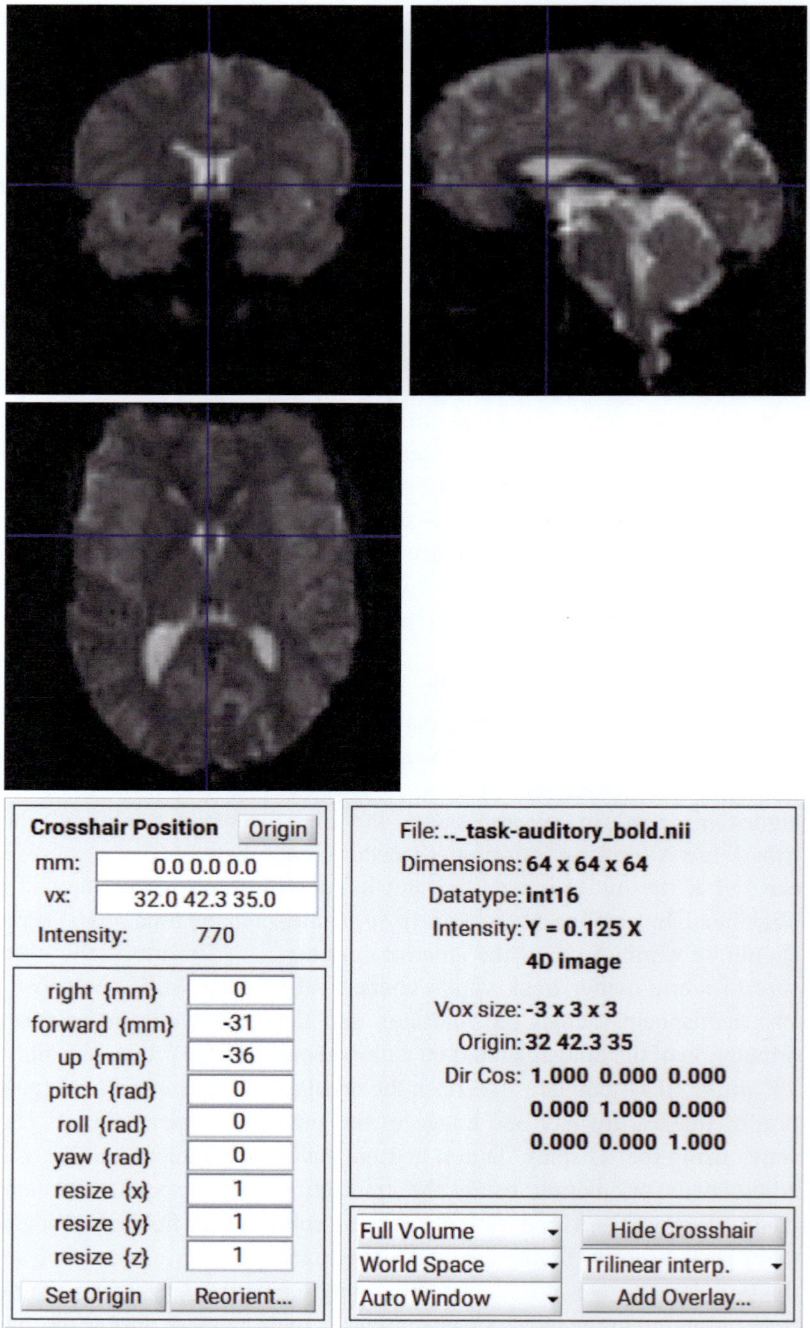

Fig. 8.4 Interface of the 'Display' option. The location of the crosshair, in *blue*, is indicated in the *bottom left panel*, both in mm and voxel. Here, a translation of [0, −31, −36] mm allows to set the origin of the image ([0, 0, 0] mm) near the anterior commissure

by susceptibility-by-movement interaction: the non-uniformity of the magnetic field is the source of geometric distortions during magnetic resonance acquisition, and the amount of distortion depends partly on the position of the head of the subject within the magnetic field; hence, large movements will result in changes in the shape of the brain in the images which cannot be captured by a rigid body transformation. The 'Realign and Unwarp' function uses a generative model that combines a model of geometric distortions and a model of subject motion to correct images. The 'Realign and Unwarp' function can be combined with the use of field maps (see the FieldMap

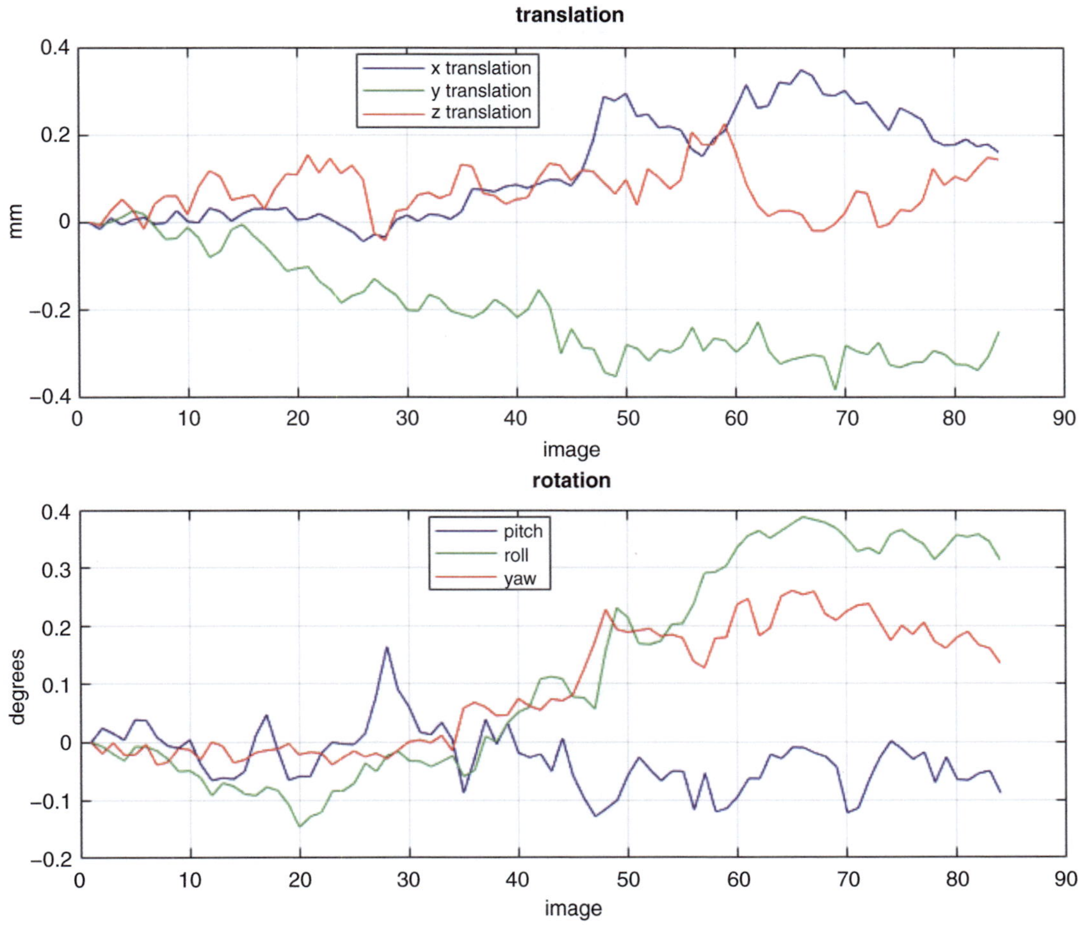

Fig. 8.5 Plot of the estimated movement parameters (three translations and three rotations) for the auditory data set as a function of time (or scan). Movements are small for this subject but we can still observe some slow drifts over time

toolbox), to further correct those geometric distortions introduced during the echo planar imaging (EPI)) acquisition (Jezzard and Balaban 1995). The resulting corrected images will have less movement-related residual variance and better matching between functional and structural images than will the uncorrected images.

For the auditory data set, functional data are motion-corrected using 'Realign: Estimate and Reslice'. Data have to be entered session by session to account for large subject movements between sessions that the algorithm is not expecting. With regard to the reslicing, it is sufficient to write out only the mean image. The output of the estimation will be encoded in the header of each image through modification of the original voxel-to-world mapping. It is best to reslice the data just once at the end of all the preprocessing steps; this ensures that all the affine transformations are taken into account in one step, preventing unnecessary interpolation of the data. The estimated movement parameters (see Fig. 8.5) are saved in a text file in the same folder as the data with an '*rp_*' prefix and will be used later in the analysis.

8.3.3 Coregistration

Coregistration is the process of registering two images of the same or different modalities from the same subject; the intensity pattern might differ between the two images, but the overall shape remains constant. Coregistration of single subject structural and functional data firstly allows functional results to be superimposed on an anatomical scan for clear visualisation. Secondly, spatial normalisation is more precise when warps are estimated from a detailed anatomical image than from functional images; if the functional and structural images are in alignment, warps estimated from the structural image can then be applied to the functional data.

As with realignment, coregistration is performed by optimising the six parameters of a rigid body transformation; however, the objective function is different as image intensities cannot be compared directly as they were with the sum of squared differences. Instead, the similarity measures that are used rely on a branch of applied mathematics called *information theory* (Collignon et al. 1995; Wells et al. 1996). The most commonly used similarity measure is called *mutual information*; this is a measurement of shared information between data sets, based on joint probability distributions of the intensities of the images. The mutual information is assumed to be maximal when the two images are perfectly aligned and will serve here as the objective function to maximise.

For the auditory data set, the structural image should be coregistered to the mean functional image (computed during realignment) using 'Coregister: Estimate'. Once again, there is no need to reslice at this stage; reslicing can be postponed until later to minimise interpolation steps. In the interface, the *reference* image (the target) is the mean functional image, while the *source* image is the structural image. Default parameters can be left as they are; they have been optimised over years and should satisfy most situations. The output of the algorithm will be stored in the header of the structural image by adjusting its voxel-to-world mapping. Figure 8.6 shows the alignment of the two images after registration.

8.3.4 Spatial Normalisation

Spatial normalisation is the process of warping images from a number of individuals into a common space. This allows signals to be compared and averaged across subjects so that common activation patterns can be identified: the goal of most functional imaging studies. Even single subject analyses usually proceed in a standard anatomical space so that regionally specific effects can be reported within a frame of reference that can be related to other studies (Fox 1995). The most commonly used coordinate system within the brain imaging community is the one described by Talairach and Tournoux (1988), although new standards based on digital atlases

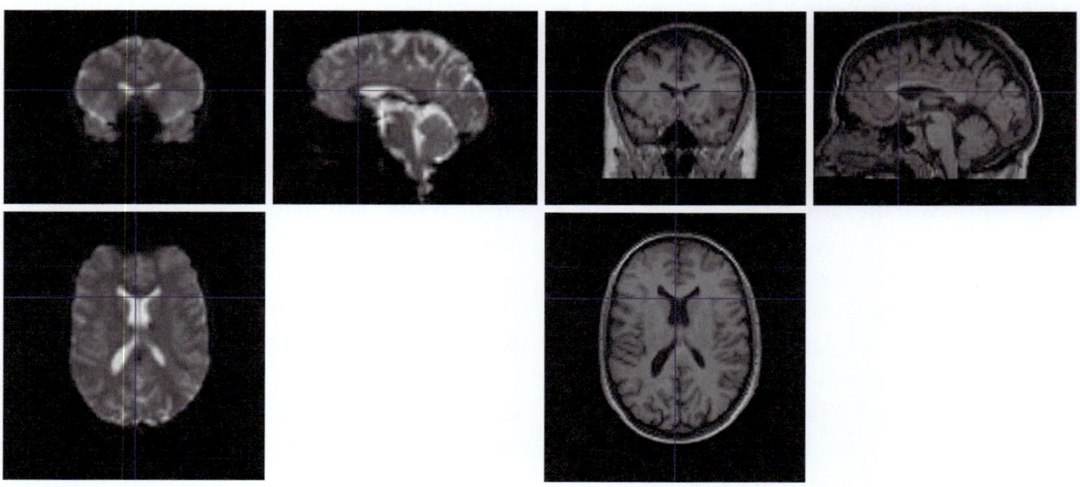

Fig. 8.6 Coregistered mean functional and structural images using mutual information. Some important dropouts in the functional data can be observed

(such as the Montreal Neurological Institute (MNI) space) are nowadays widespread (Mazziotta et al. 1995).

The rigid body approach used previously when registering brain images from the same subject is not appropriate for matching brain images from different subjects; it is insufficiently complex to deal with interindividual differences in anatomy. More complex transformations (i.e. with more degrees of freedom) such as affine or *non-linear transformations* are used instead. (Non-linear registration is also used when characterising change in a subject's brain anatomy over time, such as those due to growth, ageing, disease or surgical intervention.)

The normalisation deformation model has to be flexible enough to capture most changes in shape but must also be sufficiently constrained that realistic brain warps are generated; *a priori*, we expect the deformation to be spatially smooth. This can be nicely framed in a Bayesian setting by adding a prior term to the objective function to incorporate prior information or add constraints to the warp. For instance, consider a deformation model in which each voxel is allowed to move independently in three dimensions. There would be three times as many parameters in this model than there are voxels. To deal with this, the deformation parameters need to be regularised; the prior term enables this. Priors become more important as the number of parameters specifying the mapping increases, and they are central to high-dimensional non-linear warping schemes. The approach taken in previous versions of SPM was to parameterise the deformations by a linear combination of smooth, continuous basis functions, such as low-frequency cosine transform basis functions (Ashburner and Friston 1999). These models have a relatively small number of parameters, about 1000 (although this is of course large in comparison with 6 parameters for a rigid body transformation and 12 for an affine transformation), and allow a better description of the observed structural changes whilst providing reasonably smoothed deformations. SPM12 uses a much more refined spatial transformation model based on small deformations parameterised by over 1000,000 values (Weiskopf et al. 2011) and a more sophisticated regularisation model comprising five penalty terms (Malone et al. 2015). The optimisation procedure relies on an iterative local optimisation algorithm and needs reasonable starting estimates (hence the reorientation of the images at the very beginning of the analysis pipeline).

In practice, better alignment can be achieved by matching grey matter with grey matter and white matter with white matter. The process of classifying voxels into different tissue types is called *segmentation*, and an approach combining segmentation and normalisation will provide better results than normalisation alone. This is the strategy implemented via the 'Normalise' and 'Segment' buttons in SPM; it is referred to as *Unified segmentation* (Ashburner and Friston 2005). Unified segmentation uses a generative model which involves (1) a mixture of Gaussians to model intensity distributions, (2) a bias correction component to model smooth intensity variations in space and (3) a non-linear registration with tissue probability maps as described in the previous paragraph.

We will use the unified segmentation approach on the auditory data set through the 'Normalise' button. The normalisation/segmentation of the structural image (using, by default, tissue probability maps that can be found in the '*tpm*' folder of the SPM installation, see Fig. 8.7) will estimate the deformation field, saved in a 5D NIfTI file with a '*y_*' prefix. This file can be used to apply the deformation, that is, to normalise the functional images (as they are in the same space as the structural scan thanks to the coregistration step) with the 'Normalise: Write' button. A new 4D image will be written to disk with a '*w*' prefix (for warp). The same procedure can be applied to the structural scan in order to later superimpose the functional activations on the anatomy of the subject. In both instances, some parameters have to be updated: the voxel size of the new set of images is preferably chosen in relation to the initial resolution of the images, for example, to the nearest integer. Here we used [*3*, *3*, *3*] for the functional data and [*1*, *1*, *3*] for the structural scan. The default interpolation scheme is to use

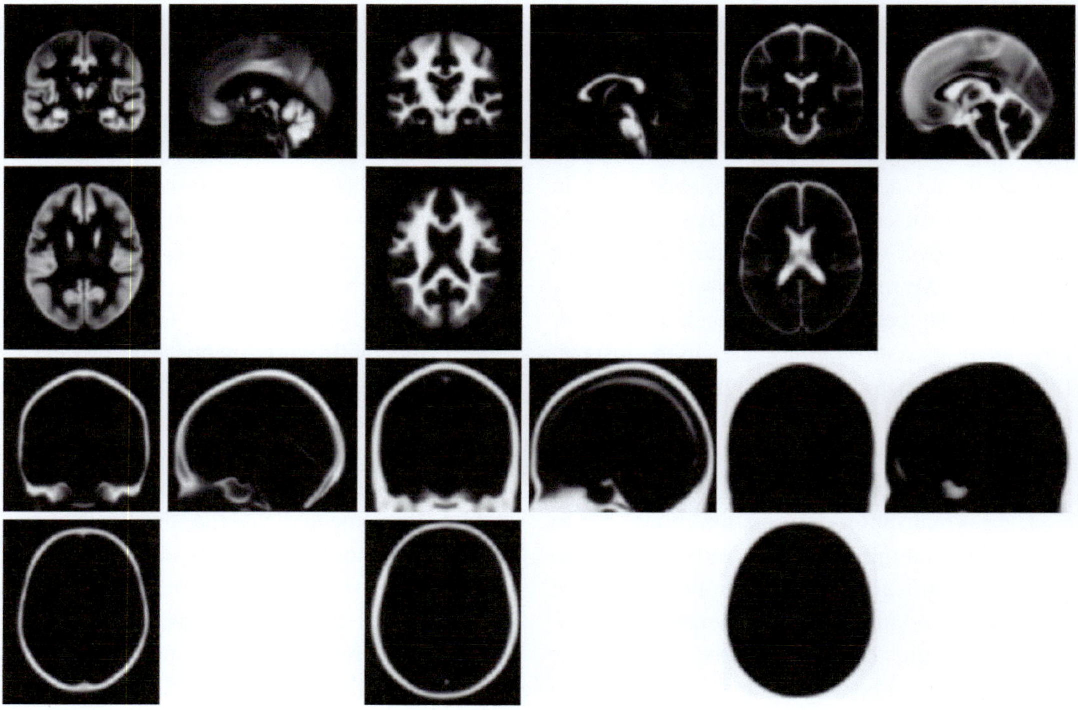

Fig. 8.7 Tissue probability maps used for segmentation/spatial normalisation. There are six tissue classes corresponding approximately to grey matter, white matter, cerebrospinal fluid, bone, soft tissue, and air/background

high-order interpolation, with a fourth-degree B-spline (Unser et al. 1993). The coordinates of locations within a normalised brain can now be reported as MNI coordinates in publications (Brett et al. 2002).

On a final note, spatial normalisation may require some extra care when dealing with patient populations with gross anatomical pathology, such as stroke lesions. This can generate a bias in the normalisation as the generative model is based on anatomically 'normal' data. Solving this usually involves imposing constraints on the warping to ensure that the pathology does not bias the deformation of undamaged tissue, for example, by decreasing the precision of the data in the region of pathology so that more importance is afforded to the anatomically normal priors. This is the principle of lesion masking (Brett et al. 2001). There is evidence, however, that the Unified Segmentation approach is actually quite robust in the presence of focal lesions (Crinion et al. 2007; Andersen et al. 2010).

8.3.5 Spatial Smoothing

Spatial smoothing consists of applying a spatial low-pass filter to the data. Typically, this takes the form of a 3D Gaussian kernel, parameterised by its full width at half maximum (FWHM)) along the three directions. In other words, the intensity at each voxel is replaced by a weighted average of itself and its neighbouring voxels, where the weights follow a Gaussian shape centred on the given voxel. The underlying mathematical operation is a convolution, and the effect of smoothing with different kernel sizes is illustrated in Fig. 8.8.

It might seem counterintuitive to reduce the resolution of fMRI data through smoothing, but there are four reasons for doing this. Firstly, smoothing increases the signal-to-noise ratio in the data. The matched filter theorem stipulates that the optimal smoothing kernel corresponds to the size of the effect that one anticipates. A kernel similar in size to the anatomical extent of the expected haemodynamic response should

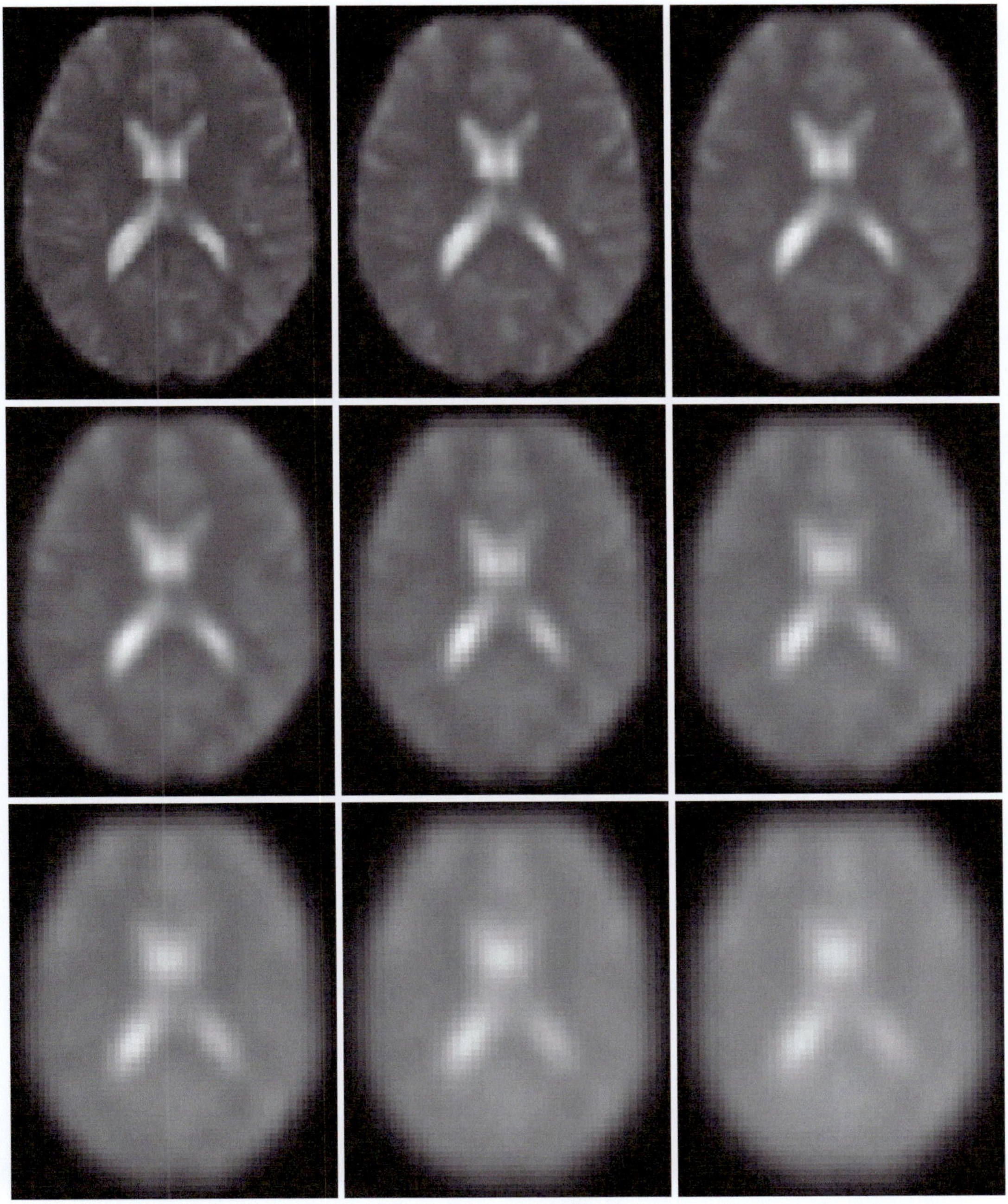

Fig. 8.8 Axial slice of a functional MRI scan smoothed with 3D Gaussian kernels of different isotropic FHWMs. From *top to bottom* and *left to right*, these show the effects of smoothing with kernels of the following FWHMs: 0, 2, 4, 6, 8, 10, 12, 14 and 16 mm

therefore be chosen. Secondly, thanks to the central limit theorem, smoothing the data will render errors, or noise, more normally distributed, and will validate the use of inference based on parametric statistics. Thirdly, as we shall see later, when using the random field theory to make inference about regionally specific effects, there are specific assumptions that require smoothness in the data to be substantially greater than the voxel size (typically, as a rule of thumb, about three times the voxel size). Fourthly, small misregistration errors are inevitable in group studies; smoothing increases the degree of anatomical and functional overlap across subjects, reduces the effects of misregistration and thereby increases the significance of ensuing statistical tests.

In practice, there is no definitive amount of smoothing that should be applied to any data set; choice of smoothing kernel depends on the resolution of the data, the regions under investigation and single subject versus group analysis amongst other things. Commonly used FWHMs are between 6- and 12-mm isotropic.

For the auditory data set, we will smooth the 84 normalised volumes with a [*6*, *6*, *6*]-mm FWHM kernel to produce a new 4D NIfTI file with an '*s*' prefix.

8.4 Modelling and Statistical Inference

Statistical parametric mapping is a voxel by voxel hypothesis testing approach through which regions that show a significant experimental effect of interest are identified (Friston et al. 1991). It relies upon the construction of statistical parametric maps (SPMs), which are images with values at each voxel that are, under the null hypothesis, distributed according to a known probability density function (usually the Student's *t*- or *F*-distributions). The parameters used to compute a standard univariate statistical test at each and every voxel in the brain are obtained from the estimation of a *general linear model* which partitions observed responses into components of interest (such as the experimental effect of interest), confounding factors (examples of such will be given later) and error (or 'noise') (Friston et al. 1994a). Hence, SPM is a *mass-univariate* approach: statistics are calculated independently at each voxel. The *random field theory* is then used to characterise the SPM and resolve the multiple comparisons problem induced by making inferences over a volume of the brain containing multiple voxels (Worsley et al. 1992, 1996; Friston et al. 1994b). 'Unlikely' topological features of the SPM, like activation peaks, are interpreted as regionally specific effects attributable to the experimental manipulation (Flandin and Friston 2015).

In this section, we will describe the general linear model in the context of fMRI time series. We will then estimate its parameters using the *maximum likelihood method* and describe how to test hypotheses by making statistical inferences on some of the parameter estimates by using *contrast*. The resulting statistical parameters are assembled into an image: this is the SPM. The random field theory provides adjusted *p* values to control false-positive rate for the search volume.

8.4.1 The General Linear Model

After the spatial preprocessing of the fMRI data, we can assume that all data from one particular voxel are derived from the same part of the brain, and that in any single subject, the data from that voxel form a sequential time series. A time series selected from a (carefully chosen) voxel in the auditory data set is shown in Fig. 8.9a: variation in the response over time can be seen. There are 84 values, or data points, or observations. The aim is now to define a generative model of these data. This involves defining a prediction of what we might expect to observe in the measured BOLD signal given our knowledge of the acquisition apparatus and the experimental design. Here, the paradigm consisted of alternating periods (or 'blocks') of rest and auditory stimulation, with each block lasting for six scans. We expect that a voxel in a brain region sensitive to auditory stimuli will show a response that alternates with the same pattern and would thus, in the absence of noise, look like the plot in Fig. 8.10a.

However, we also know that with fMRI we are not directly measuring the neuronal activity, but the brain oxygen level-dependent (BOLD)) signal with which it is associated. The observed BOLD signal corresponds to neuronally mediated haemodynamic change which can be modelled as a convolution of the underlying neuronal process by a *haemodynamic response function* (HRF)). This function is called the *impulse response function*: it is the response that would be

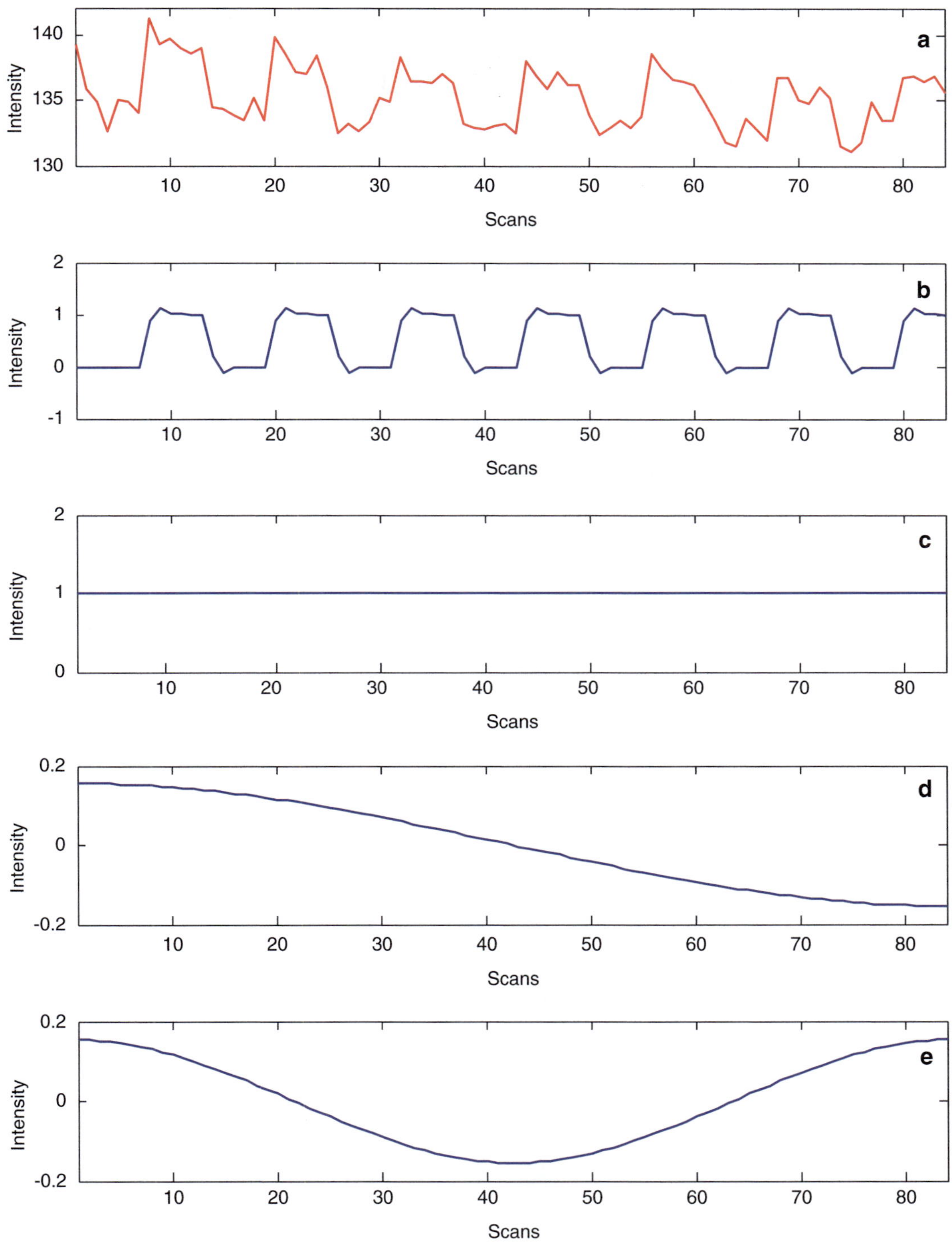

Fig. 8.9 Predictors of an fMRI time series: (**a**) raw time series at a given voxel in the brain, (**b**) stimulus function convolved with the canonical haemodynamic response function, (**c**) constant term modelling the mean whole brain activity, (**d**, **e**) the first two components of a discrete cosine basis set modelling slow fluctuations

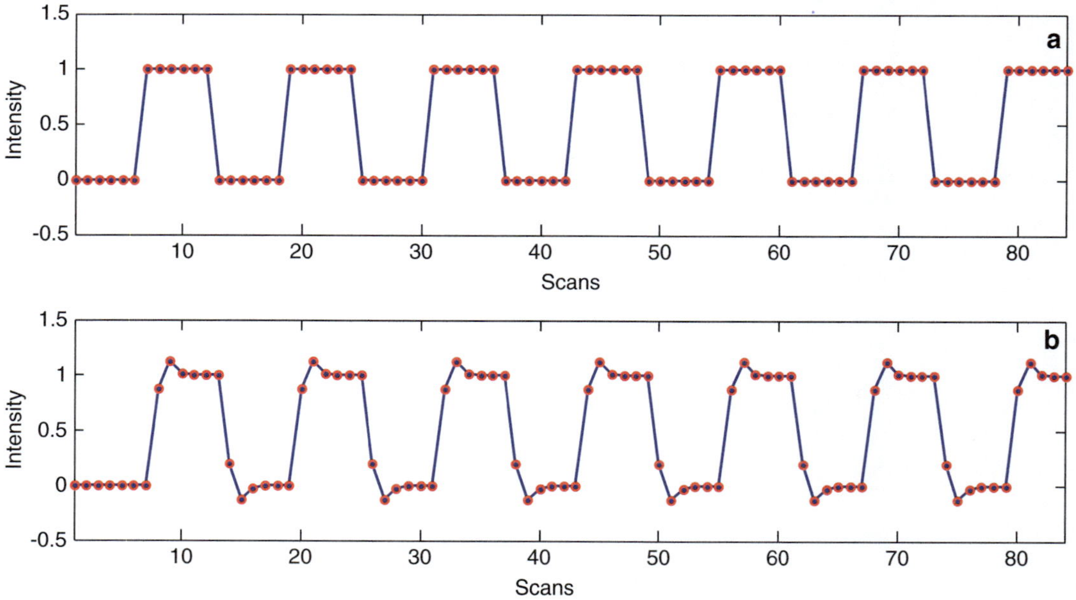

Fig. 8.10 Effect of convolution by the haemodynamic response function: (**a**) stimulus function constructed as a boxcar function and (**b**) after convolution with the canonical HRF

observed in the BOLD signal in the presence of a brief neuronal stimulation at $t = 0$. The *canonical HRF* used in SPM is depicted in Fig. 8.11. The HRF models the fact that the BOLD response peaks about 5 s after the neuronal stimulation and takes about 32 s to go back to baseline, in a slow and smooth fashion, undershooting towards the end before reaching baseline.

We can thus improve our prediction by modifying the box car stimulus function of Fig. 8.10a to take into account the shape of the HRF. This is done through convolution, by assuming a linear time-invariant model. This convolution operation is conceptually the same as the one that was used in the smoothing preprocessing step; that was a convolution in space with a Gaussian kernel, whilst here it is a convolution in time with the canonical HRF. The output of this mathematical operation is displayed in Fig. 8.10b.

Looking at the raw time series of Fig. 8.9a, we can also directly observe that the mean of the signal is not zero; this should also be part of our prediction model. We model the (non-zero) mean of the signal with a predictor that is held constant over time, as shown in Fig. 8.9c.

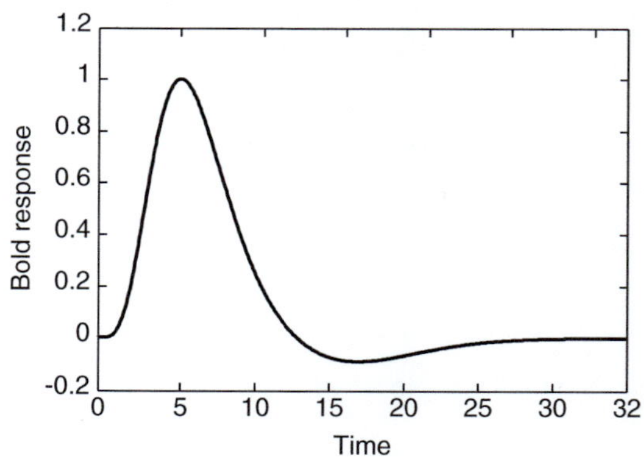

Fig. 8.11 Canonical haemodynamic response function (HRF) as used by SPM. This is the typical BOLD response to a single, impulse stimulation

Furthermore, we can also observe some slow fluctuations in the measured signal: what seems to be the response to the first block of stimulation has a higher amplitude than the response to the last one shown. There are indeed some low-frequency components in fMRI signals; these can be attributed to scanner drift (small changes in the magnetic field of the scanner over time) and/or to the effect of cardiac and respiratory cycles. As slow fluctuations are something that we expect in the data, we should also define predictors for them. A solution is to model the fluctuations through a discrete cosine transform basis set: a linear combination of cosine waves at several frequencies can accommodate a range of fluctuations. In order to remove any function with a cycle longer than 128 s (the default in SPM) and given the sampling rate and the number of scans, nine components are here required in the basis set. The first two components are displayed in Fig. 8.9d, e. Together, the set of cosine waves will effectively act as a high-pass filter with a 128-s cutoff.

Our best prediction of the observed data in Fig. 8.9a will then be a linear superposition of all the effects and confounds defined above and displayed in Fig. 8.9b–e. This is the assumption underlying the general linear model (GLM): the observed response (BOLD signal) y is expressed in terms of a linear combination of explanatory variables plus a well-behaved error term ε (Friston et al. 1994a):

$$y = X\beta + \varepsilon$$

The matrix X contains column-wise all the predictors that we have defined: everything we know about the experimental design and all potential confounds. This matrix is referred to as the *design matrix*. The one described so far is depicted in Fig. 8.12: it has 84 rows and 11 columns, each representing a predictor (or explanatory variable, covariate, regressor). This is just another way of representing conjointly the time series of Fig. 8.9 as an image where white represents a high value and black a low one.

The relative contribution of each of these columns to the response is controlled by the parameters β. These are the weights or regression coefficients of the GLM and will correspond to the size of the effects that we are measuring. β is a vector whose length is the number of regressors in the design matrix, that is, its number of columns. The β-parameters are the unknown factor in this model.

Finally, the error term ε contains everything that cannot be explained by the model; these values are also known as the residuals, that is, the difference between the data y and the model prediction $X\beta$. In the simplest case, ε is assumed to follow a Gaussian distribution with a mean of zero and a standard deviation σ.

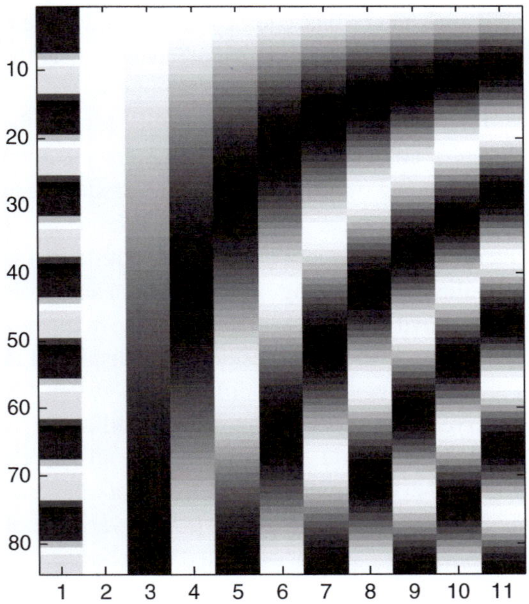

Fig. 8.12 Design matrix for the auditory data set: the first column models the condition-specific effect (boxcar function convolved with the HRF); the next column is a constant term, while the last nine columns are the components of a discrete cosine basis set modelling signal drifts over time. Note that a design matrix as displayed in SPM will not show the last nine terms

The general linear model is a very generic framework that encompasses many standard statistical analysis approaches: multiple regression, analysis of variance (ANOVA), analysis of covariance (ANCOVA)) and t tests can all be framed in the context of a GLM and correspond to a particular form of the design matrix.

Fitting the GLM, or inverting the generative model, is the process of estimating its parameters given the data that we observed. This corresponds to adjusting the β-parameters of the model in order to obtain the best fit of the model to the data. Another way of thinking of this is that we need to find the β-parameters that minimise the error term ε. It can be shown that under the assumption that the errors are normally distributed, the parameters can be estimated using the following equation:

$$\hat{\beta} = \left(X^{\mathrm{T}}X\right)^{-1} X^{\mathrm{T}} y$$

This is the ordinary least squares (OLS) equation that relates the estimated parameters $\hat{\beta}$ to the design matrix X and the observed time series y.

Figure 8.13 shows how the GLM with the design matrix shown in Fig. 8.12 fits the time series shown in Fig. 8.9a and reproduced in Fig. 8.13a in blue. The predicted time series is overlaid in red; it is a linear combination of the stimulus function (Fig. 8.13b), the mean whole brain activity (Fig. 8.13c) and the low-frequency drifts (Fig. 8.13d). The residuals are displayed in Fig. 8.13e; they are the difference between the observed time series and its model prediction.

This procedure is repeated for all voxels within the brain, generating maps of the estimated regression coefficients $\hat{\beta}$. The variance of the noise $\hat{\sigma}^2$ is also estimated voxel-wise. As mentioned above, this is essentially a mass-univariate approach: the same model (design matrix X) is fitted independently to the time series at every voxel, providing local estimates of the effect sizes.

Following on from this description of how data are modelled, there are a few more considerations that need to be taken into account:

- In practice, the low-frequency components from the discrete cosine transform (DCT)) basis set are not added to the design matrix, but the data and design are instead temporally filtered before the model is estimated. This is mathematically identical but computationally more efficient as drift effects will always be confounds of no interest that are not tested. Hence, in practice they do not appear in the design matrix as in Fig. 8.12, but they are still dealt within the background (and the degrees of freedom of the model are adjusted accordingly).
- When using the canonical HRF to model the transfer function from neuronal activity to BOLD response, we assumed that it was known and fixed. However, in practice this is not actually the case; the HRF varies across brain regions and across individuals. A solution is to use a set of basis functions rather than a single function in order to add some flexibility to the modelling of the response. The HRF will then be modelled as a linear combination of these basis functions. A popular choice, providing flexibility and parsimony, is to use the *informed* basis set: this consists of the canonical HRF and its temporal and dispersion derivatives, as shown in Fig. 8.14. According to the weight given to each of the components, the informed basis set allows us to model a shift in the latency of the response (with the temporal derivative) and changes in the width of the response (with the dispersion derivative). When using the informed basis set, each experimental condition is modelled by a set of three regressors, each of which is the neuronal activity stimulus function convolved separately with one of the three components. The predicted response for that condition will be a linear condition of these three regressors. The temporal derivative is also useful to model slice-timing issues. In multislice acquisitions, different slices are acquired at different times. A solution is to temporally realign the data as if they were acquired at the same time through interpolation. This is called slice-timing correction and is a possible option during the preprocessing of the data. Using the informed basis set is an alternative way to correct for the same effect (please see (Sladky et al. 2011) for a comparison of the two approaches).
- fMRI data exhibit short-range serial or temporal correlations. This means that the error at time t is correlated with the error at previous time points. This has to be modelled, because ignoring these correlations may lead to invalid statistical testing. An error covariance matrix must therefore be estimated by assuming some kind of non-sphericity, a departure from the independent and identically distributed assumptions of the noise (Worsley and Friston 1995). A popular model used to capture the typical form of serial correlation in fMRI data is the autoregressive model of order 1, AR(1), relating the error at time t to the error at time $t-1$ with a single parameter. It can be estimated efficiently and precisely by pooling its estimate over voxels. Once the error covariance matrix is estimated, the GLM can be

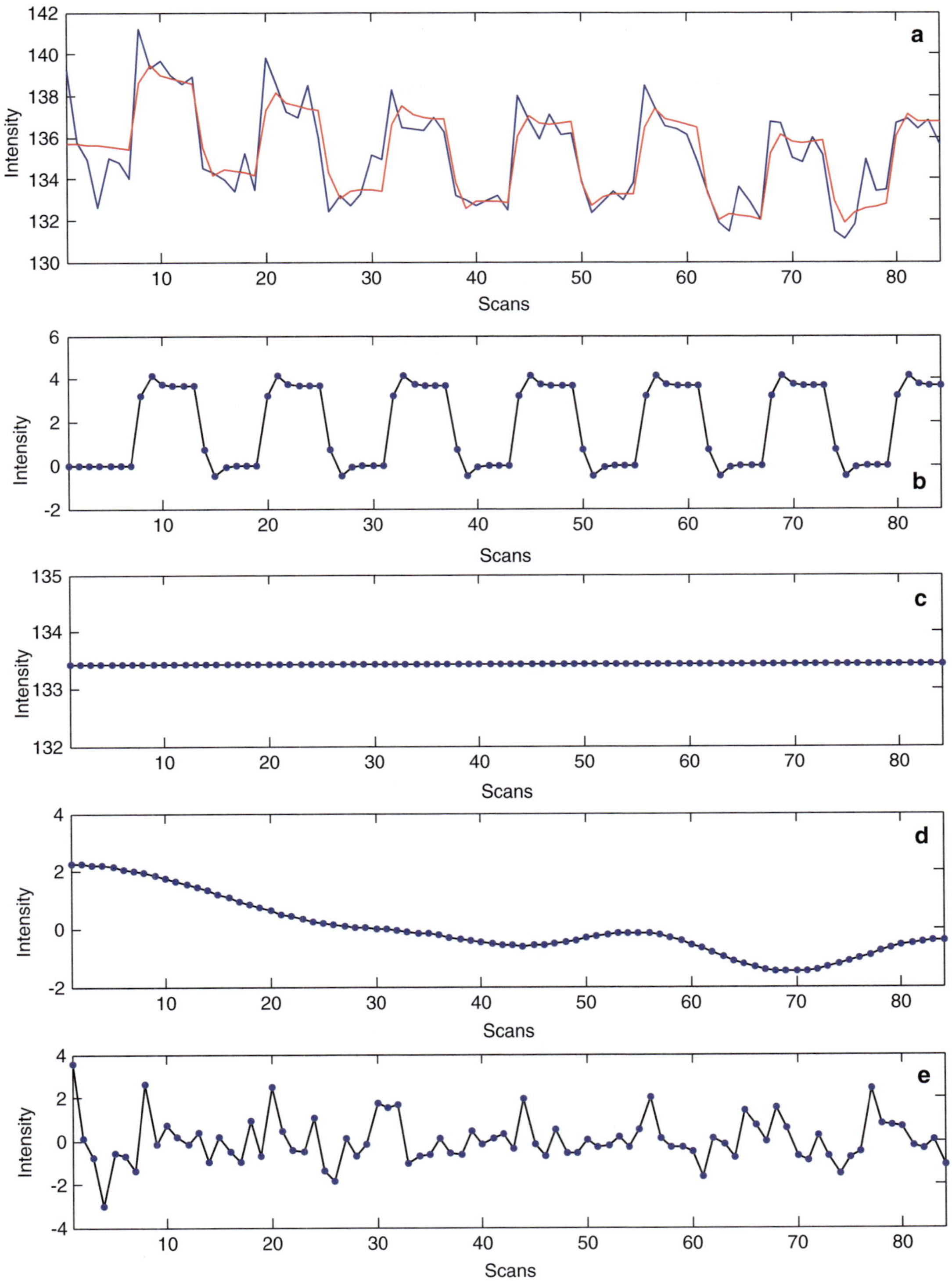

Fig. 8.13 Fit of the GLM defined earlier on the fMRI time series of Fig. 8.9: (**a**) observed fMRI time series in *blue* and model prediction in *red*, fitted predictors for the (**b**) condition-specific effect, (**c**) constant term, (**d**) slow frequency fluctuations and (**e**) residuals

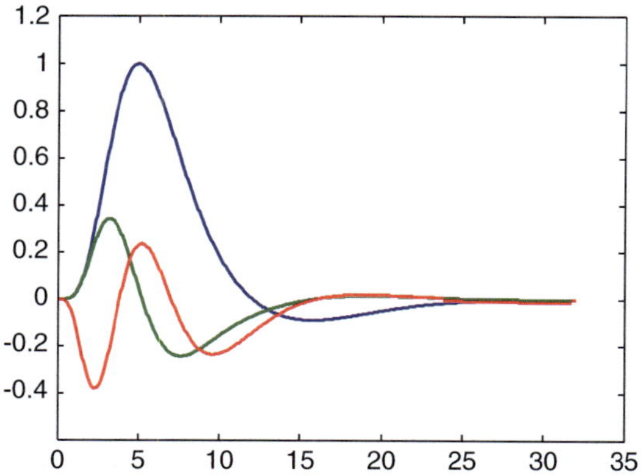

Fig. 8.14 The 'informed' basis set: the canonical HRF (*blue*) and its temporal (*green*) and dispersion (*red*) derivatives

inverted using weighted least squares (WLS)) instead of OLS; alternatively, the estimated error covariance matrix can be used to whiten data and design, that is, to *undo* the serial correlation, so that OLS can be applied again. This is the approach implemented in SPM. A more flexible model of the noise (FAST) is also available for rapidly sampled fMRI time series (Corbin et al. 2018).

- It is also possible to add regressors to the design matrix without going through the convolution process described above. An important example is the modelling of residual movement-related effects. Because movement expresses itself in the data directly and not through any haemodynamic convolution, it can be added directly as a set of explanatory variables. Similarly, in the presence of an abrupt artefact in the data corrupting one scan, a strategy is to model it as a regressor that is zero everywhere but one at that scan. This will effectively covary out that artefactual value in the time series, reducing the inflated variance that it was contributing to. This is better than manually removing that scan prior to analysis as it preserves the temporal process.
- An important distinction in experimental design for fMRI is that between event- and epoch-related designs. Event-related fMRI is simply the use of fMRI to detect responses to individual trials (Josephs et al. 1997). The neuronal activity is usually modelled as a delta function—an *event*—at the trial onset. Practically speaking, in SPM we assume that the duration of a trial is zero. In an epoch-related design, however, we assume that the duration of the trial is greater than zero. This is the case in block-design studies, in which the responses to a sequence of trials (which all evoke the same experimental effect of interest) are modelled together (as an epoch). There are otherwise no conceptual changes in the statistical analysis of event-related and epoch-related (block) designs. One of the advantages of event-related designs is that trials of different types can be intermixed instead of blocking events of the same type together, allowing the measurement of a greater range of psychological effects. There are a number of considerations which impact on the choice of an experimental design, including the constraints imposed by high-pass filtering and haemodynamic convolution of the data affecting its efficiency. We refer interested readers to Chapter 15 of (Friston et al. 2007) or its online version[11] for a thorough examination of design efficiency.

For the auditory data set, the first step is to specify the design matrix; this is done through the 'Specify first-level' button. After specifying a directory in which the results will be stored, the inputs to specify are the units in which the onsets and duration of each trial will be entered (these can be either 'scans' or 'seconds'; we will use 'scans' in this example), the TR (7 s) and the actual preprocessed data to be analysed (the 4D NIfTI file with an '*sw*' prefix). In this data set, there is just one condition to specify: the onsets are [6 18 30 42 54 66 78], corresponding to the scan number at the beginning of each auditory stimulation block, and the durations are [*6*], indicating that each auditory stimulation block lasts for six scans (with a rest block in between each one). The movement parameters can be added as extra regressors using the 'Multiple regressors' entry by selecting the '*rp_*.txt*' file that was

[11] http://imaging.mrc-cbu.cam.ac.uk/imaging/DesignEfficiency.

saved during the realignment. Other parameters can be left as default, especially the high-pass filter cut-off (128 s), the use of the canonical HRF only and the modelling of serial correlation using an AR(1) model. The output is an *SPM.mat* file; this contains all the information about the data and the model design. The design matrix is also displayed for review. As expected, it has eight columns: the first column is the block stimulus function convolved by the HRF, the following six columns are the movement parameters (three translations and three rotations, see Fig. 8.5) and the last column is a constant term modelling the whole brain activity. The 'Estimate' button then allows us to invert this GLM and estimate its parameters. A number of image files will be created, including eight maps of the estimated regression coefficients, one for each column of the design matrix (*beta_*.nii*) and one mask image (*mask.nii*), which contains a binary volume indicating which voxels were included in the analysis.

8.4.2 Contrasts

Having specified and estimated parameters of the general linear model, the next step is to make a statistical inference about those parameters. This is done by using their estimated variance. Some of the parameters will be of interest (those pertaining to the experimental conditions), while others will be of no interest (those pertaining to confounding effects). Inference allows one to test the null hypothesis that all the estimates are zero, using the F-statistic to give an *SPM{F}*, or that some particular linear combination (e.g. a subtraction) of the estimates is zero, using the t-statistic to give an *SPM{t}*. A linear combination of regression coefficients is called a *contrast*, and its corresponding vector of weights c is called a contrast vector.

The t-statistic is obtained by dividing a contrast (specified by contrast weights) of the associated parameter estimates by the standard error of that contrast. The latter is estimated using the variance of the residuals $\hat{\sigma}^2$.

$$T = \frac{c^{\mathrm{T}}\hat{\beta}}{\sqrt{\hat{\sigma}^2 c^{\mathrm{T}}\left(X^{\mathrm{T}}X\right)^{-1}c}}$$

This is essentially a signal-to-noise ratio, comparing an effect size with its precision.

An example of a contrast vector would be $c^{\mathrm{T}} = [1 \quad -1 \quad 0 \quad \ldots]$ to compare the difference in responses evoked by two conditions, modelled by the first two condition-specific regressors in the design matrix. In SPM, a t test is signed, in the sense that a contrast vector $c^{\mathrm{T}} = [1 \quad -1 \quad 0 \quad \ldots]$ is looking for a greater response in the first condition than in the second condition, while a contrast $c^{\mathrm{T}} = [-1 \quad 1 \quad 0 \quad \ldots]$ is looking for the opposite effect. In other words, it means that a t-contrast tests the null hypothesis $c^{\mathrm{T}}\beta = 0$ against the one-sided alternative $c^{\mathrm{T}}\beta > 0$. The resulting *SPM{t}* is a statistic image, with each voxel value being the value of the t-statistic for the specified contrast at that location. Areas of the *SPM{t}* with high voxel values (higher than one might expect by chance) indicate evidence for 'neural activations'.

Similarly, if you have a design where the third column in the design matrix is a covariate, then the corresponding parameter is essentially a regression slope, and a contrast with weights $c^{\mathrm{T}} = [0 \quad 0 \quad 1 \quad 0 \quad \ldots]$ tests the hypothesis of zero regression slope, against the alternative of a positive slope. This is equivalent to a test of no correlation, against the alternative of positive correlation. If there are other terms in the model beyond a constant term and the covariate, then this correlation is a partial correlation, the correlation between the data and the covariate after accounting for the other effects (Andrade et al. 1999).

Sometimes, several contrasts of parameter estimates are jointly interesting. In these instances, an *SPM{F}* is used and is specified with a matrix of contrast weights which can be thought of as a collection of t-contrasts. An F-contrast might look like this

$$c^{\mathrm{T}} = \begin{bmatrix} 1 & 0 & 0 & 0 & \ldots \\ 0 & -1 & 0 & 0 & \ldots \end{bmatrix}$$

This would test for the significance of the first or the second parameter estimates. The fact that the second weight is negative has no effect on the test because the F-statistic is blind to sign as it is based on sums of squares. The F-statistic can also be interpreted as a model comparison device, comparing two nested models using the extra sum-of-squares principle. For the F-contrast above, this corresponds to comparing the specified full model with a reduced model where the first two columns would have been removed. F-contrasts are mainly used either as two-sided tests (the *SPM{F}* then being the square of the corresponding *SPM{t}*) or to test the significance of effects modelled by several columns. Effects modelled by several columns might include the use of a multiple basis set to model the HRF, a polynomial expansion of a parametric modulated response or a contrast testing more than two levels in a factorial design.

As with the *SPM{t}*, the resulting *SPM{F}* is a statistic image, with voxel values the value of the F-statistic for the specified contrast at that location. Areas of the *SPM{F}* with high voxel values indicate evidence for 'neural activations'.

8.4.3 Topological Inference

Having computed the statistic, we need to decide whether it represents convincing evidence of the effect in which we are interested; this decision is the process of making a statistical inference. This is done by testing the statistic against the null hypothesis that there is no effect. Here, the null hypothesis is distributed according to a known parametric probability density function, a Student's t- or F-distribution. Then, by choosing a significance level (which is the level of control over the false-positive error rate, usually chosen as 0.05), we can derive a critical threshold above which we will reject the null hypothesis and accept the alternative hypothesis that there is convincing evidence of an effect. If the observed statistic is lower than the critical threshold, we fail to reject the null hypothesis and we must conclude that there is no convincing evidence of an effect. A p value can also be computed to measure the evidence against the null hypothesis: this is the probability of observing a statistic at least as large as the one observed under the null hypothesis (i.e. by chance).

The problem we face in functional imaging is that we are not dealing with a single statistic value, but with an image that comprises many thousands of voxels and their associated statistical values. This gives rise to the multiple comparisons problem, which is a consequence of the use of a mass-univariate approach: as a general rule, without using an appropriate method of correction, the greater the number of voxels tested, the greater the number of false positives. This is clearly unacceptable and requires the definition of a new null hypothesis which takes into account the whole volume, or family, of statistics contained in an image: the *family-wise* null hypothesis that there is no effect *anywhere* in the entire search volume (e.g. the brain). We then aim to control the family-wise error rate (FWER))—the probability of making one or more false positives over the entire search volume. This results in adjusted p values, *corrected* for the search volume.

A traditional statistical method for controlling FWER is to use the Bonferroni correction, in which a voxel-wise significance level simply corresponds to the family-wise significance level (e.g. 0.05) divided by the number of tests (i.e. voxels). However, this approach assumes that every test (voxel statistic) is independent and is too conservative to use in the presence of correlation between tests, such as the case with functional imaging data. Functional imaging data are intrinsically smoothed due to the acquisition process and have also been smoothed as part of the spatial preprocessing; neighbouring voxel statistics are therefore not independent. The random field theory (RFT) provides a way of adjusting the p value to take this into account (Worsley et al. 1992, 1996; Friston et al. 1994b). Providing that data are smooth, the RFT adjustment is less severe (i.e. more sensitive) than a Bonferroni correction for the number of voxels. The p value is a function of the search volume and *smoothness* (parameterised as the FWHM of the Gaussian kernel required to simulate images with the same apparent spatial smoothness as the one we observe). A description of the random field theory is well beyond the scope of this chapter (see Flandin and Friston 2015, 2017), but it is worth mentioning that one of the assumptions for its application on discrete data fields is that the observed fields are smooth. This was one of the motivations for smoothing the fMRI data as a preprocessing step. In practice, smoothness will be estimated from the data themselves (to take into account both intrinsic and explicit smoothness) (Kiebel et al. 1999). The RFT correction discounts voxel sizes by expressing the search volume in terms of smoothness or resolution elements (*resels*).

To make inferences about regionally specific effects, the SPM is thresholded using height and spatial extent thresholds that are specified by the user. Corrected p values can then be derived that pertain to topological features of the thresholded map (Friston et al. 1996a):

- The number of activated regions (i.e. the number of clusters above the height and volume threshold). These are *set-level* inferences.
- The number of activated voxels (i.e. the volume or extent) comprising a particular cluster. These are *cluster-level* inferences.
- The height of each local maxima, or peak, within that cluster. These are *peak-level* inferences.

Set-level inferences are generally more powerful than cluster-level inferences, which are themselves generally more powerful than peak-level inferences. The price paid for this increased sensitivity is a reduced localising power. Peak-level tests permit individual maxima to be identified as significant, whereas cluster and set-level inferences only allow clusters or a set of clusters to be declared significant. In some cases, however, focal activation might actually be detected with greater sensitivity using tests based on peak height (with a spatial extent threshold of zero). In practice, this is the most commonly used level of inference, reflecting the fact that characterisation of functional anatomy is generally more useful when specified with a high degree of anatomical precision.

When making inferences about regional effects in SPMs, one often has some idea *a priori* about where the activation should be. In this instance, a correction for the entire search volume is inappropriately stringent. Instead, a small search volume within which analyses will be carried out can be specified beforehand, and an RFT correction applied restricted to that region only (Worsley et al. 1996). This is often referred to as a small volume correction (SVC)).

For the auditory data set, inference is performed through the 'Results' button by selecting the *SPM.mat* file from the previous step. To test for the positive effect of passive listening to words versus rest, the t-contrast to enter is $c^{\mathrm{T}} = [1 \quad 0 \quad 0 \quad 0 \quad 0 \quad 0 \quad 0 \quad 0]$. Two files will be created on disk at this stage: a *con_0001.nii* file of the contrast image (here identical to *beta_0001.nii*) and the corresponding *SPM{T} spmT_0001.nii*. Choosing a 0.05 FWE-corrected threshold yields the results displayed in Fig. 8.15. The maximum intensity projection (MIP) image gives an overview of the activated regions, the auditory cortices. This can be overlaid on the anatomy of the subject (the normalised '*w*.nii*' image file) using the menu entry 'Overlays>Sections' of the Interactive window or on a canonical mesh by choosing the 'Render' option and selecting one of the GIfTI files ('*.*surf.gii*') from the 'canonical' directory from the SPM distribution (see Fig. 8.16). The button 'whole brain' will display the results table (see Fig. 8.17) listing the p values adjusted for the search volume (the whole brain here) for all topological features of the excursion set: local maxima height for peak-level inference, cluster extent for cluster-level inference and number of clusters for set-level inference. The footnote of the results table lists some numbers pertaining to the RFT: the estimated FWHM smoothness is [*9.9 9.9 8.4*] in mm and the number of resels is 2067 here. These are the values reflecting the size and smoothness of the search volume that are used to control for the FWER.

Guidelines for reporting an fMRI study in a publication are given in Nichols et al. (2017).

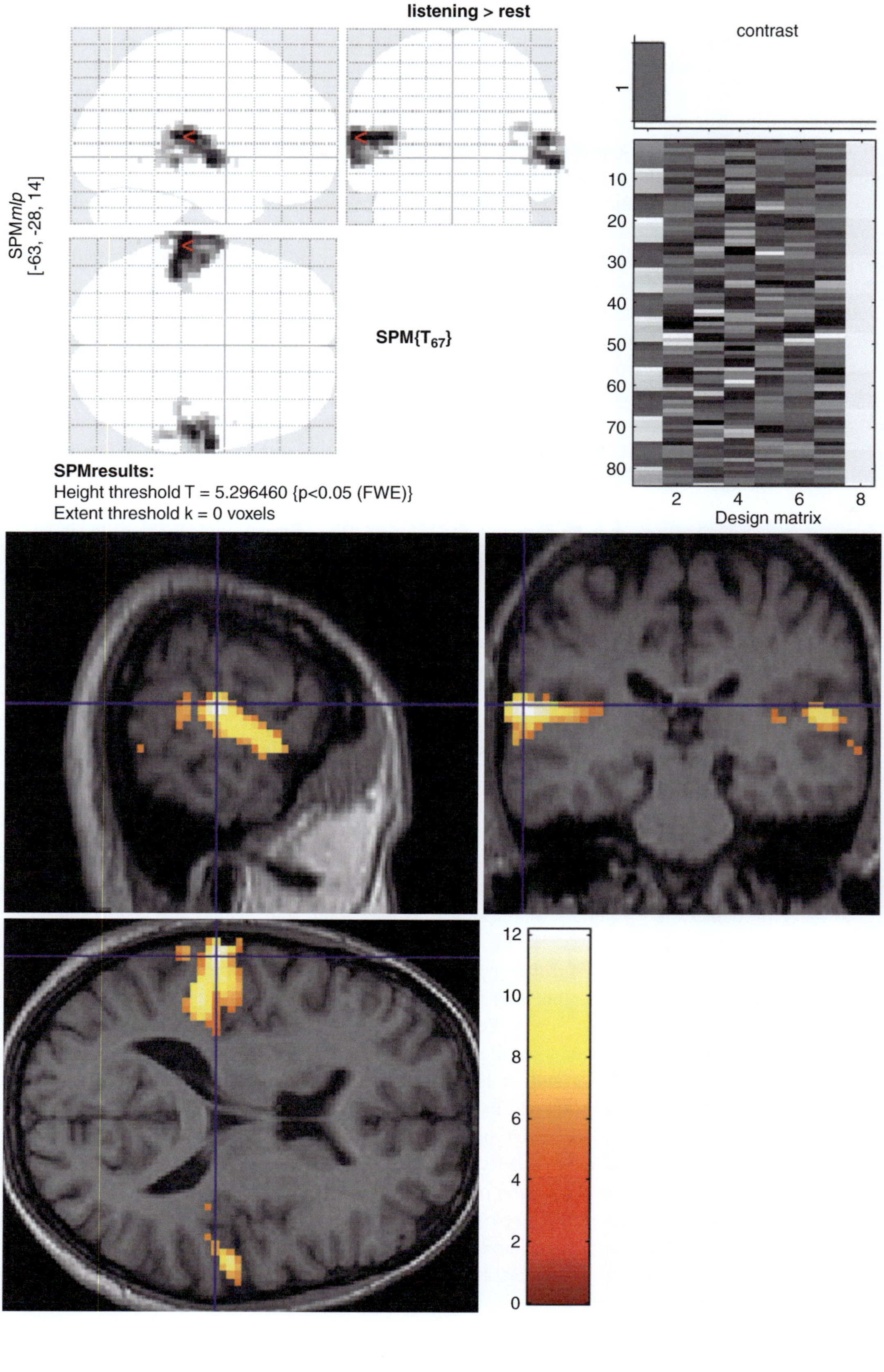

listening > rest
contrast
SPMmip
[-63, -28, 14]
SPM{T67}
SPMresults:
Height threshold T = 5.296460 {p<0.05 (FWE)}
Extent threshold k = 0 voxels
Design matrix

Fig. 8.15 Results of the statistical inference for the auditory data set when looking for regions showing an increased activity when words are passively listened to in comparison with rest. *Top right*: design matrix and contrast $c^{\mathrm{T}} = [1\ \ 0\ \ 0\ \ 0\ \ 0\ \ 0\ \ 0\ \ 0]$. *Top left*: *SPM{t}* displayed as a maximum intensity projection over three orthogonal planes. To control for $p < 0.05$ corrected, the applied threshold was $T = 5.28$. *Lower panel*: Thresholded *SPM{t}* overlaid on the normalised structural scan of that subject, highlighting the bilateral activation

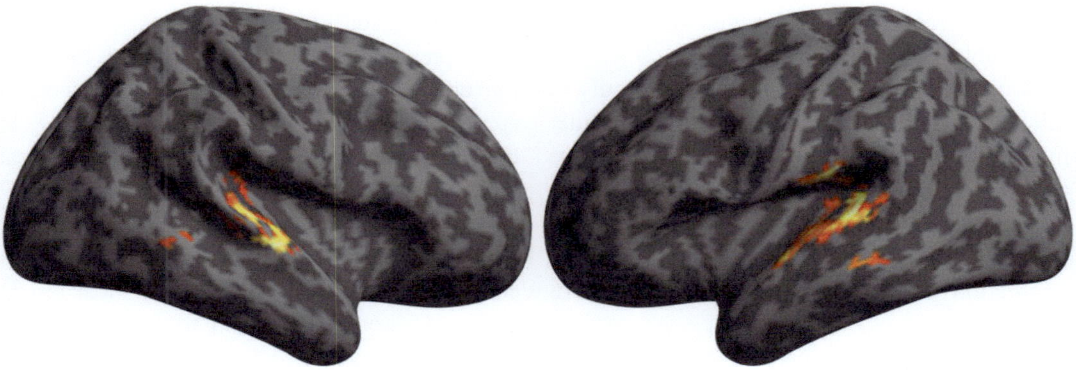

Fig. 8.16 Thresholded *SPM{t}* overlaid on a canonical mesh, also highlighting the bilateral activation following auditory stimulation

Statistics: ***p-values adjusted for search volume***

Set-level		cluster-level				peak-level					mm	mm	mm
p	c	$p_{\text{FWE-corr}}$	$q_{\text{FDR-corr}}$	k_E	p_{uncorr}	$p_{\text{FWE-corr}}$	$q_{\text{FDR-corr}}$	T	$(Z_{\equiv})$	p_{uncorr}			
0.000	6	**0.000**	**0.000**	**416**	**0.000**	**0.000**	**0.000**	**12.13**	**Inf**	**0.000**	**-63**	**-28**	**14**
						0.000	0.000	11.33	Inf	0.000	-45	-34	11
						0.000	0.000	10.12	7.84	0.000	-66	-10	-1
		0.000	**0.000**	**216**	**0.000**	**0.000**	**0.000**	**12.09**	**Inf**	**0.000**	**57**	**-22**	**11**
						0.000	0.000	11.12	Inf	0.000	66	-13	-4
						0.000	0.002	7.19	6.17	0.000	60	-37	5
		0.001	**0.024**	**5**	**0.012**	**0.007**	**0.244**	**5.79**	**5.19**	**0.000**	**66**	**-25**	**-1**
		0.015	**0.220**	**1**	**0.220**	**0.013**	**0.379**	**5.64**	**5.08**	**0.000**	**72**	**-34**	**-10**
		0.015	**0.220**	**1**	**0.220**	**0.027**	**0.614**	**5.46**	**4.95**	**0.000**	**-63**	**-58**	**-4**
		0.006	**0.136**	**2**	**0.091**	**0.035**	**0.727**	**5.39**	**4.90**	**0.000**	**51**	**5**	**-7**

table shows 3 local maxima more than 8.0mm apart

Height threshold: T = 5.30, p = 0.000 (0.050)
Extent threshold: k = 0 voxels
Expected voxels per cluster, <k> = 0.714
Expected number of clusters, <c> = 0.07
FWEp: 5.296, FDRp: 6.557, FWEc: 1, FDRc: 5

Degrees of freedom = [1.0, 67.0]
FWHM = 9.9 9.9 8.4 mm mm mm; 3.3 3.3 2.8 {voxels}
Volume: 1911168 = 70784 voxels = 2066.8 resels
Voxel size: 3.0 3.0 3.0 mm mm mm; (resel = 30.61 voxels)

Fig. 8.17 Results table summarising the inferences made with the *t*-contrast $c^{\mathrm{T}} = [1\ \ 0\ \ 0\ \ 0\ \ 0\ \ 0\ \ 0\ \ 0]$, adjusted for the search volume (the whole brain in this case). See text for description of the key elements

8.4.4 Population-Level Inference

Neuroimaging data from multiple subjects can be analysed using fixed-effects (FFX) or random-effects (RFX) analyses (Holmes and Friston 1998). FFX analysis is used for reporting case studies, while RFX is used to make inferences about the population from which the subjects were drawn. In the former, the error variance is estimated on a scan-by-scan basis and contains contributions from within-subject variance only. We are therefore not making formal inference about population effects using FFX, but are restricted to informal inferences based on separate case studies or summary images showing the average group effect. (This is implemented in SPM by concatenating data from all subjects into the same GLM, simply modelling subjects as coming from separate sessions.) Conversely, random-effects analyses take into account both sources of variance (within- and between-subject). The term '*random effect*' indicates that we have accommodated the randomness of different responses from subject to subject.

Both analyses are perfectly valid but only in relation to the inferences that are being made: inferences based on fixed-effect analyses are about the particular subjects studied. Random-effects analyses are usually more conservative but allow the inference to be generalised to the population from which the subjects were drawn.

In practice, RFX analyses can be implemented using the computationally efficient '*summary-statistic*' approach. Contrasts of parameters estimated from a *first-level* (within-subject) analysis are entered into a *second-level* (between-subject) analysis. The second-level design matrix then simply tests the null hypothesis that the contrasts are zero (and is usually a column of ones, implementing a one-sample t test). The validity of the approach rests upon the use of balanced designs (all subjects have identical design matrices and error variances) but has been shown to be remarkably robust to violations of this assumption (Mumford and Nichols 2009).

For our auditory data set, if we had scanned 16 subjects, for example, each of whom performed the same task, the group analysis would entail (1) applying the same spatial preprocessings to each of the 16 subjects, (2) fitting a first-level GLM independently to each of the 16 subjects, (3) defining the effect of interest for each subject with a contrast vector $c^{\mathrm{T}} = [1 \quad 0 \quad 0 \quad 0 \quad 0 \quad 0 \quad 0 \quad 0]$ and producing a contrast image containing the contrast of the parameter estimates at each voxel and (4) feeding each of the 16 contrast images into a second-level GLM, through which a one-sample t test could be carried out across all 16 subjects to find the activations that show significant evidence of a population effect.

8.5 Conclusions

In this chapter we have described how statistical parametric mapping can be used to identify and characterise regionally specific effects in functional MRI data. We have also illustrated the principles of SPM through the analysis of a block-design data set using the SPM software. After preprocessing the data to correct them for movement and normalise them into a standard space, the general linear model and random field theory are used to analyse and make classical inferences. The GLM is used to model BOLD responses to given experimental manipulations. The estimated parameters of the GLM are used to compute a standard univariate statistical test at each and every voxel, leading to the construction of statistical parametric maps. The random field theory is then used to resolve the multiple comparisons problem induced by inferences over a volume of the brain containing many voxels. RFT provides a method for adjusting p values for the search volume of a statistical parametric map to control false-positive rates.

We have here described the fundamental methods used to carry out fMRI analyses in SPM. There are, however, many additional approaches and tools that can be used to refine and extend analyses, such as voxel-based morphometry (VBM) to analyse structural data sets (Ashburner and Friston 2000; Ridgway et al. 2008) and dynamic causal modelling (DCM) to study effective connectivity (Friston et al. 2003; Stephan et al. 2010; Kahan and Foltynie 2013). While the key steps of the SPM approach we describe above remain broadly constant, SPM software (along with many other software analysis packages) is constantly evolving to incorporate advances in neuroimaging analysis; we encourage readers to explore these exciting new developments.

References

Andersen SM, Rapcsak SZ et al (2010) Cost function masking during normalization of brains with focal lesions: still a necessity? NeuroImage 53:78–84. https://doi.org/10.1016/j.neuroimage.2010.06.003

Andersson JLR, Hutton C et al (2001) Modeling geometric deformations in EPI time series. NeuroImage 13:903–919. https://doi.org/10.1006/nimg.2001.0746

Andrade A, Paradis AL et al (1999) Ambiguous results in functional neuroimaging data analysis due to covariate correlation. NeuroImage 10:483–486. https://doi.org/10.1006/nimg.1999.0479

Ashburner J (2011) SPM: a history. NeuroImage. https://doi.org/10.1016/j.neuroimage.2011.10.025

Ashburner J, Friston KJ (1999) Nonlinear spatial normalization using basis functions. Hum Brain Mapp 7:254–266

Ashburner J, Friston KJ (2000) Voxel-based morphometry—the methods. NeuroImage 11:805–821. https://doi.org/10.1006/nimg.2000.0582

Ashburner J, Friston KJ (2005) Unified segmentation. NeuroImage 26:839–851. https://doi.org/10.1016/j.neuroimage.2005.02.018

Brett M, Leff AP et al (2001) Spatial normalization of brain images with focal lesions using cost function masking. NeuroImage 14:486–500. https://doi.org/10.1006/nimg.2001.0845

Brett M, Johnsrude IS et al (2002) The problem of functional localization in the human brain. Nat Rev Neurosci 3:243–249. https://doi.org/10.1038/nrn756

Collignon A, Maes F et al (1995) Automated multimodality image registration based on information theory. In: Proceedings of information processing in medical imaging (IPMI), Ile de Berder, 1995

Corbin N, Todd N, Friston KJ, Callaghan MF (2018) Accurate modeling of temporal correlations in rapidly sampled fMRI time series. Hum Brain Mapping 39(10):3884–3897. https://doi.org/10.1002/hbm.24218

Crinion J, Ashburner J et al (2007) Spatial normalization of lesioned brains: performance evaluation and impact on fMRI analyses. NeuroImage 37:866–875. https://doi.org/10.1016/j.neuroimage.2007.04.065

Flandin G, Friston KJ (2008) Statistical parametric mapping (SPM). Scholarpedia 3(4):6232. https://doi.org/10.4249/scholarpedia.6232

Flandin G, Friston KJ (2015) Topological inference. In: Brain mapping: an encyclopedic reference. Academic Press, Cambridge, MA, pp 495–500

Flandin G, Friston KJ (2017) Analysis of family-wise error rates in statistical parametric mapping using random field theory. Hum Brain Mapp. https://doi.org/10.1002/hbm.23839

Fox PT (1995) Spatial normalization origins: objectives, applications, and alternatives. Hum Brain Mapp 3:161–164. https://doi.org/10.1002/hbm.460030302

Friston KJ, Frith CD et al (1991) Comparing functional (PET) images: the assessment of significant change. J Cereb Blood Flow Metab 11:690–699. https://doi.org/10.1038/jcbfm.1991.122

Friston KJ, Holmes AP et al (1994a) Statistical parametric maps in functional imaging: a general linear approach. Hum Brain Mapp 2:189–210. https://doi.org/10.1002/hbm.460020402

Friston KJ, Worsley KJ et al (1994b) Assessing the significance of focal activations using their spatial extent. Hum Brain Mapp 1:210–220. https://doi.org/10.1002/hbm.460010306

Friston KJ, Ashburner J et al (1995) Spatial registration and normalization of images. Hum Brain Mapp 3:165–189. https://doi.org/10.1002/hbm.460030303

Friston KJ, Holmes A et al (1996a) Detecting activations in PET and fMRI: levels of inference and power. NeuroImage 4:223–235. https://doi.org/10.1006/nimg.1996.0074

Friston KJ, Williams S et al (1996b) Movement-related effects in fMRI time-series. Magn Reson Med 35:346–355

Friston KJ, Harrison L et al (2003) Dynamic causal modelling. NeuroImage 19:1273–1302

Friston K, Ashburner J et al (2007) Statistical parametric mapping: the analysis of functional brain images. Elsevier/Academic, Amsterdam/Boston

Gorgolewski KJ, Auer T, Calhoun VD, Craddock RC, Das S, Duff EP et al (2016) The brain imaging data structure, a format for organizing and describing outputs of neuroimaging experiments. Scientific Data 3:160044

Holmes A, Friston K (1998) Generalisability, random effects and population inference. NeuroImage 7:S754

Jezzard P, Balaban RS (1995) Correction for geometric distortion in echo planar images from B0 field variations. Magn Reson Med 34:65–73

Josephs O, Turner R et al (1997) Event-related fMRI. Hum Brain Mapp 5:243–248

Kahan J, Foltynie T (2013) Understanding DCM: ten simple rules for the clinician. NeuroImage 83:542–549. https://doi.org/10.1016/j.neuroimage.2013.07.008

Kiebel SJ, Poline JB et al (1999) Robust smoothness estimation in statistical parametric maps using standardized residuals from the general linear model. NeuroImage 10:756–766. https://doi.org/10.1006/nimg.1999.0508

Malone IB, Leung KK, Clegg S, Barnes J, Whitwell JL, Ashburner J et al (2015) Accurate automatic estimation of total intracranial volume: a nuisance variable with less nuisance. NeuroImage 104:366–372

Mazziotta JC, Toga AW et al (1995) A probabilistic atlas of the human brain: theory and rationale for its development. The international consortium for brain mapping (ICBM). NeuroImage 2:89–101

Mumford JA, Nichols T (2009) Simple group fMRI modeling and inference. NeuroImage 47:1469–1475. https://doi.org/10.1016/j.neuroimage.2009.05.034

Nichols TE, Das S, Eickhoff SB, Evans AC, Glatard T, Hanke M et al (2017 Feb 23) Best practices in data analysis and sharing in neuroimaging using MRI. Nat Neurosci 20:299–303

Ridgway GR, Henley SMD et al (2008) Ten simple rules for reporting voxel-based morphometry studies. NeuroImage 40:1429–1435. https://doi.org/10.1016/j.neuroimage.2008.01.003

Sladky R, Friston KJ et al (2011) Slice-timing effects and their correction in functional MRI. NeuroImage 58:588–594. https://doi.org/10.1016/j.neuroimage.2011.06.078

Stephan KE, Penny WD et al (2010) Ten simple rules for dynamic causal modeling. NeuroImage 49:3099–3109. https://doi.org/10.1016/j.neuroimage.2009.11.015

Talairach J, Tournoux P (1988) Co-planar stereotaxic atlas of the human brain: an approach to medical cerebral imaging. Thieme Medical, New York

Unser M, Aldroubi A et al (1993) B-spline signal processing. I. Theory. IEEE Trans Signal Process 41:821–833. https://doi.org/10.1109/78.193220

Weiskopf N, Lutti A, Helms G, Novak M, Ashburner J, Hutton C (2011) Unified segmentation based correction of R1 brain maps for RF transmit field inhomogeneities (UNICORT). NeuroImage 54(3):2116–2124

Wells WM 3rd, Viola P et al (1996) Multi-modal volume registration by maximization of mutual information. Med Image Anal 1:35–51

Worsley KJ, Friston KJ (1995) Analysis of fMRI time-series revisited—again. NeuroImage 2:173–181. https://doi.org/10.1006/nimg.1995.1023

Worsley K, Evans A et al (1992) A three-dimensional statistical analysis for CBF activation studies in human brain. J Cereb Blood Flow Metab 12:900–918

Worsley KJ, Marrett S et al (1996) A unified statistical approach for determining significant signals in images of cerebral activation. Hum Brain Mapp 4:58–73

9 Meta-Analyses in Basic and Clinical Neuroscience: State of the Art and Perspective

Simon B. Eickhoff, Julius Kernbach, and Danilo Bzdok

9.1 An Introduction to Quantitative Meta-Analysis in Neuroimaging Science

While a major overarching goal of systems neuroscience research is to unveil the dysfunctional neural mechanisms that underlie neurological and psychiatric disorders, such endeavor will be futile without a profound understanding of the physiological organization of brain functions. That is, to appreciate the relationship between localized changes in brain structure or function and pathological mental states or functional impairments, we have to elucidate the regionally specific localization of mental processes. Until about 20 years ago, the most common approaches to localize human brain functions consisted in lesion studies and direct brain stimulation during neurosurgical interventions. The beginning of the functional neuroimaging era by positron emission tomography (PET) and functional magnetic resonance imaging (fMRI) then enabled the non-invasive, in vivo investigation of functional specialization in the human brain. Based on local changes in cerebral blood flow, glucose or oxygen metabolism, these techniques allow the identification of regional increases in neural activation during the performance of specific tasks. Usually, the neural correlates of a given task (reflecting a mental process of interest) are isolated by subtraction of the activation measured during a closely related task (i.e., control task) that is supposed not to evoke the psychological process of interest. Evidently, the spectrum of neuroimaging-compatible tasks is practically only limited by the scanner surroundings and the interdiction of head movements. In fact, the constantly increasing publication rate currently counts more than 1000 new neuroimaging articles per year (Derrfuss and Mar 2009). PubMed searches for PET and (f)MRI studies likewise revealed a permanently expanding number of published studies. In 2015, the total papers amounted to more than ~24,000 published neuroimaging experiments (Eickhoff et al. 2016). Functional neuroimaging has hence provided a wealth of

S. B. Eickhoff (✉)
Institute of Systems Neuroscience, Medical Faculty, Heinrich Heine University Düsseldorf, Düsseldorf, Germany

Institute of Neuroscience and Medicine, Brain & Behaviour (INM-7), Research Centre Jülich, Jülich, Germany
e-mail: s.eickhoff@fz-juelich.de

J. Kernbach
Department of Psychiatry, Psychotherapy and Psychosomatics, RWTH Aachen University, Aachen, Germany

D. Bzdok
Department of Psychiatry, Psychotherapy and Psychosomatics, RWTH Aachen University, Aachen, Germany

Parietal Team, INRIA, Gif-sur-Yvette, France

JARA-BRAIN, Jülich-Aachen Research Alliance, Aachen, Germany

S. Ulmer, O. Jansen (eds.), *fMRI*, https://doi.org/10.1007/978-3-030-41874-8_9

information on the cerebral localization of sensory processing, motor actions, as well as cognitive and affective functions.

In spite of its success in revealing the location of regionally specific effects in health and disease, however, functional neuroimaging using PET or fMRI suffers from several limitations that restrict the amount of knowledge that may be gained from each individual imaging experiment:

First, there is the small sample size. Usually, between 15 and 30 subjects participate in a neuroimaging study. Although this denotes a remarkable increase since the beginnings of neuroimaging science, it is still a rather small sample size comparing to other scientific disciplines, such as social sciences, population genetics, or clinical trials. Moreover, in contrast to, for example, experimental psychology, the considerable logistical and financial efforts of each neuroimaging study discourage replication studies as well as the combination of several studies into one paper, leading at times to the publication of isolated findings. It must be remembered that both PET and fMRI scanners measure neuronal activity in an indirect way by the triggered regional increases of metabolic respectively hemodynamic brain activity. On the one hand, the recorded signals are thus potentially confounded by a vast range of biological, technical, and methodological factors, which reduce the reliability of the obtained results. In fact, the underlying relationship between neuronal activity and measured signals is currently not exhaustively understood. On the other hand, PET and fMRI yield relative, rather than absolute, signals related to neuronal activity. The neural correlates underlying a given psychological task thus need to be derived by subtraction between two experimental conditions rendering the resulting activation pattern context dependent. In fact, it has repeatedly been questioned that conclusions on general physiological or pathological mechanisms can be drawn if relying on the neuroimaging-inherent subtraction logic (Stark and Squire 2001). In other words, even though frequently discussed in terms of general mechanisms, the results of a particular neuroimaging study actually just impart the difference of the two specifically chosen conditions.

These diverse limitations of any neuroimaging study thus severely lessen the amount of knowledge that may be gained from each individual neuroimaging study. This consideration has consequently prompted a need for synthesizing and integrating existing research. By judging concordance and variability across a high number of studies, the limitation of each individual PET or fMRI experiment may be overcome, and a synoptic view on published isolated findings can be acquired. Therefore, the sheer abundance of available neuroimaging studies encouraged the development of quantitative meta-analysis approaches. Such model-based neuroinformatic methods allow statistically summarizing hundreds of neuroimaging studies across a large number of participants and diverse experimental settings, which considerably strengthens ensuing conclusions on the organizational principles of the healthy and diseased brain. In the course of the last years, the field of quantitative meta-analysis has been increasingly dominated by methods for coordinate-based meta-analysis (CBMA). Image-based meta-analysis (Schilbach et al. 2008), on the other hand, draws on the full statistic images and, thus, acknowledges the entirety of the spatial information of each neuroimaging experiment. Yet, these approaches usually rely on a much smaller experiment samples, as the original data is often considerably more difficult to obtain than activation coordinates and only comparable contrast images are eligible. Rather than pooling raw data or complete activation maps of previous neuroimaging experiments, CBMA only assesses convergence of the reported peak coordinates. As algorithms for CBMA hence rest on the model-based integration of published activation coordinates, they can potentially be applied to the entirety of the available literature. Applying CBMA to the published neuroimaging experiments on a specific topic (e.g., the brain areas related to grammar processing) thus permits to identify the quintessence of emergent knowledge in that entire field in an unbiased fashion without being skewed by experimental idiosyncrasies or neuroanatomical variability.

To this end, CBMA tries to answer the following question: where in the brain do the included activation foci cluster more tightly than it would be expected if they were randomly distributed? In statistical terms, the assumption of random distribution of the considered activation foci will be rejected in those voxels where the amount of convergence between reported foci is greater than expected by chance, yielding statistically defensible inference on the integration of previous findings. Taken together, CBMA is able to objectively synthesize large amounts of neuroimaging data and overcome the limitations of each individual experiment raised above.

9.2 Preconditions and Preliminaries of Quantitative Meta-Analysis

The feasibility and potential of quantitative integration for functional neuroimaging results is greatly aided by the high standardization for the reporting of neuroimaging data, which is brought upon by two important preconditions that thus paved the way for the emergence of meta-analyses. First, almost from the beginning of neuroimaging research, investigators adopted common stereotactic coordinate systems for specifying localization information, rather than relying purely on neuroanatomical nomenclatures. That is, most neuroimaging articles report significant activation foci according to either the Talairach and Tournoux (1988) or Montreal Neurological Institute [MNI; (Evans et al. 1992)] 3D reference space, which can be easily converted into each other (Lancaster et al. 2007). A common coordinate system is crucial because neuroimaging data is formally processed by cubical "voxels" and not by brain regions. The variably sized and shaped "native" brains of the participants therefore need to be warped to a "standard" brain space to enable comparison within and across neuroimaging studies. Second, results of functional imaging experiments are conventionally reported as coordinates for local maxima in standard coordinates provided in tables grouped by the contrast experiment from which they were derived. That is, tables usually provide all peak coordinates of significant differences in brain activity for each comparison between two conditions. These early established standards for spatial normalization to common reference systems and for communicating activation results as coordinates in these reference spaces greatly contributed to the accessibility of existing neuroimaging studies.

Any meta-analysis starts out by a thorough literature search for relevant publications pertaining to the research question. Literature databases, such as PubMed (www.ncbi.nlm.nih.gov), ISI Web of Knowledge (apps.webofknowledge.com), and PsycINFO (www.apa.org/pubs/databases/psycinfo), are powerful tools to find relevant papers by means of keywords search. Such a database search should be complemented by means of tracing the citations in the thus retrieved papers and review articles. Moreover, coordinate databases, BrainMap currently being the most comprehensive one (www.brainmap.org), allow searching relevant papers by means of brain locations or paradigm classes.

Quanititative meta-analyses are increasingly applied to summarise and integrate the expanding amount of neuroimaging experiments ranging from basic to clinical neuroscience (Bludau et al. 2015; Chase et al. 2015; Kohn et al. 2014). Given the expansion of ALE analyses into always more fields of research, neuroimaging investigators need to be conscious of the strengths and weaknesses of this methodological approach. Müller and colleagues recently provided best-practice recommendations (Müller et al. 2018) as guideline for conducting meta-analyses to help researchers from different disciplines make informed choices. At the beginning of every meta-analysis, investigators need to define the number of eligible experiments to include into the stuedy. However, we always face a trade-off between the gain in statistical power and additionally introducing heterogeneity into the data as we increase the number of experiments (Müller et al. 2018). Eickhoff and colleagues conducted an empirical simulation analysis to provide a quantitative answer to that question of minimal amount of necessary studies to be meta-analyzed (Eickhoff et al. 2016). The authors characterized the behavior of the ALE analysis approach across 120,000 simulated meta-analyses datasets. They concluded that a minimum of 20 experiments should be included in any conducted meta-analyses to obtain robust results.

As for any meta-analysis, the thoughtful choice of judicious inclusion criteria is a crucial step of the analysis, given their obvious impact on the outcome of the analysis. Absolute inclusion criteria embrace considering only either neurotypicals (i.e., healthy subjects) or a specific clinical population (but not mixing these two), either focusing on or completely excluding pharmacological manipulation, exclusive consideration of studies that report coordinates provided in a standard reference space (Talairach/Tournoux, MNI), and reliance on full-brain coverage (versus analyses based on ROIs or functional localizers). Relative inclusion criteria, however, depend on the actual research question and may embrace specific contrast analyses, paradigms, stimulus material, or experimental instructions. For instance, only including target-versus-baseline contrasts would aim at identifying *all* the neural correlates underlying a given psychological process, while only including target-versus-control contrasts would aim at identifying only the *specific* neural correlates underlying a given psychological process.

Please note that within the realms of coordinate-based meta-analysis (CBMA), the term "experiment" usually refers to any single analysis on imaging data yielding localization information, while the term "study" usually refers to a scientific publication reporting one or more "experiments." Following this definition, a contrast analysis between two conditions and a correlation of brain activity with participants' reaction times would, for instance, make up two "experiments" whose activation coordinates are summarized in the tables of the one "study" publishing these results. The coordinates collected from all the eligible studies on a given topic are then to be summarized in a table, which forms the input for the CBMA algorithm.

9.3 Activation Likelihood Estimation

The most important algorithm for coordinate-based meta-analysis is activation likelihood estimation (ALE), proposed by Turkeltaub et al. (2002). The key idea behind ALE resides in considering each included activation focus as a center of probability distribution instead of a dimensionless point in the voxel-scaled brain (Fig. 9.1a). This accounts for the spatial uncertainty associated with neuroimaging results, as it assumes that the true location of an activation is most likely at the reported coordinate but it may also be with finite possibility in its vicinity. Hence, the unit reflecting activation information in that 3D space is not binary (i.e., activated or not) but dimensional (i.e., more or less probable activation). In other words, the probability of "true" activation is regarded to diminish gradually with increasing distance from a reported activation peak.

As a first step, ALE therefore models foci as centers for 3D Gaussian probability distributions that capture the spatial uncertainty associated with each focus. This probability distribution acknowledges the uncertainty that arises mainly from between-subject variances, attributable in large extent to neuroanatomical variability and small sample sizes, as well as between-laboratory variances, attributable in large extent to different normalization strategies and brain templates across laboratories. These two sources of uncertainty used to be gauged subjectively by the investigator, which has recently been replaced by empirical estimates (Eickhoff et al. 2009). Moreover, the width of the spatial uncertainty of any focus is adjusted by the number of subjects that participated in the corresponding experiment. Put concretely, the more participants contributed to a study, the bigger the likelihood of "true" activation near the foci reported in that study; hence, the modeled spatial uncertainty around this studies' foci becomes smaller and the influence of those foci on the outcome of the meta-analysis larger.

In a second step, the probability distributions of all activation foci in a given experiment are

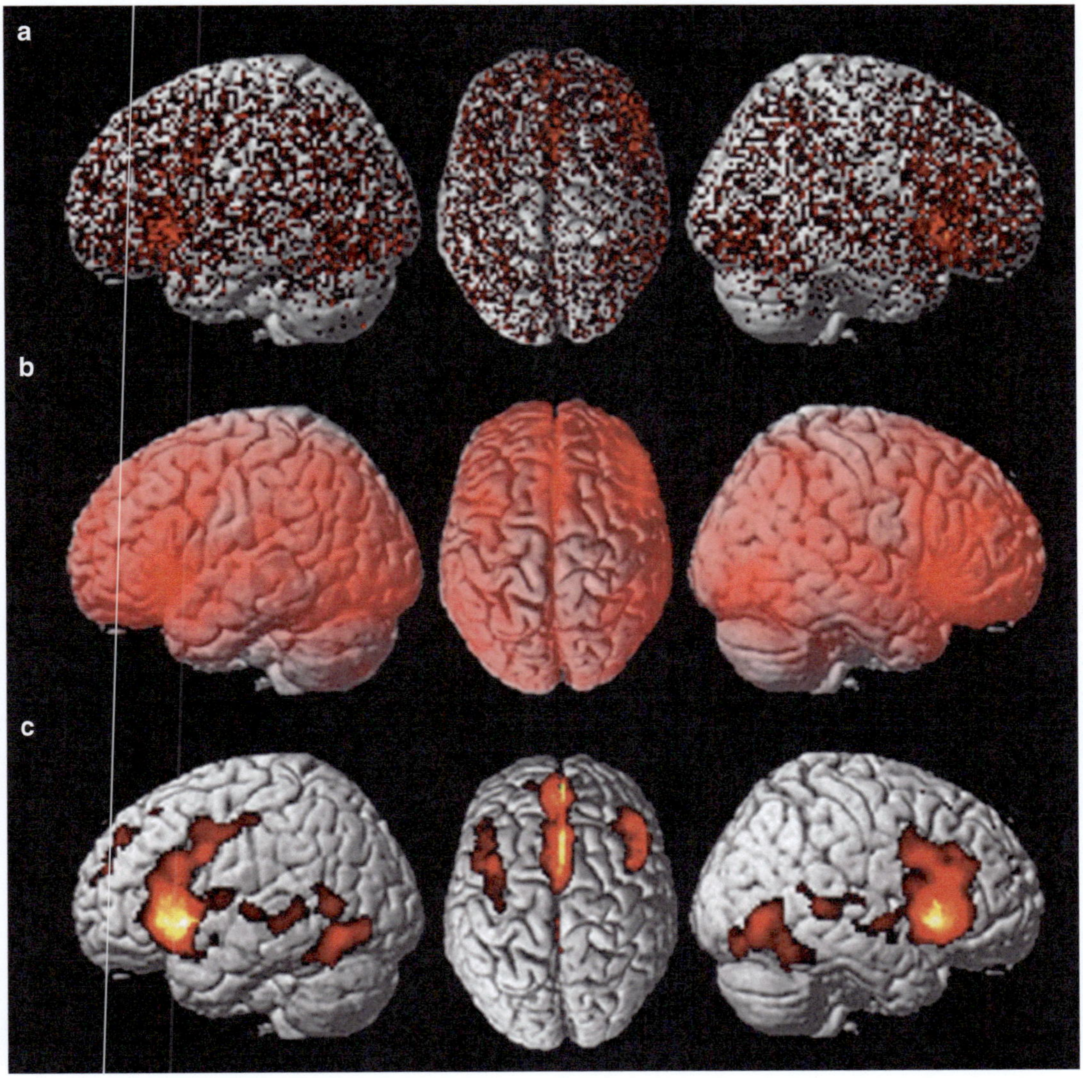

Fig. 9.1 (**a**) Reported peak locations of 2393 individual neuroimaging experiments in 35,386 healthy participants related to the neural correlates involved in various paradigms on emotion processing (experiments provided by the BrainMap database). (**b**) Shows the unified "activation likelihood estimations" (i.e., union of modeled probability distributions) which describes the local convergence across the included neuroimaging experiments. (**c**) Significant voxels are determined as a function of whether the corresponding ALE score is higher than it would be expected if all included neuroimaging experiments converged completely by chance. This panel shows the significant convergence across experiments after correction for multiple comparisons

combined for each voxel, yielding a so-called modeled activation map (MA map). The MA map can hence be thought of as a 3D summary of the results reported in that experiment, taking into account the spatial uncertainty associated with the reported coordinates. The final ALE map, comprising the voxel-wise ALE scores, then results from the union across these MA maps (Fig. 9.1b). The ALE map thus indicates the convergence across experiments at each particular location, which is subsequently assessed for statistical significance. More specifically, the original implementation of the ALE approach (Turkeltaub et al. 2002) was designed to test for above-chance clustering of individual *foci* instead of results from different *experiments*, invoking a fixed-effects analysis. In the current implementation (Eickhoff et al. 2009), the within-experiment distribution of foci is regarded to be fixed, hence testing for above-chance clustering of *experiments*, rather than *foci*, invoking a random-effects analysis. Importantly, only random-effects analyses allow extrapolation of the findings beyond the considered data set (Penny and Holmes 2004). Put differently, obsolete testing for convergence between *foci* only allowed conclusions about the very neuroimaging studies included in the meta-analysis, while testing for convergence between *experiments* allows conclusions about studies not included in the meta-analysis as well as about the investigated psychological state per se. Taken together, the ALE approach represents each included experiment as a modeled activation probability map (i.e., MA map) that was derived from the union of the Gaussian probabilities of that experiment's activation foci. These MA maps are then combined voxel-wise to yield the final ALE maps that indicate the likelihood of convergence between the considered experiments.

The third and last step distinguishes between random and "true" convergence by comparing the computed ALE map against a null distribution that reflects a random spatial association between the experiments' MA maps. That is, the null distribution indicates the voxel-wise ALE values that would be observed if the considered experiments converged entirely by chance. While most CBMA approaches proposed so far rely on a computationally expensive permutation procedure to obtain the null distribution (Wager et al. 2007), ALE recently adopted a faster and more accurate analytical solution to the problem (Eickhoff et al. 2011). Rather than considering each voxel individually, all voxels showing the same MA value in a particular experiment are joined into and represented as a single bin in a histogram. The entire histogram thus holds the occurrences of all possible MA values disregarding spatial information. The null distribution is then computed from successive integration of the probabilities stored in the histograms across the possible combinations. Finally, spatial inference is drawn by identifying those voxels where the experiments (i.e., MA maps) converged more robustly (reflected by the ALE scores) than expected if the results were independently distributed (reflected by the null distribution) (Fig. 9.1c).

Importantly, the ALE algorithm is readily available to the neuroimaging community in form of the operation-system-independent GingerALE desktop application (http://brainmap.org/ale). GingerALE is part of the BrainMap project devoted to create tools for large-scale data mining and meta-analysis of the neuroimaging literature (Laird et al. 2009, 2011). The GingerALE software allows performing a quantitative meta-analysis based on the most recent version of the ALE algorithm on either the coordinates retrieved from automated queries to the BrainMap database or tabular-formatted list of coordinates retrieved by manual search of the literature. Many best-practice recommendations, including guidelines for image- and coordinate-based meta-analyses, are further detailed elsewhere (Müller et al. 2018).

9.4 Applying Quantitative Meta-Analysis

The ALE procedure has been illustrated above by depicting the three major steps of the analysis on a pool of neuroimaging experiments pertaining to emotion processing tasks in healthy participants (Fig. 9.1a–c). Converging brain activity across various emotional tasks included the bilateral amygdala, fusiform gyrus, posterior superior temporal sulcus, basal ganglia, dorsal anterior cingulate cortex/supplementary motor cortex (dACC/SMA), and the anterior insula/inferior frontal gyrus (AI/IFG) (Fig. 9.2, left column). Concurrently, the amygdala has been linked with processing various aspects of emotional and social environmental information as well as the shaping of respondent behavior. The fusiform gyrus is consistently accredited importance in processing mainly stable properties of facial stimuli, while the posterior superior temporal sulcus is consistently discussed as processing mainly variable properties of facial stimuli. The

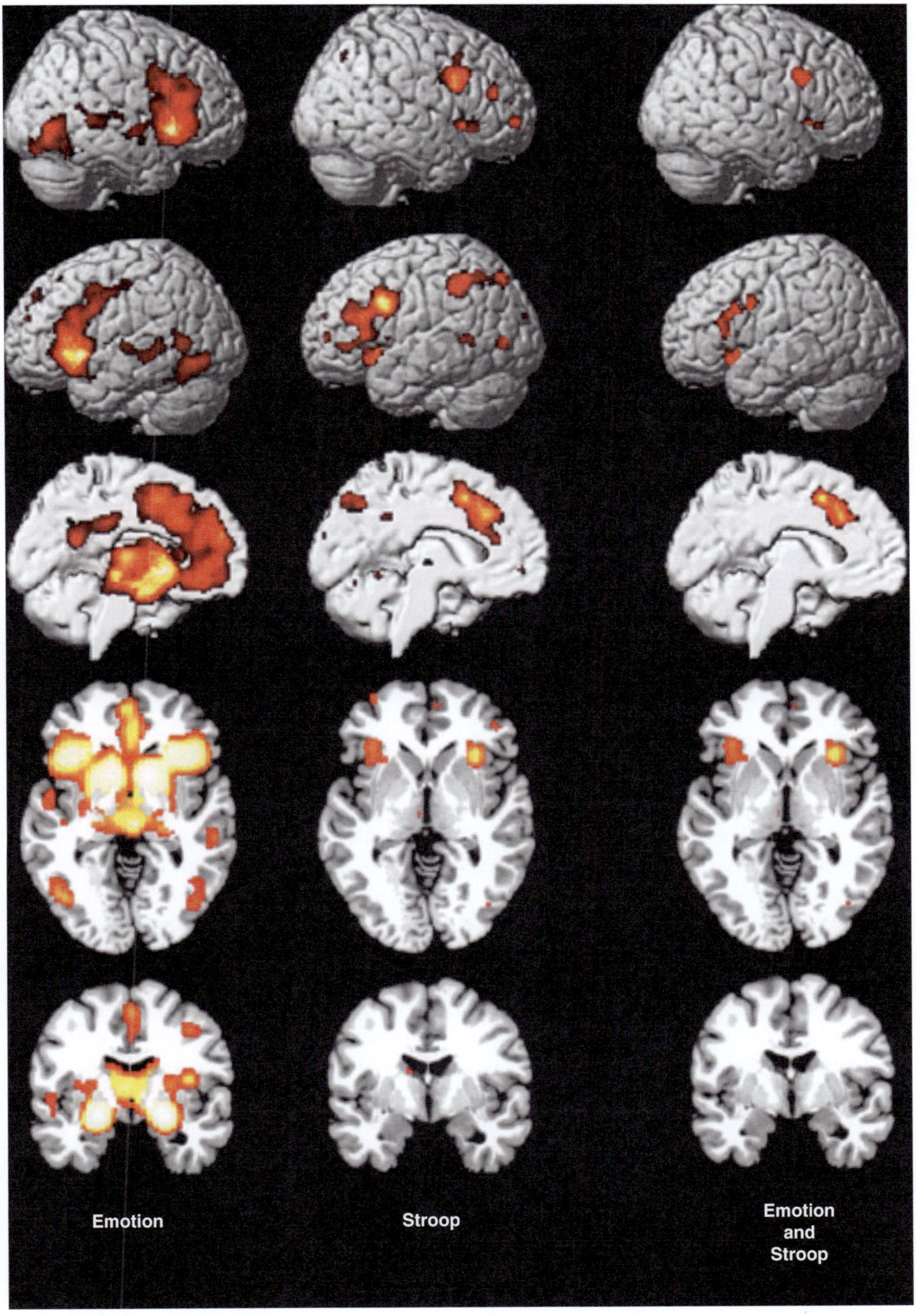

Fig. 9.2 Whole-brain renderings as well as sagittal, axial, and coronal slices depicting the results of the ALE meta-analyses on neuroimaging experiments related to emotion tasks in the *left column* (cf. Fig. 9.1) and related to the Stroop tasks in the *middle column* (219 individual neuroimaging experiments in 2850 healthy participants). The *right column* shows significant convergence across both these individual ALE meta-analyses by performing an AND conjunction (all experiments provided by the BrainMap database)

convergence in these two areas is meaningful in that most considered neuroimaging experiments employed facial pictures as stimulus material. The robust engagement of the basal ganglia in appraising emotional faces is believed to reflect the representation of motor programs for the facial musculature, which plays a crucial role in realizing emotional and social gestures. Similarly, the dACC/SMA and AI/IFG form a network that is believed to represent both one's own and others' emotional states regardless of the actual affective or sensory modality. This functional concept usually serves to explain the concomitant involvement of the dACC/SMA and AI/IFG in neuroimaging experiments on empathy. Taken together, the observed neural activation pattern underlying emotion processing is in line with the notion that similar brain regions are recruited in experiencing own and recognizing others' emotional states.

Another research question that can be addressed using ALE meta-analysis is the quantitative juxtaposition of the neural correlates that pertain to different psychological entities. This is exemplified here by computing the overlap between the coherent brain activity during emotion processing and the Stroop task. The latter refers to a classical paradigm in psychology for inducing cognitive conflict by asking participants to read aloud single words of colors whose letters are, however, colored incongruently. Put differently, we here compared the neural networks that subserve emotion processing and cognitive interference (Fig. 9.2, left and middle column), hence, two a priori rather unrelated psychological constructs. The conjunction analysis across the ALE meta-analysis on emotional tasks and Stroop tasks yielded robust convergence in the bilateral dACC/SMA and AI/IFG (Fig. 9.2, right column). In fact, increased brain activity in the bilateral dACC/SMA and AI/IFG in tandem is considered to be typical in the neuroscientific literature on both empathy (Lamm et al. 2011) and switching between cognitive sets (Dosenbach et al. 2006), notwithstanding they seldom cross-reference each other. The observed neural overlap across these two heterogeneous tasks epitomizes the urgent need for impartial integration of knowledge from intuitively unconnected, yet neurobiologically related, research areas in neuroimaging science.

The biggest potential of ALE might however rely in quantitatively summarizing neuroimaging data from clinical populations. That is because the above mentioned downsides of neuroimaging methods show the biggest effect for diagnosed participants, considering recruiting difficulties, the clinical exclusion/inclusion criteria, and the frequent occurrence of aborted measurements due to noncompliance, as well as often incongruent treatment within the clinical sample and interindividual variability of a same disease. As a consequence, clinical neuroimaging research tends to be based on rather small sample sizes.

The aptitude of ALE to determine the neural substrates related to pathological brain function is exemplified here by a quantitative meta-analysis on differential brain activity in depressive patients during emotion processing (Fig. 9.3). Any ALE meta-analysis based on data from clinical populations necessarily rests on neuroimaging experiments that compare a group of patients versus a parallel group of healthy control subjects. This approach yields consistent convergence between cerebral hypo- or hyperactivity in patients comparing to normal subjects. Figure 9.3 thus depicts the localization of deviant brain activity in depressed patients across a vast variety of subjects, paradigms, and experimental circumstances. Please appreciate that all the brain areas found to differ in brain metabolism during emotion processing in depression (Fig. 9.3) have also been determined to be part of the normal neural network engaged in emotion processing in a separate pool of subjects and experiment (Figs. 9.1c and 9.2, left column). This emphasizes the ability of ALE meta-analysis to identify the aberrant network nodes associated with a given mental condition within the neural network related to a given psychological process in healthy individuals.

Differences in brain metabolism in diseased populations cannot always be interpreted straightforwardly. For instance, more activity in the patient group could be read as reflecting an increased effort that is needed to compensate for

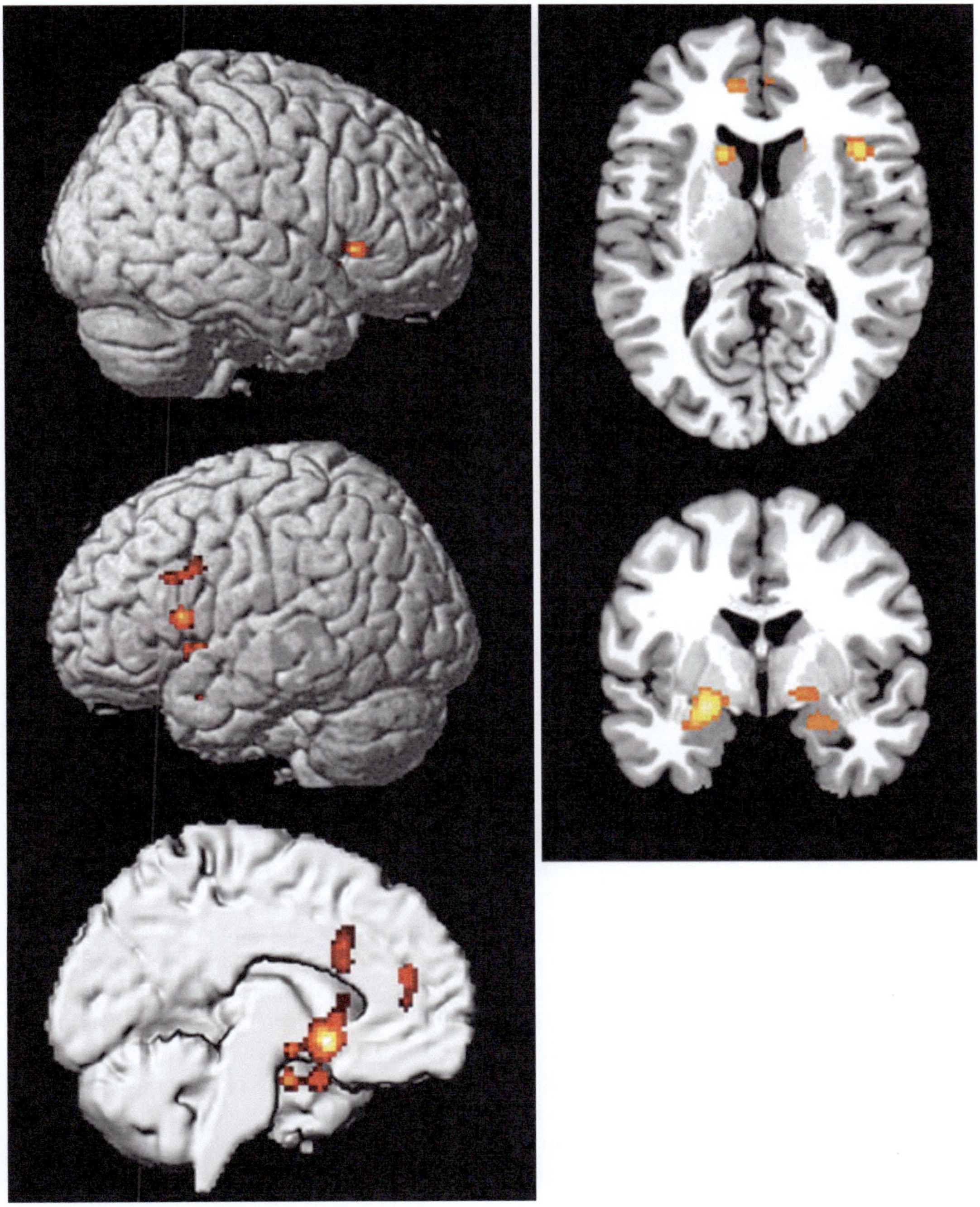

Fig. 9.3 Whole-brain renderings as well as sagittal, axial, and coronal slices depicting the results of the ALE meta-analysis of 131 individual neuroimaging experiments in 1893 depressive patients that reported differential brain activity during various paradigms on emotion processing in comparison to healthy controls (experiments provided by the BrainMap database)

deficient processing. Contrarily, less activity in the patient group could also be read as reflecting deficient processing due to lowered neural recruitment. This dilemma can be addressed by integrating the observed altered brain activity with prior evidence that was preferentially obtained using a different methodological modality, such as behavioral data or lesion studies. Furthermore, aberrant brain activity evidently raises the question of the underlying pathological process. One should be cautious to claim regional metabolic aberration as causal for the dysfunction of a specific psychological process. This line of thought implicitly assumes that psychological processes can be identified from mere topography of brain activity, termed "reverse inference" (Poldrack 2006). This type of induction might, however, be limited in that one-to-one mapping between a certain brain region and a given psychological process is probably rare, if not inexistent.

9.5 Perspectives and Future Directions

Coordinate-based meta-analysis enables the quantitative localization of above-chance convergence across multiple neuroimaging experiments in a 3D reference space. This integration and synthesis of neuroimaging data thus permits statistically defensible generalizations on the neural basis of psychological processes in health and disease, which far exceeds the knowledge that may be gained from a single neuroimaging study. It also allows relating different tasks or processes to each other by performing meta-analyses on different neuropsychological phenomena, such as inhibition, attention, or working memory, which is often not feasible in a single experiment due to logistic expenses and the natural time limits of any scanner session. Moreover, CBMA offers a unique opportunity to weigh concordance between neuroimaging results without the implicit assumptions of neuroanatomical terminologies, which are frequently used in an inconsistent, if not competitive, manner. For instance, the temporoparietal junction is commonly referenced as angular gyrus, inferior parietal lobule, posterior superior temporal sulcus, supramarginal gyrus, BA 39, PGa/PGp, as well as "pli courbe" ("curved gyrus" in French). Another example is the long-standing debate about the constituent nodes of the limbic system. Consequently, conveying verbalized localization information may entail confusion by the same brain area being associated with discrepant neuroanatomical terms respectively the same neuroanatomical term being associated with discrepant groups of brain areas. Therefore, impartial comparison between neuroimaging studies using CBMA can possibly resolve conflicting views by reliance on location probabilities instead of neuroanatomical nomenclature.

Descriptive review articles are a commonly and eagerly employed mean to juxtapose and integrate distributed neuroimaging findings. However, those critical verbal analyses tend to focus on a limited number of preselected aspects and tend to be biased by the authors' own adherence to a specific research area. In contrast to classical review articles, CBMA is hypothesis-free, data-driven, and, hence, objective by algorithmically weighing all results equally. As the CBMA method is not skewed by subjectivity, it precludes overinterpretation of expected, easily interpretable findings and neglect of unexpected, barely reconcilable findings in neuroimaging research. CBMA might therefore help to point out consistent yet frequently ignored findings. For instance, cerebellar activation is typically overlooked in neuroimaging studies on non-motor topics, although cerebellar lesion does entail a variety of cognitive deficits, including language, visual-spatial, affective, and executive dysfunction (Stoodley and Schmahmann 2009). In this way, CBMA might be valuable in identifying previously unidentified brain regions or network nodes, respectively.

Moreover, it is increasingly acknowledged that the relationship between brain areas and psychological processes is best explained by a many-to-many rather than a one-to-one mapping (Price and Friston 2005). Said differently, a single brain region can be involved in several cognitive processes, and a single cognitive process may increase activity in several brain regions. These circumstances typically favor the development of parallel yet independent research trends that interpret activity in a same brain region according to completely diverging sets of theories and references. For instance, brain activity in the (left) inferior frontal gyrus is often read as specific for language processing by many authors yet specific for representation of (observed) motor action by others. By performing a rigorous summary of existing neuroimaging evidence, CBMA allows to unveil neurotopographical co-occurrences of a priori unrelated psychological processes and to, thereby, potentially reconcile domain-centered research niches in an unbiased fashion. The ensuing meta-analytic convergence, in turn, might help to generate testable hypotheses for targeted neuroimaging studies to come.

CBMA can, however, not only be used for retrospective purposes, but also as a preliminary step to guide analysis in newly acquired experimental data. In particular, formal meta-analysis on a prespecified psychological state may yield reliable regions of interest (ROIs) that can be employed as a cornerstone for a variety of consecutive neuroimaging analyses. Functional ROIs constrained by prior meta-analysis can, for instance, readily inform seed-based structural and functional connectivity analyses. Sets of such meta-analytically constructed regions provide a solid basis for targeted follow-up analyses. In one example, a meta-analytic set of ROIs underlying the mirror neuron system were used in a combined computational and experimental study (Horoufchin et al. 2018). First, previously published ALE maps were successfully exploited to reduce the search space to a readily interpretable set of involved regions. These identified neuroimaging foci were then successfully used as seeds in an innovative machine-learning pattern analysis.

Generally, meta-analytically seed-regions can be used in analyses of various different imaging modalities. On the one hand, diffusion-weighted imaging (DWI) in concert with tractography algorithms has become popular as a measure of structural connectivity that delineates white-matter tracts in the human brain in vivo. On the other hand, resting-state neuroimaging data (rsMRI) is currently widely employed as a measure of functional connectivity based on correlations between spontaneous fluctuations of brain activity in the absence of an externally structured task. In both approaches, meta-analysis-derived ROIs can serve as a starting point for structural and functional connectivity analyses to reveal the whole-brain connectivity pattern of such functionally constrained seed regions (Eickhoff and Grefkes 2011). In a similar vein, approaches for effective connectivity aim at modeling the interactions within a predefined set of ROIs based on explicit a priori assumptions about their mutually related functional relationships. Such effective connectivity analyses, including psychophysiological interactions (PPI), structural equation models (SEM)), dynamic causal modeling (DCM)), and Granger causality mapping (GCM)), infer the directionality in the information flow between the designated network nodes based on the ROI-defined fMRI signals (Eickhoff and Grefkes 2011). Evidently, the validity of the emerging interaction patterns critically hinges on the proper fit of the initially defined ROIs. Approaches for effective connectivity can thus take advantage of meta-analysis-defined ROIs that constitute a topographical consensus across numerous previous experiments. That is, ALE meta-analyses can be used to build domain-specific atlases underlying specific cognitive processes. A recent ALE investigation allowed to derive a first robust consensus definition of the neural correlates underlying social-affective behaviour. This quantified definition of the social brain then provided as data-derived basis of seeds underlying social-affective processing for further analyses (Alcalá-López et al. 2017). This bottom-up approach allowed to derive an atlas of the social brain without relying on preselected brain regions or only a restricted experimental set of cognitive processes. From a broader perspective, any neuroimaging technique reliant on preselected ROIs (e.g., even including transient brain lesion by transcranial magnetic stimulation) may enhance their potency by introducing coordinate-based meta-analysis as a complementary methodological step.

Today, the field of neuroscience is undergoing fast changes as big data repositories are becoming more accessible and richer in detail. Increasingly embraced state-of-the-art modeling approaches are needed to succeed in such a data-rich setting (Bzdok & Yeo 2017). The continuous stream of newly developed methods also provide the opportunity for currently under-appreciated methological combinations. Advanced methods can then be joined to investigate clinical research questions (Kernbach et al. 2018). Particularily meta-analyses, such as ALE, represent a powerful utility to gain a synoptic view of distributed neuroimaging findings in a quantitative and impartial fashion. Retrospectively, CBMA might thus potentially remedy conflicting views that arose from inconsistent neuroanatomical labeling or domain-centered interpretation conventions. Prospectively, meta-analysis-derived regions of interest can serve as a solid basis for a variety of neuroimaging methods, including functional and effective connectivity analyses.

References

Alcalá-López D, Smallwood J, Jefferies E, Van Overwalle F, Vogeley K, Mars RB, Turetsky BI, Laird AR, Fox PT, Eickhoff SB, Bzdok D (2017) Computing the social brain connectome across systems and states. Cereb Cortex:1–26

Bludau S, Bzdok D, Gruber O, Kohn N, Riedl V, Sorg C, Palomero-Gallagher N, Müller VI, Hoffstaedter F, Amunts K (2015) Medial prefrontal aberrations in major depressive disorder revealed by cytoarchitectonically informed voxel-based morphometry. Am J Psychiatr 173(3):291–298

Bzdok D, Yeo BTT (2017) Inference in the age of big data: Future perspectives on neuroscience. NeuroImage 155:549–564

Chase HW, Kumar P, Eickhoff SB, Dombrovski AY (2015) Reinforcement learning models and their neural correlates: An activation likelihood estimation meta-analysis. Cogn Affect Behav Neurosci 15:435–459

Derrfuss J, Mar RA (2009) Lost in localization: the need for a universal coordinate database. NeuroImage 48:1–7

Dosenbach NU, Visscher KM et al (2006) A core system for the implementation of task sets. Neuron 50:799–812

Eickhoff SB, Grefkes C (2011) Approaches for the integrated analysis of structure, function and connectivity of the human brain. Clin EEG Neurosci 42:107–121

Eickhoff SB, Laird AR et al (2009) Coordinate-based activation likelihood estimation meta-analysis of neuroimaging data: a random-effects approach based on empirical estimates of spatial uncertainty. Hum Brain Mapp 30:2907–2926

Eickhoff SB, Bzdok D et al (2011) Activation likelihood estimation meta-analysis revisited. NeuroImage 59(3):2349–2361

Eickhoff SB, Nichols TE, Laird AR, Hoffstaedter F, Amunts K, Fox PT, Bzdok D, Eickhoff CR (2016) Behavior, sensitivity, and power of activation likelihood estimation characterized by massive empirical simulation. NeuroImage 137:70–85

Evans AC, Collins DL et al (1992) An MRI-based stereotactic atlas from 250 young normal subjects. Soc Neurosci Abstr 18:408

Horoufchin H, Bzdok D, Buccino G, Borghi AM, Binkofski F (2018) Action and object words are differentially anchored in the sensory motor system-A perspective on cognitive embodiment. Sci Rep 8:1–11

Kernbach, J., Satterthwaite, T., Bassett, D., Smallwood, J., Margulies, D., Krall, S., Shaw, P., Varoquaux, G., Thirion, B., Konrad, K., Bzdok, D., 2018. Shared Endo-phenotypes of Default Mode Dysfunction in Attention Deficit/Hyperactivity Disorder and Autism Spectrum Disorder. Transl Psychiatry

Kohn N, Eickhoff SB, Scheller M, Laird AR, Fox PT, Habel U (2014) Neural network of cognitive emotion regulation—an ALE meta-analysis and MACM analysis. NeuroImage 87:345–355

Laird AR, Eickhoff SB et al (2009) ALE meta-analysis workflows via the brainmap database: progress towards a probabilistic functional brain atlas. Front Neuroinform 3:23

Laird AR, Eickhoff SB et al (2011) The BrainMap strategy for standardization, sharing, and meta-analysis of neuroimaging data. BMC Res Notes 4:349

Lamm C, Decety J et al (2011) Meta-analytic evidence for common and distinct neural networks associated with directly experienced pain and empathy for pain. NeuroImage 54:2492–2502

Lancaster JL, Tordesillas-Gutierrez D et al (2007) Bias between MNI and Talairach coordinates analyzed using the ICBM-152 brain template. Hum Brain Mapp 28:1194–1205

Müller VI, Cieslik EC, Laird AR, Fox PT, Radua J, Mataix-Cols D, Tench CR, Yarkoni T, Nichols TE, Turkeltaub PE, Wager TD, Eickhoff SB (2018) Ten simple rules for neuroimaging meta-analysis. Neurosci Biobehav Rev 84:151–161

Penny WD, Holmes AP (2004) Random effects analysis. In: Frackowiak RSJ, Friston KJ, Frith R, Dolan KJ, Price CJ, Zeki S, Ashburner J, Penny WD (eds) Human brain function. Academic, San Diego, pp 843–850

Poldrack RA (2006) Can cognitive processes be inferred from neuroimaging data? Trends Cogn Sci 10:59–63

Price C, Friston K (2005) Functional ontologies for cognition: the systematic definition of structure and function. Cogn Neuropsychol 22:262–275

Schilbach L, Eickhoff SB et al (2008) Minds at rest? Social cognition as the default mode of cognizing and its putative relationship to the "default system" of the brain. Conscious Cogn 17:457–467

Stark CE, Squire LR (2001) When zero is not zero: the problem of ambiguous baseline conditions in fMRI. Proc Natl Acad Sci U S A 98:12760–12766

Stoodley CJ, Schmahmann JD (2009) Functional topography in the human cerebellum: a meta-analysis of neuroimaging studies. NeuroImage 44:489–501

Talairach J, Tournoux P (1988) Co-planar stereotaxic atlas of the human brain. Thieme, New York

Turkeltaub PE, Eden GF et al (2002) Meta-analysis of the functional neuroanatomy of single-word reading: method and validation. NeuroImage 16:765–780

Wager TD, Lindquist M et al (2007) Meta-analysis of functional neuroimaging data: current and future directions. Soc Cogn Affect Neurosci 2:150–158

Part II

Clinical Applications

10 Special Issues in fMRI Involving Children

Lucie Hertz-Pannier and Marion Noulhiane

10.1 Introduction

Anatomo-functional brain imaging methods have considerably developed recently, leading to new advances in *noninvasive* exploration of children with various neurological disorders. In addition, fMRI is a unique method to study healthy children because it does not require any exogenous tracer and has no reported side effects. It thus gives us access to normative data of functional brain development and to the assessment of networks reorganization following focal anatomical or functional abnormality, which is particularly relevant in the child's immature and plastic brain.

In children, like in adults, the main (if not only) clinical application of fMRI is to provide reliable presurgical mapping of eloquent cortices (mostly motor areas and lateralized language areas) and of their relationship with the planned resection (tumor or epilepsy surgery), in order to select patients, tailor resection, and avoid postoperative deficits referring to Chap. 15. Staudt in the same book! When combined with clinical, neuropsychological, and neurophysiological data, anatomo-functional MRI techniques offer the possibility of a noninvasive presurgical work-up, therefore reducing the need for invasive techniques and impacting on patient management (Petrella et al. 2006). In that context, all methods implemented must reach a high sensitivity for detecting activated areas at the individual level, and high reproducibility, especially in young children. Thus, most teams use validated tasks amenable to patients with variable abilities, in robust block paradigms, and with individual analyses involving adapted statistical thresholds. Still most needed here are further validation and standardization of the whole process across clinical teams.

Beside this unique clinical application, a number of studies have been performed recently to unravel the neural correlates of various cognitive developmental pathologies (learning disorders, ADHD, autism) and of brain plasticity in children with brain lesions, such as motor plasticity in cerebral palsy, or language plasticity in focal epilepsies. These clinical research studies do involve very different experimental conditions with dedicated and often elaborated paradigms in homogeneous populations of children (patients and controls), which are analyzed as groups to extract differences over the whole groups with increased statistical power, but do not usually provide clinically relevant individual results.

However, the mere comparison between the explosive number of fMRI studies in adults (both cognitive and clinical studies) and the still limited studies in children highlights the intrinsic difficulties of studying children. While all methods and tools have been developed for analyses of healthy adult brains, there are numerous

L. Hertz-Pannier (✉) · M. Noulhiane
UMR 663, INSERM, Paris Descartes University, Neurospin, I2BM, DSV, CEA, Paris, France
e-mail: lucie.hertz-pannier@cea.fr

S. Ulmer, O. Jansen (eds.), *fMRI*, https://doi.org/10.1007/978-3-030-41874-8_10

specific limitations and constraints pertaining to data acquisition and analysis in the pediatric population that all remain to be solved to make these tools fully adapted to a wide range of clinical pediatric applications. Recently, the possibility of studying brain functional connectivity with fMRI *during rest* (rs-fcMRI for resting-state functional connectivity MRI) has opened new research avenues and makes it possible to overcome a number of those limitations, to assess the development of neuronal networks from birth on, in health and in disease.

10.2 Issues Pertaining to the Developing Brain

Several characteristics of the developing brain are prone to influencing signal in fMRI studies in children, especially in neonates and infants, and are the field of intense research using multimodal imaging with fMRI, DTI, morphometric analyses, and most recently resting-state functional connectivity studies.

10.2.1 Brain Maturation

The main biological characteristics of the developing brain is a succession of progressive and regressive events, with intense synaptic growth from birth on leading to synaptic overproduction and redundancy in the primary school years, and then slow progressive synaptic pruning with stabilization of efficient networks during adolescence and young adulthood (Huttenlocher and Dabholkar 1997). This triphasic process is common to all functional systems but occurs with different time windows in different networks (earlier in primary systems and later into the second decade for associative networks), and is accompanied by changes in glucose consumption and blood flow, according to the known steps of psychomotor development (Chugani et al. 1987; Chiron et al. 1992). At a macroscopic level, these biological events can be seen as local/regional variations of cortical thickness (Faria et al. 2012; Sowell et al. 2003), chapters of both white matter signal and volume and of DTI parameters (decrease in mean and radial diffusivity, increase in fractional anisotropy (Faria et al. 2012)) and finally in global and regional brain growth (Giedd and Rapoport 2010).

Ongoing myelination is accompanied by a longer latency of electrical induction which speeds up rapidly during the first year of life, and more slowly thereafter, during the specification and maturation of functional networks.

10.2.2 Evolution of BOLD Signal According to Age

These combined biological events in immature networks have been associated with changes in oxidative metabolism and vascular reactivity during neuronal firing that may contribute to the negative BOLD response during visual and sensorimotor stimulations described in neonates and infants (Marcar et al. 2004; Morita et al. 2000). Part of this negative response might however also be attributed to sedation, which is commonly used at this age. In a study of nonsedated and sometimes awake 3-month-old infants, using ecological auditory stimuli, we found a hemodynamic response largely comparable to adults (Dehaene-Lambertz et al. 2002). Beyond the first weeks of life, BOLD hemodynamic response is very stable across ages, although with possible increase in amplitude until adulthood (Shapiro et al. 2007), and some variations across tasks (Brauer et al. 2008). Finally, physiological noise is increased in children due to larger cardiovascular and respiratory dynamics, although with no clearly demonstrated effect on BOLD signal.

10.3 Experimental Design of Pediatric fMRI Studies

10.3.1 Paradigm Design

So far, all fMRI clinical applications in children have used "block paradigms" in which the patient performs the tasks repeatedly over the activation and reference periods (usually 20–40 s each), repeated several times in a single trial. This approach is the most robust and reproducible, because of good statistical power per unit time, and therefore is used when individual assessment is required in clinical applications such as presurgical motor or language mapping. It can also be usefully applied in clinical research programs where children are to be pooled in groups for comparing activation differences according to a clinical marker.

More sophisticated single-event paradigms, which allow monitoring brain response during processing of a single stimulus, may prove very useful in patients, since they avoid using a control task (thus reducing a possible confounding factor); they permit to account for response variability; and they offer extended possibilities of experimental designs (e.g., for memory studies). But their implementation remains difficult in clinical environments (especially in children), due to long acquisition times, lower sensitivity, very large data volumes, and the need for customized analyses.

10.3.2 Choice of Tasks

In children like in adults, the most critical part of fMRI studies resides in the choice of activation and reference tasks, as data analysis most often relies on "cognitive subtraction" (Binder et al. 1995), that is, the resulting activated areas are thought to sustain the cognitive components that are involved in the activated state but *not* in the reference one. For example, the comparison of an auditorily cued semantic decision task and a simple tone discrimination task shows mainly regions involved in semantic processes (Humphries et al. 2006). On the other hand, the comparison of a more global language task (such as sentence generation to a given noun) compared to simple "rest" will show a larger functional network that includes numerous modules of receptive and expressive language (phonemic discrimination, phonological encoding, lexical retrieval, semantic analysis, and syntax, along with verbal working memory and pre-articulatory processing). However, the underlying assumptions of cognitive subtraction may not be fulfilled in all cases because of nonlinearity of many brain processes (interactions may also be studied).

The experimental constraints of fMRI are particularly demanding for children, as tasks paradigms are designed in a very rigid manner, according to a priori models of BOLD contrast time course. In addition, the intrinsically low BOLD contrast/noise ratio requires the repetition of events to gain statistical power. In that context, task complexity is a critical issue, in terms of temporal sequence of both stimuli and responses and of cognitive/attentional demands. According to the research question, the age, and the cognitive level of the subjects, block paradigms with simple tasks may be suited, for example, alternating hand movements with rest for motor mapping. It must be noted that in all cases, tasks can be adapted to the performance level (even in motor paradigms, from complex sequential finger tapping to simple grasp movement, or passive wrist flexion-extension). In cognitive paradigms, explicit tasks are most often used and adapted to subject's abilities and performance. In children, this means using tasks adapted from age-validated neuropsychological tests and appropriately testing them prior to MRI. Implicit tasks can be implemented, especially when there is strong a priori on the localization of signal changes, by the presentation of visual and/or auditory stimuli not requiring any particular response (e.g., Monzalvo et al. 2012). In such paradigms, it is important however to drive the child's attention to the stimuli, usually by the means of a simple additional task (e.g., button press on the detection of a particular visual or auditory stimulus), which also allows to monitor the compliance, but will not be analyzed further.

Strictly passive tasks are also used in particular cases, such as passive movements in patients with motor deficits, or presentation of auditory stimuli in neonates, and asleep infants and toddlers (Dehaene-Lambertz et al. 2002; Redcay et al. 2007). While these tasks may reveal interesting activation often grossly comparable to that of active ones, they obviously do not provide the same level of functional assessment. Sedation can be occasionally used to assess basic functions for clinical purposes (e.g., auditory stimulation before cochlear implantation (Altman and Bernal 2001)), but with a careful choice of anesthetic drugs and dosages (Heinke and Koelsch 2005).

Multiple tasks are required when testing complex cognitive functions such as language (Wilke et al. 2008) in order to highlight the different processes involved and to increase the robustness of lateralization assessment by combining the different tasks in individual subjects (Rutten et al. 2002). In some instances, lateralization may vary according to the type of task, either as a normal pattern (e.g., left semantic vs. right prosody) or related to mixed language representation secondary to left focal epilepsy or lesion (e.g., with left dominance for expressive language and right dominance for receptive one).

The use of "rest" as reference task is being debated because of the uncertainty regarding what children do while resting. In all cases, giving clues to the child on "rest" instruction (listening to the scanner noise, concentrating on its own breathing…) may help him/her to comply. On the one hand, it has the advantage of simplicity for very young or disabled children that may have difficulties in rapidly alternating different tasks. On the other hand, children may involuntarily not stop the "activation task" (resulting in falsely negative results) , and there are no means of controlling ongoing cognitive activity during rest. Some experimenters therefore use very simple tasks as references such as finger tapping or tone listening in children with sufficient mental flexibility.

10.3.3 Control of Task Performance

A precise monitoring of task performance is desirable for fully analyzing and interpreting activation maps, as the latter reflect what has been actually done during scanning. This may be obtained using computer-based paradigms with visual or audio presentation of items, by monitoring responses of the patient pressing on joystick or buttons. In that case, balancing the side of responding hand may be useful to avoid systematic bias in brain activation. However, this right-left shift may complicate the paradigm for young children not fully acquainted with their own right and left side. In language fMRI studies, most tasks are performed silently, producing similar activation as overt ones, but avoiding artifacts due to face movements. Not only this precludes any performance control, but it may also not be amenable to deficient children. Some experimenters have used oral responses (with on line response recording), associated to adapted MR sequences with no image acquisition during the response interval to avoid articulation-related motion artifacts while taking benefit from the delayed hemodynamic response. Nowadays, eye-tracking devices are being increasingly used to monitor eye movements during cognitive tasks, but the experimental setup is very demanding for children and currently remains largely beyond the possibilities of a clinical environment.

10.3.4 Group Studies in Children

In the context of clinical research, it is often desirable to compare two selected groups to unravel a relevant biomarker. Reference data in healthy children can be helpful to understand the spatiotemporal sequence of the development of cognitive systems and to assess brain plasticity in various early pathologies. In the majority of cases, group comparison is thus made with typical children that must be carefully matched to the patient population. However, the criteria for matching pediatric populations are not straightforward, and depend on research goals: while in most studies, the control population is composed by age and gender-matched typical children, this might not prove appropriate in other cases, for example, the study of intellectual deficiencies, where it might be more relevant to use "developmental age" (or associated parameter) as matching criterion. Indeed, gross differences in performance between groups are likely to be accompanied by different strategies and activation patterns, with no particular insight on the specific neural substrates underlying them. In addition, there is very often a recruitment bias in the control population of published studies, with children with high IQ and/or of high socioeconomic status. One way to alleviate the constraints on group selection is to select "implicit tasks" that do not require active responses (Monzalvo et al. 2012). Still, many other parameters are likely to influence the comparison between two groups with variable cognitive abilities, such as motion artifacts, performance on the reference task, attentional resources, and level of anxiety.

In many developmental studies, the variables of interest strongly depend on age and learning and therefore constitute continuous variables, making it arbitrary to split the population into age groups. Correlation analysis can be performed over the entire group, to demonstrate developmental patterns and their differences between typical and nontypical children (Fair et al. 2008).

Most developmental studies use a cross-sectional design to gather a sample of selected children in a limited period of time, sometimes in multicenter studies (e.g., the NIH pediatric database, http://pediatricmri.nih.gov/nihpd/info/index.html). While having definitive advantages in terms of efficiency, such designs suffer from many confounding factors associated to intersubject variability. The ideal way of studying development is to design longitudinal studies (e.g., Szaflarski et al. 2006), but such designs pose multiple ethical, technical, and methodological questions that make them very challenging, especially when planned on a relatively long term. In particular, the recruitment and follow-up of children over several years, and the maintenance of the methodological setup to keep sequential data comparable despite technical upgrades, are constraints extremely difficult to deal with.

10.3.5 Age Versus Performance

Finally, a critical goal in developmental studies is to disentangle the effects of age and of performance, which are obviously strongly correlated in children. Different approaches can be used (Church et al. 2010), such as the constitution of groups with different ages but similar performances (e.g., Schlaggar et al. 2002), or the post hoc grouping of subjects with equivalent performances. Alternatively, regressing performance variables in the analysis can be helpful if the age regressors are not collinear.

10.4 Technical Issues

As BOLD contrast to noise ratio increases with field strength, the use of higher fields (3 T vs. 1.5 T) increases the sensitivity of functional MRI, despite aggravation of various artifacts (which can be corrected in most cases). This better sensitivity to BOLD contrast can be used to either shorten acquisition time or increase spatial resolution to improve localization of activated clusters, which can be valuable in young children with small heads, all while maintaining adequate signal-to-noise ratio. High-field MR imaging is being considered by the FDA as minimal-risk procedure up to 8 T for adults and children and up to 4 T for neonates below 1 month of age. Nowadays, 3 T fMRI has become standard in babies and children as in adults, including in healthy subjects.

Multichannel coils with parallel imaging have further improved the signal-to-noise ratio, but have made it even more critical to use coils adapted to the head size. In neonates and infants, smaller coils such as knee coils provide better signal and improve the sensitivity of fMRI. MR-compatible incubators are needed to prevent hypothermia in neonates (especially premature babies), but they are expensive and cumbersome. Smaller dedicated 1.5 T MR systems are being designed to be placed in NICU and improve the feasibility of MRI and fMRI in neonates.

One issue often neglected in fMRI is the acoustic noise created by Lorentzian forces secondary to gradient switching in EPI images (in functional imaging as well as in DTI). Not only may noise prevent children to remain still because of anxiety and/or difficulty to sleep, but the risk of acoustic trauma must also not be underestimated, as functional MRI sequences often reach 110-dB levels at peak frequencies. As noise depends upon multiple sequence parameters (type of sequence, spatial and temporal resolutions, parallel imaging), acoustic measurements should be performed for each sequence, whenever possible. Careful prevention must always be undertaken, including in asleep or sedated infants and children, with a whole variety of devices (earplugs, headphones, foams). Some companies offer hardware options reducing acoustic noise of various sequences by modifying gradients shape and strength.

Temporal resolution of fMRI is mainly dependent upon the shape of the hemodynamic response, which is comparable to adults after the first few months of life (see above). Shortening TR from standard 3–5 to 2–2.5 s provides better sampling of subtle variations of the hemodynamic response and increases statistical power (Beware of acoustic noise!).

Spatial resolution can strongly benefit from higher fields, and it is current standard practice to acquire 3 T EPI data with 3 × 3 × 3-mm^3 voxels. Although this nominal resolution is not clearly reflected in the results due to numerous steps of spatial filtering, it permits better localization of activated clusters in small anatomical regions (e.g., in neonates and infants) by reducing partial volume effects. On the other hand, motion artifacts are more conspicuous and problematic in highly resolved scans.

Finally, "real-time fMRI" may be of particular value in children, as it provides continuous monitoring of the acquisition, by reconstructing and analyzing the images "online," and providing a constant update of the quality of the functional study. This is especially relevant in clinical studies, where paradigms are being kept simple, with reasonable datasets and standard statistical analyses. This might prove a challenge in more sophisticated studies with event-related paradigms, large datasets, and analyses requiring heavy post-processing.

10.5 Feasibility

The constitution of appropriate groups in pediatric clinical research fMRI studies has been partly discussed above. Recruitment of minor subjects (especially when healthy) poses specific ethical questions, requiring to justify the enrolment of children instead of adults in all steps of the research and to ensure full agreement of parents (written consent) and of the child (oral or written consent whenever possible, after providing extended and adapted information). Globally, like in adults, fMRI is recognized worldwide as noninvasive minimal-risk procedure for pediatric studies, even at high field and in neonates and infants, after ruling out the usual contraindications of MRI (intracorporeal ferromagnetic bodies, which are much rarer in children than in adults). Research on healthy fetuses remains not authorized in most countries.

In fMRI activation studies, gaining child's cooperation is critical. However, MR imagers remain very child-unfriendly experimental devices, and strict immobility is mandatory to avoid motion artifacts. Obtaining compliance to the tasks is therefore a challenge in young or deficient children and requires extra time and resources with at best a dedicated visit before the study with the child and the parents. This visit with the experimenter(s) that will perform the fMRI study (such as radiologist, neurologist, or neuropsychologist) is necessary to show the child the imager and explain the tasks, to train him/her to remain still in a mock scanner if available, and to practice the fMRI tasks, but with different stimuli than those used in the fMRI session (to avoid test-retest effects). It also makes it possible to adapt the paradigm in case of deficiency or poor compliance to optimize feasibility of clinical studies, and sometimes to cancel the study, when sufficient compliance cannot be obtained, thus optimizing scanner occupancy.

During scanning, many adaptations can be implemented to improve child's comfort and quietness, such as having the experimenter and the parents in the magnet room, interacting very often to the child through intercom, playing movies during anatomical scans, monitoring child's movements through an MR-compatible camcorder, and providing him/her a feedback along scanning. In all cases is good head immobilization necessary to discourage movements. Providing the child with visual inputs also decreases head motion artifacts (Yuan et al. 2009).

Time issues are critical in fMRI as statistical power depends directly on the number of scan repetitions thus on scanning duration. On the one hand, it is necessary to keep paradigms long enough to get reliable contrast to noise, on the other hand, attentional resources and compliance of children cannot be maintained during too long scans. Higher-field acquisitions (3 T) do contribute to alleviate these constraints. Still, unlike in adults where 20-min runs are commonly acquired, in most children the whole acquisition is preferably segmented in shorter runs of 3–5 min. It is cautious to repeat similar runs during a single session, given the high rate of poor quality data in younger children due to motion or transient incompliance. A whole study must be completed in 20 min in babies or poorly compliant children and in up to 1 h in older school-age children with no significant cognitive or behavioral impairments. Acquisition may also be split in two or more sessions separated by a break, even on separate days, as there are no limitations given the absence of known side effects. In that case, images from different sessions must be coregistered during analysis.

Eventually, cooperation can be obtained for adapted paradigms from children with a developmental age of around 5–6 years and/or IQs around 60, provided there are no behavioral disorders. Passive tasks can be used in sleeping or quiet neonates, infants, and children (either with or without sedation), using receptive language tasks or sensory stimulations.

However, as obtaining cooperation is not possible in younger children, and because sedation cannot be performed in healthy children (for obvious ethical reasons), there is nowadays only a couple of fMRI studies in healthy children between 6 months and 5–6 years (Redcay et al. 2007), since getting natural sleep in such a noisy environment remains a challenge. The emergence of resting-state functional connectivity studies, which require no cooperation from the child, has made it recently possible to get new insights on brain development during early life (see below). Overall, the attrition rate of fMRI studies in children is much higher than in adults, especially in activation studies. It is thus common practice when designing a pediatric study, to plan the inclusion of 10–30% more children than needed, to account for the risk of failure and/or missing data.

10.6 Data Analysis

Head motion remains a critical limiting factor, especially in uncooperative, young, or debilitated patients, and is more frequent and pronounced in boys than in girls (Yuan et al. 2009). The use of dedicated registration algorithms is most often necessary, but the choice of registration method is rather empirical, depending upon the type and amplitude of movements. Motion parameters can be introduced as regressors of noninterest in the analysis to reduce variance. Some algorithms are based on data interpolation to replace heavily corrupt images; others take into account discarded thus missing data. Overall, the resulting corrected images must be checked carefully, as a significant amount of registered data must eventually be discarded due to insufficient correction, therefore reducing the statistical power of the analysis.

The choice of anatomical template for pediatric group studies is conditioned by the children's age range. Indeed, brain growth and maturation in the first years of life make it inappropriate to use adult templates for normalization and tissue segmentation. Generating dedicated templates (Dehaene-Lambertz et al. 2002; Wilke et al. 2008) provides a common spatial referential to compare children. However, in our experience, it is possible to use adult templates for studies from 6–7 years of age on.

Statistical analysis of pediatric datasets follows the same rules and constraints as in adults and strongly depends upon the goal of the study: in group comparisons, the most frequent goal is to reach high specificity to demonstrate a difference between groups in which individual datasets are analyzed with strictly similar thresholds, often resulting in low sensitivity at the individual level. In pediatric data, analysis must also take into account the frequency of small samples and of missing data within functional runs, given the high attrition rate. Hemodynamic models adapted for temporal sequences with occasional missing data and nonparametric tests of small samples that may not follow a normal distribution are useful in challenging studies of poorly compliant infants and children (e.g., Dehaene-Lambertz et al. 2006).

Finally, as pediatric studies very often contain continuous variables associated with learning and development (age, performance level, and any associated co-variable), correlation studies are useful to avoid the arbitrary constitution of age groups and to unravel the continuous dynamics of specific learning (Ghetti et al. 2010).

By contrast, in presurgical studies of patients, the main goal is to optimize at the individual level the sensitivity of the detection of activated areas, which may depend upon multiple factors (i.e., age, efficiency, attention, pathology, medications). In such circumstances, testing multiple thresholds and taking into account the performance level is likely to increase the sensitivity of detection of activated networks, especially in children. Overall, in presurgical studies, thresholding and interpretation of activation maps still depend heavily on the expertise of the investigator, especially for datasets containing residual motion artifacts.

10.7 Multimodal Imaging

Multimodality is an exquisite asset of MRI, as comprehensive assessment of brain anatomy, microstructure, function, and biochemistry can be obtained within a single session using different techniques, giving access to structural, functional, and effective brain connectivity during normal and abnormal development. Beyond anatomical imaging for localization of activated clusters, 3D T1 images can be used for morphometric studies of gyration/sulcation development and organization (Dubois et al. 2008) for quantification of gray and white matter volumes (e.g., Giedd et al. 2006). DTI can demonstrate the structural connectivity of involved regions, by tracking the main fascicles (i.e., corticospinal tracts, optic radiations, arcuate and uncinate fasciculi) and monitoring their maturation (Bassi et al. 2008; Dubois et al. 2008). Functional connectivity can be studied in fMRI acquisitions during rest (see below, and Fransson et al. 2009).

10.8 Clinical Research Applications: Studying Plastic Changes of Functional Systems

In the recent years, fMRI has emerged as a unique tool to study the exquisite plasticity of the immature brain, which sustains both normal learning and memory acquisition, and recovery following a focal insult or abnormality with an incomparably better functional outcome as compared to adults with similar condition. As the maturation of functional networks is asynchronous, starting with "lower-level" primary functions such as vision and motricity, and followed by elaborated cognitive functions (i.e., language, memory, executive functions), it can be anticipated that pathological plasticity will strongly depend upon the maturation stage of the involved network, among other parameters.

The general pattern of functional maturation of a specific network has been shown as regional specialization of activated clusters with age, starting from a more widespread activation in earlier ages (Gaillard et al. 2000, 2003), and associating progressive and regressive changes in different regions (Brown et al. 2005). These focal changes are associated with changes in short- and long-range connectivity, as recently discovered by functional connectivity studies (see below).

Importantly, fMRI has also demonstrated that some malformations of cortical development (i.e., heterotopias, polymicrogyrias) may retain functional cortical organization (i.e., vision, motor, language) with a risk of postoperative deficit in case of a resection of the malformed cortex (Liegeois et al. 2004). By contrast, it seems that Taylor-type focal cortical dysplasias do not retain functional activity within the area containing balloon cells (hypersignal on FLAIR or T2 images; Marusic et al. 2002).

10.8.1 Motor Cortex

Plasticity of the primary motor cortex has been probed in several series of adult and pediatric patients with tumors, epilepsy foci, or perinatal lesions located in the central region. These studies have shown consistent activation in regions predicted by the electrophysiological data (Penfield's homonculus), when the lesion was relatively remote from the functional areas. However, plastic changes of the cortical organization could also be demonstrated in cases of lesions within the motor cortex, in excellent agreement with the results of cortical stimulation. Motor plasticity has been extensively studied with fMRI and transcranial magnetic stimulation (TMS)) in children with congenital hemiplegia, showing that the central and precentral cortex contralateral to the lesion can take over the impaired function and that the presumed date of the prenatal injury is critical to the development of functional compensation and plasticity (Staudt et al. 2003). Those children with earlier insults (first trimester) had the best motor recovery, sustained by the persistence of the ipsilateral corticospinal tract. This type of reorganization was however much less observed in children with later lesions (around birth). Overall, these results confirm the good localizing power of motor fMRI in children as well as in adults and its utility in the surgical planning of focal lesions of the central region.

10.8.2 Language

It has been long known that morphological brain asymmetries present from fetal life on are related to speech dominance of the left hemisphere (Dehaene-Lambertz et al. 2006). Recently, fMRI studies in 3-month-old infants showed that the leftward asymmetry of language networks is detectable in early infancy, before oral language development has started (Dehaene-Lambertz et al. 2002, 2010), in agreement with behavioral data in newborns and infants. Longitudinal fMRI studies of healthy children and adolescents have demonstrated that asymmetry is weaker in early childhood (Redcay et al. 2007; Szaflarski et al. 2006) and strengthens over the years toward the adult left dominant pattern, with increasing activation of the frontal lateral cortex (Broca's area) and to a lesser degree of the left posterior temporal region (Wernicke's area) and the angular gyrus (Ressel et al. 2008; Szaflarski et al. 2006) and with differential regional effects of both age and performance (Brown et al. 2005).

In adults with early left hemisphere injury or epilepsy, the capacity of language networks to reorganize either by interhemispheric shift (Rasmussen and Milner 1977) or by intrahemispheric displacement of eloquent areas (Ojemann et al. 1989) is known to depend on many variables such as handedness, type and location of the lesion, age at onset and duration of epilepsy, and baseline of cognitive status. In children, language develops quite similarly in the case of left or right hemispheric lesions, although a slight and transient difference in performances can be disclosed (Vargha-Khadem et al. 1985). Recent data have demonstrated subtle language deficits in children suffering from left hemisphere lesions (MacWhinney et al. 2000) further highlighting the early left hemisphere superiority for language development. The clear deleterious effect of early epilepsy has been demonstrated (Vargha-Khadem and Polkey 1992). However, electrical stimulation in children has shown that developmental lesions and early-onset seizures do not displace language cortex from prenatally determined sites, whereas lesions acquired before the age of 5 years may cause language to relocate to the opposite hemisphere only when language cortex is destroyed (Duchowny and Harvey 1996).

In children with left temporal lobe epilepsy (LTLE), we found that atypical expressive language organization depends on handedness and epilepsy duration and that right-handed children usually retain left dominance, even more so children with mesial TLE, by contrast to adults. These results suggest that early LTLE hampers the normal progression of left hemispheric specialization of expressive, but not receptive, language during childhood, especially in left-handers, supporting the hypothesis of a long-term effect of epilepsy on the organization of language that is strongly linked with the plasticity of the motor system.

In a series of 100 adults (Woermann et al. 2003), the discordance between invasive gold standard Wada test and fMRI in terms of language dominance remained low (9% of cases). As the only "gold standard" for testing the function of a specific cortical area would be an unexpected postoperative deficit, which is fortunately rare, it is most often impossible to conclude on language dominance in such cases. In fact, in both tests do results depend on the nature and multiplicity of language tasks and of subject's compliance. Expressive tasks such as sentence or word generation seem to lateralize better and have a better correlation with invasive methods like the Wada test (Lehericy et al. 2000). Even though fMRI assessment of language dominance is now everyday practice in adults, fMRI is not yet fully accepted as a standard of care in pediatric epilepsy because of the limited number of published studies validating the method in children (Hertz-Pannier et al. 1997, 2002; Liegeois et al. 2006).

Presurgical cortical mapping of regions sustaining language functions may be needed when surgery is to be performed in the dominant hemisphere, but these techniques carry significant risks and are difficult to perform. Direct intraoperative cortical stimulation, considered the gold standard in adults, is not feasible in most children. More recently, perioperative stimulation using subdural grids and depth electrodes has been challenged because of its insufficient sensitivity in children. This may result from reorganized language distribution, limited testing capacity, and incomplete myelination leading to higher stimulation thresholds. Concordance between intraoperative stimulations and fMRI has been assessed in both isolated cases and case series in adults and children (de Ribaupierre et al. 2012; FitzGerald et al. 1997; Roux et al. 2003; Ruge et al. 1999; Rutten et al. 2002). Co-localization of fMRI activated regions and significant stimulation sites have been reported within 1–2 cm in several preliminary reports. Overall, in these studies the sensitivity of fMRI varied from 38 to 100%, and the specificity from 65 to 97% (de Ribaupierre et al. 2012). However, strict comparison of both techniques remains difficult, since cortical stimulation discloses only limited regions critical to language functions, whereas fMRI does not provide hierarchical information on the numerous activated regions, which may not all be essential to language (low specificity).

Finally, fMRI is a unique tool for longitudinal studies to follow the postoperative reorganization of functional networks. For example, the longitudinal observation of a case of left hemisphere disconnection in a 10-year-old boy suffering from Rasmussen encephalitis demonstrated the late ability of the nondominant hemisphere to take over main language functions in a network mirroring that of the left hemisphere before surgery (Hertz-Pannier et al. 2002).

10.8.3 Reading

Reading may be broken down into two components that are distinct from functional, anatomical, and developmental points of view. First, the visual word form area (VWFA), in the mid-portion of the left occipitotemporal sulcus, encodes the abstract identity of strings of visual letters (Cohen and Dehaene 2004). This system reaches its adult properties by the age of 10, although it is already left lateralized at the time of reading acquisition (Monzalvo et al. 2012). Second, children learn how to translate letter strings into phonological and lexical representations subtended by left perisylvian language areas. An fMRI study of reading has shown a dissociated reorganization of both components in a child with early left inferotemporal epilepsy before reading acquisition, who maintained a left perisylvian language network, with an elective contralateral plasticity of the VWFA allowing to resect the left epileptic focus without creating any postoperative reading deficit (Cohen et al. 2004).

10.8.4 Memory Functions

Nowadays, researches have convincingly demonstrated that temporal lobe epilepsy can cause specific memory deficit in children with distinct patterns of deficiencies according to the lateralization of seizures (Jambaque et al. 1993, 2007; Kelly et al. 2009; Lehericy et al. 2000; Liegeois et al. 2004, 2006; Lin et al. 2008; Liu et al. 2008; Mabbott and Smith 2003). Children with left temporal lobe epilepsy (LTLE) are mostly impaired on verbal episodic memory, whereas children with right temporal lobe epilepsy (RTLE) are mostly impaired on visuospatial episodic memory. Overall children tend to recover from memory deficits better than adults suggesting that the developing brain may benefit from compensatory cognitive and neurofunctional mechanisms (Jambaque et al. 2007). Whereas fMRI exploration of episodic memory is just emerging in pediatric TLE and preliminary data suggest that a fronto-hippocampo-parietal network may be bilaterally impaired in left TLE, studies in adults with TLE show that mesio-temporal structures are asymmetrically impaired: activations are greater contralaterally to the epilepsy, in good concordance with individual results of the memory Wada test (Detre et al. 1998).

To investigate the role of medial temporal lobe structures in episodic memory, recent fMRI studies have concerned healthy children. These structures, that is, hippocampus and surrounding cortices including entorhinal, perirhinal, parahippocampal, and temporopolar cortices, are known to distinctly contribute to recognition memory in adults (Montaldi and Mayes 2010; Wixted and Squire 2011). Recognition memory network also includes the prefrontal cortex and thalamus, which are both highly connected with the hippocampus and parahippocampal gyrus (Wixted and Squire 2011). Using fMRI, authors have reported discrepant results on age-related changes from childhood to adulthood in these structures (Ghetti et al. 2010; Maril et al. 2010, 2011; Menon et al. 2005) Besides, the structural maturation of medial temporal lobe structures is nonlinear, which leads to distinctly consider hippocampal subregions in developmental studies.

10.9 Resting-State fMRI and Development

As shown above, investigating the maturation of functional networks underlying brain development continues to present unique scientific and methodological challenges. Recent advances in MRI methodology have qualified precise measurements of correlated activity throughout the brain, leading to the first comprehensive descriptions of functional brain networks in humans. In this vein, a growing literature deals with the development of functional networks, from infancy through adolescence, as measured by resting-state functional connectivity MRI (for reviews, see Power et al. 2012; Uddin et al. 2010). This method is now increasingly used to complement traditional task-based fMRI, but its use in developmental studies is still in its infancy.

10.9.1 Functional Connectivity

Functional connectivity is defined as the temporal coherence, or statistical dependence, between measurements of activity in different neurons or neural ensembles. rsfMRI has emerged as a novel framework for investigating the development of large-scale organization of the developing brain by measuring spontaneous, high-amplitude, low-frequency (<0.1 Hz) BOLD signal fluctuations in subjects at rest (i.e., performing no explicit task). These spontaneous fluctuations are posited to organize, coordinate, and maintain functional brain systems (Fox and Raichle 2007; Raichle 2010).

The advantages of using rsfMRI in pediatric and clinical populations are that functional brain organization can be examined independently of task performance, and a full dataset can be collected in as little as 5 min (Van Dijk et al. 2009). Indeed, rsfMRI involves collecting functional imaging data from participants as they lay in the MRI scanner, typically with eyes closed or fixating gaze on a crosshair, without any specific cognitive demand. Because the rsfMRI procedure implies insignificant cognitive load on the participant and requires relatively little time in the scanner compared to task related fMRI studies, data can be collected from low-functioning and very young populations. Functional connectivity measures derived from rsfMRI data are particularly useful in studying age-related variations in the wiring of neural networks (Supekar et al. 2009). For example, Lin et al. (2008) suggested that sensorimotor networks emerge early in infancy and appear to develop well before visual networks.

10.9.2 Methodological Aspects

Two main methodological approaches are considered here: seed-ROI-based correlation and independent component analysis (ICA)), each making significant contributions to the study of intrinsic brain architecture, and they can be used in a complementary method to clarify global and functional properties of the developing brain. Region-of-interest (ROI) seed-based analysis is the most widely used method of analysis of rsfMRI. This hypothesis-driven approach typically involves choosing one or more ROIs and investigating their whole-brain functional connectivity, often using a regression or correlation model. Unlike ROI-based analysis, independent component analysis (ICA) is a model-free data-driven approach whereby four-dimensional fMRI data is decomposed into a set of independent one-dimensional time series and associated three-dimensional spatial maps, which all describe the temporal and spatial characteristics of the underlying signal or components (Beckmann et al. 2005). ICA is currently a widely used method for analyzing rsfMRI data (Calhoun et al. 2008). Within- and between-subject measures computed from rsfMRI are quite consistent and reproducible (Damoiseaux et al. 2006; Shehzad et al. 2009). However, the methods remain to be fully validated.

Graphs are data structures, which have nodes and edges between the nodes (Bondy and Murty 1976). Graph theoretical metrics such as clustering coefficient, path length, degree, and centrality provide quantitative measures to characterize large-scale networks represented as a graph (Bullmore and Sporns 2009). In a graphical representation of a brain network, a node reflects the functional interactions between two brain regions. Developmental studies are beginning to examine how these network metrics change with age and cognitive skills (Gao et al. 2009; Spreng et al. 2009; Uddin et al. 2007).

10.9.3 Typical Development: From Infancy to Adolescence

Studies investigating functional connectivity in infants, children, and adolescents have revealed consistent findings with respect to the development of long-distance connectivity and regional functional specialization (Uddin et al. 2010). Many of the developmental studies have captured the functional connectivity of the default mode network (DMN) over development. The DMN is so named due to its uniquely high metabolic resting activity (Raichle 2010) and characteristic deactivation during challenging cognitive tasks (Shulman et al. 1997).

Initial developmental studies have shown in neonates five unique resting-state networks in the infant brain that encompassed the primary visual cortex, bilateral sensorimotor areas, bilateral auditory cortex, a network including the precuneus area, lateral parietal cortex, and cerebellum, as well as an anterior network that incorporated the medial and dorsolateral prefrontal cortex. These results suggest that resting-state networks driven by spontaneous signal fluctuations are present already in the infant brain. Further studies have suggested that this intrinsic organization can be demonstrated in awake, asleep, sedated, and event-anesthetized subjects. Beyond infancy, multiple studies agree that by age 7–9, children manifest a similar "small-world" type of functional architecture as adults (Fair et al. 2008; Supekar et al. 2009) although the organizations of individual functional subnetworks as well as their interactions have a protracted developmental course (Supekar et al. 2009).

10.9.4 Neurodevelopmental Disorders: Studies in Children

rsfMRI has been used to investigate potentially altered functional connectivity associated with neurodevelopmental studies, in particular attention-deficit/hyperactivity disorder (ADHD; Cao et al. 2006; Zhu et al. 2008), autism spectrum disorders (e.g., Weng et al. 2010), or other neurodevelopmental disorders and genetics effects. However, its clinical relevance is still unknown.

In summary, rsfMRI studies contribute to elucidate and reveal key principles of functional brain development, including a shift from diffuse to focal activation patterns, simultaneous pruning of local connectivity, and strengthening of long-range connectivity with age. Nevertheless, most of the studies have been conducted in older children, adolescents, and adults, and thus, to date little is known regarding how global or local network organization changes during the important developmental period from infancy to early childhood. And the clinical impact of this new approach remains to be demonstrated.

10.10 Conclusion

These techniques are constantly evolving and open new avenues to further understand a variety of pathological conditions in infancy and childhood. They also promises to extent the field of clinical applications to the longitudinal evaluation of cognitive rehabilitation methods and the assessment of cognitive side effects of neurotropic drugs and of postoperative plasticity during brain development and maturation. Combined with advances in other related fields such as DTI and morphometric studies, these techniques are likely to profoundly influence the way various neurodevelopmental disorders will be diagnosed and treated in the future.

References

Altman NR, Bernal B (2001) Brain activation in sedated children: auditory and visual functional MR imaging. Radiology 221:56–63

Bassi L, Ricci D et al (2008) Probabilistic diffusion tractography of the optic radiations and visual function in preterm infants at term equivalent age. Brain 131:573–582

Beckmann CF, DeLuca M et al (2005) Investigations into resting-state connectivity using independent component analysis. Philos Trans R Soc Lond Ser B Biol Sci 360:1001–1013

Binder JR, Rao SM et al (1995) Lateralized human brain language systems demonstrated by task subtraction functional magnetic resonance imaging. Arch Neurol 52:593–601

Bondy JA, Murty USR (1976) In: Co AEP (ed) Graph theory with applications. New York, Elsevier Science Ltd

Brauer J, Neumann J et al (2008) Temporal dynamics of perisylvian activation during language processing in children and adults. NeuroImage 41:1484–1492

Brown TT, Lugar HM et al (2005) Developmental changes in human cerebral functional organization for word generation. Cereb Cortex 15:275–290

Bullmore E, Sporns O (2009) Complex brain networks: graph theoretical analysis of structural and functional systems. Nat Rev Neurosci 10:186–198

Calhoun VD, Kiehl KA et al (2008) Modulation of temporally coherent brain networks estimated using ICA at rest and during cognitive tasks. Hum Brain Mapp 29:828–838

Cao Q, Zang Y et al (2006) Abnormal neural activity in children with attention deficit hyperactivity disorder: a resting-state functional magnetic resonance imaging study. Neuroreport 17:1033–1036

Chiron C, Raynaud C et al (1992) Changes in regional cerebral blood flow during brain maturation in children and adolescents. J Nucl Med 33:696–703

Chugani HT, Phelps ME et al (1987) Positron emission tomography study of human brain functional development. Ann Neurol 22:487–497

Church JA, Petersen SE et al (2010) The "task B problem" and other considerations in developmental functional neuroimaging. Hum Brain Mapp 31:852–862

Cohen L, Dehaene S (2004) Specialization within the ventral stream: the case for the visual word form area. NeuroImage 22:466–476

Cohen L, Jobert A et al (2004) Distinct unimodal and multimodal regions for word processing in the left temporal cortex. NeuroImage 23:1256–1270

Damoiseaux JS, Rombouts SA et al (2006) Consistent resting-state networks across healthy subjects. Proc Natl Acad Sci U S A 103:13848–13853

de Ribaupierre S, Fohlen M et al (2012) Presurgical language mapping in children with epilepsy: clinical usefulness of functional magnetic resonance imaging for the planning of cortical stimulation. Epilepsia 53:67–78

Dehaene-Lambertz G, Dehaene S et al (2002) Functional neuroimaging of speech perception in infants. Science 298:2013–2015

Dehaene-Lambertz G, Hertz-Pannier L et al (2006) Functional organization of perisylvian activation during presentation of sentences in preverbal infants. Proc Natl Acad Sci U S A 103:14240–14245

Dehaene-Lambertz G, Montavont A et al (2010) Language or music, mother or Mozart? Structural and environmental influences on infants' language networks. Brain Lang 114:53–65

Detre JA, Maccotta L et al (1998) Functional MRI lateralization of memory in temporal lobe epilepsy. Neurology 50:926–932

Dubois J, Benders M et al (2008) Primary cortical folding in the human newborn: an early marker of later functional development. Brain 131:2028–2041

Duchowny M, Harvey AS (1996) Pediatric epilepsy syndromes: an update and critical review. Epilepsia 37(Suppl 1):S26–S40

Fair DA, Cohen AL et al (2008) The maturing architecture of the brain's default network. Proc Natl Acad Sci U S A 105:4028–4032

Faria AV, Zhang J et al (2012) Atlas-based analysis of neurodevelopment from infancy to adulthood using diffusion tensor imaging and applications for automated abnormality detection. NeuroImage 52:415–428

FitzGerald DB, Cosgrove GR et al (1997) Location of language in the cortex: a comparison between functional MR imaging and electrocortical stimulation. AJNR Am J Neuroradiol 18:1529–1539

Fox MD, Raichle ME (2007) Spontaneous fluctuations in brain activity observed with functional magnetic resonance imaging. Nat Rev Neurosci 8:700–711

Fransson P, Skiöld B et al (2009) Spontaneous brain activity in the newborn brain during natural sleep–an fMRI study in infants born at full term. Pediatr Res 66:301–305

Gaillard WD, Hertz-Pannier L et al (2000) Functional anatomy of cognitive development: fMRI of verbal fluency in children and adults. Neurology 54:180–185

Gaillard WD, Balsamo LM et al (2003) FMRI identifies regional specialization of neural networks for reading in young children. Neurology 60:94–100

Gao W, Zhu H, Giovanello KS et al (2009) Evidence on the emergence of the brain's default network from 2-week-old to 2-year-old healthy pediatric subjects. Proc Natl Acad Sci U S A 106:6790–6795

Ghetti S, DeMaster DM et al (2010) Developmental differences in medial temporal lobe function during memory encoding. J Neurosci 30:9548–9556

Giedd JN, Rapoport JL (2010) Structural MRI of pediatric brain development: what have we learned and where are we going? Neuron 67:728–734

Giedd JN, Clasen LS et al (2006) Puberty-related influences on brain development. Mol Cell Endocrinol 254–255:154–162

Heinke W, Koelsch S (2005) The effects of anesthetics on brain activity and cognitive function. Curr Opin Anaesthesiol 18:625–631

Hertz-Pannier L, Gaillard WD et al (1997) Noninvasive assessment of language dominance in children and adolescents with functional MRI: a preliminary study. Neurology 48:1003–1012

Hertz-Pannier L, Chiron C et al (2002) Late plasticity for language in a child's non-dominant hemisphere: a pre- and post-surgery fMRI study. Brain 125:361–372

Humphries C, Binder JR et al (2006) Syntactic and semantic modulation of neural activity during auditory sentence comprehension. J Cogn Neurosci 18:665–679

Huttenlocher PR, Dabholkar AS (1997) Regional differences in synaptogenesis in human cerebral cortex. J Comp Neurol 387:167–178

Jambaque I, Dellatolas G et al (1993) Verbal and visual memory impairment in children with epilepsy. Neuropsychologia 31:1321–1337

Jambaque I, Dellatolas G et al (2007) Memory functions following surgery for temporal lobe epilepsy in children. Neuropsychologia 45:2850–2862

Kelly AM, Di Martino A et al (2009) Development of anterior cingulate functional connectivity from late childhood to early adulthood. Cereb Cortex 19:640–657

Lehericy S, Cohen L et al (2000) Functional MR evaluation of temporal and frontal language dominance compared with the Wada test. Neurology 54:1625–1633

Liegeois F, Connelly A et al (2004) Language reorganization in children with early-onset lesions of the left hemisphere: an fMRI study. Brain 127:1229–1236

Liegeois F, Cross JH et al (2006) Role of fMRI in the decision-making process: epilepsy surgery for children. J Magn Reson Imaging 23:933–940

Lin W, Zhu Q et al (2008) Functional connectivity MR imaging reveals cortical functional connectivity in the developing brain. AJNR Am J Neuroradiol 29(10):1883–1889

Liu WC, Flax JF et al (2008) Functional connectivity of the sensorimotor area in naturally sleeping infants. Brain Res 1223:42–49

Mabbott DJ, Smith ML (2003) Memory in children with temporal or extra-temporal excisions. Neuropsychologia 41:995–1007

MacWhinney B, Feldman H et al (2000) Online measures of basic language skills in children with early focal brain lesions. Brain Lang 71(3):400–431

Marcar VL, Strassle AE et al (2004) The influence of cortical maturation on the BOLD response: an fMRI study of visual cortex in children. Pediatr Res 56:967–974

Maril A, Davis PE et al (2010) Developmental fMRI study of episodic verbal memory encoding in children. Neurology 75:2110–2116

Maril A, Avital R et al (2011) Event congruency and episodic encoding: a developmental fMRI study. Neuropsychologia 49:3036–3045

Marusic P, Najm IM et al (2002) Focal cortical dysplasias in eloquent cortex: functional characteristics and correlation with MRI and histopathologic changes. Epilepsia 43:27–32

Menon V, Boyett-Anderson JM et al (2005) Maturation of medial temporal lobe response and connectivity during memory encoding. Brain Res Cogn Brain Res 25:379–385

Montaldi D, Mayes AR (2010) The role of recollection and familiarity in the functional differentiation of the medial temporal lobes. Hippocampus 20:1291–1314

Monzalvo K, Fluss J et al (2012) Cortical networks for vision and language in dyslexic and normal chil-

dren of variable socio-economic status. NeuroImage 61:258–274
Morita T, Kochiyama T et al (2000) Difference in the metabolic response to photic stimulation of the lateral geniculate nucleus and the primary visual cortex of infants: a fMRI study. Neurosci Res 38:63–70
Ojemann G, Ojemann J et al (1989) Cortical language localization in left, dominant hemisphere. An electrical stimulation mapping investigation in 117 patients. J Neurosurg 71:316–326
Petrella JR, Shah LM et al (2006) Preoperative functional MR imaging localization of language and motor areas: effect on therapeutic decision making in patients with potentially resectable brain tumors. Radiology 240:793–802
Power JD, Fair AD et al (2012) The development of human functional brain networks. Neuron 67:735
Raichle ME (2010) Two views of brain function. Trends Cogn Sci 14:180–190
Rasmussen T, Milner B (1977) The role of early left-brain injury in determining lateralization of cerebral speech functions. Ann N Y Acad Sci 299:355–369
Redcay E, Kennedy DP et al (2007) FMRI during natural sleep as a method to study brain function during early childhood. NeuroImage 38:696–707
Ressel V, Wilke M et al (2008) Increases in language lateralization in normal children as observed using magnetoencephalography. Brain Lang 106:167–176
Roux FE, Boulanouar K et al (2003) Language functional magnetic resonance imaging in preoperative assessment of language areas: correlation with direct cortical stimulation. Neurosurgery 52:1335–1345. discussion 1345–7
Ruge MI, Victor J et al (1999) Concordance between functional magnetic resonance imaging and intraoperative language mapping. Stereotact Funct Neurosurg 72:95–102
Rutten GJ, Ramsey NF et al (2002) FMRI-determined language lateralization in patients with unilateral or mixed language dominance according to the Wada test. NeuroImage 17:447–460
Schlaggar BL, Brown TT et al (2002) Functional neuroanatomical differences between adults and school-age children in the processing of single words. Science 296:1476–1479
Shapiro KL, Johnston SJ et al (2007) Increased functional magnetic resonance imaging activity during nonconscious perception in the attentional blink. Neuroreport 18:341–345
Shehzad Z, Kelly AM et al (2009) The resting brain: unconstrained yet reliable. Cereb Cortex 19:2209–2229
Shulman GL, Fiez JA et al (1997) Common blood flow changes across visual tasks: II. Decreases in cerebral cortex. J Cogn Neurosci 9(5):648–663
Sowell ER, Peterson BS et al (2003) Mapping cortical change across the human life span. Nat Neurosci 6:309–315
Spreng RN, Mar RA et al (2009) The common neural basis of autobiographical memory, prospection, navigation, theory of mind, and the default mode: a quantitative meta-analysis. J Cogn Neurosci 21(3):489–510
Staudt M, Pavlova M et al (2003) Pyramidal tract damage correlates with motor dysfunction in bilateral periventricular leukomalacia (PVL). Neuropediatrics 34:182–188
Supekar K, Musen M et al (2009) Development of large-scale functional brain networks in children. PLoS Biol 7:e1000157. https://doi.org/10.1371/journal.pbio.1000157
Szaflarski JP, Holland SK et al (2006) FMRI study of language lateralization in children and adults. Hum Brain Mapp 27:202–212
Uddin LQ, Iacoboni M et al (2007) The self and social cognition: the role of cortical midline structures and mirror neurons. Trends Cogn Sci 11:153–157
Uddin LQ, Supekar K et al (2010) Typical and atypical development of functional human brain networks: insights from resting-state fMRI. Front Syst Neurosci 4:1–12
Van Dijk KR, Hedden T et al (2009) Intrinsic functional connectivity as a tool for human connectomics: theory, properties, and optimization. J Neurophysiol 103(1):297–321
Vargha-Khadem F, Polkey CE (1992) A review of cognitive outcome after hemidecortication in humans. Adv Exp Med Biol 325:137–151
Vargha-Khadem F, O'Gorman AM et al (1985) Aphasia and handedness in relation to hemispheric side, age at injury and severity of cerebral lesion during childhood. Brain 108:677–696
Weng SJ, Wiggins JL et al (2010) Alterations of resting state functional connectivity in the default network in adolescents with autism spectrum disorders. Brain Res 1313:202–214
Wilke M, Holland SK et al (2008) Template-O-Matic: a toolbox for creating customized pediatric templates. NeuroImage 41:903–913
Wixted JT, Squire LR (2011) The medial temporal lobe and the attributes of memory. Trends Cogn Sci 15:210–217
Woermann FG, Jokeit H et al (2003) Language lateralization by Wada test and fMRI in 100 patients with epilepsy. Neurology 61:699–701
Yuan W, Altaye M et al (2009) Quantification of head motion in children during various fMRI language tasks. Hum Brain Mapp 30:1481–1489
Zhu CZ, Zang YF et al (2008) Fisher discriminative analysis of resting-state brain function for attention-deficit/hyperactivity disorder. NeuroImage 40:110–120

Multimodal Brain Mapping in Patients with Early Brain Lesions

11

Martin Staudt

11.1 Introduction

The developing human brain possesses a superior potential of functional reorganization after lesions compared with the adult brain. Because of such reorganizational processes, children with early brain lesions often show abnormally located cortical representations of certain brain functions, e.g. of motor representations (Carr et al. 1993; Staudt et al. 2002a, 2004a) or of language functions (Rasmussen and Milner 1977; Staudt et al. 2002b). Nowadays, these abnormally located representations can be identified non-invasively using techniques such as functional MRI (fMRI), transcranial magnetic stimulation (TMS) or magnetoencephalography (MEG). Thus, these techniques not only can contribute to our general understanding of the processes involved in the reorganization of the developing human brain but can also be used clinically in the pre-surgical evaluation of children who have to undergo brain surgery, e.g. for the relief of pharmaco-refractory epilepsies originating from their lesions (Hertz-Pannier et al. 2001; Staudt et al. 2001, 2004a, b; Liégeois et al. 2006).

The clinical application of these mapping techniques in this context is particularly challenging: first, most of these patients are children, often with various degrees of cognitive impairments so that their ability to comply with the experimental requirements is often reduced; second, the brain lesions often destroy or distort anatomical landmarks, which can normally be used for the identification of eloquent brain regions; and third, the cortical representations of brain functions may have shifted because of reorganizational processes following lesions acquired during ongoing brain development. This chapter gives typical examples of examinations of children, mostly in the pre-surgical evaluation before epilepsy surgery, highlighting a number of important aspects.

11.2 Example 1

A 3-year-old boy suffered from therapy-refractory focal seizures originating from a cortical dysplasia (yellow arrows in Fig. 11.1) in the central (Rolandic) region of the right hemisphere. On clinical examination, left-hand function was normal. Prior to possible epilepsy surgery, fMRI during a simple active hand motor task (repetitive squeezing of a toy) was used to visualize the spatial relation between the dysplasia and the primary sensorimotor representation of the contralateral hand.

Based on these findings of fMRI activation in the immediate vicinity of the dysplasia, no total resection of the dysplasia was performed.

M. Staudt (✉)
Center for Pediatric Neurology, Neurorehabilitation and Epileptology, Schön Clinic, Vogtareuth, Germany
e-mail: martin.staudt@med.uni-tuebingen.de

S. Ulmer, O. Jansen (eds.), *fMRI*, https://doi.org/10.1007/978-3-030-41874-8_11

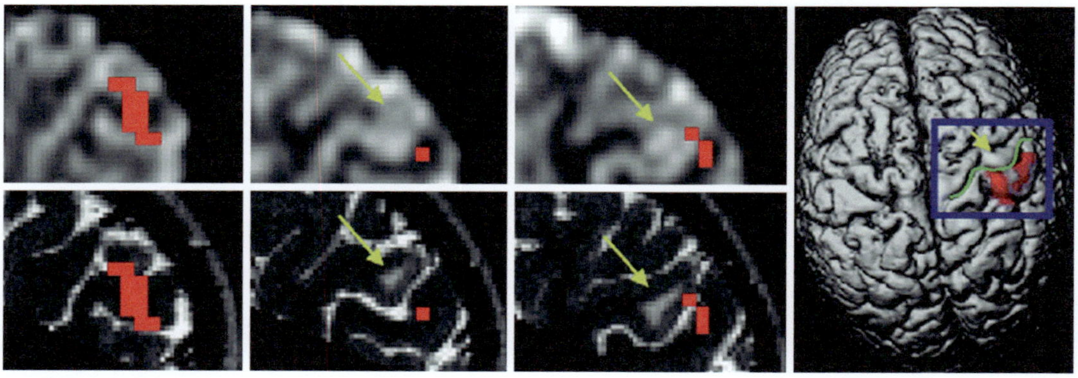

Fig. 11.1 fMRI during active left-hand movement in a 3-year-old boy with a focal cortical dysplasia (hyperintense on T2, *yellow arrows*) of the right central (Rolandic) region. The fMRI activation (in *red*) is superimposed directly on the (functional) EPI images (yielding the most reliable topographical localization since no coregistration is involved, *upper row*) after co-registration, to high-resolution structural T2-weighted images acquired in general anaesthesia during a separate session (*lower row*, courtesy of Prof. Winkler, Schön Klinik Vogtareuth), as well as onto a 3D surface reconstruction (*right*). *Green line* = central sulcus, *blue rectangle* = position of the enlarged details on the *left*

fMRI can be used even in pre-school children to localize the primary sensorimotor region (S1M1) in the vicinity of epileptogenic lesions.

11.3 Example 2

A 16-year-old girl with congenital hemiparesis due to a perinatally acquired cortico-subcortical infarct in the territory of the middle cerebral artery (MCA) showed a striking discrepancy between a large cystic lesion and relatively well-preserved sensorimotor functions (preserved grasp) of the contralateral (paretic) hand (Staudt et al. 2006b). On neurophysiological examination, TMS revealed preserved crossed cortico-spinal projections from the affected hemisphere to the paretic hand, and MEG identified the first cortical response to repetitive tactile stimulation of the paretic thumb (N20m) in the affected hemisphere, indicating the presence of preserved crossed spino-thalamocortical somatosensory projections. Accordingly, diffusion tensor imaging (DTI) tractography with a seed region positioned in the small bridge of preserved white matter between the enlarged lateral ventricle and the cystic lesion visualized extensive connectivity provided by this area (Fig. 11.2).

Small areas of preserved white matter can provide surprisingly extensive connectivity in patients with early brain lesions. Such projections can be visualized by DTI tractography.

11.4 Example 3

A 20-year-old young man with congenital right hemiparesis due to a large polymicrogyria in the left frontoparietal region shows partially preserved sensorimotor functions (preserved individual finger movements) of the contralateral (paretic) right hand (Staudt et al. 2004b). On neurophysiological examination, TMS revealed preserved crossed cortico-spinal projections from the affected hemisphere to the paretic hand. Accordingly, fMRI during a simple active hand motor task (repetitive opening/closing of the paretic hand) revealed activation in the polymicrogyric cortex. Thus, both TMS and fMRI demonstrate that, in this patient, the polymicrogyric cortex harbours the primary motor representation of the paretic hand (Fig. 11.3).

Dysgenic cortex (here: polymicrogyria) can fulfil primary motor functions, with normal descending corticospinal motor projections. This can be confirmed by a combination of fMRI and TMS.

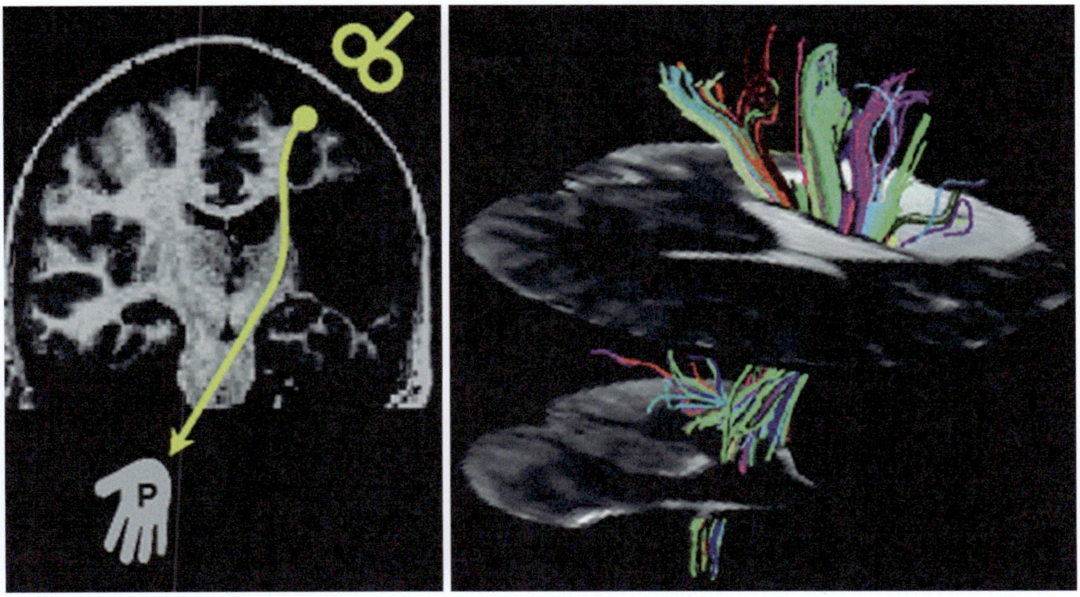

Fig. 11.2 MRI and TMS findings of a 16-year-old girl with congenital hemiparesis due to a large cortico-subcortical infarct. *Left*: coronal T1-weighted image depicting the cystic lesion. TMS (indicated by the *yellow figure-eight-coil symbol*) of the affected hemisphere elicited normal motor-evoked potentials in the paretic hand (P), confirming the presence of preserved crossed cortico-spinal projections (*yellow arrow*). *Right*: MR diffusion tensor tractography (in random colours on unweighted diffusion images; tilted axial planes, anterior-lateral-superior view) visualized numerous fibre trajectories passing through the small bridge of preserved white matter between the cystic lesion and the lateral ventricle. (Adapted from Staudt et al. (2006b) with permission)

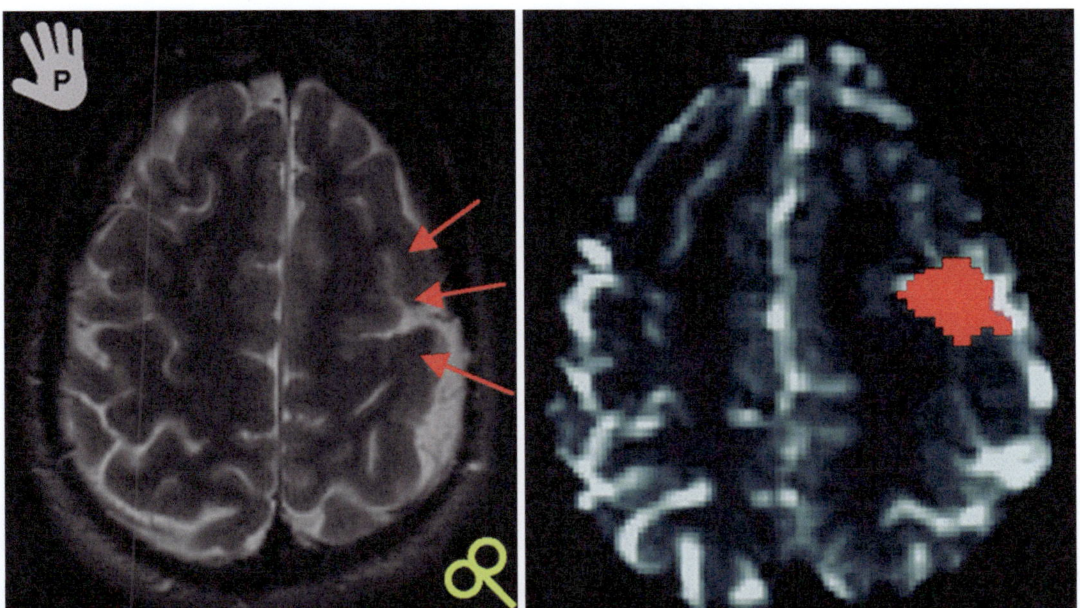

Fig. 11.3 MRI and TMS findings of a 20-year-old man with congenital hemiparesis due to a large polymicrogyria. *Top*: axial T2-weighted image depicting the polymicrogyria in the left frontoparietal region (*red arrows*). TMS (indicated by the *yellow figure-eight-coil symbol*) of the affected hemisphere elicited normal motor-evoked potentials in the paretic hand (P), confirming the presence of preserved crossed cortico-spinal projections. *Bottom*: fMRI activation (in *red*, superimposed on the functional EPI) during active movement of the paretic hand revealed activation in the polymicrogyria, approximately opposing the Rolandic region in the contra-lesional hemisphere

11.5 Example 4

A 6-year-old boy with congenital right hemiparesis due to a complex hemispheric malformation suffered from pharmaco-refractory seizures (Staudt et al. 2001). Clinical examination showed preserved individual finger movements in the paretic hand and massive mirror movements during voluntary movements of both the paretic and the non-paretic hand. Prior to epilepsy surgery, fMRI and TMS were performed to identify the primary motor representation of the paretic hand. TMS of the affected hemisphere did not elicit any response, whereas TMS of the contra-lesional hemisphere elicited bilateral responses with similar latencies. This indicated the presence of fast-conducting ipsilateral cortico-spinal projections, allowing the contra-lesional hemisphere to exert motor control over the paretic hand. Accordingly, fMRI during a simple active hand motor task (repetitive opening/closing of the paretic hand) revealed activation in the 'hand knob' area of the contra-lesional hemisphere, not different from the fMRI activation elicited by movements of the non-paretic hand. Active grasping was still possible after functional hemispherectomy (Fig. 11.4).

Early brain lesions (malformations but also defective lesions) can induce shifting of the primary motor representation (M1) of the paretic hand to the contra-lesional hemisphere (with ipsilateral cortico-spinal tracts).

11.6 Example 5

A 19-year-old woman with congenital right hemiparesis due to a large unilateral periventricular brain lesion showed preserved individual finger movements in the paretic hand and massive mirror movements during voluntary movements of both the paretic and the non-paretic hand (Staudt et al. 2006a). As in the patient in Example 4, TMS of the affected hemisphere did not elicit any response, but TMS of the contra-lesional hemisphere elicited bilateral responses with similar latencies. This indicated the presence of ipsilateral cortico-spinal projections, allowing the contra-lesional hemisphere to exert

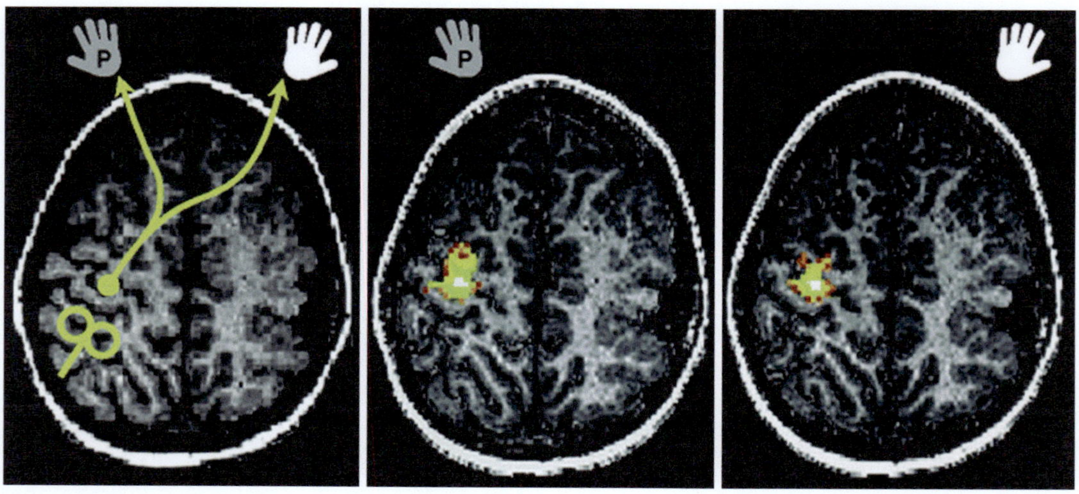

Fig. 11.4 MRI and TMS findings of a 6-year-old boy with congenital hemiparesis due to a complex hemispheric malformation. *Left*: axial T1-weighted image depicting the malformation of almost the entire hemisphere. TMS (indicated by the *yellow figure-eight-coil symbol*) of the contra-lesional hemisphere elicited not only the normal contralateral responses in the non-paretic hand but also ipsilateral motor-evoked potentials in the paretic hand (P), demonstrating the presence of ipsilateral cortico-spinal projections. fMRI during active movement of the paretic hand (*middle*) revealed activation in the hand knob area of the contra-lesional (ipsilateral) hemisphere, not different from the activation elicited by active movement of the non-paretic hand (*right*)

motor control over the paretic hand. Accordingly, fMRI during a simple active hand motor task (*active* opening/closing of the paretic hand) revealed not only activation in the 'hand knob' area of the contra-lesional hemisphere but also activation in the contralateral Rolandic region, an area from which no motor-evoked potentials could be elicited by TMS. fMRI during *passive* hand movement also elicited activation in the contralateral Rolandic region (i.e. of the affected hemisphere), suggesting preserved somatosensory functions in this region. And indeed, MEG recorded the first cortical response to repetitive tactile stimulation of the paretic thumb (N20m) in the contralateral Rolandic region, confirming this region to harbour the primary somatosensory representation (S1) of the paretic hand. Finally, DTI with a seed region in the dorsal brainstem (tegmentum pontis) visualized ascending spino-thalamocortical projections bypassing the lesion on their way to this preserved somatosensory representation of the paretic hand. This observation can be explained by the fact that developing thalamocortical somatosensory projections had not yet reached their cortical target areas by the time of the insult (the early third trimester of pregnancy; Kostovic and Judas 2002) so that these outgrowing fibres could find an alternative route in the preserved tissue, thus forming 'axonal bypasses' around the defective areas (Staudt et al. 2006a).

This example and similar cases (Thickbroom et al. 2001; Staudt et al. 2006a) teach important lessons for the application of non-invasive imaging techniques in children with early brain lesions:

1. Different mechanisms are available for the reorganization of primary motor and primary somatosensory representations (shifting to the contra-lesional hemisphere for motor functions, forming axonal bypasses around a lesion for somatosensory functions).
2. This can lead to a 'hemispheric dissociation' between the primary motor (M1) and the primary somatosensory (S1) representations of a paretic hand.
3. fMRI of passive hand movement alone is not suited to identify the 'sensorimotor representation' of a paretic hand (see Fig. 11.5); the reorganization of the primary motor representation in Example 5 would have been missed with the 'normal-looking' result for passive hand movement!

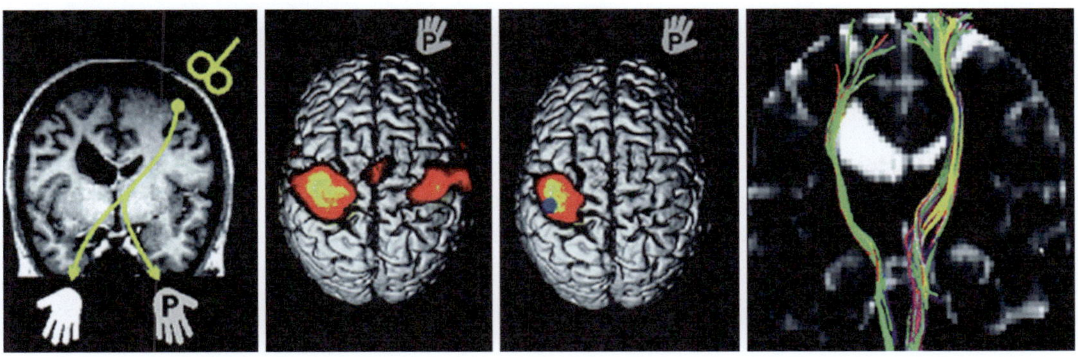

Fig. 11.5 MRI, TMS, fMRI, MEG and DTI tractography findings of a 19-year-old female with congenital hemiparesis due to a unilateral periventricular brain lesion. *Left*: coronal T1-weighted image depicting the periventricular lesion. TMS (indicated by the *yellow figure-eight-coil symbol*) of the contra-lesional hemisphere elicited not only the normal contralateral responses in the non-paretic hand but also ipsilateral motor-evoked potentials in the paretic hand (P), demonstrating the presence of ipsilateral cortico-spinal projections. *Middle*: fMRI during active (*middle left*) and passive (*middle right*) movement of the paretic hand. The *blue circle* indicates the position of the dipole reconstruction from MEG recording of the first cortical response to tactile stimulation of the paretic thumb. *Right*: diffusion tensor imaging (DTI) tractography of ascending spino-thalamocortical projections, with seed regions in the dorsal brainstem (tegmentum pontis) and in the subcortical Rolandic white matter of both hemispheres. (From Staudt et al. (2006a) with permission)

11.7 Example 6

A 7-year-old girl with right-hemispheric polymicrogyria showed congenital hemiparesis (with preserved grasp function of the paretic hand) and pharmaco-refractory epilepsy, so that a surgical disconnection of the malformed right hemisphere (hemispherotomy) for the relief of the epilepsy was considered. TMS and fMRI showed exactly the same constellation as in the patient in Example 5, so that the phenomenon of 'M1-S1-dissociation' was apparently present in this girl as well, with a reorganized primary motor (M1) representation of the paretic hand in the contra-lesional (ipsilateral) hemisphere and a contralateral primary somatosensory representation (S1) of the paretic hand in the polymicrogyria. Accordingly, color-coded fractional anisotropy (DTI) of the pons revealed symmetrical ascending tracts in the tegmentum (including the medial lemniscus carrying the somatosensory projections), while in the basis pontis, cortico-spinal projections were only seen in the contra-lesional side of the brainstem. And as predicted by this pattern (Küpper et al. 2016), when hemispherotomy was performed, the girl showed preserved grasp function but reduced tactile discrimination with her paretic hand.

11.8 Conclusions

Non-invasive mapping techniques such as fMRI, TMS, MEG and DTI tractography are useful techniques in the pre-surgical diagnostic workup of children with early brain lesions. These situations often require a combined use of complementary techniques.

The combination of fMRI (during active movements) and TMS is well suited to identify motor representations, with TMS being specific for areas from where cortico-spinal projections originate and fMRI visualizing the entire sensorimotor network with a high spatial resolution in three dimensions (Thickbroom et al. 2001; Staudt et al. 2002a, 2004a, b). This is important for the identification of (a) the spatial relation between M1 and an epileptogenic lesion (as in Example 1; Fig. 11.1), (b) a preserved M1 in dysgenic cortex (as in Example 3; Fig. 11.3) and (c) a reorganization of M1 into the contra-lesional hemisphere (as in Examples 4, 5, and 6; Figs. 11.4, 11.5 and 11.6). In this respect, patients with a 'hemispheric dissociation' between M1 and S1 (Thickbroom et al. 2001; Staudt et al. 2006a) are particularly challenging since, here, fMRI of active hand movements typically yields bilateral Rolandic activation.

The combination of fMRI (during passive movements) and MEG is well suited to identify somatosensory representations, with MEG (due to its high temporal resolution) being specific for primary somatosensory representations (i.e. the cortical projection areas of somatosensory fibres) and fMRI visualizing the somatosensory network with a high spatial resolution in three dimensions (Staudt et al. 2006a; Wilke et al. 2008). Similar to the motor system, this combination can identify (a) preserved somatosensory projections in preserved white-matter bridges (as in Example 2; Fig. 11.2), (b) a preserved S1 in Rolandic cortex overlying even large lesions (as in Example 5; Fig. 11.5) and (c) a preserved S1 in dysgenic cortex (as in example 6; Fig. 11.6).

DTI tractography can visualize preserved projections in the vicinity of a lesion (as in Example 2; Fig. 11.2) or 'axonal bypasses' around a lesion (as in Example 5; Fig. 11.5). Because of the uncertainties involved in this new technique, we still recommend to use such information only when additional evidence (e.g. neurophysiological evidence from TMS or MEG) for the existence of such projections is available. Finally, DTI fractional anisotropy maps of the brainstem, when showing marked asymmetries of the cortico-spinal tracts in the basis pontis, help to predict preserved grasp function of the paretic hand after hemispherotomies (Küpper et al. 2016).

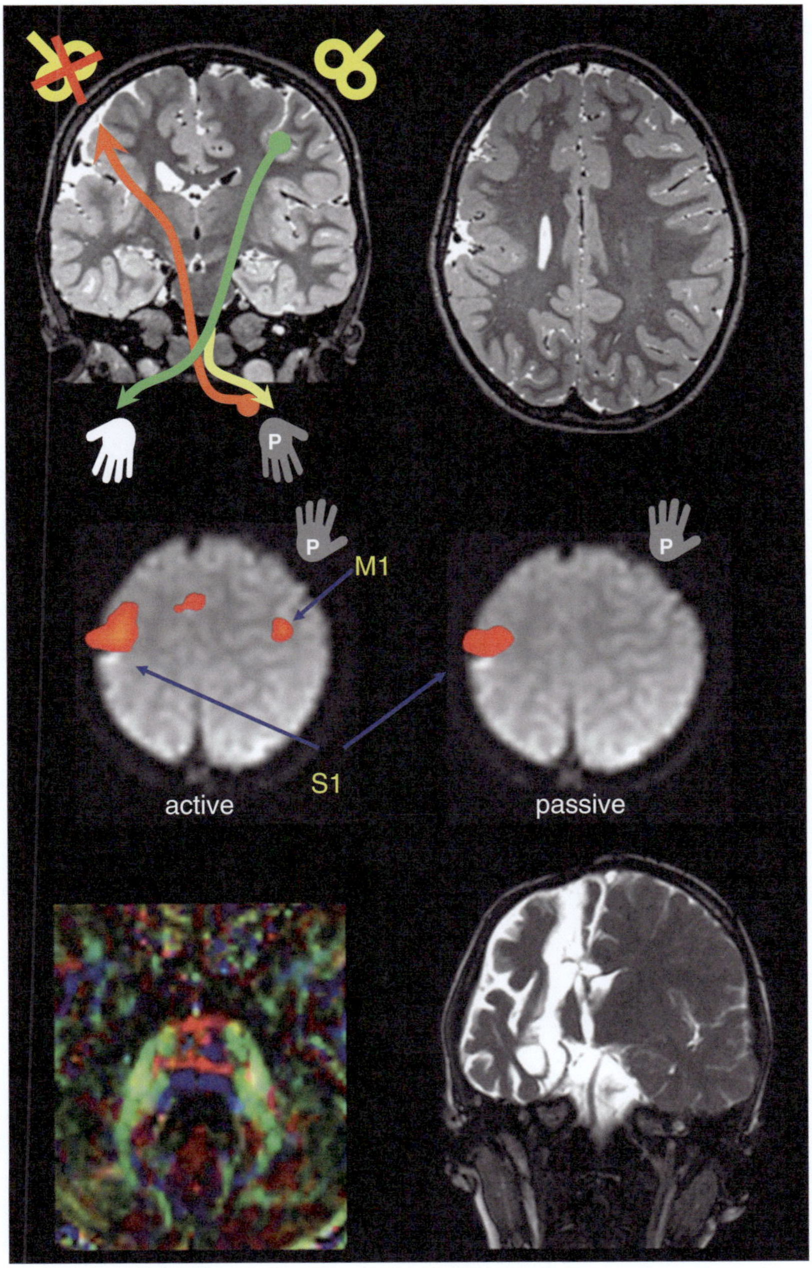

Fig. 11.6 MRI, TMS, fMRI and color-coded DTI (fractional anisotropy map) findings of a 7-year-old girl with congenital hemiparesis and pharmaco-refractory epilepsy due to polymicrogyria of the right hemisphere. *Top*: coronal (*left*) and axial (*right*) T2-weighted images depicting the polymicrogyria. TMS (indicated by the *yellow figure-eight-coil symbol*) of the contra-lesional hemisphere elicited not only the normal contralateral responses in the non-paretic hand (*green arrow*) but also ipsilateral motor-evoked potentials in the paretic hand (P), demonstrating the presence of ipsilateral cortico-spinal projections (*yellow arrow*). The *orange arrow* symbolizes crossed ascending somatosensory projections to the primary somatosensory representation of the paretic hand in the polymicrogyria (*see below*). *Middle*: fMRI during active (*middle left*) and passive (*middle right*) movement of the paretic hand. *Bottom left*: axial diffusion tensor imaging (DTI) fractional anisotropy map of the brainstem, depicting symmetrical ascending fibres in the tegmentum pontis, whereas the basis pontis shows cortico-spinal projections only in the left (healthy) side (*all coded in blue*). *Bottom right*: post-operative MRI (coronal T2 weighted) shows the vertical parasagittal hemispherotomy. (Performed by M. Kudernatsch, Schön Klinik Vogtareuth)

References

Carr LJ, Harrison LM et al (1993) Patterns of central motor reorganization in hemiplegic cerebral palsy. Brain 116:1223–1247

Hertz-Pannier L, Chiron C et al (2001) Functional imaging in the work-up of childhood epilepsy. Childs Nerv Syst 17:223–228

Kostovic I, Judas M (2002) Correlation between the sequential ingrowth of afferents and transient patterns of cortical lamination in preterm infants. Anat Rec 267:1–6

Küpper H, Kudernatsch M, Pieper T, Groeschel S, Tournier JD, Raffelt D, Winkler P, Holthausen H, Staudt M (2016) Predicting hand function after hemidisconnection: a study on 102 patients. Brain 139:2456–2468

Liégeois F, Cross JH et al (2006) Role of fMRI in the decision-making process: epilepsy surgery for children. J Magn Reson Imaging 23:933–940

Rasmussen T, Milner B (1977) The role of early left-brain injury in determining lateralization of cerebral speech functions. Ann N Y Acad Sci 30:355–369

Staudt M, Pieper T et al (2001) Functional MRI in a 6-year-old boy with unilateral cortical malformation: concordant representation of both hands in the unaffected hemisphere. Neuropediatrics 32:159–161

Staudt M, Grodd W et al (2002a) Two types of ipsilateral reorganization in congenital hemiparesis: a TMS and fMRI study. Brain 125:2222–2237

Staudt M, Lidzba K et al (2002b) Right-hemispheric organization of language following early left-sided brain lesions: functional MRI topography. Neuroimage 16:954–967

Staudt M, Gerloff C et al (2004a) Reorganization in congenital hemiparesis acquired at different gestational ages. Ann Neurol 56:854–863

Staudt M, Krägeloh-Mann I et al (2004b) Searching for motor functions in dysgenic cortex: a clinical TMS and fMRI study. J Neurosurg 101:69–77

Staudt M, Braun C et al (2006a) Developing somatosensory projections bypass periventricular brain lesions. Neurology 67:522–525

Staudt M, Erb M et al (2006b) Extensive peri-lesional connectivity in congenital hemiparesis. Neurology 66:771

Thickbroom GW, Byrnes ML et al (2001) Differences in sensory and motor cortical organization following brain injury early in life. Ann Neurol 49:320–327

Wilke M, Staudt M et al (2008) Somatosensory system in two types of motor reorganization in congenital hemiparesis: topography & function. Hum Brain Mapp 30:776–788

12 Combining Transcranial Magnetic Stimulation with (f)MRI

Gesa Hartwigsen, Tanja Kassuba, and Hartwig R. Siebner

12.1 Introduction

Transcranial magnetic stimulation (TMS) is a noninvasive and painless tool for the electrical stimulation of the human cortex (Barker et al. 1985). TMS depolarizes cortical neurons and can evoke measurable electrophysiological and behavioral effects. TMS is usually applied to one cortical area but can also be given to two or more areas (i.e., multisite TMS). Single or paired stimuli and short stimulus trains (i.e., high-frequency bursts) provide a means of transiently disrupting ongoing neuronal processing in the stimulated cortex. Repetitive TMS (rTMS) refers to the application of prolonged trains of stimuli, which are given either continuously as long trains at a constant rate (continuous rTMS) or intermittently as repetitive bursts (i.e., intermittent or burst-like rTMS). rTMS can modify the excitability of the cerebral cortex at the stimulated site and also at remote interconnected brain regions, beyond the time of stimulation. Its neuromodulatory effects make rTMS a valuable tool for studying the functional plasticity of neuronal networks and may be used therapeutically in patients with neurological and psychiatric disorders.

G. Hartwigsen (✉)
Lise Meitner Research Group Cognition and Plasticity, Max Planck Institute for Human Cognitive and Brain Sciences, Leipzig, Germany
e-mail: hartwigsen@cbs.mpg.de

T. Kassuba
Department of Psychology, Center for the Study of Brain, Mind & Behavior, Princeton University, Princeton, NJ, USA

H. R. Siebner
Danish Research Center for Magnetic Resonance, Center for Functional and Diagnostic Imaging, Copenhagen University Hospital Hvidovre, Hvidovre, Denmark

12.1.1 How Does TMS Excite Cortical Neurons?

TMS causes inductive (electro-magneto-electric) stimulation of neuronal axons. A brief, high-current pulse is produced in a stimulating coil. The time-varying electrical field produces a time-varying magnetic field with lines of flux oriented perpendicularly to the plane of the coil. The pulsed magnetic field is not attenuated by the skull and induces an electric field in the superficial brain tissue (i.e., cortex), which runs parallel to the plane of the coil but has a direction that is opposite to the electric field in the coil. Hence, the pulsed magnetic field is only used as a means to generate an electric field in the brain that is suprathreshold for exciting cortical axons.

How does the time-varying electrical field induced in the cortex excite neurons? The electrical field induced in the neuronal tissue drives transmembraneous ionic currents. The most relevant parameter is the rate of change of the electric field along the nerve. Depending on the gradient and the orientation of the electric field

S. Ulmer, O. Jansen (eds.), *fMRI*, https://doi.org/10.1007/978-3-030-41874-8_12

gradient relative to the course of the axon, the pulsed electrical field may generate an outward current and local depolarization at distinct sites of neuronal axons. If the outward current causes sufficient membrane depolarization, this will trigger an action potential. This action potential propagates along the axon and may cause a trans-synaptic excitation of postsynaptic neurons. Crucial for an efficient depolarization of an axon is the spatial gradient of the induced electric field in relation to the orientation of the axon. At the cellular level, the events that lead to neuronal excitation are still poorly understood. For instance, the relevance of cellular and gyral shapes, the gray matter boundaries, the local variations in tissue conductivity, and the role of background neuronal activity for neuronal stimulation are largely unknown (for recent reviews, see Miniussi et al. 2010; Sandrini et al. 2011; Siebner et al. 2009b).

The majority of studies have investigated the physiological mechanisms of TMS in the human primary motor cortex (M1) because its effects can be quantified by recording the TMS-evoked motor potential (MEP). For other brain regions, such direct quantification is difficult to obtain. Therefore, researchers have used neuroimaging techniques such as positron emission tomography (PET), electroencephalography (EEG), or functional magnetic resonance imaging (fMRI) to map TMS-evoked changes in regional neuronal activity throughout the brain (Bestmann et al. 2003b; Ilmoniemi et al. 1997; Lee et al. 2003; Massimini et al. 2005; Siebner et al. 2003). These studies have revealed that the TMS-induced changes in regional neuronal activity are not restricted to the stimulated cortex but give rise to functional changes in connected cortical areas, including subcortical brain regions (Bestmann et al. 2003b; Lee et al. 2003; Siebner et al. 2003).

Regarding fMRI, a critical question is whether the blood-oxygen-level-dependent (BOLD) signal really captures the TMS-induced changes in regional neuronal activity. Allen et al. (2007) combined optical imaging with electrophysiological recordings of neuronal activity in cat visual cortex to show that TMS-induced changes in neural activity are readily reflected by cerebral hemodynamics. Further, the quantitative coupling between TMS-evoked neural activity and cerebral hemodynamics was present over a range of stimulation parameters. These results demonstrate the usefulness of combined TMS–fMRI studies in humans showing that TMS-induced neural changes are "faithfully reflected in hemodynamic signals" (Allen et al. 2007).

12.1.2 Some Physical Aspects of Transcranial Magnetic Stimulation

The induced magnetic and electric field decreases rapidly with increasing distance from the coil. The maximal depth of penetration depends on the shape and size of the coil, the employed stimulation intensity, and the responsiveness of the targeted tissue. The decrease with distance is more rapid for small coils than for large ones. The coil should be placed tangentially on the skin to minimize the coil–cortex distance. Commercially used coils reach a penetration depth of approximately 2–3 cm. This implies that only cortical neuronal tissue is within the range of TMS, while deep cerebral gray matter nuclei cannot be stimulated directly with TMS.

In general, TMS does not produce a focal stimulation of neuronal tissue at a small predictable site. The geometry of the coil is an important factor in determining the magnitude and spatial extent of cortical stimulation. The two most commonly used coil shapes are circular (i.e., referred to as round coil) and figure of eight (referred to as figure-of-eight-shaped coil or butterfly coil). The circular coil induces a concentric circular electric field. If the coil is placed with its entire surface tangentially to the skin, neuronal structures in the tissue underlying the circular coil will be activated. It should be noted that neuronal stimulation is minimal in the brain tissue underlying the center of the coil when the flat surface of the circular coil is placed on the scalp tangentially to the skin (Weyh and Siebner 2007). The other coil design has a figure-of-eight configuration. Figure-of-eight coils consist of two circular coils placed side by side and are wired such that the current from the stimulator passes in opposite directions in each. This produces a relatively clear-defined maximum of the induced current where the two coils approach each other (i.e., in the geometrical center of the coil). With a spatial resolution of approximately 1–1.5 cm, the figure-of-eight coil is substantially more focal than the circular coil. This explains why the figure-of-eight coil is preferred to the round coil when TMS is used to map cortical functions (Walsh and Rushworth 1999). It needs to be borne in mind that commercially available stimulation devices may differ in terms of coil design. This may alter the characteristics of neuronal stimulation, including the heating properties during rTMS and the hardware design (Lang et al. 2006; Weyh et al. 2005).

12.1.3 Clinical and Neuroscientific Applications of TMS

TMS can be used in several ways to study human brain function. Single-pulse or paired-pulse TMS can be applied to probe the excitability of intracortical inhibitory and facilitatory circuits in the motor and visual cortex. Since the action potentials induced by TMS spread along preexisting axonal connections, TMS-induced neuronal excitation is not limited to the stimulated cortex but leads to a transsynaptic spread of excitation to interconnected cortical areas. This renders TMS a very powerful means of studying functional and effective connectivity in the intact human brain (Kobayashi and Pascual-Leone 2003). For instance, TMS has been extensively used to probe corticocortical and corticospinal connectivity in the motor system. In clinical neurology, TMS is commonly used as a routine evaluation of the excitability and conductivity of corticospinal pathways.

TMS can induce a transient dysfunction in the stimulated cortex, sometimes referred to as "virtual lesion" (Pascual-Leone et al. 2000). When being applied in its "virtual lesion" mode during an experimental task, TMS may produce measurable changes in task performance. These changes in behavior can be used to make inferences about the importance of the stimulated brain area for a specific cognitive, sensory, or motor function (Walsh and Cowey 2000; Walsh and Rushworth 1999; see Siebner et al. 2009b for a review). Various rTMS protocols are being increasingly used by clinicians and neuroscientists to induce lasting changes in the status of the human brain (Siebner and Rothwell 2003). Conventional rTMS protocols consist of a continuous series of pulses with constant repetition rates. In the "continuous mode" of rTMS, stimulation rates of around 1 Hz are referred to as *low-frequency rTMS* and stimulation rates between 5 and 50 Hz as *high-frequency rTMS*. Most studies regarding the motor cortex suggest inhibitory effects of low-frequency rTMS and facilitatory effects of high-frequency rTMS (Berardelli et al. 1998; Chen et al. 1997a; Pascual-Leone et al. 1998). Recent protocols use more complex temporal stimulation patterns such as double-pulse rTMS (Thickbroom et al. 2006), quadro-pulse rTMS (Hamada et al. 2007), or theta burst stimulation (TBS), which gives short, high-frequent *bursts* of pulses every 0.2 s (Huang et al. 2005). Ongoing research addresses the question on whether the neuromodulatory effects of these rTMS protocols may have a therapeutic application in neurological and psychiatric disorders (Wassermann and Lisanby 2001).

TMS can be applied while subjects perform an experimental task (*online TMS*) or shortly before they perform the task (*offline TMS*). Offline TMS usually involves an rTMS protocol that induces a lasting alteration of cortical excitability, while online TMS may consist of single pulses or short high-frequency trains that are given at distinct points in time during task performance. Both approaches allow the testing of the functional relevance of the targeted brain area by measuring the acute (*online TMS*) or conditioning (*offline TMS*) effects of TMS on electrophysiological measures (e.g., MEP amplitude), on behavioral measures (e.g., response latencies or error rate), or more directly on regional brain activity using brain mapping techniques such as EEG, PET, or fMRI (Siebner et al. 2009a). While conventional paradigms apply uni-site TMS over a single cortical area, more recent studies have also started to include multisite TMS over two or more areas simultaneously (Hartwigsen et al. 2010a, b).

12.1.4 Adverse Effects and Safety Precautions

TMS has the capability of producing adverse effects, especially if rTMS is used. These side effects are extensively discussed in a recent review (Wassermann 2008). The most relevant adverse effect is the induction of epileptic seizures. Since rTMS induces stronger and more persistent effects on cortical excitability and function than single-pulse TMS, it bears a higher risk of provoking epileptic seizures even in healthy individuals. Therefore, safety guidelines were established that specify the maximal number of pulses per session, stimulus intensity, and frequency that are considered to be safe in terms of seizure induction (Chen et al. 1997b; Rossi et al. 2009; Rossini et al. 2015; Wassermann 1998). Since the introduction of the safety guidelines, only a few cases of accidental seizures with TMS have been reported worldwide, and none of the individuals who had experienced rTMS-induced seizures has suffered lasting physical sequelae.

The rapid discharge through the coil produces a characteristic clicking sound in the frequency range of 2–7 kHz. The click is caused by mechanical deformation of the coil during strong magnetic pulses. Peak sound pressure has been reported to be 120–130 dB at a distance of 10 cm from the coil (Starck et al. 1996). Sound levels will be higher when TMS is given inside the MRI bore because of the additional magnetic field generated by the MR scanner. Therefore, individuals who receive rTMS or are examined in the MR scanner should always wear earplugs (cf. Sect. 12.3.2.1).

12.2 Placement of the Coil Over the Cortical Target Area

Accurate placement of the TMS coil over the cortex area that is to be stimulated with TMS is crucial. The motor response that is evoked by TMS can be used to localize the primary motor cortex. A similar approach can be chosen for TMS of the visual cortex by positioning the coil at the site where TMS most reliably elicits a phosphene. In both instances, TMS produces an overt response that can be used to functionally determine the appropriate site of stimulation. For most remaining cortical areas, no such responses can be elicited, and other strategies have to be used to accurately place the coil over the cortical target.

Some researchers use the optimal site to stimulate the primary motor cortex as "anchor point" for the stimulation of pericentral cortical areas such as premotor or somatosensory areas (Gerschlager et al. 2001; Koch et al. 2006; Lee and van Donkelaar 2006). However, this method is not sufficiently accurate for targeting more distant areas such as the dorsolateral prefrontal cortex (Bohning et al. 2003b).

The international 10–20 system for the placement of EEG electrodes (Jasper 1958) is often used for the positioning of the TMS coil. The 10–20 system offers a grid of electrode sites located on the scalp that is derived from standard cranial landmarks, i.e., the inion, nasion, or preauricular points. This method assumes a consistent correlation between scalp locations and underlying brain structures across subjects. Greater accuracy can be obtained by acquiring structural MR images of the brain, together with capsules containing a high-contrast marker attached to the head (Terao et al. 1998). The placement of the coil can then be referenced to the position of the marker.

Neuronavigated TMS guided by frameless stereotaxy represents the method of choice as it allows both the exact placement and monitoring of the coil throughout the TMS experiment (Denslow et al. 2005a; Herwig et al. 2003a; Neggers et al. 2004; Sack et al. 2006; Schonfeldt-Lecuona et al. 2005). Optical (infrared-based) and acoustic (ultrasound-based) devices are available for neuronavigation. These systems use passive (reflecting) or active (emitting) markers that are attached to the subject's head and to the TMS coil (Ettinger et al. 1998). Sparing et al. (2008) compared different methods for the placement of the TMS coil over the primary motor cortex in terms of accuracy. The least accurate results were obtained when the 10–20 EEG system or function-guided procedures were used, although there was a great variation among different electrode positions as some can be located more reliably than others. In that study, fMRI-guided neuronavigated stimulation yielded the highest spatial accuracy in the range of a few millimeters. Other studies have confirmed these results (Denslow et al. 2005a; Herwig et al. 2003b; Schonfeldt-Lecuona et al. 2005).

Neuronavigation requires a T1-weighted, high-resolution image of the subject's brain. The anatomical images have to be transferred into three-dimensional space. Optionally, individual fMRI activation maps can be overlaid on the structural images. Predefined anatomical landmarks are marked on the individual structural MRI with special neuronavigation software. Usually, the nasion, the nibs of the tragus of both ears, and the internal angle of the eyes are used. A headband is then strapped around the subject's head. A tracker with at least three passive spheres or ultrasound reflecting transmitters is firmly attached to the headband, indicating the position of the subject's head. Another tracker is fixed onto the TMS coil. These dynamic reference systems provide online information about the location of the head and the coil in space. A camera system detects the position of the dynamic reference systems and displays this information on a computer screen using navigation software for visual localization of the coil (see Fig. 12.1).

The subject's head and the structural MR scans are coregistered by touching the predefined landmarks on the subject's face using a pointer equipped with trackers. An accurate coregistration procedure is crucial to the exact placement of the coil. The position of the coil is visualized in real time on a computer screen relative to the individual three-dimensional anatomy of the brain. The exact position of the cortical target area can be defined either anatomically based on the gyral anatomy or functionally on the basis of activation maps that have been obtained with fMRI. In addition to the individual activation map, one can also use the stereotactic coordinates of a peak activation that has been identified in a group of subjects. In this instance, the coordinates from standardized space (MNI, Talairach) have to be transformed to the subject's "native" space.

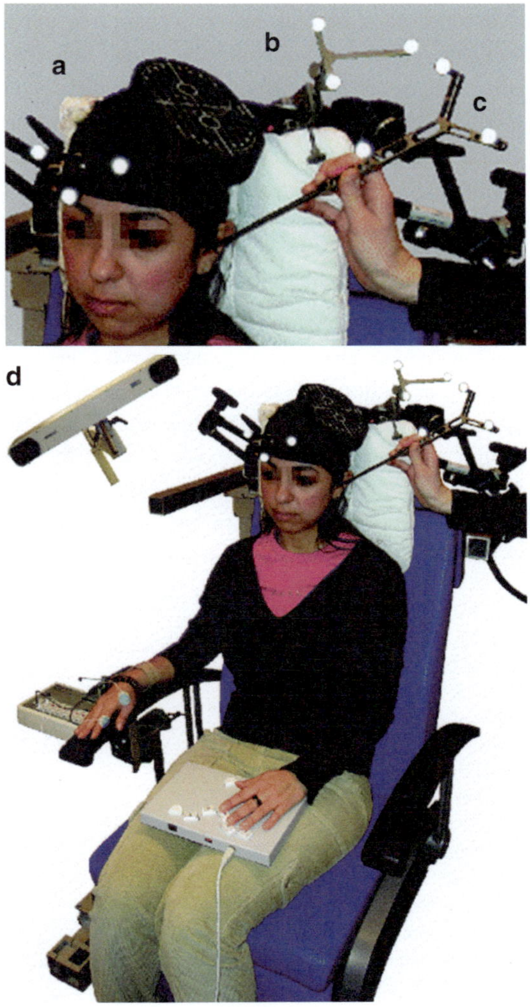

Fig. 12.1 Neuronavigated TMS guided by frameless stereotaxy. A tracker with three passive spheres is attached to the headband of the subject (**a**) and to the TMS coil (**b**) and fixed on a pointer (**c**). These dynamic reference systems provide online information about the location of the head and the coil in space. A camera system (**d**) detects the position of the dynamic reference systems and displays this information on a computer screen using navigation software for visual localization of the coil

12.3 Combinations of fMRI with TMS

12.3.1 Why Combine TMS with fMRI?

fMRI provides a sensitive means of identifying brain regions where regional neuronal activity correlates with behavior. Due to its correlative nature, fMRI-based activation maps cannot establish whether such activation makes a relevant contribution to the behavior. By temporarily disrupting ongoing neural activity, TMS permits to make causal inferences regarding the contribution of the stimulated cortex to a specific brain function. Since single-pulse TMS offers a high temporal resolution, it can also be used to identify the period during which the stimulated area makes a critical contribution to the experimental task. Thus, a combined TMS and fMRI gives access to noninvasive measuring of stimulation effects on the brain with a high spatial (fMRI: spatial resolution in the millimeter range) and temporal (single-pulse TMS: temporal resolution in the order of milliseconds) resolution.

The temporal relationship between TMS and fMRI defines which question can be addressed using a combined TMS–fMRI approach. TMS can be given in the MR scanner during fMRI data acquisition (online approach) to investigate the immediate effects of TMS on brain activity and behavior. Alternatively, TMS and fMRI may be separated in space and time (offline approach). In this case, TMS is given outside the MRI suite before or after fMRI (see Fig. 12.2).

12.3.2 TMS in the MR Scanner During fMRI (Online TMS–fMRI Approach)

TMS during fMRI (interleaved TMS–fMRI) enables the researcher to probe the immediate impact of TMS on regional neuronal activity

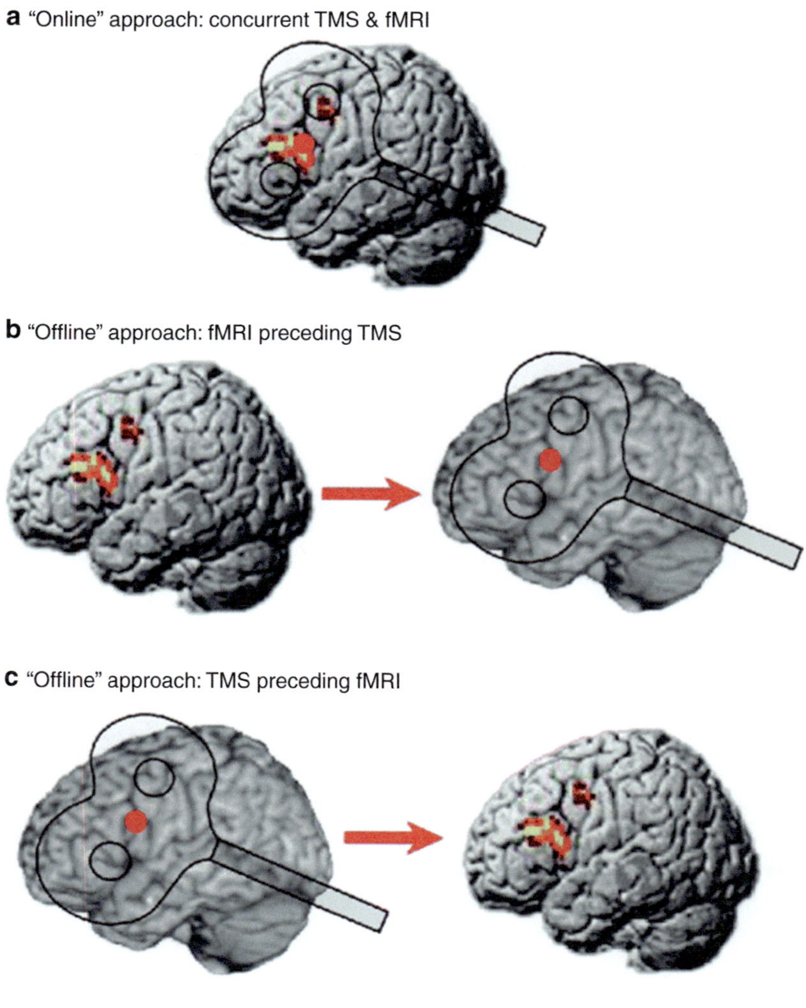

Fig. 12.2 Relative timing of TMS and fMRI determines the application of combined TMS–fMRI. TMS and fMRI can be performed interleaved (i.e., "online" approach) to investigate immediate effects of TMS on brain functions (**a**). In the "offline" approach, fMRI precedes or follows TMS. fMRI preceding TMS is usually used to identify appropriate sites for focal TMS (**b**), while TMS preceding fMRI can be used to probe the lasting effects of TMS conditioning on brain functions (**c**)

across the whole brain. By applying TMS during different functional states of the brain, the online TMS–fMRI approach can explore how the TMS influences on neuronal activity in the stimulated and distant areas vary with task demands.

12.3.2.1 Methodological Issues

Although the prerequisites to apply TMS during fMRI were already introduced by Bohning et al. (1997, 1998, 1999) approximately 10 years ago, interleaved TMS–fMRI failed to become a routine procedure yet. At present, most of the studies that used interleaved TMS–fMRI were carried out by three research groups in Charleston (North Carolina, USA), Göttingen (Germany), and London (UK; for details, see Table 12.1). A simple implementation of TMS in the MRI environment is precluded by problems originating from the application of magnetic pulses in the static magnetic field of the MR scanner and in the presence of magnetic field gradients required for image acquisition (Baudewig et al. 2001). Therefore, nonferromagnetic coils have to be used that are mechanically strengthened to prevent coils from breaking during fMRI. Subjects have to wear earplugs and headphones because mechanical interactions between the TMS-evoked local magnetic field and the static magnetic field of the MR scanner result in a louder click when the coil is discharged inside the scanner. The presence of the MR-compatible TMS coil may cause geometric image distortions (Baudewig et al. 2000; Bestmann et al. 2003a). These can be reduced by a shorter readout time of echoplanar imaging (EPI) sequences, the use of stronger imaging gradients, and parallel imaging.

The ferromagnetic stimulation device must be placed at sufficient distance from the magnetic field of the MR scanner, outside the scanner room, or in a radio-frequency-shielded cabinet inside the scanner room. This requires a longer cable to connect the coil with the stimulator.

MR-compatible TMS coil holders help to ensure accurate placement of the coil inside the scanner. Yet spatial limitations imposed by the MR head coil may restrict access to some cortical areas, especially in the basal, frontal, and temporal lobes. TMS also evokes twitches of cranial muscles and somatosensory and auditory stimulation, which may cause discomfort and movement artifacts and contribute to functional brain activation. Nonspecific auditory and somatosensory stimulation as well as the unpleasantness of TMS complicate the interpretation of TMS-induced brain activation by causing BOLD signal changes in subcortical and cortical areas involved in sensory or affective processing (Bestmann et al. 2005). It is therefore advisable to include a control condition that matches the auditory and somatosensory stimulation but does not cause transcranial cortical stimulation. Alternatively, the same TMS protocol might be applied to a control area in a separate fMRI session.

Dynamic artifacts pose a major problem to concurrent TMS during fMRI. Radio-frequency (RF) noise can markedly reduce the signal-to-noise ratio of MR images. TMS stimulators may themselves produce RF noise, and the antenna-like properties of the TMS coil cable can additionally guide RF noise into the scanner, which can be reduced by customized RF filters. Leakage currents that originate from the high-voltage capacitors of the TMS stimulator may induce additional image distortions and artifacts. Of note, these leakage currents change with the intensity of TMS and can give rise to intensity-dependent BOLD signal changes. Remote-controlled high-voltage relay-diode systems reduce leakage currents flowing between the stimulator and the TMS coil and can thus be used to resolve this problem (Bestmann et al. 2007).

The strong magnetic pulses induced by TMS can severely distort MR images depending on TMS coil orientation, TMS pulse intensity, and MR magnetic field strength (Bestmann et al. 2003a; Shastri et al. 1999). Therefore, a direct interference between TMS pulse and EPI excitation pulses should be avoided, and images being perturbed by TMS pulses must be replaced (Bestmann et al. 2008). A feasible solution to this problem is to introduce a sufficiently long temporal gap between TMS pulses and subsequent MR image acquisition (for more technical details, see Baudewig and Bestmann 2007; Bestmann et al. 2008).

Table 12.1 Studies using interleaved TMS–fMRI in healthy volunteers

Target area	Task	TMS–fMRI protocol (frequency, % MT, total no. of pulses per train/session)	Reference
Left M1	Rest	0.83 Hz, 110, 20/session	Bohning et al. (1998)
Left M1	Rest	1 Hz, 80/110, 18/session	Bohning et al. (1999)
Left M1	Rest/finger movements	1 Hz, 110, 21/train	Bohning et al. (2000a)
Left M1	Rest	SP, 120, 15/session	Bohning et al. (2000b)
Left M1	Rest/finger movements	10 Hz, 110, 10/train	Baudewig et al. (2001)
Left PMd		10 Hz, 90/110, 10/train	
Left PFC	Rest	1 Hz, 80/100/120, 21/train	Nahas et al. (2001)
Left M1/S1	Rest	4 Hz, 90/110/110 AMT, 40/train	Bestmann et al. (2003b)
Left M1	Rest	1 Hz, 110, *not reported*	Bohning et al. (2003a)
Left M1	Rest	1 Hz; 120; 1, 2, 4, 8, 16, 24/train	Bohning et al. (2003c)
Left M1	Rest	4 Hz, 150, 4/train	Kemna and Gembris 2003
Left M1	Rest	1 Hz, 110, 21/train	McConnell et al. (2003)
Left M1	Rest	3.1 Hz, 90/110 AMT, 30/session	Bestmann et al. (2004)
Left M1/S1	Rest/finger movements	1 Hz, 110, 21/train	Denslow et al. (2004)
Left PFC	Rest	1 Hz, 100, 21/session	Li et al. (2004a)[a]
Left M1	Rest	1 Hz, 110/120, *not reported*	Li et al. (2004b)
Left PFC			
Left PMd	Rest/finger movements	3 Hz, 90/110 AMT, *not reported*	Bestmann et al. (2005)
Left M1	Rest/finger movements	1 Hz, 110, 21/train	Denslow et al. (2005a)
Left M1	Rest	1 Hz, 110, 21/train	Denslow et al. (2005b)
Left M1	Rest	SP; ~90;98/102;110 SoM; 20; 40/session	Bestmann et al. (2006)[b]
Right FEF	Rest/visual judgment	9 Hz; 40/55/70/85 TOP	Ruff et al. (2006)
		10 Hz; 65 TOP; 5/train	
Left PMd	Isometric left-hand grips	11 Hz, 70/110, 5/train	Bestmann et al. (2007)
Left/right SPL	Visuospatial tasks	13.3 Hz, 100 TOP, 5/train	Sack et al. (2007)
Right IPS/FEF	Visual task (moving stimuli)	9 Hz, 40/55/70/85 TOP, 5/train	Ruff et al. (2008)

AMT active motor threshold, *FEF* frontal eye field, *IPS* intraparietal sulcus, *M1* primary motor cortex, *PFC* prefrontal cortex, *PMd* dorsal premotor cortex, *RMT* resting motor threshold, *SoM* sense of movement, *SP* single pulse, *TOP* total output

[a]Depressive patients

[b]Amputee patient

12.3.2.2 Applications of Interleaved TMS–fMRI

Several researchers applied TMS over the motor cortex during rest and showed that TMS-induced acute changes in BOLD signal are a dose-dependent fashion (Baudewig et al. 2001; Bestmann et al. 2003a, 2004; Bohning et al. 1998, 1999, 2000b). A single TMS pulse evoked regional increases in BOLD signal that were similar to those evoked by volitional movements (Bohning et al. 2000b). Such BOLD signal increases were only observed at suprathreshold intensities, which evoked a muscle twitch in the contralateral hand. Hence, it remains unclear whether the observed activation was directly induced by cortical stimulation or resulted from somatosensory feedback activation caused by the TMS-induced movement. However, Bestmann et al. (2005) applied short trains of 3 Hz rTMS over the left premotor cortex, which produced an increase in BOLD signal in the stimulated cortex and connected areas. Since the premotor TMS train did not produce overt muscle movements, it was concluded that these BOLD signal changes resulted from cortical stimulation rather than from somatosensory feedback activation.

Interleaved TMS–fMRI studies revealed that TMS can evoke changes in neural activity in connected cortical and subcortical areas (Baudewig et al. 2001; Bestmann et al. 2004, 2005; Bohning et al. 1998, 1999, 2000a; Ruff et al. 2008). These distant BOLD signal changes can occur even in the absence of consistent signal changes in the area that was directly targeted by TMS (Bestmann et al. 2004). This suggests that transsynaptic spread of excitation from the stimulated to connected brain areas makes a major contribution to neuronal stimulation that is induced by TMS in the human brain.

Interleaved TMS–fMRI opens up the possibility to examine how TMS interacts with intrinsic task-related activation and how these TMS-induced changes in task-related activity relate to changes in behavior. In a recent study, parietal rTMS was performed during fMRI to map TMS-induced changes in task-related brain activity that underlies the TMS-induced impairment of visuospatial judgments (Ruff et al. 2008). Concurrent TMS–fMRI was employed to investigate the influences of a short high-frequency rTMS train over the right frontal eye field (FEF) or intraparietal sulcus on the BOLD response in occipital activity to visual stimulation. The authors showed that TMS-induced changes in occipital activity critically depend on the actual state of the visual system at the time of TMS. Increased activity over visual area V5/MT+ was only found if moving stimuli were concurrently presented. Conversely, visual areas V1–V4 were specifically activated during the absence of input.

So far, very few interleaved TMS–fMRI studies have been carried out in patients. In a case study, Bestmann et al. (2006) investigated TMS-induced activity changes in distinct cortical areas of an amputee. At an intermediate stimulus intensity, TMS over the motor hand representation contralateral to amputation elicited a phantom sensation of movement in half of the trials without producing overt activity in the remaining muscles. The authors compared event-related BOLD signal changes in trials with a phantom sensation of movement to trials without a sensation. Because the settings of TMS were identical, this comparison subtracted any nonspecific TMS effects on regional neuronal activity. The sensation of a phantom movement was associated with increased activity in the primary motor cortex, dorsal premotor cortex, anterior intraparietal sulcus, and caudal supplementary motor area. Based on these results, it was argued that activity in these frontoparietal areas represents the neuronal correlate of the phantom sense of movement (see Fig. 12.3 for details). Concurrent TMS–fMRI may also be of value to study how "therapeutic" rTMS protocols acutely change neuronal activity in functional brain networks. For instance, fMRI has been used to probe the immediate effects of continuous 1 Hz TMS at 100% MT

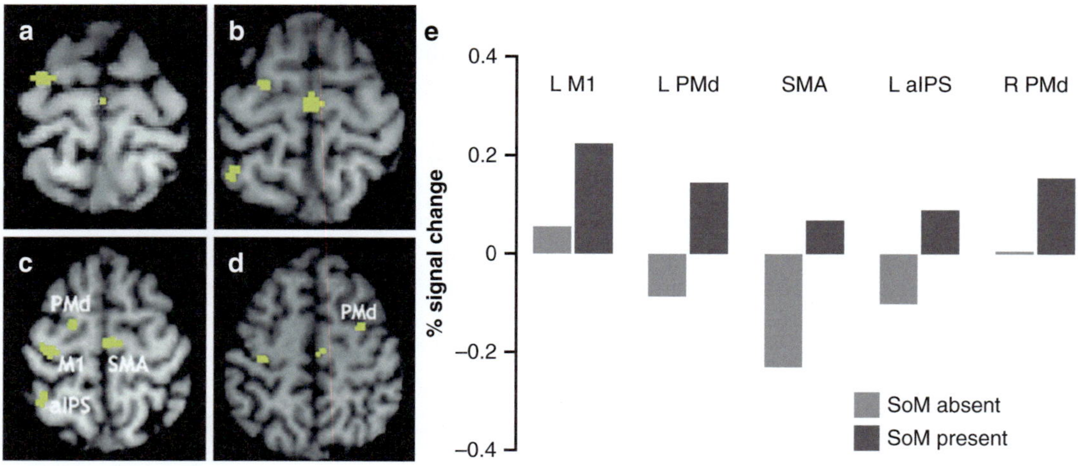

Fig. 12.3 Activity changes for the comparison of trials with versus without SoM reported, at intermediate TMS intensities (SPM(T) thresholded at $T \geq 3$). When a conscious phantom SoM was perceived, activity increases were observed in several motor-related regions, including the left (stimulated) M1, left and right PMd, left anterior intraparietal sulcus (aIPS), and caudal SMA. Note that the intermediate stimulation intensities applied were held constant in this contrast and were below threshold for evoking peripheral muscle responses. The results are displayed on the patient's anatomical T1-weighted MRI: (**a**) transverse section, $z = 72$; (**b**) $z = 67$; (**c**) $z = 62$; (**d**) $z = 57$; (**e**) fMRI percent signal change with respect to the session mean in peaks from these five motor-related regions (left M1, left and right PMd, SMA, left aIPS) for trials with or without evoked phantom SoM experienced. (Reprinted from Bestmann et al. (2006) with permission from Elsevier)

over the left dorsolateral prefrontal cortex in 14 patients with major depression (Li et al. 2004a; see also Vink et al. 2018).

12.3.3 Offline Combination of TMS and FMRI

12.3.3.1 TMS Following FMRI

There is consensus that fMRI can reliably identify brain regions in which increases in BOLD signal are correlated with the performance of an experimental task. Yet the correlational nature of fMRI provides no information about the functional contribution of any activated brain region to the task. This question can be addressed using TMS. TMS can be applied over the area of interest to disrupt neuronal processing while participants perform the same experimental task. If the TMS-induced local perturbation affects task performance, this is taken as evidence that the stimulated cortical area is functionally relevant.

An elegant illustration of this approach was provided by Cohen and colleagues in a TMS study on blind subjects (Cohen et al. 1997). Previous neuroimaging studies had shown that Braille reading consistently activated visual cortical areas in blind subjects but not in those with sight. To investigate the significance of task-related activation in the occipital cortex, short trains of 10 Hz rTMS were given to several brain regions time locked to Braille reading. Occipital rTMS induced errors and distorted the tactile perceptions of congenitally blind subjects but had no effects on tactile performance in normal sighted. This finding proved that the occipital visual cortex makes a relevant contribution to the processing of tactile input in blind subjects.

Across the last decade(s), an increasing number of studies used TMS to test the functional relevance of task-related activity for different cognitive functions, including memory, attention, auditory cognition, as well as speech and language functions, higher social cognition, and music perception (e.g., Davey et al. 2015; Mottonen et al. 2014; Rushworth et al. 2001; Andoh et al. 2018; Donaldson et al. 2018; Hartwigsen 2015 for review). In general, most of these studies reported behavioral impairment (i.e., delayed response times or decreased accuracy) with TMS over key regions for specific cognitive functions. However, some studies also found (paradoxical) facilitation when TMS was applied during or immediately before a task (e.g., Mottaghy et al. 1999, 2006; Sparing et al. 2001). These findings might be best explained in terms of the *state-dependency* concept (Pasley et al. 2009; Silvanto et al. 2017; Silvanto and Cattaneo 2017), arguing that the direction and strength of a TMS-induced effect may crucially depend on the task-induced neural activity or brain state. The TMS-induced activity or "neural noise" is unlikely to be completely random (Ruzzoli et al. 2010) and might be synchronized with the ongoing relevant signal, thereby rendering the signal stronger and providing an "optimum" level of noise for a specific task (Miniussi et al. 2013). As a consequence, the impact of a TMS-induced perturbation effect might also change with varying task conditions and complexity.

Notably, the application of TMS to investigate causal structure-function relationships is not restricted to single brain regions. For instance, we used a multifocal TMS approach to investigate whether right hemisphere brain regions critically contribute to specific language functions (Hartwigsen et al. 2010a). This study was based on previous fMRI investigations that had shown activation of the supramarginal gyri (SMG) in both hemispheres for phonological word processing. To test the functional relevance of these phonological activation patterns, we applied 10 Hz rTMS trains to left, right, or bilateral SMG, while participants performed phonological and semantic word decisions. The results of this study showed that TMS relative to an ineffective sham procedure impaired phonological decisions but did not affect semantic decisions independent of the stimulated hemisphere. Moreover, performance was not worse for dual-site TMS as opposed to uni-site TMS. Together, these findings provide evidence that both hemispheres equally contribute to accurate and efficient phonological decisions in the healthy brain, without any evidence for an acute compensation of a "virtual lesion" induced in the homologous area in the opposite hemisphere.

Several studies further combined TMS before a task (i.e., offline) with TMS during a task (online) to investigate functional interactions within networks for different cognitive processes (e.g., Hartwigsen et al. 2012, 2016). Such "condition-and-perturb" approaches are particularly suited to test compensation between different network nodes, especially if space restrictions preclude the use of simultaneous online perturbation of several regions.

Functional MRI can be used to functionally localize the optimal site for TMS. In a study by Neggers et al. (2007), participants first performed a saccade task during fMRI. In each subject, the individual peak activation in the precentral sulcus was identified and superimposed on the structural image of the subject's brain. Then frameless stereotaxy was used to place the coil over the fMRI-defined FEF. This fMRI-guided stereotactic approach is likely to be more precise than relying on structural anatomical landmarks because it takes into account the interindividual variability of the functional representation of the FEF in the precentral cortex. An alternative strategy uses the results of a previous fMRI study that has used the same or a similar experimental task. The stereotactic coordinates of task-related peak activation in the area of interest define the site of stimulation. The individual site of stimulation is determined by using the inverse of the normalization transformation and transforming the coordinates from standard to "individual" space (e.g., Hartwigsen et al. 2010a, b). Considering the high interindividual variability of the therapeutic effects of rTMS in psychiatric and neurological disorders (e.g., Gross et al. 2007; Lefaucheur et al. 2007; Ridding and Rothwell 2007), the use of fMRI-guided TMS, which takes into account the functional neuroanatomy of each individual, may also increase the efficacy of rTMS as a therapeutic tool.

12.3.3.2 fMRI Following TMS

Another way to combine rTMS and fMRI is to apply rTMS before fMRI. Here, rTMS is used to induce an acute reorganization in the human brain (Siebner and Rothwell 2003). After rTMS, fMRI is performed to map the lasting functional impact of rTMS on task-related neuronal activity at a system level (O'Shea et al. 2007; Rounis et al. 2007). Performing fMRI after rTMS outside the scanner does not require specific methodological precautions because rTMS and fMRI are separated in space and time. This *condition-and-map approach* can be used to study the changeability of functional brain networks. Preferably, fMRI should start as quickly as possible after rTMS to capture the transient effects of rTMS (Baudewig and Bestmann 2007). The conditioning effects of rTMS on regional neuronal activity can be detected by comparing task-related activation before and after rTMS. It is important to control unspecific changes in task-related activity that are simply due to the repetition of the experimental task in the MR scanner. This can be achieved by introducing a second session during which sham rTMS is given to the cortical target area. Sham rTMS should match real rTMS in terms of auditory and somatosensory stimulation but without inducing transcranial stimulation of the cortex. Alternatively, the same effective rTMS protocol might be applied to a second (control) area. A change in the pattern of activation after rTMS but not after control rTMS indicates a true reorganization in response to rTMS conditioning. Task specificity of functional reorganization can be shown by having participants perform a control task during the same fMRI session.

The condition-and-map approach has mostly been applied to study functional plasticity in healthy volunteers (see Table 12.2). For example, a recent study investigated the modulation and reorganization of networks associated with sensory perception and motor performance after subthreshold high-frequency (10 Hz, 90% resting motor threshold) rTMS of the right primary motor hand area (Yoo et al. 2008). Using a sham-controlled within-subject design, BOLD signal change during a sequential finger motor task and noxious tactile stimulation of the left hand were assessed before and after real and sham rTMS. Compared to sham rTMS, real rTMS led to increased activation in the motor network, which was associated with enhanced motor performance. On the other hand, real rTMS caused deactivation in the sensory network, which correlated with an increase in tactile sensory threshold. In another study, fMRI used in healthy right handers to probe short-term reorganization in right PMd after 1-Hz rTMS induced a lasting disruption of neuronal processing in the dominant left PMd specialized for action selection (O'Shea et al. 2007). Moreover, 1-Hz rTMS specifically increased activity in right PMd and connected medial premotor areas during action selection without affecting behavior. Based on additional experiments, it was claimed that this increase in activity reflects compensatory short-term reorganization that helps to preserve behavior after the "neuronal challenge" induced by rTMS.

More recently, the condition-and-map approach has also been used to investigate short-term reorganization and adaptive plasticity for cognitive functions, including higher auditory cognition (Andoh and Zatorre 2013) and language (Andoh and Paus 2011; Binney and Lambon Ralph 2015; Hallam et al. 2016; Hartwigsen et al. 2013, 2017; Jung and Lambon Ralph 2016; see Hartwigsen et al. 2016 for review). Some studies used modeling of neuroimaging data to map TMS-induced changes in the effective connectivity (i.e., the functional interactions) (Friston et al. 2003) between key regions for specific language functions. These studies have provided converging evidence that focal rTMS can consistently change effective connectivity in specific neural networks, including brain regions that are not directly targeted by rTMS (Grefkes et al. 2010; Hartwigsen et al. 2017; Herz et al. 2014).

Two recent studies combined focal perturbation of the left anterior temporal lobe (ATL) with subsequent fMRI to map compensatory reorganization in the semantic system (Binney and Lambon Ralph 2015; Jung and Lambon Ralph 2016). Binney and Lambon Ralph (2015) found that continuous theta burst stimulation (cTBS) over the left ATL suppressed task-related semantic activity not only at the stimulated site but also in other areas of the semantic network, including the ventral ATL and ventrolateral prefrontal and posterolateral temporal cortex. In turn, ATL suppression led to an extended, compensatory upregulation of the contralateral homologous region, indicating a high degree of adaptive plasticity in the semantic network. Congruent with the

Table 12.2 Example studies performing fMRI after a conditioning session of rTMS

Target area	Task during fMRI	TMS protocol (frequency, % RMT, total no. of pulses/session)	Reference
Left S1	Rest	5 Hz; 90; 2500	Tegenthoff et al. (2005)
Left IFG	Semantic object classification	10 Hz, 110, 300	Wig et al. (2005)
Left S1	Tactile frequency discrimination	5 Hz; 90; 1250	Pleger et al. (2006)
Right vs. left DLPFC	Cued choice reaction	5 Hz; 90 AMT; 1800	Rounis et al. (2006)
Left PFC	Face-name memory	5 Hz, 80, 500	Sole-Padulles et al. (2006)[a]
Right PFC	Tower of London	1 Hz; 110; 720 vs. 10 Hz; 100; 1500	Fitzgerald et al. (2007)[b]
Left PMd, left SM	Action selection	1 Hz, 90 AMT, 900	O'Shea et al. (2007)
Left DLPFC	Emotional stimuli	5 Hz; 120; 3750	Cardoso et al. (2008)[c]
Right FEF	Saccade-fixation	30 Hz TBS, 80, 600	Hubl et al. (2008)
Contrales. M1	Hand grip movements	1 Hz, 100, 600	Nowak et al. (2008)[d]
Right M1	Sequential finger motor task, noxious tactile stimuli	10 Hz; 90; 1000	Yoo et al. (2008)
Right M1	Fist closure movements	1 Hz, 100, 600	Grefkes et al. (2010)[d]
Left PMd	Action reprogramming	1 Hz, 90, 1800	Ward et al. (2010)
L/R MTP	Word recognition	10 Hz, 100, 450	Andoh and Paus (2011)
L/R HGa	Melody discrimination	cTBS, 80 AMT, 600	Andoh and Zatorre (2013)
Left pIFG	Overt pseudoword repetition	50 Hz cTBS, 80 AMT, 600	Hartwigsen et al. (2013)
Pre-SMA	Modified Simon task	1 Hz, 100, 1800	Herz et al. (2014)
Left ATL	Semantic judgements	1 Hz, 120, 660	Binney and Lambon Ralph (2015)
Left vATL	Semantic judgements	cTBS, 80, 600	Jung and Lambon Ralph (2016)
Left IFG	Semantic relatedness judgements	1 Hz, 100 AMT, 900	Hallam et al. (2016)
Left AG/SMG	Semantic and phonological decisions	50 Hz cTBS, 80 AMT, 600	Hartwigsen et al. (2017)

AG angular gyrus, *AMT* active motor threshold, *(v)ATL* ventral anterior temporal lobe, *DLPFC* dorsolateral prefrontal cortex, *FEF* frontal eye field, *L/R HGa* left/ right anterolateral Heschl's gyrus, *(p)IFG* (posterior) inferior frontal gyrus, *M1* primary motor cortex, *L/R MTP* left/right posterior temporal area (Wernicke), *PFC* prefrontal cortex, *PMd* dorsal premotor cortex, *pre-SMA* presupplementary motor area, *RMT* resting motor threshold, *S1* primary somatosensory cortex, *SM* sensorimotor cortex, *SMG* supramarginal gyrus, *(c)TBS* continuous theta burst stimulation

[a]Elderly subjects with memory complaints

[b]Patients with treatment-resistant depression

[c]Depressive patients with Parkinson's disease

[d]Stroke patients

reported flexible adaptation of the semantic network, a second study from the same group (Jung and Lambon Ralph 2016) also found decreased activity in the left ventrolateral ATL after cTBS induced suppression of this region (relative to a control site in the occipital pole) and compensatory upregulation of the contralateral homologue. The upregulation of the right ATL was negatively correlated with task speed, indicating that subjects with shorter response latencies showed stronger right ATL activation. Additionally, effective connectivity analysis revealed that, after cTBS, the right ATL increased its intrinsic facilitatory influence on the left ATL, demonstrating a flexible, bilateral organization of the semantic system with a strong degree of adaptive plasticity.

In a behavioral experiment, cTBS also delayed task performance during synonym judgements, providing evidence for the functional relevance of this area for semantic processes. In line with other TMS–fMRI studies in the language domain (e.g., Hallam et al. 2016; Hartwigsen et al. 2013, 2017), these results provide evidence for a flexible, compensatory redistribution between key regions for language processing.

To date, patients have been rarely studied with the offline combination of rTMS and fMRI (see Cardoso et al. 2008; Fitzgerald et al. 2007; Nowak et al. 2008; Grefkes et al. 2010; Hartwigsen et al. in press for some examples). However, a large number of condition-and-map studies used offline rTMS followed by PET in patients with neurological and psychiatric disorders such as tinnitus (Richter et al. 2006; Smith et al. 2007), depression (Kuroda et al. 2006; Peschina et al. 2001; Speer et al. 2000), schizophrenia (Langguth et al. 2006), dystonia (Siebner et al. 2003), or Parkinson's disease (Strafella et al. 2005). These studies have shown that the condition-and-map approach is important to advance our understanding of the therapeutic effects of rTMS, as well as the underlying pathological brain mechanisms, and should encourage investigators to perform fMRI after rTMS in patients. More recently, some studies combined offline rTMS with PET or fMRI to map changes in language function after rTMS had been combined with speech and language therapy (e.g., Heiss et al. 2013; see Chap. 17). These studies show that such treatment approaches may result in a reshift of language activity toward the dominant left hemisphere. Future studies are necessary to make more specific predictions about the network effects of rTMS on aphasia recovery and identify effective treatment protocols that may change across the time course of language recovery after stroke (Hartwigsen and Saur 2019).

12.4 Conclusion

TMS can be used concurrently with fMRI (online approach), or it can be given before or after fMRI (offline approach). While online TMS during fMRI is technically demanding and requires specific safety precautions, the offline TMS before or after fMRI approach outside the MR scanner can be easily performed. The relative timing between TMS and fMRI defines the scientific and clinical questions that can be tackled with the combined TMS–fMRI approach. This approach provides unique opportunities to explore the dynamic aspects of functional neuronal networks in space and time and how these functional interactions are affected by disease. It also bears great potential for studying the physiological impact of TMS on the human brain. This knowledge will be crucial to the increased efficacy of TMS as a therapeutic tool.

References

Allen EA, Pasley BN et al (2007) Transcranial magnetic stimulation elicits coupled neural and hemodynamic consequences. Science 317:1918–1921

Andoh J, Paus T (2011) Combining functional neuroimaging with off-line brain stimulation: modulation of task-related activity in language areas. J Cogn Neurosci 23:349–361

Andoh J, Zatorre RJ (2013) Mapping interhemispheric connectivity using functional MRI after transcranial magnetic stimulation on the human auditory cortex. Neuroimage 79:162–171

Andoh J, Matsushita R et al (2018) Insights into auditory cortex dynamics from non-invasive brain stimulation. Front Neurosci 12:469

Barker AT, Jalinous R et al (1985) Non-invasive magnetic stimulation of human motor cortex. Lancet 1:1106–1107

Baudewig J, Bestmann S (2007) Transkranielle Magnetstimulation und funktionelle Magnetresonanztomographie [Transcranial magnetic stimulation and functional magnetic resonance tomography]. In: Siebner HR, Ziemann U (eds) Das TMS-Buch [The TMS book]. Springer, Heidelberg

Baudewig J, Paulus W et al (2000) Artifacts caused by transcranial magnetic stimulation coils and EEG electrodes in T(2)*-weighted echo-planar imaging. Magn Reson Imaging 18:479–484

Baudewig J, Siebner HR et al (2001) Functional MRI of cortical activations induced by transcranial magnetic stimulation (TMS). Neuroreport 12:3543–3548

Berardelli A, Inghilleri M et al (1998) Facilitation of muscle evoked responses after repetitive cortical stimulation in man. Exp Brain Res 122:79–84

Bestmann S, Baudewig J et al (2003a) On the synchronization of transcranial magnetic stimulation and functional echo-planar imaging. J Magn Reson Imaging 17:309–316

Bestmann S, Baudewig J et al (2003b) Subthreshold high-frequency TMS of human primary motor cortex modulates interconnected frontal motor areas as detected by inter-leaved fMRI-TMS. Neuroimage 20:1685–1696

Bestmann S, Baudewig J et al (2004) Functional MRI of the immediate impact of transcranial magnetic stimulation on cortical and subcortical motor circuits. Eur J Neurosci 19:1950–1962

Bestmann S, Baudewig J et al (2005) BOLD MRI responses to repetitive TMS over human dorsal premotor cortex. Neuroimage 28:22–29

Bestmann S, Oliviero A et al (2006) Cortical correlates of TMS-induced phantom hand movements revealed with concurrent TMS-fMRI. Neuropsychologia 44:2959–2971

Bestmann S, Swayne O et al (2007) Dorsal pre-motor cortex exerts state-dependent causal influences on activity in contralateral primary motor and dorsal premotor cortex. Cereb Cortex 18(6):1281–1291

Bestmann J, Ruff CC et al (2008) Concurrent TMS and functional magnetic resonance imaging: methods and current advances. In: Wassermann EM, Epstein CM, Ziemann U (eds) The Oxford handbook of transcranial stimulation. Oxford University Press, New York

Binney RJ, Lambon Ralph MA (2015) Using a combination of fMRI and anterior temporal lobe rTMS to measure intrinsic and induced activation changes across the semantic cognition network. Neuropsychologia 76:170–181

Bohning DE, Pecheny AP et al (1997) Mapping transcranial magnetic stimulation (TMS) fields in vivo with MRI. Neuroreport 8:2535–2538

Bohning DE, Shastri A et al (1998) Echoplanar BOLD fMRI of brain activation induced by concurrent transcranial magnetic stimulation. Investig Radiol 33:336–340

Bohning DE, Shastri A et al (1999) A combined TMS/fMRI study of intensity-dependent TMS over motor cortex. Biol Psychiatry 45:385–394

Bohning DE, Shastri A et al (2000a) Motor cortex brain activity induced by 1-Hz transcranial magnetic stimulation is similar in location and level to that for volitional movement. Investig Radiol 35:676–683

Bohning DE, Shastri A et al (2000b) BOLD-f MRI response to single-pulse transcranial magnetic stimulation (TMS). J Magn Reson Imaging 11:569–574

Bohning DE, Denslow S et al (2003a) Interleaving fMRI and rTMS. Suppl Clin Neurophysiol 56:42–54

Bohning DE, Denslow S et al (2003b) A TMS coil positioning/holding system for MR image-guided TMS interleaved with fMRI. Clin Neurophysiol 114:2210–2219

Bohning DE, Shastri A et al (2003c) BOLD-fMRI response vs. transcranial magnetic stimulation (TMS) pulse-train length: testing for linearity. J Magn Reson Imaging 17:279–290

Cardoso EF, Fregni F et al (2008) rTMS treatment for depression in Parkinson's disease increases BOLD responses in the left prefrontal cortex. Int J Neuropsychopharmacol 11:173–183

Chen R, Classen J et al (1997a) Depression of motor cortex excitability by low-frequency transcranial magnetic stimulation. Neurology 48:1398–1403

Chen R, Gerloff C et al (1997b) Safety of different inter-train intervals for repetitive transcranial magnetic stimulation and recommendations for safe ranges of stimulation parameters. Electroencephalogr Clin Neurophysiol 105:415–421

Cohen LG, Celnik P et al (1997) Functional relevance of cross-modal plasticity in blind humans. Nature 389:180–183

Davey J, Cornelissen PL et al (2015) Automatic and controlled semantic retrieval: TMS reveals distinct contributions of posterior middle temporal gyrus and angular gyrus. J Neurosci 35:15230–15239

Denslow S, Lomarev M et al (2004) A high resolution assessment of the repeatability of relative location and intensity of transcranial magnetic stimulation-induced and volitionally induced blood oxygen level-dependent response in the motor cortex. Cogn Behav Neurol 17:163–173

Denslow S, Bohning DE et al (2005a) An increased precision comparison of TMS-induced motor cortex BOLD fMRI response for image-guided versus function-guided coil placement. Cogn Behav Neurol 18:119–126

Denslow S, Lomarev M et al (2005b) Cortical and subcortical brain effects of transcranial magnetic stimulation (TMS)-induced movement: an interleaved TMS/functional magnetic resonance imaging study. Biol Psychiatry 57:752–760

Donaldson PH, Kirkovski M et al (2018) Autism-relevant traits interact with temporoparietal junction stimulation effects on social cognition: a high-definition transcranial direct current stimulation and electroencephalography study. Eur J Neurosci 47:669–681

Ettinger GJ, Leventon ME et al (1998) Experimentation with a transcranial magnetic stimulation system for functional brain mapping. Med Image Anal 2:133–142

Fitzgerald PB, Sritharan A et al (2007) A functional magnetic resonance imaging study of the effects of low frequency right prefrontal transcranial magnetic stimulation in depression. J Clin Psychopharmacol 27:488–492

Friston KJ, Harrison L et al (2003) Dynamic causal modelling. Neuroimage 19:1273–1302

Gerschlager W, Siebner HR et al (2001) Decreased corticospinal excitability after subthreshold 1 Hz rTMS over lateral premotor cortex. Neurology 57:449–455

Grefkes C, Nowak DA et al (2010) Modulating cortical connectivity in stroke patients by rTMS assessed with fMRI and dynamic causal modeling. Neuroimage 50:233–242

Gross M, Nakamura L et al (2007) Has repetitive transcranial magnetic stimulation (rTMS) treatment for depression improved? A systematic review and meta-analysis comparing the recent vs. the earlier rTMS studies. Acta Psychiatr Scand 116:165–173

Hallam GP, Whitney C et al (2016) Charting the effects of TMS with fMRI: modulation of cortical recruitment within the distributed network supporting semantic control. Neuropsychologia 93:40–52

Hamada M, Hanajima R et al (2007) Quadropulse stimulation is more effective than paired-pulse stimulation for plasticity induction of the human motor cortex. Clin Neurophysiol 118:2672–2682

Hartwigsen G (2015) The neurophysiology of language: insights from non-invasive brain stimulation in the healthy human brain. Brain Lang 148:81–94

Hartwigsen G, Saur D (2019) Neuroimaging of stroke recovery from aphasia – insights into plasticity of the human language network. Neuroimage 190:14–31

Hartwigsen G, Baumgaertner A et al (2010a) Phonological decisions require both the left and right supramarginal gyri. Proc Natl Acad Sci U S A 107:16494–16499

Hartwigsen G, Price CJ et al (2010b) The right posterior inferior frontal gyrus contributes to phonological word decisions in the healthy brain: evidence from dual-site TMS. Neuropsychologia 48:3155–3163

Hartwigsen G, Bestmann S et al (2012) Left dorsal premotor cortex and supramarginal gyrus complement each other during rapid action reprogramming. J Neurosci 32:16162–16171

Hartwigsen G, Saur D et al (2013) Perturbation of the left inferior frontal gyrus triggers adaptive plasticity in the right homologous area during speech production. Proc Natl Acad Sci U S A 110:16402–16407

Hartwigsen G, Weigel A et al (2016) Dissociating parieto-frontal networks for phonological and semantic word decisions: a condition-and-perturb TMS study. Cereb Cortex 26:2590–2601

Hartwigsen G, Bzdok D et al (2017) Rapid short-term reorganization in the language network. Elife 6: pii: e25964

Hartwigsen G, Stockert S et al (in press) Short-term modulation of the lesioned language network. eLife.

Heiss WD, Hartmann A et al (2013) Noninvasive brain stimulation for treatment of right- and left-handed poststroke aphasics. Cerebrovasc Dis 36:363–372

Herwig U, Abler B et al (2003a) Verbal storage in a premotor-parietal network: evidence from fMRI-guided magnetic stimulation. Neuroimage 20:1032–1041

Herwig U, Satrapi P et al (2003b) Using the international 10–20 EEG system for positioning of transcranial magnetic stimulation. Brain Topogr 16:95–99

Herz DM, Christensen MS et al (2014) Motivational tuning of fronto-subthalamic connectivity facilitates control of action impulses. J Neurosci 34:3210–3217

Huang YZ, Edwards MJ et al (2005) Theta burst stimulation of the human motor cortex. Neuron 45:201–206

Hubl D, Nyffeler T et al (2008) Time course of blood oxygenation level-dependent signal response after theta burst transcranial magnetic stimulation of the frontal eye field. Neuroscience 151:921–928

Ilmoniemi RJ, Virtanen J et al (1997) Neuronal responses to magnetic stimulation reveal cortical reactivity and connectivity. Neuroreport 8:3537–3540

Jasper HH (1958) The ten-twenty electrode system of the International Federation. Electroencephalogr Clin Neurophysiol 10:367–380

Jung J, Lambon Ralph MA (2016) Mapping the dynamic network interactions underpinning cognition: a cTBS-fMRI study of the flexible adaptive neural system for semantics. Cereb Cortex 26:3580–3590

Kemna LJ, Gembris D (2003) Repetitive transcranial magnetic stimulation induces different responses in different cortical areas: a functional magnetic resonance study in humans. Neurosci Lett 336:85–88

Kobayashi M, Pascual-Leone A (2003) Transcranial magnetic stimulation in neurology. Lancet Neurol 2:145–156

Koch G, Franca M, Albrecht UV et al (2006) Effects of paired pulse TMS of primary somatosensory cortex on perception of a peripheral electrical stimulus. Exp Brain Res 172:416–424

Kuroda Y, Motohashi N et al (2006) Effects of repetitive transcranial magnetic stimulation on [11C]raclopride binding and cognitive function in patients with depression. J Affect Disord 95:35–42

Lang N, Harms J et al (2006) Stimulus intensity and coil characteristics influence the efficacy of rTMS to suppress cortical excitability. Clin Neurophysiol 117:2292–2301

Langguth B, Eichhammer P et al (2006) Neuronavigated transcranial magnetic stimulation and auditory hallucinations in a schizophrenic patient: monitoring of neurobiological effects. Schizophr Res 84:185–186

Lee JH, van Donkelaar P (2006) The human dorsal premotor cortex generates on-line error corrections during sensorimotor adaptation. J Neurosci 26:3330–3334

Lee L, Siebner HR et al (2003) Acute remapping within the motor system induced by low-frequency repetitive transcranial magnetic stimulation. J Neurosci 23:5308–5318

Lefaucheur JP, Brugieres P et al (2007) The value of navigation-guided rTMS for the treatment of depression: an illustrative case. Neurophysiol Clin 37:265–271

Li X, Nahas Z et al (2004a) Acute left prefrontal transcranial magnetic stimulation in depressed patients is associated with immediately increased activity in prefrontal cortical as well as subcortical regions. Biol Psychiatry 55:882–890

Li X, Teneback CC et al (2004b) Interleaved transcranial magnetic stimulation/functional MRI confirms that lamotrigine inhibits cortical excitability in healthy young men. Neuropsychopharmacology 29:1395–1407

Massimini M, Ferrarelli F et al (2005) Breakdown of cortical effective connectivity during sleep. Science 309:2228–2232

McConnell KA, Bohning DE et al (2003) BOLD fMRI response to direct stimulation (transcranial magnetic stimulation) of the motor cortex shows no decline with age. J Neural Transm 110:495–507

Miniussi C, Ruzzoli M et al (2010) The mechanism of transcranial magnetic stimulation in cognition. Cortex 46:128–130

Miniussi C, Harris JA et al (2013) Modelling non-invasive brain stimulation in cognitive neuroscience. Neurosci Biobehav Rev 37:1702–1712

Mottaghy FM, Hungs M et al (1999) Facilitation of picture naming after repetitive transcranial magnetic stimulation. Neurology 53:1806–1812
Mottaghy FM, Sparing R et al (2006) Enhancing picture naming with transcranial magnetic stimulation. Behav Neurol 17:177–186
Mottonen R, van de Ven GM et al (2014) Attention fine-tunes auditory-motor processing of speech sounds. J Neurosci 34:4064–4069
Nahas Z, Lomarev M et al (2001) Unilateral left prefrontal transcranial magnetic stimulation (TMS) produces intensity-dependent bilateral effects as measured by interleaved BOLD fMRI. Biol Psychiatry 50: 712–720
Neggers SF, Langerak TR et al (2004) A stereotactic method for image-guided transcranial magnetic stimulation validated with fMRI and motor-evoked potentials. Neuroimage 21:1805–1817
Neggers SF, Huijbers W et al (2007) TMS pulses on the frontal eye fields break coupling between visuospatial attention and eye movements. J Neurophysiol 98:2765–2778
Nowak DA, Grefkes C et al (2008) Effects of low-frequency repetitive transcranial magnetic stimulation of the contralesional primary motor cortex on movement kinematics and neural activity in subcortical stroke. Arch Neurol 65:741–747
O'Shea J, Johansen-Berg H et al (2007) Functionally specific reorganization in human premotor cortex. Neuron 54:479–490
Pascual-Leone A, Tormos JM et al (1998) Study and modulation of human cortical excitability with transcranial magnetic stimulation. J Clin Neurophysiol 15:333–343
Pascual-Leone A, Walsh V et al (2000) Transcranial magnetic stimulation in cognitive neuroscience—virtual lesion, chronometry, and functional connectivity. Curr Opin Neurobiol 10:232–237
Pasley BN, Allen EA et al (2009) State-dependent variability of neuronal responses to transcranial magnetic stimulation of the visual cortex. Neuron 62:291–303
Peschina W, Conca A et al (2001) Low frequency rTMS as an add-on antidepressive strategy: heterogeneous impact on 99 mTc-HMPAO and 18F-FDG uptake as measured simultaneously with the double isotope SPECT technique. Pilot study. Nucl Med Commun 22:867–873
Pleger B, Blankenburg F et al (2006) Repetitive transcranial magnetic stimulation-induced changes in sensorimotor coupling parallel improvements of somatosensation in humans. J Neurosci 26:1945–1952
Richter GT, Mennemeier M et al (2006) Repetitive transcranial magnetic stimulation for tinnitus: a case study. Laryngoscope 116:1867–1872
Ridding MC, Rothwell JC (2007) Is there a future for therapeutic use of transcranial magnetic stimulation? Nat Rev Neurosci 8:559–567
Rossi S, Hallett M et al (2009) Safety, ethical considerations, and application guidelines for the use of transcranial magnetic stimulation in clinical practice and research. Clin Neurophysiol 120(12):2008–2039
Rossini PM, Burke D et al (2015) Non-invasive electrical and magnetic stimulation of the brain, spinal cord, roots and peripheral nerves: basic principles and procedures for routine clinical and research application. An updated report from an I.F.C.N. Committee. Clin Neurophysiol 126:1071–1107
Rounis E, Stephan KE et al (2006) Acute changes in frontoparietal activity after repetitive transcranial magnetic stimulation over the dorsolateral prefrontal cortex in a cued reaction time task. J Neurosci 26:9629–9638
Rounis E, Yarrow K et al (2007) Effects of rTMS conditioning over the frontoparietal network on motor versus visual attention. J Cogn Neurosci 19:513–524
Ruff CC, Blankenburg F et al (2006) Concurrent TMS-fMRI and psychophysics reveal frontal influences on human retinotopic visual cortex. Curr Biol 16:1479–1488
Ruff CC, Bestmann S et al (2008) Distinct causal influences of parietal versus frontal areas on human visual cortex: evidence from concurrent TMS-fMRI. Cereb Cortex 18:817–827
Rushworth MF, Ellison A et al (2001) Complementary localization and lateralization of orienting and motor attention. Nat Neurosci 4:656–661
Ruzzoli M, Marzi CA et al (2010) The neural mechanisms of the effects of transcranial magnetic stimulation on perception. J Neurophysiol 103:2982–2989
Sack AT, Kohler A et al (2006) The temporal characteristics of motion processing in hMT/V5+: combining fMRI and neuronavigated TMS. Neuroimage 29:1326–1335
Sack AT, Kohler A et al (2007) Imaging the brain activity changes underlying impaired visuospatial judgments: simultaneous FMRI, TMS, and behavioral studies. Cereb Cortex 17:2841–2852
Sandrini M, Umilta C et al (2011) The use of transcranial magnetic stimulation in cognitive neuroscience: a new synthesis of methodological issues. Neurosci Biobehav Rev 35:516–536
Schonfeldt-Lecuona C, Thielscher A et al (2005) Accuracy of stereotaxic positioning of transcranial magnetic stimulation. Brain Topogr 17:253–259
Shastri A, George MS et al (1999) Performance of a system for interleaving transcranial magnetic stimulation with steady state magnetic resonance imaging. Electroencephalogr Clin Neurophysiol Suppl 51:55–64
Siebner HR, Rothwell J (2003) Transcranial magnetic stimulation: new insights into representational cortical plasticity. Exp Brain Res 148:1–16
Siebner HR, Filipovic SR et al (2003) Patients with focal arm dystonia have increased sensitivity to slow-frequency repetitive TMS of the dorsal premotor cortex. Brain 126:2710–2725
Siebner HR, Bergmann TO et al (2009a) Consensus paper: combining transcranial stimulation with neuroimaging. Brain Stimul 2:58–80
Siebner HR, Hartwigsen G et al (2009b) How does transcranial magnetic stimulation modify neuronal activity in the brain? Implications for studies of cognition. Cortex 45:1035–1042

Silvanto J, Cattaneo Z (2017) Common framework for "virtual lesion" and state-dependent TMS: the facilitatory/suppressive range model of online TMS effects on behavior. Brain Cogn 119:32–38

Silvanto J, Bona S et al (2017) Initial activation state, stimulation intensity and timing of stimulation interact in producing behavioral effects of TMS. Neuroscience 363:134–141

Smith JA, Mennemeier M et al (2007) Repetitive transcranial magnetic stimulation for tinnitus: a pilot study. Laryngoscope 117:529–534

Sole-Padulles C, Bartres-Faz D et al (2006) Repetitive transcranial magnetic stimulation effects on brain function and cognition among elders with memory dysfunction. Cereb Cortex 16:1487–1493

Sparing R, Mottaghy FM et al (2001) Repetitive transcranial magnetic stimulation effects on language function depend on the stimulation parameters. J Clin Neurophysiol 18:326–330

Sparing R, Buelte D et al (2008) Transcranial magnetic stimulation and the challenge of coil placement: a comparison of conventional and stereotaxic neuronavigational strategies. Hum Brain Mapp 29:82–96

Speer AM, Kimbrell TA et al (2000) Opposite effects of high and low frequency rTMS on regional brain activity in depressed patients. Biol Psychiatry 48:1133–1141

Starck J, Rimpilainen I et al (1996) The noise level in magnetic stimulation. Scand Audiol 25:223–226

Strafella AP, Ko JH et al (2005) Corticostriatal functional interactions in Parkinson's disease: a rTMS/[11C] raclopride PET study. Eur J Neurosci 22:2946–2952

Tegenthoff M, Ragert P et al (2005) Improvement of tactile discrimination performance and enlargement of cortical somatosensory maps after 5 Hz rTMS. PLoS Biol 3:e362

Terao Y, Ugawa Y et al (1998) Localizing the site of magnetic brain stimulation by functional MRI. Exp Brain Res 121:145–152

Thickbroom GW, Byrnes ML et al (2006) Repetitive paired-pulse TMS at I-wave periodicity markedly increases corticospinal excitability: a new technique for modulating synaptic plasticity. Clin Neurophysiol 117:61–66

Vink JJT, Mandija S et al (2018) A novel concurrent TMS-fMRI method to reveal propagation patterns of prefrontal magnetic brain stimulation. Hum Brain Mapp 39:4580

Walsh V, Cowey A (2000) Transcranial magnetic stimulation and cognitive neuroscience. Nat Rev Neurosci 1:73–79

Walsh V, Rushworth M (1999) A primer of magnetic stimulation as a tool for neuropsychology. Neuropsychologia 37:125–135

Ward NS, Bestmann S et al (2010) Low-frequency transcranial magnetic stimulation over left dorsal premotor cortex improves the dynamic control of visuospatially cued actions. J Neurosci 30:9216–9223

Wassermann EM (1998) Risk and safety of repetitive transcranial magnetic stimulation: report and suggested guidelines from the international workshop on the safety of repetitive transcranial magnetic stimulation, 5–7 June, 1996. Electroencephalogr Clin Neurophysiol 108:1–16

Wassermann EM (2008) The motor-evoked potential in health and disease. In: Wassermann EM, Epstein CM, Ziemann U (eds) The oxford handbook of transcranial stimulation. Oxford University Press, New York

Wassermann EM, Lisanby SH (2001) Therapeutic application of repetitive transcranial magnetic stimulation: a review. Clin Neurophysiol 112:1367–1377

Weyh T, Siebner HR (2007) Hirnstimulation – Technische Grundlagen [Stimulation of the brain – technical basics]. In: Siebner HR, Ziemann U (eds) Das TMS-Buch [the TMS book]. Springer, Heidelberg

Weyh T, Wendicke K et al (2005) Marked differences in the thermal characteristics of figure-of-eight shaped coils used for repetitive transcranial magnetic stimulation. Clin Neurophysiol 116:1477–1486

Wig GS, Grafton ST et al (2005) Reductions in neural activity underlie behavioral components of repetition priming. Nat Neurosci 8:1228–1233

Yoo WK, You SH et al (2008) High frequency rTMS modulation of the sensorimotor networks: behavioral changes and fMRI correlates. Neuroimage 39:1886–1895

13 Simultaneous EEG and fMRI Recordings (EEG–fMRI)

Friederike Moeller, Michael Siniatchkin, and Jean Gotman

Abbreviations

AAS	Averaged artefact subtraction
BOLD	Blood oxygenation level-dependent
EEG	Electroencephalography
fMRI	Functional magnetic resonance imaging
GSW	Generalised spike-wave discharges
HRF	Haemodynamic response function
IGE	Idiopathic generalised epilepsy

13.1 Introduction

Scalp EEG is an important tool for the investigation of patients with epilepsy. It can help to diagnose and classify epilepsy and localise the source of epileptic activity. However, a disadvantage of EEG is its low spatial resolution and the weakness to detect epileptic activity from deep brain structures. In contrast, fMRI is characterised by a good spatial resolution and is equally sensitive to signals of deep and superficial brain structures. By combining EEG with fMRI, it is possible to detect BOLD signal changes associated with EEG patterns detected on the scalp EEG, even if deep brain structures are involved.

Epileptic patients usually show specific EEG patterns, allowing EEG–fMRI studies to delineate the epileptogenic zone non-invasively. Furthermore, EEG–fMRI studies have contributed to the understanding of the pathophysiological mechanisms of epilepsy. In this chapter, the methodological background is described and an overview about EEG–fMRI studies in the fields of focal and generalised epilepsy and paediatric epilepsy is given.

13.2 Methods

It is challenging to record an EEG in an MRI environment of changing electromagnetic fields that interfere with EEG. In 1993, Ives and colleagues demonstrated that it is possible to record an EEG during an fMRI investigation (Ives et al. 1993). The first EEG–fMRI recordings were performed in a spike-triggered manner: if epileptic activity was observed in the EEG, fMRI acquisition was started. This way, the images were acquired approximately 4 s after the event, obscuring the EEG with gradient artefacts during the scanning.

F. Moeller (✉)
Department of Neurophysiology, Great Ormond Street Hospital for Children, London, UK
e-mail: Friederike_moeller@gosh.nhs.uk

M. Siniatchkin
Clinic of Child and Adolescents Psychiatry and Psychotherapy, Ev. Hospital Bethel, Bielefeld, Germany
e-mail: michael.siniatchkin@evkb.de

J. Gotman
Montreal Neurological Institute, McGill University, Montreal, QC, Canada
e-mail: jean.gotman@mcgill.ca

S. Ulmer, O. Jansen (eds.), *fMRI*, https://doi.org/10.1007/978-3-030-41874-8_13

This approach is possible since the haemodynamic response function peaks several seconds after an event (Krakow et al. 1999; Seeck et al. 1998). However, with this approach, the correct identification of the spikes by an experienced observer during the scanning is necessary and the time course of the spike-associated BOLD signal changes is not detected. Since the EEG is obscured by gradient artefacts during the scanning, it cannot be excluded that spikes occurred during the acquisition. The development of gradient artefact correction algorithms made it possible to perform fMRI scanning continuously while also recording the EEG continuously (Allen et al. 2000; Hoffmann et al. 2000; Lemieux et al. 2001), which is the standard method used in EEG–fMRI studies today. The scanning time for EEG–fMRI studies varies from 20 min in children up to 90 min in adults. In some studies, sedation (for example with chloral hydrate) is needed for children undergoing EEG–fMRI recordings (Jacobs et al. 2007, 2008; Moeller et al. 2008a; Siniatchkin et al. 2007b, 2010, 2011). A child-friendly setting with movie viewing during the study may reduce movements and avoid the need for sedation (Centeno et al. 2016).

13.2.1 How to Do It?

Figure 13.1 summarises the different steps of an EEG–fMRI investigation. In order to record the EEG inside the scanner, the following points need to be considered.

13.2.1.1 Equipment

An MRI-compatible EEG recording system is needed. The electrodes and wires need to be non-

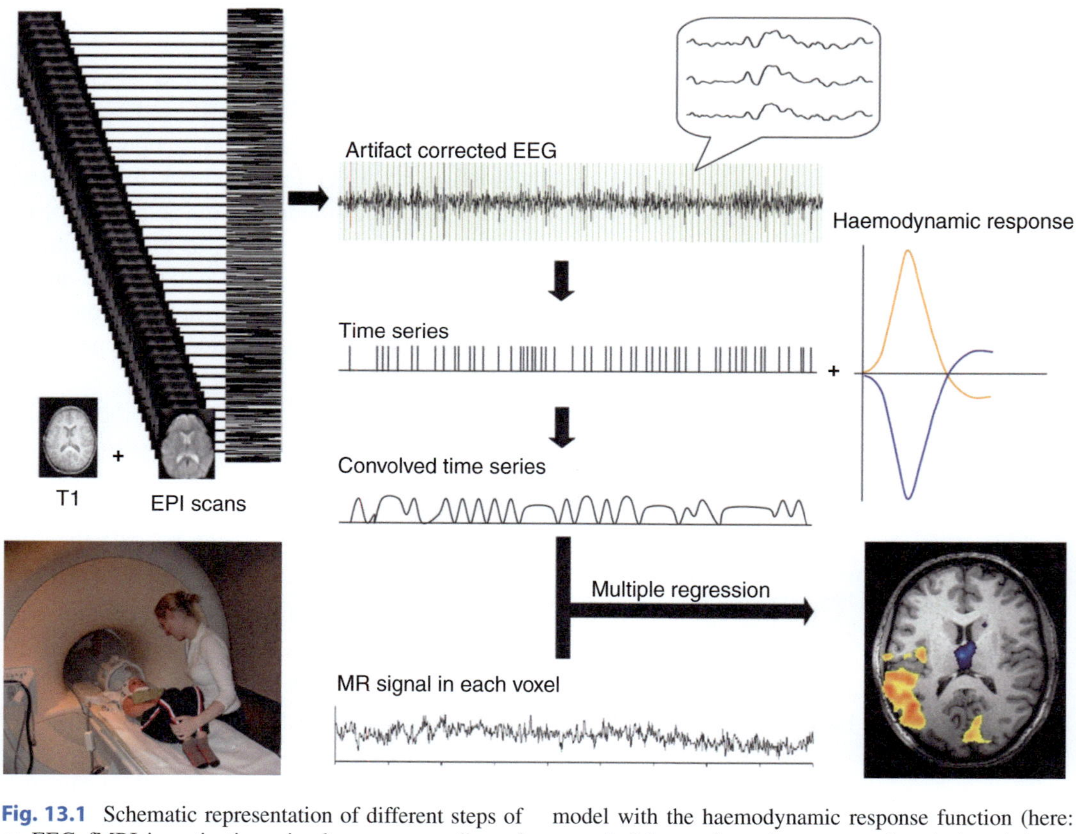

Fig. 13.1 Schematic representation of different steps of an EEG–fMRI investigation: simultaneous recording of EEG and functional MRI, artefact correction of the EEG, identification of the events (e.g. spikes) in the corrected EEG, building a spike-related model, convolution of the model with the haemodynamic response function (here: canonical haemodynamic response function) and detection of spike-related BOLD signal changes. (Taken from Moeller et al. (2013c))

magnetic, which is the case for Ag/AgCl or gold electrodes. It is possible to use whole-head caps or single electrodes. Using caps reduces the time needed to attach electrodes, which is an important factor if working with children. Individual electrodes allow a tight wrapping of all electrode wires with a bandage.

Loops in the wires or movement of the wires could cause heating or artefacts and should be avoided. Foam pads and vacuum pillows can be used to help secure the EEG leads, minimise motion and improve patient comfort. The wires are connected to an MRI-compatible high-input impedance amplifier, which is placed inside the scanner room either directly behind the head coil (e.g. MR-compatible EEG recording system "BrainAmp-MR" by Brain Products Co., Munich, Germany) or beside the subject (MR System Electrical Geodesics, EGI Co., Memphis, USA) in most cases. The data are transmitted via a fibre optic cable to a computer located outside the scanner room. In some cases, MR-compatible caps are used and connected via a long cable with an EEG system placed outside the scanner room (MagLink system, Neuroscan/Compumedics Co.).

13.2.1.2 Artefact Correction

During the scanning, the rapidly changing magnetic field induces a strong current, which results in a high-amplitude gradient artefact in simultaneous EEG recordings. These artefacts can be removed after the scanning by artefact correction software so that the EEG is free from artefacts and events can be identified. The most commonly applied artefact correction uses an averaged artefact subtraction (AAS) method described by Allen et al. (2000). This method estimates the gradient artefact and subtracts it from each frame. For this step, a high sampling rate (several kHz) as well as a large amplitude dynamic range are needed to fully capture the shape of the gradient artefact. Furthermore, the scanner (10-MHz sampling rate) can be synchronised with the EEG amplifier (5-kHz sampling rate) to ensure identical sampling of the artefact for each frame, which optimises artefact correction. The EEG data are corrected relative to the gradient artefact onset, which is indicated by a trigger received from the MR system and recorded with the EEG for which commercial software is available (e.g. BrainVision Analyzer software, Brain Products Co., Munich, Germany). Corrected EEG data are filtered using a high-pass filter at 0.03 Hz and a low-pass filter at 75 Hz and down sampled to 250 Hz. For a comprehensive review about different artefact correction approaches, see Abreu et al. (2018).

In addition to gradient artefacts, many EEG data sets are affected by heartbeat synchronous artefacts. These so-called pulse or ballistocardiographic artefacts are caused by subtle pulse synchronous movements of the head and can be removed by the same AAS method (Allen et al. 1998) or independent component analysis-based procedures (Bénar et al. 2003; Srivastava et al. 2005). Correcting motion-induced voltages and gradient artefacts in the EEG using an fMRI prospective motion correction system can facilitate spike identification further (Körbl et al. 2016; Maziero et al. 2016). Figure 13.2 illustrates the different steps for artefact correction of the EEG.

To enable a visual inspection of the EEG during the EEG–fMRI recording, an online correction of gradient artefacts is possible.

13.2.2 Statistical Analysis of fMRI Data

The preprocessing of the fMRI images does not differ from a standard fMRI analysis and includes realignment, smoothing and normalisation in the case of group analyses. Removal of non-physiological signal changes such as movements can be used to reduce spurious false positive results and increase sensitivity, especially in children (Tierney et al. 2016). Since many analyses are based on single-subject analysis, normalisation is omitted in many studies on focal epilepsy. The classical analysis uses the event-related general linear model-based approach. For building the statistical model, the artefact-corrected EEG is reviewed, and all events (e.g. spikes) are marked. The timing of each event is

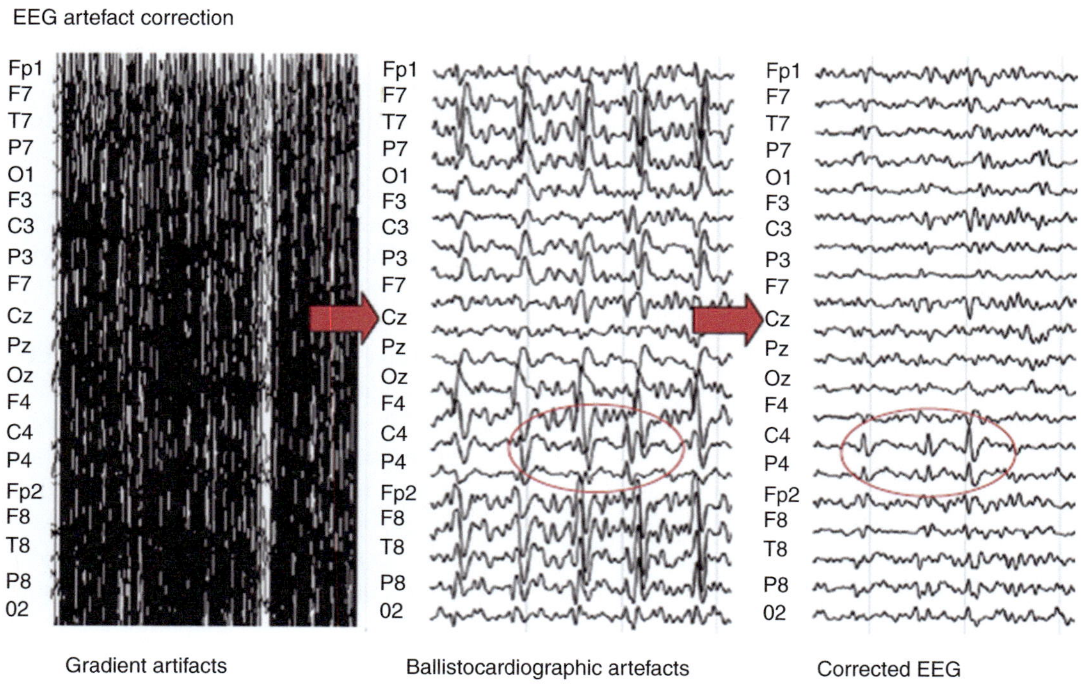

Fig. 13.2 Artefact correction of the EEG recorded during the fMRI investigation. Examples of the same segment of the EEG without artefact correction, after gradient artefact correction and after removal of the ballistocardiographic artefacts are shown

then used to build time series for the statistical analysis. In the standard analysis, the timing of the events is convolved with the standard haemodynamic response function, which is derived from a response to brief auditory stimuli and peaks approximately 5 s after the event (Glover 1999). Statistical maps are computed, showing voxels significantly correlated with the marked event in the EEG (Friston et al. 1996). However, taking a standard HRF does not take into account that shape and latency of the HRF might vary with age, different brain regions or altered response in epilepsy. Several studies have shown that the EEG–fMRI results can be improved if a more flexible HRF is applied. A more variable shape of the HRF can be achieved by including the derivative of the HRF in addition to the standard HRF (Hamandi et al. 2006) or by estimating non-canonical HRFs (Lemieux et al. 2007; van Houdt et al. 2010b) or using a set of four HRFs with peaks at 3, 5, 7 and 9 s to capture BOLD responses with different latencies (Bagshaw et al. 2004; Lu et al. 2007).

13.2.3 Methodological Refinements

Alternative modelling approaches: in many EEG–fMRI studies, only few spikes were recorded during the EEG–fMRI investigation, leading to inconclusive results. Instead of marking spikes in the scanner EEG, Groullier et al. built scalp voltage maps of averaged spike recorded during clinical long-term monitoring and computed the correlation of this map with the intra-MR topography at each EEG time frame. In 12 patients (~65%) with previously inconclusive studies, BOLD changes concordant with intracranial EEG or the resection area were detected. This voltage map-based analysis also yielded conclusive results when no clear spike in the scanner EEG was detected (Grouiller et al. 2011). By modelling sleep-specific activity (Moehring et al. 2011) or by modelling pulse height variability, eye blinks, swallowing and other video-EEG-detected physiological confounds (van Houdt et al. 2010a; LeVan et al. 2010a; Chaudhary et al. 2012) the sensitivity of detecting of spike related

BOLD signal changes could be increased. Lopes and colleagues showed that it might be possible to detect epileptic activity in the fMRI data without the help of an EEG: based on a wavelet model of the fMRI data, the authors could detect in a few cases similar results compared to an EEG-based fMRI analysis (Lopes et al. 2012). It is also possible to perform an analysis by using only the timing of spikes but making no assumption regarding the shape of the HRF (Lu et al. 2007). Another approach, which involves neither a priori models of HRF shape nor knowledge about the timing of interictal epileptiform discharge (IED) events, was proposed by Caballero-Gaudes and colleagues, who analysed EEG–fMRI data based on mutual information between the presence of spikes on EEG and the fMRI data (Caballero-Gaudes et al. 2013).

Advances of MRI scanners and sequences: scanning at 3 T rather than at 1.5 T also improves sensitivity (Gholipour et al. 2011; Pittau et al. 2012a). First studies have shown that EEG–fMRI is feasible even in a 7 T scanner but is challenged by more prominent ballistocardiogram (BCG) artefacts in the EEG (Jorge et al. 2015a, b; Abreu et al. 2016). And finally, also new sequences with improved temporal resolution of the BOLD signal have been developed. A so-called magnetic-resonance-encephalography (MREG) sequence allows temporal resolution of around 100 ms instead of seconds in conventional EPI (echo planar imaging) sequences. This higher sampling of the BOLD signal leads to improved statistic and significant BOLD responses even if only few spikes occurred during the investigation (Jacobs et al. 2014; Safi-Harb et al. 2015).

13.3 EEG–fMRI in Focal Epilepsy

13.3.1 Interictal Activity

The development of EEG–fMRI was clinically motivated to localise the region presumably generating focal interictal spikes. But does the spike-associated BOLD signal represent the spike generator?

To answer this question, BOLD signal changes were compared to intracranial EEG recordings preformed after the EEG–fMRI investigation. In a study by Bénar et al. (2006), active electrodes on the intracranial EEG recordings were close to the areas of spike-associated BOLD response. Furthermore, there are several cases in EEG–fMRI studies in focal epilepsy in which the concordance between spike-associated BOLD signal changes and the seizure onset determined by intracranially recorded seizures were detected (Bagshaw et al. 2004; Laufs et al. 2006; Grova et al. 2008; Tyvaert et al. 2008; Khoo et al. 2017b). While these studies compared EEG–fMRI results and intracranial recordings, which were recorded on different days, it is now possible to perform an EEG–fMRI recording in patients with intracranial electrodes (Carmichael et al. 2012; Boucousis et al. 2012). Studies in single patients showed BOLD response close to the electrodes from which spikes were recorded and also in remote areas (Vulliemoz et al. 2011; Cunningham et al. 2012). This pattern of BOLD signal changes in the presumed epileptogenic zone and also in remote areas is frequently detected in both single-subject analyses and group analyses in EEG–FMRI studies (Kobayashi et al. 2006a, 2009; Laufs et al. 2007). These remote BOLD signal changes may be remote the effects of the epileptic spikes. Combined source analysis and EEG–fMRI studies suggests that distant BOLD signal changes might be explained by propagated epileptic activity (Vulliemoz et al. 2009; Groening et al. 2009). This was confirmed in a recent study which showed that intracranial spikes in contacts close to the area of maximum BOLD responses (investigated in an EEG-fMRI study prior to implantation) preceded spikes in remote locations (Khoo et al. 2018). The same group demonstrated that intracranial electrodes in areas that had shown BOLD responses in a previous EEG–fMRI study displayed synchrony with other areas of BOLD responses. This study supports the existence of a neuronally based interictal epileptic network, which can be investigated non-invasively with EEG–fMRI (Khoo et al. 2017a).

In most studies, both positive and negative BOLD responses were observed. While positive BOLD responses reflect increased neuronal activity compared to baseline (Logothetis et al. 2001), negative BOLD responses have been shown to reflect suppressed neuronal activity (Devor et al. 2007). Spike-associated BOLD deactivation might be caused by remote inhibition (Gotman et al. 2005; Laufs et al. 2007). Negative BOLD responses in the area presumably generating the discharges are less common and may be explained by the presence of a slow wave, which is the likely electrographic correlate of prolonged inhibition (Pittau et al. 2013).

13.3.1.1 Can EEG–fMRI Be Used as a Non-invasive Tool in Pre-surgical Evaluation?

A study in patients with medically intractable epilepsy suggested that EEG–fMRI may add useful information in the preoperative workup (Zijlmans et al. 2007). In patients with non-lesional frontal lobe epilepsy, a concordance between positive BOLD signal changes and post-operative pathological analysis or other imaging modalities was found (Moeller et al. 2009a). An example of a comparison between EEG–fMRI results and methods of pre-surgical evaluation in a patient with focal epilepsy is depicted in Fig. 13.3. Post-surgical studies showed that a surgical removal including the areas of positive BOLD response was associated with a good post-surgical outcome, whereas widespread or discordant BOLD responses were associated with poor post-surgical outcome (Thornton et al. 2010, 2011). EEG–fMRI results may therefore predict post-surgical outcome (An et al. 2013). This was also described in patients with temporal lobe epilepsy who seem to show a better post-operative outcome if surgical resection included regions of haemodynamic changes (Coan et al. 2016). EEG–fMRI combined with electrical source imaging may predict surgical outcome better than each individual test (Centeno et al. 2017). And also combining results from EEG–fMRI and high-frequency oscillation (HFO) analysis yields additional information: HFOs are a well-studied promising biomarker for the epileptogenic zone from intracranial recordings. A recent study combined results from EEG–fMRI studies and intracranial HFO analysis and demonstrated that in patients with unifocal epilepsy, the maximum haemodynamic response related to scalp interictal discharges overlaps with the tissue generating high-frequency oscillations at high rates. Higher HFO rates inside than outside the maximum response indicates that the patient has indeed a focal epileptogenic zone, whereas similar rates inside and outside may indicate a widespread epileptogenic zone or an epileptogenic zone not covered by the implantation (González Otárula et al. 2018).

If a method is used for clinical purposes, it has to yield reproducible results. Gholipour and colleagues showed a good reproducibility of EEG–fMRI results, supporting its validity for clinical use (Gholipour et al. 2011). One study evaluated the new localising information generated by EEG–fMRI compared to traditional EEG and found that this occurred in a large proportion of patients (Pittau et al. 2012a). In a prospective EEG–FMRI study, Markoula et al. (2018) investigated the impact of EEG–fMRI results on a pre-surgical clinical decision-making process and reported that the EEG–fMRI results resulted in a modification of the initial surgical plan in 77% of the patients.

In summary, it is important that results are interpreted carefully since EEG–fMRI does not only show areas of the presumed epileptogenic zone but also areas that might be indirectly influenced by the spikes, also in distant areas. If EEG–fMRI results are considered in the context of other investigations of the pre-surgical evaluation, they can contribute to a better understanding of the epileptic zone in a specific patient.

13.3.1.2 Beyond the Focus

Several studies go beyond the analysis of the epileptogenic zone by investigating the functional connectivity of patients with mesial temporal lobe epilepsy. Functional connectivity studies measure how different brain areas are interconnected during the resting state of the brain (for

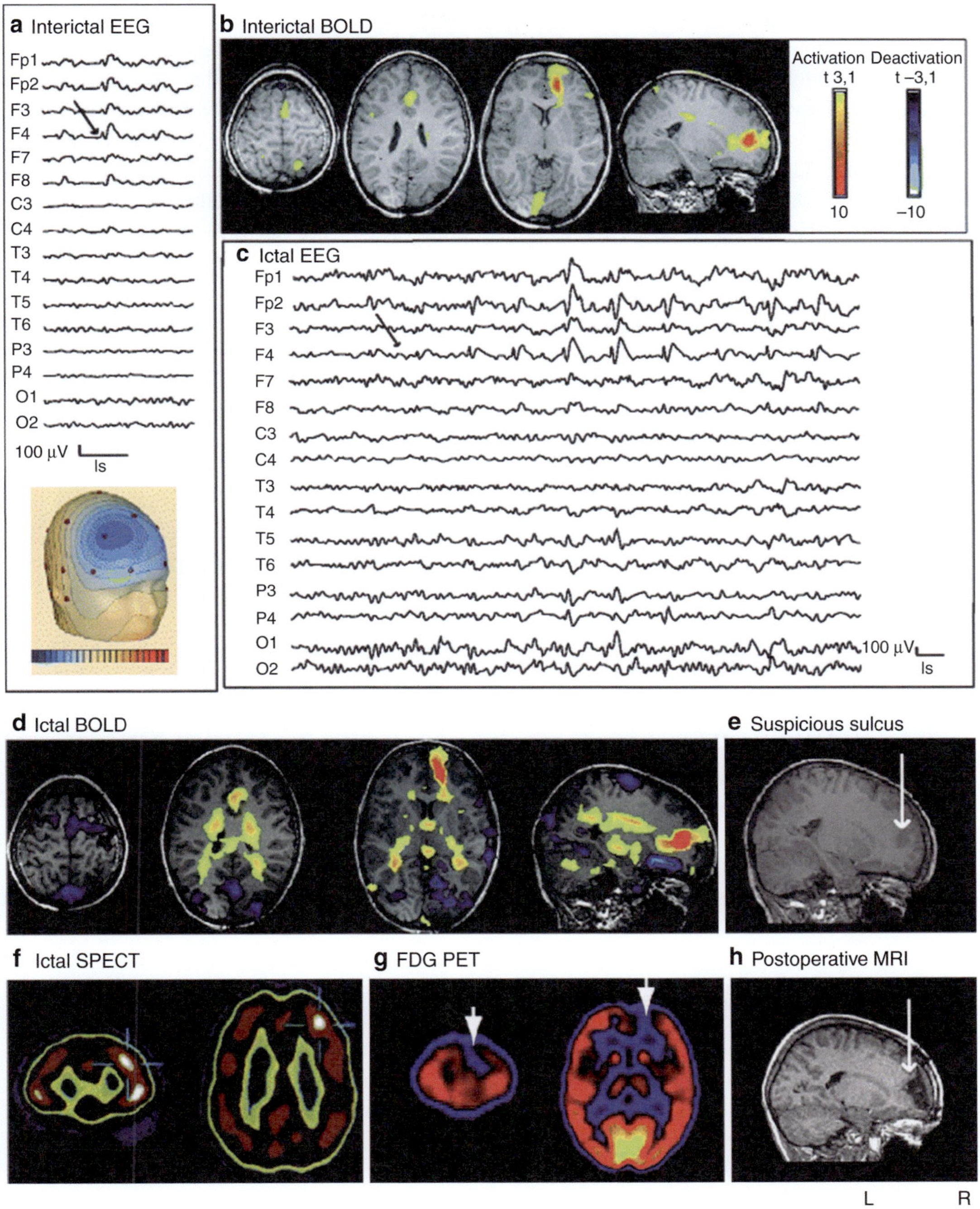

Fig. 13.3 Comparison between EEG–fMRI and methods of the pre-surgical evaluation in a patient with focal epilepsy. (**a**) Interictal EEG (average montage): focus F4 (*black arrow*). (**b**) Interictal fMRI: positive BOLD response frontopolar, no negative BOLD response. (**c**) Ictal EEG: rhythmic spike and wave F4 (*black arrow*). (**d**) Ictal fMRI: positive BOLD response frontopolar, negative BOLD response: frontal and posterior cingulate. (**e**) MRI: suspicious deep right middle frontal sulcus (*white arrow*). (**f**) Ictal SPECT: hyperperfusion frontal right. (**g**) FDG-PET: hypometabolism frontal right (*white arrows*). (**h**) Post-operative MRI (*white arrow* indicates resected area). (Taken from Moeller et al. (2009a))

details, please read the chapter on resting-state fluctuations in this book). Studies of patients with mesial temporal lobe epilepsy show that the functional connectivity in the diseased hippocampus, as well as in default mode areas, is decreased, indicating that this localisation-related epilepsy is also a network disease (Bettus et al. 2009; Pereira et al. 2010; Liao et al. 2011; Zhang et al. 2010; Pittau et al. 2012b). Various intrinsic connectivity networks of the brain have frequently been found to be compromised in patients with epilepsy, as demonstrated across many resting-state fMRI studies (for review, see Centeno and Carmichael 2014) suggesting a reduction in functional connectivity within these intrinsic networks as a feature of epilepsy. Negishi et al. (2011) demonstrated that altered functional connectivity can be used as a predictor for the surgical outcome of epilepsy. The appearance of new networks in temporal lobe epilepsy has also been observed (Lee et al. 2018).

13.3.2 Seizures

It is challenging to record seizures inside the scanner. The occurrence of a seizure cannot be predicted, and it is very rare that a seizure is captured during the short time of EEG–fMRI recording. If a seizure is recorded, it is often accompanied by head movements that make the data analysis difficult. To avoid seizure-induced motion problems, Federico et al. (2005) analysed the BOLD signal prior to the beginning of the clinical seizure in three patients with focal epilepsy and found BOLD signal changes in the pre-ictal state. However, over the years, several seizures without associated head movements were recorded. These studies were analysed in a block design and showed extensive seizure-associated BOLD signal changes, which also included the presumed seizure onset zone (Salek-Haddadi et al. 2002; Kobayashi et al. 2006b). In a study on malformation of cortical development, interictal and ictal BOLD signal changes differed in some patients (Tyvaert et al. 2008). By new techniques, the dynamics of seizure-associated BOLD signal changes can also be analysed. In studies where a sequential analysis of the BOLD signal or an independent component analysis was applied, the regions of seizure onset and propagation could be mapped (Tyvaert et al. 2009; Donaire et al. 2009; LeVan et al. 2010b). A case report in a 2-year-old patient with hypothalamic hamartoma suggests that seizure propagation pathways can be investigated by dynamic causal modelling. The authors discussed that the knowledge of propagation pathways might contribute to decision-making in the pre-surgical evaluation (Murta et al. 2012). Chaudhary et al. (2016) were able to record a seizure during intracranial EEG–fMRI and demonstrated BOLD signal changes in the seizure onset zone associated with beta and gamma activity in the amygdala and hippocampus.

13.4 EEG–fMRI in Idiopathic Generalised Epilepsy (IGE)

While in focal epilepsy the main aim is to identify the brain area of spike generation, in patients with IGE the aim is to identify networks to better understand the pathophysiological background of these epilepsies. IGE is characterised by EEG with generalised spike-wave discharges (GSW) typically arising from normal background activity. Animal models of IGE show that thalamocortical loops play an important role in the generation of GSW (Gloor 1968; Meeren et al. 2002; Slaght et al. 2004; Timofeev and Steriade 2004; Paz et al. 2005). Early EEG–fMRI studies investigated adult patients with idiopathic generalised epilepsy who showed short GSW paroxysms in the EEG (Aghakhani et al. 2004; Gotman et al. 2005; Hamandi et al. 2006). These studies confirmed that the thalamus is activated during GSW and also showed a deactivation in default mode areas (Raichle and Mintun 2006). The GSW-associated decrease in BOLD signal in default mode areas may indicate a disturbance of this physiological resting activity (Gotman et al. 2005) and, as shown in focal epilepsy with subsequent stereoelectroencephalography (SEEG) exploration, is associated with a decrease in gamma activity and increase in lower frequencies (Fahoum et al. 2013). While these studies were performed on adult patients with long-standing medically treated epilepsy, Moeller et al. (2008a) investigated absences in drug-naïve children with newly diagnosed epilepsy and confirmed a thalamic activation, along with deactivation, in default mode areas and the caudate nucleus. But how are absences initiated? Animal studies in genetic models of absence epilepsy strongly suggest that GSW are triggered in a restricted region of the somatosensory cortex (Meeren et al. 2002; Klein et al. 2004; Manning et al. 2004; Polack et al. 2007). A sliding window analysis of human absences showed that default mode areas and the caudate nucleus were involved significantly earlier than the thalamus. Early patient-specific BOLD signal changes could mirror a cortical focus (Moeller et al. 2010a). An example of a sliding window analysis of absences can be found in Fig. 13.4.

In a dynamic group analysis of absence seizure, Bai et al. (2010) showed that BOLD signal changes in the orbitofrontal cortex preceded the onset of absence seizures by up to 14 s, whereas negative BOLD signal changes in default mode areas were seen up to 20 s after the end of absence seizures. This analysis indicated that there are long-lasting BOLD signal changes that are not detectable by conventional HRF modelling in many regions. There are inconsistent results regarding the question on whether BOLD signal changes might occur prior to GSW: while preceding BOLD signal changes are reported in some adult patients with GSW, children with polyspike-wave paroxysms and a group analysis of absences (Hawco et al. 2007; Moeller et al. 2008b; Bai et al. 2010), no preceding BOLD signal changes are detected in other studies (Moeller et al. 2008a, 2011b). Early parietal BOLD signal changes prior to absences (Carney et al. 2010, 2012) support the hypothesis that changes in activity within the default mode areas could facilitate the occurrence of GSW (Vaudano et al. 2009). One might assume that conflicting results may be explained by different analysis techniques and different groups of patients. One study tried to specifically investigate the termination of absence seizures and found BOLD signal

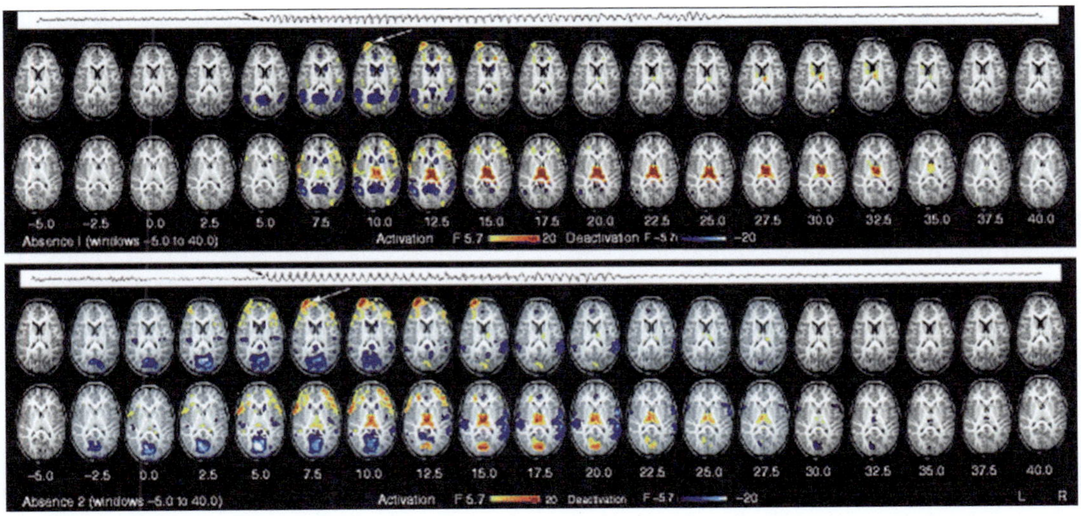

Fig. 13.4 Sliding window analysis for two absences of the same patient (windows −5–40 s). The duration of the absence is indicated by one EEG channel (Fp2 with average reference); the onset is indicated by a *black arrow*. Please note that the EEG onset of the absence is shifted 5 s to account for the haemodynamic delay of the BOLD response and to allow a direct comparison of absence duration and associated BOLD signal changes. First activation consistent for both absences was found in the left frontopolar cortex (*white arrows*). In the first absence, this activation started 10 s after onset; for the second, it started 5 s after onset. The thalamic activation started 7.5 s after onset in both, deactivation in the caudate nucleus 5 s after onset and deactivation in default mode areas 5 s after onset in the first and 2.5 s before onset in the second. BOLD signal changes in the thalamus and default mode areas exceeded the duration of the absence by several windows. In the second absence, thalamic activation was followed by thalamic deactivation. (Taken from Moeller et al. (2010a))

increase over the precuneus-posterior cingulate region bilaterally, as well as decreased neural activity of lateral prefrontal cortex at GSW termination. Whether these structures play a role in the offset of discharges remains unclear (Benuzzi et al. 2015).

Myoclonic astatic epilepsy (MAE) is a difficult to treat subgroup of IGE of early childhood. An EEG–fMRI study in patients with MAE showed involvement of the motor network and putamen associated with generalised spike-wave discharges (Moeller et al. 2014). This may indicate that a dysfunction in the motor network may lead to myoclonic seizures observed in these groups of patients.

13.4.1 Absences and Cognitive Impairment

EEG–fMRI studies with simultaneous testing during absences suggest that absences that are associated with a stronger cognitive impairment are associated with more widespread BOLD signal changes than absences with no or mild cognitive impairment (Berman et al. 2010). However, in a case report in a girl with long-lasting GSW paroxysms without concomitant cognitive impairment, the same networks were activated as in absences with clinical manifestation (Moeller et al. 2010b). Recently, it was shown that impaired consciousness in absence seizures seems to be related to the intensity of physiological changes in GSW-associated networks of the brain. Increased EEG and fMRI amplitude at the onset of seizures are associated with behavioral impairment. These findings suggest that a vulnerable state may exist at the initiation of some seizures leading to greater physiological changes and altered consciousness (Guo et al. 2016).

13.4.2 IGE and Functional Connectivity

As mentioned before, GSW are characterised by a thalamocortical interaction. But are there also pathological thalamocortical interactions in periods free from GSW discharges? Studying children with absence seizures, Bai et al. (2010) found increased interhemispheric connectivity in the orbitofrontal cortex, indicating increased synchronous activity between both hemispheres at rest. Increased connectivity was also found in the network of the basal ganglia when compared to healthy controls. This increased connectivity was even more pronounced during periods with GSW (Luo et al. 2012). However, decreased functional connectivity was described for the thalamus (Masterton et al. 2012; Wang et al. 2012), the default mode network (DMN) (Luo et al. 2011) and the attention network (Killory et al. 2011) in children with absence seizures. These findings might explain impaired interictal attention in these children. Decreased connectivity in the (DMN) areas was negatively correlated with epilepsy duration (Luo et al. 2011; Maneshi et al. 2012). Furthermore, Yang et al. (2013) showed that this decreased connectivity within the DMN, the cognitive control network, and the attention network was more pronounced during interictal GSW. In patients with juvenile myoclonic epilepsy, GSW seem to compromise various networks such as the default mode network, self-reference network and basal ganglia (Dong et al. 2016). However, not all studies showed changes in functional connectivity: in adult patients with different types of IGE, one functional connectivity study did not show pathological connectivity in areas that are known to interact during GSW, which could underline the paroxysmal character of GSW discharges (Moeller et al. 2011a, b). Functional connectivity analysis may also be used to predict treatment outcome: Tenney et al. (2018) demonstrated that pretreatment ictal connectivity differences in children with childhood absence epilepsy (CAE) were associated with response to anti-epileptic treatment. One study investigated functional connectivity before GSW and found a pro-ictal, "GSW permissive" network state lasting at least 1 min before onset characterised by increased sensorimotor connectivity and decreased posterior network connections, followed by a pre-ictal network state lasting several seconds characterised by a steadily increasing widespread synchrony (Tangwiriyasakul et al. 2018).

13.4.3 EEG–fMRI Studies in Generalised Photoparoxysmal Responses

Photoparoxysmal response (PPR) is an electroencephalographic trait characterised by the occurrence of epileptiform discharges in response to visual stimulation. Studying this trait helps to learn about the mechanisms of epileptogenicity. An EEG–fMRI study showed an involvement of the parietal and frontal cortex but not the thalamus in most of the subjects during a generalised PPR (Moeller et al. 2009b). In contrast to spontaneous GSW in which a thalamic involvement is commonly found, PPR seems to be mainly a cortical phenomenon. However, in a patient in whom photic stimulation evoked a generalised seizure, an excessive increase in BOLD signal in the visual cortex, together with thalamic increase in BOLD signal, was detected (Moeller et al. 2009c). These results were confirmed in a source analysis study in which dynamic imaging of coherent sources (DICS) was performed in the EEG studies recorded in the above-mentioned EEG–fMRI studies in absences and PPR (Moeller et al. 2008b, 2009a). Re-normalised partial directed coherence (RPDC) in these data sets suggested that in absences, cortical sources were influenced by the thalamic source; in PPR, however, an information flow from the occipital cortex was found (Moeller et al. 2013a).

Functional connectivity in PPR shows decreased alpha-related inhibition of the visual cortex and sensory-motor networks at rest. These findings could represent the substrate of the clinical manifestation of myoclonus, which can be associated with PPR (Vaudano et al. 2017).

13.5 Paediatric EEG–fMRI Studies

Childhood epilepsies differ from adult epilepsies with regard to aetiology, pathogenesis, seizure semiology and EEG patterns and prognosis (Roger et al. 2005). The immature brain is more prone to develop seizures, and epileptic discharges are more frequent and less localised in children than in adults (Holmes 1997). The clinical manifestations are also age correlated and can vary within patients throughout their maturation process (Ben-Ari 2006). The following section will give an overview about differences in HRFs observed in children and EEG–fMRI studies in different paediatric epilepsy syndromes. Paediatric EEG–fMRI studies in IGE are discussed in Sect. 13.4.

13.5.1 Modelling Spike-Related BOLD Changes in Children

Jacobs et al. (2007, 2008) underlined the impact of age on spike-related BOLD changes and demonstrated that children with focal lesional epilepsy show deactivations more frequently than activations in the epileptogenic zone compared to adults; the shape of the HRF especially differed in young children. Modelling spike-related BOLD signal changes in children might be even more complex since BOLD signal changes that precede the spike can be found in paediatric patients (Jacobs et al. 2009). These preceding BOLD signal changes were more localised than later BOLD signal changes (Jacobs et al. 2009). The question of why BOLD signal changes might precede the spike detected on the scalp EEG is still unanswered. Preceding BOLD signal changes might be explained by synchronised discharges detectable with depth electrodes but not visible on the scalp EEG (Pittau et al. 2011) in some patients only.

13.5.2 Self-Limited Focal Epilepsies

Early applications of EEG–fMRI in children were carried out in cases with benign focal epilepsies. Benign focal epilepsies represent a group of epileptic disorders that are related to well-localised focal EEG patterns of centro-temporal spikes (Dalla Bernardina et al. 2005). Seizures in benign epilepsy with centro-temporal spikes (BECTS) typically begin with paraesthesia or jerking in the mouth, face and hand, usually with a preserved level of consciousness, supporting their origin in the sensorimotor cortex. EEG–fMRI studies in patients with BECTS showed spike-related BOLD signal changes in the sensorimotor cortex (Archer et al. 2003; Boor et al. 2003, 2007; Lengler et al. 2007; Siniatchkin et al. 2007b; Masterton et al. 2010), whereas distant BOLD signal changes were interpreted as propagated activity, as shown by source analysis (Boor et al. 2007). The BOLD response to spikes in BECTS was different from the canonical shape of the HRF, underscoring the importance of more variable HRF in pediatric studies (Masterton et al. 2010, 2013a, b). Functional connectivity analysis in children with BECTS prior to spikes, during spikes and post spikes suggests that spikes directly disrupt the functional brain networks responsible for language, behaviour and cognition (Xiang et al. 2016). In other benign epilepsies (benign occipital lobe epilepsies), Leal et al. (2006, 2007) found an activation pattern in different cortical occipital and parietal areas corresponding well to the localisation of interictal epileptiform discharges. A study in atypical benign partial epilepsy demonstrated patterns similar to studies in BECTS (focal BOLD signal changes in the spike field), as well as patterns observed in continuous spikes and waves during slow sleep (CSWS) (distant BOLD signal changes in cortical and subcortical structures), thereby underscoring that idiopathic focal epilepsies of childhood form a spectrum of overlapping syndromes (Moeller et al. 2013b).

13.5.3 Epileptic Encephalopathies

West syndrome is a prototype of severe epileptic encephalopathies of infancy, consisting of tonic spasms, psychomotor developmental delay and the characteristic electroencephalographic pattern of hypsarrhythmia. The EEG features are characterised by a multifocal spike and sharp-wave activity and high-voltage slow-wave activity (Dulac 2001; Hrachovy and Frost 2003). In an EEG–fMRI study, Siniatchkin and colleagues showed that interictal spikes were associated with positive BOLD changes in the cerebral cortex (especially in occipital areas), whereas high-amplitude slow-wave activity in hypsarrhythmia was commonly associated with BOLD signal changes in the brainstem, putamen, thalamus and different cortical areas (Siniatchkin et al. 2007a). When applying source analysis (DICS) to the same data sets, the same key structures were detected with the brainstem driving putamen and cortical sources (Japaridze et al. 2013). These results are in line with previous PET studies that had shown metabolic changes in the cortex, putamen and brainstem in West syndrome patients (Chugani et al. 1992; Chiron et al. 1993; Metsähonkala et al. 2002).

West syndrome often evolves into *Lennox–Gastaut syndrome*, an epileptic encephalopathy characterised by different types of seizures (tonic, tonic-clonic and atonic seizures, as well as atypical absences), typical EEG changes (slow spike-wave complexes ranging from 1 to 2.5/s, generalised paroxysmal fast activity) and accompanying mental retardation (Arzimanoglou et al. 2009). An EEG–fMRI study in children with Lennox–Gastaut syndrome showed activation of the brainstem and thalamus associated with epileptiform discharges pointing to common pathogenetic pathways of West syndrome and Lennox–Gastaut syndrome (Siniatchkin et al. 2007a, 2011). When analysing different EEG patterns, Pillay and colleagues demonstrated that paroxysmal fast activity is associated with coactivation of the default mode and attention network, as well as subcortical structures (brainstem, thalamus and basal ganglia). By comparison, the slow spike-wave complexes showed predominantly deactivations in cortical and subcortical areas, which often show a non-canonical haemodynamic response (Pillay et al. 2013; Archer et al. 2014). Functional connectivity studies demonstrate abnormal cognitive network interactions, which the author proposed to lead to epileptic encephalopathy (Warren et al. 2016). Increased connectivity of specific thalamocortical circuits could potentially be a target for thalamic deep brain stimulation (Warren et al. 2017).

Epileptic encephalopathy with *continuous spike and waves during slow sleep* is an age-related disorder characterised by the presence of interictal epileptiform discharges during at least >85% of sleep and cognitive deficits associated with this EEG pattern. An EEG–fMRI study showed that despite aetiological heterogeneity, patients with continuous spike and waves during slow sleep were characterised by the activation of a similar neuronal network: perisylvian region, insula and cingulate gyrus. A comparison with the electrical source analysis results suggested that the activations corresponded to both initiation and propagation pathways. Deactivations in structures of the default mode network are consistent with the concept of epileptiform activity impacting on normal brain function by inducing repetitive interruptions of neurophysiological function (Siniatchkin et al. 2010).

13.6 Conclusion

Combining EEG and fMRI has opened a new window into the exploration of epileptic discharges, allowing the investigation of the whole brain non-invasively. It combines the high spatial resolution of fMRI and the specificity of the EEG for epileptic patterns. It has now become a clinical tool in the localisation of the epileptic focus, which is also able to help predict post-surgical outcome. EEG–fMRI has uncovered unexpected mechanisms in both focal and generalised epilepsies. It is not an easy tool because of the complexity of recording the EEG in the MR scanner and removing the resulting artefacts, but it is unique in its ability to study epileptic discharges non-invasively in the whole brain.

References

Abreu R, Leite M et al (2016) Ballistocardiogram artefact correction taking into account physiological. Neuroimage 135:45–63

Abreu R, Leal A et al (2018) EEG-informed fMRI: a review of data analysis methods. Front Hum Neurosci 12:29

Aghakhani Y, Bagshaw AP et al (2004) fMRI activation during spike and wave discharges in idiopathic generalized epilepsy. Brain 127:1127–1114

Allen PJ, Polizzi G et al (1998) Identification of EEG events in the MR scanner: the problem of pulse artifact and a method for its subtraction. Neuroimage 8:229–239

Allen PJ, Josephs O et al (2000) A method for removing imaging artifact from continuous EEG recorded during functional MRI. Neuroimage 12:230–239

An D, Fahoum F et al (2013) Electroencephalography/functional magnetic resonance imaging responses help predict surgical outcome in focal epilepsy. Epilepsia 54:2184–2194

Archer JS, Briellman RS et al (2003) Benign epilepsy with Centro-temporal spikes: spike triggered fMRI shows somato-sensory cortex activity. Epilepsia 44:200–204

Archer JS, Warren AE et al (2014) Lennox-Gastaut syndrome and phenotype: secondary network epilepsies. Epilepsia 55:1245–1254

Arzimanoglou A, French J et al (2009) Lennox-Gastaut syndrome: a consensus approach on diagnosis, assessment, management, and trial methodology. Lancet Neurol 8:82–93

Bagshaw AP, Aghakhani Y et al (2004) EEG-fMRI of focal epileptic spikes: analysis with multiple haemodynamic functions and comparison with gadolinium-enhanced MR angiograms. Hum Brain Mapp 22:179–192

Bai X, Vestal M, Berman R et al (2010) Dynamic time course of typical childhood absence seizures: EEG, behavior, and functional magnetic resonance imaging. J Neurosci 30:5884–5893

Bénar C, Aghakhani Y et al (2003) Quality of EEG in simultaneous EEG-fMRI for epilepsy. Clin Neurophysiol 114:569–580

Bénar CG, Grova C et al (2006) EEG-fMRI of epileptic spikes: concordance with EEG source localization and intracranial EEG. Neuroimage 30:1161–1170

Ben-Ari Y (2006) Basic developmental rules and their implication for epilepsy in the immature brain. Epileptic Disord 8:91–102

Benuzzi F, Ballotta D et al (2015) An EEG-fMRI study on the termination of generalized spike-and-wave discharges in absence epilepsy. PLoS One 10:e0130943

Berman R, Negishi M et al (2010) Simultaneous EEG, fMRI, and behavior in typical childhood absence seizures. Epilepsia 51:2011–2022

Bettus G, Guedj E et al (2009) Decreased basal fMRI functional connectivity in epileptogenic networks and contralateral compensatory mechanisms. Hum Brain Mapp 30:1580–1591

Boor S, Vucurevic G et al (2003) EEG-related functional MRI in benign childhood epilepsy with centrotemporal spikes. Epilepsia 44:688–692

Boor R, Jacobs J et al (2007) Combined spike-related functional MRI and multiple source analysis in the non-invasive spike localization of benign rolandic epilepsy. Clin Neurophysiol 118(4):901–909

Boucousis SM, Beers CA et al (2012) Feasibility of an intracranial EEG-fMRI protocol at 3T: risk assessment and image quality. Neuroimage 63:1237–1248

Caballero-Gaudes C, Van de Ville D et al (2013) Mapping interictal epileptic discharges using mutual information between concurrent EEG and fMRI. Neuroimage 68:248–262

Carmichael DW, Vulliemoz S et al (2012) Simultaneous intracranial EEG-fMRI in humans: protocol considerations and data quality. Neuroimage 63:301–309

Carney PW, Masterton RA et al (2010) The core network in absence epilepsy. Differences in cortical and thalamic BOLD response. Neurology 75:904–911

Carney PW, Masterton RA et al (2012) The frontal lobe in absence epilepsy: EEG-fMRI findings. Neurology 78(15):1157–65.

Centeno M, Carmichael DW (2014) Network connectivity in epilepsy: resting state fMRI and EEG-fMRI contributions. Front Neurol 5:93

Centeno M, Tierney TM et al (2016) Optimising EEG-fMRI for localisation of focal epilepsy in children. PLoS One 11:e0149048

Centeno M, Tierney TM et al (2017) Combined electroencephalography-functional magnetic resonance imaging and electrical source imaging improves localization of pediatric focal epilepsy. Ann Neurol 82:278–287

Chaudhary UJ, Rodionov R, Carmichael DW, Thornton RC, Duncan JS, Lemieux L (2012) Improving the sensitivity of EEG-fMRI studies of epileptic activity by modelling eye blinks, swallowing and other video-EEG detected physiological confounds. Neuroimage 61:1383–1393

Chaudhary UJ, Centeno M et al (2016) Mapping human precital and ictal haemodynamic networks using simultaneous intracranial EEG-fMRI. Neuroimage Clin 11:486–493

Chiron C, Dulac O et al (1993) Study of regional cerebral blood flow in West syndrome. Epilepsia 34:707–715

Chugani HT, Shewmon DA et al (1992) Infantile spasms: II. Lenticular nuclei and brain stem activation on positron emission tomography. Ann Neurol 31:212–219

Coan AC, Chaudhary UJ et al (2016) EEG-fMRI in the presurgical evaluation of temporal lobe epilepsy. J Neurol Neurosurg Psychiatry 87:642–649

Cunningham CB, Goodyear BG et al (2012) Intracranial EEG-fMRI analysis of focal epileptiform discharges in humans. Epilepsia 53:1636–1648

Dalla Bernardina B, Sgro V et al (2005) Epilepsy with centro-temporal spikes and related syndromes. In: Roger J, Bureau M, Dravet C, Genton P, Tassinari CA, Wolf P (eds) Epileptic syndromes in infancy, childhood and adolescence. John Libbey Eurotext Ltd, Montrouge, pp 203–226

Devor A, Tian P et al (2007) Suppressed neuronal activity and concurrent arteriolar vasoconstriction may explain negative blood oxygenation level-dependent signal. J Neurosci 27:4452–4459

Donaire A, Bargallo N et al (2009) Identifying the structures involved in seizure generation using sequential analysis of ictal-fMRI data. Neuroimage 47:173–183

Dong L, Luo C et al (2016) Complex discharge-affecting networks in juvenile myoclonic epilepsy: a simultaneous EEG-fMRI study. Hum Brain Mapp 37:3515–3529

Dulac O (2001) What is west syndrome? Brain Dev 23:447–452

Fahoum F, Zelmann R et al (2013) Epileptic discharges affect the default mode network—FMRI and intracerebral EEG evidence. PLoS One 8:e68038

Federico P, Abbott DF et al (2005) Functional MRI of the pre-ictal state. Brain 128:1811–1817

Friston KJ, Williams S et al (1996) Movement-related effects in fMRI time-series. Magn Reson Med 35:346–355

Gholipour T, Moeller F et al (2011) Reproducibility of interictal EEG-fMRI results in epilepsy patients. Epilepsia 52:433–434

Gloor P (1968) Generalized cortico-reticular epilepsies, some considerations on the pathophysiology of generalized bilaterally synchronous spike and wave discharge. Epilepsia 9:249–263

Glover GH (1999) Deconvolution of impulse response in event-related BOLD fMRI. Neuroimage 9:416–419

González Otárula KA, Khoo HM et al (2018) Spike-related haemodynamic responses overlap with high frequency oscillations in patients with focal epilepsy. Brain 141(3):731–743

Gotman J, Grova C et al (2005) Generalized epileptic discharges show thalamocortical activation and suspension of the default state of the brain. Proc Natl Acad Sci U S A 102:15236–15240

Groening K, Brodbeck V et al (2009) Combination of EEG-fMRI and EEG source analysis improves interpretation of spike-associated activation networks in paediatric pharmacoresistant focal epilepsies. Neuroimage 46:827–833

Grouiller F, Thornton RC et al (2011) With or without spikes: localization of focal epileptic activity by simultaneous electroencephalography and functional magnetic resonance imaging. Brain 134:2867–2886

Grova C, Daunizeau J et al (2008) Concordance between distributed EEG source localization and simultaneous EEG-fMRI studies of epileptic spikes. Neuroimage 39:755–774

Guo JN, Kim R et al (2016) Impaired consciousness in patients with absence seizures investigated by functional MRI, EEG, and behavioural measures: a cross-sectional study. Lancet Neurol 1:1336–1345

Hamandi K, Salek-Haddadi A et al (2006) EEG-fMRI of idiopathic and secondary generalized epilepsies. Neuroimage 31:1700–1710

Hawco CS, Bagshaw AP et al (2007) BOLD changes occur prior to epileptic spikes seen on scalp EEG. Neuroimage 35:1450–1458

Hoffmann A, Jäger L et al (2000) Electroencephalography during functional echo-planar imaging: detection of epileptic spikes using post-processing methods. Magn Reson Med 44:791–798

Holmes GL (1997) Epilepsy in the developing brain: lessons from the laboratory and clinic. Epilepsia 38:12–30

van Houdt PJ, Ossenblok PP et al (2010a) Correction for pulse height variability reduces physiological noise in functional MRI when studying spontaneous brain activity. Hum Brain Mapp 31:311–325 van Houdt PJ, de Munck JC et al (2010b) Comparison of analytical strategies for EEG-correlated fMRI data in patients with epilepsy. Magn Reson Imaging 28:1078–1086

Hrachovy RA, Frost JD (2003) Infantile epileptic encephalopathy with hypsarrhythmia. J Clin Neurophysiol 20:408–425

Ives JR, Warach S et al (1993) Monitoring the patient's EEG during echo planar MRI. Electroencephalogr Clin Neurophysiol 87:417–420

Jacobs J, Kobayashi E et al (2007) Hemodynamic responses to interictal epileptiform discharges in children with symptomatic epilepsy. Epilepsia 48:2068–2078

Jacobs J, Hawco C et al (2008) Variability of the hemodynamic response function with age in children with epilepsy. Neuroimage 40:601–614

Jacobs J, Levan P et al (2009) Hemodynamic changes preceding the interictal EEG spike in patients with focal epilepsy investigated using simultaneous EEG-fMRI. Neuroimage 45:1220–1231

Jacobs J, Stich J et al (2014) Fast fMRI provides high statistical power in the analysis of epileptic networks. Neuroimage 88:282–294

Japaridze N, Muthuraman M et al (2013) Neuronal networks in west syndrome as revealed by source analysis and renormalized partial directed coherence. Brain Topogr 26:157–170

Jorge J, Grouiller F et al (2015a) Simultaneous EEG-fMRI at ultra-high field: artifact prevention and safety assessment. Neuroimage 2015(105):132–144

Jorge J, Grouiller F et al (2015b) Towards high-quality simultaneous EEG-fMRI at 7 T: detection and reduction of EEG artifacts due to head motion. Neuroimage 120:143–153

Khoo HM, von Ellenrieder N et al (2017a) Epileptic networks in action: synchrony between distant hemodynamic responses. Ann Neurol 82:57–66

Khoo HM, Hao Y et al (2017b) The hemodynamic response to interictal epileptic discharges localizes the seizure-onset zone. Epilepsia 58:811–823

Khoo HM, von Ellenrieder N et al (2018) The spike onset zone: the region where epileptic spikes start and from where they propagate. Neurology 91(7):e666–e674

Killory BD, Bai X et al (2011) Impaired attention and network connectivity in childhood absence epilepsy. Neuroimage 56:2209–2217

Klein JP, Khera DS et al (2004) Dysregulation of sodium channel expression in cortical neurons in a rodent model of absence epilepsy. Brain Res 1000:102–109

Kobayashi E, Bagshaw AP et al (2006a) Temporal and extratemporal BOLD responses to temporal lobe interictal spikes. Epilepsia 47:343–354

Kobayashi E, Hawco CS et al (2006b) Widespread and intense BOLD changes during brief focal electrographic seizures. Neurology 66:1049–1055

Kobayashi E, Grova C et al (2009) Structures involved at the time of temporal lobe spikes revealed by interindividual group analysis of EEG/fMRI data. Epilepsia 50:2549–2556

Körbl K, Jacobs J et al (2016) Marker-based ballistocardiographic artifact correction improves spike identification in EEG-fMRI of focal epilepsy patients. Clin Neurophysiol 127:2802–2811

Krakow K, Woermann FG et al (1999) EEG-triggered functional MRI of interictal epileptiform activity in patients with partial seizures. Brain 122:1679–1688

Laufs H, Hamandi K et al (2006) EEG-fMRI mapping of asymmetrical delta activity in a patient with refractory epilepsy is concordant with the epileptogenic region determined by intracranial EEG. Magn Reson Imaging 24:367–371

Laufs H, Hamandi K et al (2007) Temporal lobe interictal epileptic discharges affect cerebral activity in "default mode" brain regions. Hum Brain Mapp 28:1023–1032

Leal A, Dias A et al (2006) The BOLD effect of interictal spike activity in childhood occipital lobe epilepsy. Epilepsia 47:1536–1542

Leal A, Nunes S et al (2007) Brain mapping of epileptic activity in a case of idiopathic occipital lobe epilepsy (Panayiotopoulos Syndrome). Epilepsia 48:1179–1183

Lee K, Khoo HM et al (2018) Disruption, emergence and lateralization of brain network hubs in mesial temporal lobe epilepsy. Neuroimage Clin 20:71–84

Lemieux L, Salek-Haddadi A et al (2001) Event-related fMRI with simultaneous and continuous EEG: description of the method and initial case report. Neuroimage 14:780–787

Lemieux L, Salek-Haddadi A et al (2007) Modelling large motion events in fMRI studies of patients with epilepsy. Magn Reson Imaging 25:894–901

Lengler U, Kafadar I et al (2007) fMRI correlates of interictal epileptic activity in patients with idiopathic benign focal epilepsy of childhood. A simultaneous EEG-functional MRI study. Epilepsy Res 75:29–38

LeVan P, Tyvaert L et al (2010a) Modulation by EEG features of BOLD responses to interictal epileptiform discharges. Neuroimage 50:15–26

LeVan P, Tyvaert L et al (2010b) Independent component analysis reveals dynamic ictal BOLD responses in EEG-fMRI data from focal epilepsy patients. Neuroimage 149:366–378

Liao W, Zhang Z et al (2011) Default mode network abnormalities in mesial temporal lobe epilepsy: a study combining fMRI and DTI. Hum Brain Mapp 32:883–895

Logothetis NK, Pauls J et al (2001) Neurophysiological investigation of the basis of the fMRI signal. Nature 412:150–157

Lopes R, Lina JM et al (2012) Detection of epileptic activity in fMRI without recording the EEG. Neuroimage 60(3):1867–1879

Lu Y, Grova C et al (2007) Using voxel-specific hemodynamic response function in EEG-fMRI data analysis: an estimation and detection model. Neuroimage 34:195–203

Luo C, Li Q et al (2011) Altered functional connectivity in default mode network in absence epilepsy: a resting-state fMRI study. Hum Brain Mapp 32:438–449

Luo C, Li Q et al (2012) Resting state basal ganglia network in idiopathic generalized epilepsy. Hum Brain Mapp 33:1279–1294

Maneshi M, Moeller F et al (2012) Resting-state connectivity of the sustained attention network correlates with disease duration in idiopathic generalized epilepsy. PLoS One 7:e50359

Manning JP, Richards DA et al (2004) Cortical-area specific block of genetically determined absence seizures by ethosuximide. Neuroscience 123:5–9

Markoula S, Chaudhary UJ et al (2018) The impact of mapping interictal discharges using EEG-fMRI on the epilepsy presurgical clinical decision making process: a prospective study. Seizure 61:30–37

Masterton RA, Harvey AS et al (2010) Focal epileptiform spikes do not show a canonical BOLD response in patients with benign rolandic epilepsy (BECTS). Neuroimage 51:252–260

Masterton RA, Carney PW et al (2012) Cortical and thalamic resting-state functional connectivity is altered in childhood absence epilepsy. Epilepsy Res 99:327–334

Masterton RA, Jackson GD et al (2013a) Mapping brain activity using event-related independent components analysis (eICA): specific advantages for EEG-fMRI. Neuroimage 70:164–174

Masterton RA, Carney PW et al (2013b) Absence epilepsy subnetworks revealed by event-related independent components analysis of functional magnetic resonance imaging. Epilepsia 54:801–808

Maziero D, Velasco TR et al (2016) Towards motion insensitive EEG-fMRI: correcting motion-induced voltages and gradient artefact instability in EEG using an fMRI prospective motion correction (PMC) system. Neuroimage 138:13–27.

Meeren HK, Pijn JP et al (2002) Cortical focus drives widespread corticothalamic networks during spontaneous absence seizures in rats. J Neurosci 22:1480–1495

Metsähonkala L, Gaily E et al (2002) Focal and global cortical hypometabolism in patients with newly diagnosed infantile spasms. Neurology 58:1646–1651

Moehring J, Coropceanu D et al (2011) Improving sensitivity of EEG-fMRI studies in epilepsy: the role of sleep-specific activity. Neurosci Lett 505(2):211–215

Moeller F, Siebner H et al (2008a) EEG-fMRI in children with untreated childhood absence epilepsy. Epilepsia 49:1510–1519

Moeller F, Siebner H et al (2008b) Changes in activity of striato-thalamo-cortical network precede generalized spike wave discharges. Neuroimage 39:1839–1849

Moeller F, Tyvaert L et al (2009a) EEG-fMRI: adding to standard evaluations of patients with nonlesional frontal lobe epilepsy. Neurology 73:2023–2030

Moeller F, Siebner HR et al (2009b) FMRI activation during spike and wave discharges evoked by photic stimulation. Neuroimage 48:682–695

Moeller F, Siebner HR et al (2009c) Mapping brain activity on the verge of a photically induced generalized tonic-clonic seizure. Epilepsia 50:1632–1637

Moeller F, Levan P et al (2010a) Absence seizures: individual patterns revealed by EEG-fMRI. Epilepsia 51:2000–2010

Moeller F, Muhle H et al (2010b) EEG-fMRI study of generalized spike and wave discharges without transitory cognitive impairment. Epilepsy Behav 18:313–316

Moeller F, Maneshi M et al (2011a) Functional connectivity in patients with idiopathic generalized epilepsy. Epilepsia 52:515–522

Moeller F, Levan P et al (2011b) Independent component analysis (ICA) of generalized spike wave discharges in fMRI: comparison with general linear model-based EEG-fMRI. Hum Brain Mapp 2:209–217

Moeller F, Muthuraman M et al (2013a) Representation and propagation of epileptic activity in absences and generalized photoparoxysmal responses. Hum Brain Mapp 34:1896–1909

Moeller F, Moehring et al (2013b) EEG-fMRI in atypical benign partial epilepsy. Epilepsia 54(8):e103–e108

Moeller F, Stephani U et al (2013c) Simultaneous EEG and fMRI recordings (EEG-fMRI) in children with epilepsy. Epilepsia 54:971–982

Moeller F, Groening K et al (2014) EEG-fMRI in myoclonic astatic epilepsy (Doose syndrome). Neurology 82:1508–1513

Murta T, Leal A et al (2012) Dynamic causal modelling of epileptic seizure propagation pathways: a combined EEG-fMRI study. Neuroimage 62:1634–1642

Negishi M, Martuzzi R et al (2011) Functional MRI connectivity as a predictor of the surgical outcome of epilepsy. Epilepsia 52:1733–1740

Paz JT, Deniau JM et al (2005) Rhythmic bursting in the cortico-subthalamo-pallidal network during spontaneous genetically determined spike and wave discharges. J Neurosci 25:2092–2101

Pereira FR, Alessio A et al (2010) Asymmetrical hippocampal connectivity in mesial temporal lobe epilepsy: evidence from resting state fMRI. BMC Neurosci 11:66

Pillay N, Archer JS et al (2013) Networks underlying paroxysmal fast activity and slow spike and wave in Lennox-Gastaut syndrome. Neurology 817:665–673

Pittau F, Levan P et al (2011) Changes preceding interictal epileptic EEG abnormalities: comparison between EEG/fMRI and intracerebral EEG. Epilepsia 52:1120–1129

Pittau F, Dubeau F et al (2012a) Contribution of EEG/fMRI to the definition of the epileptic focus. Neurology 78(19):1479–1487

Pittau F, Grova C et al (2012b) Patterns of altered functional connectivity in mesial temporal lobe epilepsy. Epilepsia 536:1013–1023

Pittau F, Fahoum F et al (2013) Negative BOLD response to interictal epileptic discharges in focal epilepsy. Brain Topogr 264:627–640

Polack PO, Guillemain I et al (2007) Deep layer somatosensory cortical neurons initiate spike-and-wave discharges in a genetic model of absence seizures. J Neurosci 27:6590–6599

Raichle ME, Mintun MA (2006) Brain work and brain imaging. Annu Rev Neurosci 29:449–476

Roger J, Bureau M et al (2005) Epileptic syndromes in infancy, childhood and adolescence. John Libbey Eurotext Ltd, Montrouge

Safi-Harb M, Proulx S et al (2015) Advantages and disadvantages of a fast fMRI sequence in the context of EEG-fMRI investigation of epilepsy patients: a realistic simulation study. Neuroimage 119:20–32

Salek-Haddadi A, Merschhemke M et al (2002) Simultaneous EEG-correlated ictal fMRI. Neuroimage 16:32–40

Seeck M, Lazeyras F et al (1998) Non-invasive epileptic focus localization using EEG-triggered functional MRI and electromagnetic tomography. Electroencephalogr Clin Neurophysiol 106:508–512

Siniatchkin M, van Baalen A et al (2007a) Different neuronal networks are associated with spikes and slow activity in hypsarrhythmia. Epilepsia 48:2312–2321

Siniatchkin M, Moeller F et al (2007b) Spatial filters and automated spike detection based on brain topographies improve sensitivity of EEG-fMRI studies in focal epilepsy. Neuroimage 37:834–843

Siniatchkin M, Groening K et al (2010) Neuronal networks in children with continuous spikes and waves during slow sleep. Brain 133:2798–2813

Siniatchkin M, Coropceanu D et al (2011) EEG-fMRI reveals activation of brainstem and thalamus in patients with Lennox-Gastaut syndrome. Epilepsia 52(4):766–774

Slaght SJ, Paz T et al (2004) On the activity of the corticostriatal networks during spike-and-wave discharges in a genetic model of absence epilepsy. J Neurosci 24:6816–6825

Srivastava G, Grottaz-Herbette S et al (2005) ICA-based procedures for removing ballistocardiogram artifacts from EEG data acquired in the MRI scanner. Neuroimage 24:50–60

Tangwiriyasakul C, Perani S et al (2018) Dynamic brain network states in human generalized spike-wave discharges. Brain 141:2981–2994

Tenney JR, Kadis DS et al (2018) Ictal connectivity in childhood absence epilepsy: associations with outcome. Epilepsia 59(5):971–981

Thornton R, Laufs H et al (2010) EEG correlated functional MRI and postoperative outcome in focal epilepsy. J Neurol Neurosurg Psychiatry 81: 922–927

Thornton R, Vulliemoz S et al (2011) Epileptic networks in focal cortical dysplasia revealed using electroencephalography-functional magnetic resonance imaging. Ann Neurol 2011(70):822–837

Tierney TM, Weiss-Croft LJ et al (2016) FIACH: a biophysical model for automatic retrospective noise control in fMRI. Neuroimage 124:1009–1020

Timofeev I, Steriade M (2004) Neocortical seizures: initiation, development and cessation. Neuroscience 123:299–336

Tyvaert L, Hawco C et al (2008) Different structures involved during ictal and interictal epileptic activity in malformations of cortical development: an EEG-fMRI study. Brain 131:2042–2060

Tyvaert L, Levan P et al (2009) Noninvasive dynamic imaging of seizures in epileptic patients. Hum Brain Mapp 30:3993–4011

Vaudano AE, Laufs H et al (2009) Causal hierarchy within the thalamo-cortical network in spike and wave discharges. PLoS One 4:e6475

Vaudano AE, Ruggieri A et al (2017) Photosensitive epilepsy is associated with reduced inhibition of alpha rhythm generating networks. Brain 140:981–997

Vulliemoz S, Thornton R et al (2009) The spatio-temporal mapping of epileptic networks: combination of EEG-fMRI and EEG source imaging. Neuroimage 46:834–843

Vulliemoz S, Carmichael DW et al (2011) Simultaneous intracranial EEG and fMRI of interictal epileptic discharges in humans. Neuroimage 54:182–190

Wang Z, Zhang Z et al (2012) Impairments of thalamic nuclei in idiopathic generalized epilepsy revealed by a study combining morphological and functional connectivity MRI. PLoS One 7(7):e39701

Warren AE, Abbott DF et al (2016) Abnormal cognitive network interactions in Lennox-Gastaut syndrome: a potential mechanism of epileptic encephalopathy. Epilepsia 57:812–822

Warren AEL, Abbott DF et al (2017) Thalamocortical functional connectivity in Lennox-Gastaut syndrome is abnormally enhanced in executive-control and default-mode networks. Epilepsia 58:2085–2097

Xiao F, An D et al (2016) Real-time effects of centrotemporal spikes on cognition in rolandic epilepsy: an EEGfMRI study. Neurology 86(6):544–51

Yang T, Luo C et al (2013) Altered resting-state connectivity during interictal generalized spike-wave discharges in drug-naïve childhood absence epilepsy. Hum Brain Mapp 34:1761–1767

Zhang Z, Lu G et al (2010) Altered spontaneous neuronal activity of the default-mode network in mesial temporal lobe epilepsy. Brain Res 1323:152–160

Zijlmans M, Huiskamp G et al (2007) EEG-fMRI in the preoperative work-up for epilepsy surgery. Brain 130:2343–2353

14 Imaging Epileptic Seizures Using fMRI

David N. Vaughan and Graeme D. Jackson

14.1 Introduction

In the study of epilepsy, functional MRI has become a major tool for both research and clinical practice over the last 25 years. Beginning in the 1990s, structural MRI revolutionized the diagnosis of focal epilepsy by enabling the identification of small anatomical lesions. The subsequent development of functional MRI methods has continued this advance through the ability to identify localized abnormalities even where macroscopic anatomy appears normal and through the delineation of overlapping cognitive functions. Arguably, the greatest conceptual impact of fMRI in epilepsy has been through the modeling and demonstrated involvement of large-scale brain networks during seizures as this perspective contributed to the 2010 redefinition of seizures by the International League Against Epilepsy (ILAE) as "occurring in and rapidly engaging … either discretely localized or more widely distributed networks" (Berg et al. 2010).

With acknowledgement to Simon M. Glynn and John A. Detre for their work on the first edition of this chapter, which provided a framework for this revised material.

D. N. Vaughan (✉) · G. D. Jackson
Florey Institute of Neuroscience and Mental Health, University of Melbourne, Parkville, VIC, Australia

Department of Neurology, Austin Health, Heidelberg, VIC, Australia
e-mail: david.vaughan@florey.edu.au; graeme.jackson@florey.edu.au

The current spectrum of applications of fMRI in epilepsy is rapidly increasing. The main validated clinical use has been the interictal localization of eloquent cortex prior to epilepsy surgery using language and motor-task paradigms. In more specialized centers, fMRI with simultaneous acquisition of electroencephalography (EEG) is being used clinically to identify the location of interictal epileptic discharges. For more details about interictal EEG-fMRI we refer to reviews by Flanagan et al. (2014), Gotman and Pittau (2011), and Murta et al. (2015). The research applications of fMRI in epilepsy are even more broad, ranging from analyses of network connectivity in specified epilepsy subtypes and identifying the alteration of specific cognitive processes to the modulation of epileptic networks by medications within "pharmaco-fMRI."

Seizures are the defining characteristic of epilepsy and recognizing specific network involvement and the temporal evolution of each paroxysmal event is central to our understanding of this disease. While obtaining fMRI recordings of seizures is both clinically and technically challenging and is unlikely to ever become part of standard clinical care, more than 50 papers reporting individuals or case series including this data have now been published. In this chapter, we take the opportunity to focus in detail on the insights that have been gained through the recording of seizures directly. We review how this has informed the development of fMRI methodology and our growing understanding of epileptic

S. Ulmer, O. Jansen (eds.), *fMRI*, https://doi.org/10.1007/978-3-030-41874-8_14

syndromes and the underlying pathophysiology of the epileptic discharge.

14.2 Imaging Epileptic Seizures

Functional imaging of seizures is challenging because they mostly occur spontaneously, at irregular times, and in most patients are relatively infrequent. This means that most fMRI of seizures is captured fortuitously, during recordings intended to capture baseline or interictal discharges. The exceptions are people who have seizures triggered by specific stimuli (induced seizures and reflex epilepsies) or people who have such frequent seizures that fMRI can be arranged with a high expectation of a seizure occurring.

The second challenge is clinical safety of patients during the seizure. Stereotyped events that are brief, have little motor manifestation, and have preserved autonomic functions (for example, absence seizures) can be easily managed in the scanner environment. On the other hand, focal or generalized seizures that involve tonic-clonic movements pose a real risk of injury, and it is clearly necessary to remove the patient from the scanner to provide appropriate care.

For all seizure types, the technical handling of subject head motion is critical. For some seizures, the degree of head motion precludes any meaningful analysis once the clinical expression has begun. Even far less extreme movements, such as the automatisms of focal or absence seizures, can confound the analysis as they are highly correlated with the seizure's timing. Ideally, acquisition sequences would be used that are relatively resistant to the effects of head motion, but this is not a common practice so far.

14.3 Functional MRI of Focal Seizures

Focal seizures are defined as originating within networks limited to one hemisphere. The epileptic discharge may be exquisitely localized or be more widely distributed and may originate in cortical or subcortical structures (Fisher et al. 2017).

The earliest fMRI of human seizures was achieved in the mid-1990s. Obvious and high-amplitude blood-oxygen-level-dependent (BOLD) changes were detected, even though the investigators did not use concurrent EEG or sophisticated statistical analysis. In the first case, a child with frequent focal motor seizures was imaged on a 1.5 T clinical MRI system, and ictal changes were identified simply by subtraction of the signal from baseline. Marked BOLD increases were seen over and surrounding the affected motor cortex during each seizure, up to 40% above baseline at some regions (Fig. 14.1; Jackson et al. 1994). In a similar case, subclinical seizures without obvious signs were detected by a BOLD signal increase of 3–4% above baseline at the motor cortex (Detre et al. 1995).

The development of EEG-correlated fMRI in the early 2000s enabled a much broader range of seizures to be identified as this no longer relies on visible signs to identify the timing. The first demonstration of this technique was in an electrographic temporal lobe seizure (Salek-Haddadi et al. 2002).

To date, focal seizures during fMRI have been reported by more than 25 papers (see Chaudhary et al. (2013) for a detailed review of earlier cases). A few centers have published their overall experience of seizures captured during planned interictal EEG-fMRI, with the rate of seizures recorded being surprisingly high at 11% (nine of 83 patients in presurgical workup) (Thornton et al. 2010) and 18% respectively (17 of 93 patients) (Tyvaert et al. 2009). Recently, the recording of seizures with intracranial EEG and concurrent fMRI has been a major advance (Chaudhary et al. 2016), which has enabled further insights into the pathophysiology of focal seizures.

14.3.1 Hemodynamic and Metabolic Responses During Focal Seizures

The BOLD response is mediated through both metabolic (oxygen utilization) and hemodynamic (changes in perfusion) mechanisms, so it is important to understand how these both

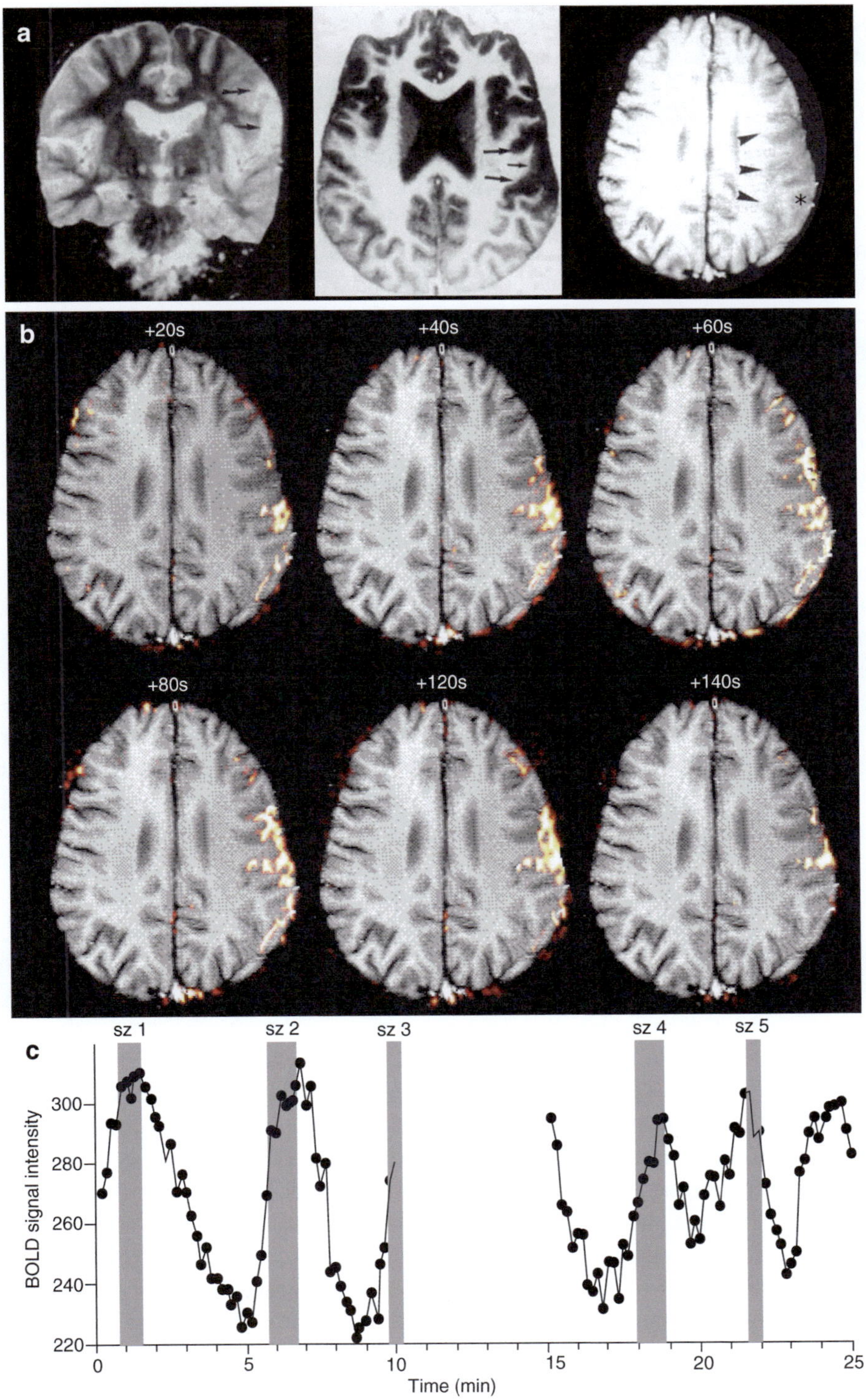

Fig. 14.1 Focal motor seizures in a four-year-old boy with Rasmussen's encephalitis. (**a**) T2, inversion-recovery, and T1-weighted images showing abnormally thickened cortex over the left hemisphere (arrows). (**b**) Spatial progression of BOLD changes during seizure #4. Clonic face movement began prior to +80s and continued until after +120 s. (**c**) Time course at left parietal cortex (at asterisk in panel A right) showing BOLD increase with each seizure and in a further subclinical event. (Adapted from Jackson et al. (1994) with permission)

progress during seizures. Regional increases in perfusion are one of the most striking changes during a seizure and can even be seen visually if the brain is exposed, as recounted by Penfield in the 1930s for seizures occurring during epilepsy surgery (Penfield 1933). This "functional hyperemia" occurs in response to the supra-physiological metabolic demand of the seizure and can be quantified as increased cerebral blood flow (CBF) and cerebral blood volume (CBV). These parameters, together with the cerebral metabolic rate of oxygen utilization ($CMRO_2$), then determine the ictal BOLD signal.

An ongoing debate is whether the intense utilization of oxygen during a focal seizure may outstrip the available perfusion, with the decoupling of this usually linear relationship. In this situation, neuronal activity would not be reflected by a proportionate BOLD increase. Findings have been contradictory, with earlier studies (which compared percentage increases in CBF and CMRO2) suggesting that perfusion is adequate (Franck et al. 1986), while others have argued that a drop in oxygenation can be observed in seizures if the rise in CBF was not sufficient (Kreisman et al. 1991). More recent multimodal approaches have used optical imaging with electrical recordings in animal models (for example, using 4-aminopyridine microinjection to induce focal seizures). These seizures show an increase in both local field power and CBV, but with a nonlinear relationship that has a ceiling effect for CBV during intense activity at the epileptic focus (Harris et al. 2014). As the seizure evolves and the region of functional hyperemia expands, this progression can become transiently uncoupled from the region of membrane depolarization (Ma et al. 2013). Another animal model (with induced cortical malformations) that may better represent the situation in chronic epilepsy shows an even stronger functional hyperemic response (Song et al. 2016).

At seizure onset, an *epileptic dip* in hemoglobin oxygenation may be seen in these animal models, caused by the initial increase in metabolic demand before adequate perfusion responds (Zhao et al. 2009) (see also Shariff et al. (2006) for a detailed review). Unlike the hemodynamic response to a physiological stimulus where there is a brief *initial dip*, during focal seizures, this early drop in hemoglobin oxygenation may last up to several seconds. Surprisingly, the magnitude of this dip is correlated with subsequent seizure duration, which may reflect more intense initial neural activity at the onset of longer seizures (Zhang et al. 2015). Similar patterns were recorded in humans using gold electrodes in the 1970s, where mild temporal lobe seizures showed a CBF increase but little change in pO2, whereas intense seizures showed a precipitous drop in tissue oxygen pressure at the onset (Dymond and Crandall 1976). More recent optical recording methods applied in human cases have also shown this initial drop in hemoglobin saturation despite increases in CBV (Zhao et al. 2007).

Specifics of the neurovascular response also depend on the cortical layer at which the seizure begins. Seizures chemically induced in deep layers show greater tissue hypoxia than seizures induced from middle cortical lamina (Harris et al. 2018). This fits with the known variation of physiological neurovascular coupling across the cortical layers that has been detected using high-resolution fMRI (Goense et al. 2012).

14.3.2 Statistical Modeling of the BOLD Signal in Focal Seizures

Functional MRI analysis of focal seizures is complicated by the variability between events in duration, multiphasic evolution, and clinical expression. The earliest papers used visual observation or patient reporting (by button press) to detect seizures, with analysis by visual inspection and percentage BOLD change from baseline. Concurrent acquisition of EEG enables more reliable detection of seizures, particularly when they have little or no obvious clinical expression, but also poses several technical challenges. Reviews of preprocessing methods for EEG-fMRI data have been published by Chaudhary et al. (2013) and Abreu et al. (2018).

Univariate parametric mapping of the seizure using a general linear model (GLM) (Salek-

Haddadi et al. 2002) adds statistical rigor to the analysis and allows physiological variables to be included as regressors of no interest. The question then becomes how the time course of the seizure event should be modeled. The simplest approach is to designate the whole period of the seizure using a boxcar function, which is then convolved with the conventional hemodynamic response function. However, this relies on the assumption of preserved neurovascular coupling for seizures (see below), constrains detection to one common time course, and neglects the multiple phases that some focal seizures express.

An advance on this simple GLM approach is to designate several phases to the seizure and model each phase using separate regressors. For example, Chaudhary et al. defined four phases: "pre-ictal" (30 s before the first clinical or EEG change), "ictal onset" (building EEG seizure rhythms before clinical expression), "ictal established" (once clinical signs occur), and "late ictal" phases (corresponding to EEG slowing) (Chaudhary et al. 2012).

To gain even more flexibility for modeling the evolving BOLD time course, an expanded basis set of regressors can be used, such as a Fourier set (Chaudhary et al. 2012), sequential boxcar functions (e.g., each 10 s long) (Donaire et al. 2009a), or a sequential set of 2-sec-wide gamma functions (Tyvaert et al. 2009). The advantage of the latter two approaches is that activation emerging in sequential epochs (as voxels with significant beta weights for a given regressor) can be interpreted as the areas showing seizure-related activation at that time.

Data-driven analysis approaches, such as spatial independent component analysis (ICA), avoid placing any constraints on the shape of the seizure-related hemodynamic response. The challenge then is to identify which of the decomposed maps/time courses are relevant to the seizure, rather than representing artifact or noise. LeVan et al. tackled this by selecting components with time courses that showed a significant change at seizure onset, through deconvolution with a flexible basis set (LeVan et al. 2010).

Comparison of these methods (GLM with seizure phases, GLM with Fourier basis set, and ICA) shows that GLM-based approaches are most effective when seizure onset can be reliably detected on scalp EEG. However, ICA can contribute additonal information when reliable timings from EEG are not available (Thornton et al. 2010).

The analysis of intracranial EEG poses new challenges because of the difficulty of accurate manual identification of frequent interictal discharges (which are not seen at the scalp) and the complex seizure patterns that can be recorded. Automated EEG metrics (such as band power) or data-driven approaches (such as principal components analysis) may therefore lead to better results than visual demarcation of the EEG (Chaudhary et al. 2016).

14.3.3 Pathology Affects the Nature of the BOLD Response in Focal Seizures

In cases of focal epilepsy due to a known cortical structural lesion, fMRI recordings of the seizure generally confirm that ictal activity occurs within and/or adjacent to the lesion (Chaudhary et al. 2012). Other regions also show activation in most cases, presumably corresponding to areas of propagation or an extended seizure network. Examples of lesion-related BOLD activation include a case of a small focal cortical dysplasia causing epileptic foot jerking (Archer et al. 2006), a case of hypothalamic hamartoma that was driving gelastic seizures (Kokkinos et al. 2012), a case of posttraumatic encephalomalacia causing posttraumatic epilepsy (Storti et al. 2015), and activation at the abnormal heterotopic gray matter in cases of double cortex (Tyvaert et al. 2008). Several cases of fMRI in focal epilepsy due to brain tumors have also been reported, with BOLD activation being seen adjacent to the tumor (Krings et al. 2000; Kubota et al. 2000; Sonmezturk et al. 2011).

However, other pathologies may not lead to such consistent BOLD patterns. In cases of periventricular nodular heterotopia (PVNH), seizures show some involvement of the lesion, but the maximal statistical BOLD activation is often found in the overlying cortex and not the heterotopic nodule itself. A similar pattern is seen with the interictal discharges of PVNH, where activation at the lesion itself is inconsistent and seen in only around half of cases (Kobayashi et al. 2006; Tyvaert et al. 2008). This suggests that seizures in this pathology predominantly involve a regional network engaging the overlying cortex.

Still other lesions may show little activation during epileptic discharges at all. This occurs in cases of "secondary network epilepsy," where the effect of the structural abnormality is to destabilize large-scale intrinsic networks, which may then autonomously express seizures independently of the lesion (Archer et al. 2014b). Lennox–Gastaut syndrome, due to a focal structural malformation, is the archetype for this idea (discussed further under tonic seizures below).

14.3.4 Comparing BOLD Patterns in Focal Seizures to Interictal Discharges

Surprisingly, few studies have compared the BOLD response of an interictal discharge to the BOLD response of a corresponding focal seizure. Overall, fMRI data indicate that activation patterns are spatially similar, although some authors have claimed that ictal and interictal discharges are generated by different mechanisms and neuronal populations (Murta et al. 2015).

For example, Epilepsy due to malformations of cortical development interictal discharges do involve the same regions as the seizures by visual comparison (Tyvaert et al. 2008). The statistical significance score is generally greater for the ictal events, probably reflecting higher signal-to-noise ratio as a consequence of greater percentage BOLD signal increase during seizures. Similarly, in the case of nonlesional frontal lobe epilepsy, fMRI activity during the seizure was congruent with interictal discharges, but the seizure also showed additional distant regions of both increased and decreased BOLD (Meletti et al. 2015), probably reflecting network activation or propagation.

Comparison of seizure-related hyperperfusion (recorded by ictal single-photon emission computed tomography (SPECT)) to BOLD activation with interictal discharges also shows a significant overlap in the majority of cases (Tousseyn et al. 2015). This is observed not only at the epileptogenic zone but also at distant sites not involved in seizure onset, such as the basal ganglia or cerebellum, supporting the idea that seizures and interictal discharges engage common networks and that epileptic activity is often not confined to a single "focus."

14.3.5 Identifying the Region of Focal Seizure Onset with fMRI

Identifying the primary region of seizure onset is often the critical clinical question when epilepsy surgery is being considered. If multiple regions are highlighted by fMRI, it is important to distinguish seizure initiation from areas of later propagation. This technical problem has been approached in several ways:

1. When multiple regions of positive BOLD are detected during the seizure, the cluster that is most likely to correspond to seizure onset can often be identified by its concordance with other clinical data. This approach is practical but diminishes the utility of fMRI as an independent predictor.
2. When using a linear model, some authors have argued that the cluster with the highest peak *t* score is likely to reflect the generator of the epileptic event (Tyvaert et al. 2008). Although appealing, this common assertion does not appear to have been rigorously tested.
3. Simply searching for the first voxels that show a relatively large BOLD increase from baseline may be sufficient in some cases. Using a threshold of 3% increase in the case of occipital lobe epilepsy, this method identified the earliest BOLD change adjacent to the known tumor (Sonmezturk et al. 2011)
4. When the dynamic time course of seizures is modeled by a GLM with multiple sequential

gamma function regressors, the region of onset can be identified from the earliest significant regressor. This approach identified a single cluster in 70% of cases, and the cluster typically had a volume greater than 2 cm^3 (Tyvaert et al. 2009). A subset of these patients later had intracranial EEG recordings, and electrographic seizure onset was confirmed at the first region of fMRI activation in two out of three cases (in the third case, intracranial EEG was not informative). A similar idea was applied in the case of seizures consisting of a throat sensation and mouth clonus, by sequentially estimating cross-correlation of the BOLD signal to a prespecified reference curve, shifted across time. This approach plausibly detected activation of the insular cortex more than 1 min before the onset of mouth clonus, congruent with the clinical impression (Auer et al. 2008).

5. Similarly, the time period covering the seizure can be modeled with sequential 10-s-long regressors and seizure onset identified by the earliest significant contrast between two consecutive blocks (Donaire et al. 2009a; Donaire et al. 2009b). One advantage of this approach is that it does not require concurrent EEG. Using this approach, the region identified was congruent with intracranial EEG localization of seizure onset (in the two patients who had this performed) and was also congruent with ictal SPECT data (in four of five cases).
6. When seizures are divided into phases (such as EEG onset, clinical, and late blocks) and each modeled within the GLM, activation detected in the first rather than later phases is more indicative of seizure onset. With this approach, Thornton et al. found a single localized cluster at the first phase in 22% of cases (two of nine) and multiple regions or extensive activation in 33% (Thornton et al. 2010). Activation was judged to be concordant with seizure onset on intracranial EEG in 57% of cases when a BOLD response was detected (four of seven cases). Discordant cases in this series were best explained by obscuration of the EEG signal due to large head motions. In another case series using the seizure-phase approach, ictal-onset phase BOLD changes were found to be concordant (or had partial concordance) with the seizure onset in 85% of cases (17 of 20). Concordance was significantly higher for the ictal-onset phase than for later seizure phases (Chaudhary et al. 2012). In patients who went on to have invasive EEG ($n = 6$), the cluster with the maximum t score was always found close to the electrode of seizure onset (less than 3.5 cm away).
7. A more data-driven approach is to apply ICA and then identify early components that best correspond to the timing of seizure onset. However, these maps have demonstrated widespread activation, on average involving more than 20% of brain volume. The presumed seizure onset zone (on clinical grounds) was included in these extensive regions in 13 of 15 patients (LeVan et al. 2010). While the relative timing of different components may indicate regions of propagation, directly interpreting the data in this way neglects the confounding effect of spatial variability in neurovascular responses. Nevertheless, this type of analysis may be particularly useful when scalp EEG is noninformative as regional hemodynamic time courses can still be extracted for manual interpretation.

Beyond these modeling approaches, using scalp EEG to define seizure onset has an important limitation. When electrical epileptic activity begins deep in the brain, an ictal rhythm may not be seen on the scalp until many seconds later. This problem can be overcome by the specialized technique of plancing an intracranial EEG electrode into the seizure onset zone, allowing the timing of seizure onset to be precisely determined. This of course requires that the seizure onset zone is already suspected or known before electrode insertion.

The first example of fMRI acquired with concurrent intracranial EEG was in a patient with mesial temporal lobe epilepsy (Chaudhary et al. 2016). Seizure onset was recognized by 6.4 s of beta activity at the right amygdala, before bilateral gamma rhythms developed. The fMRI correlate of this interval was a BOLD increase at the right fusiform gyrus, temporal pole, middle temporal gyrus, and cingulate. This pattern was judged as "concordant plus" to the electrographically defined seizure onset zone in the amygdala/hippocampus, demonstrating that epileptic activity may often be more spatially extensive on fMRI than can be recognized with the limited spatial sampling of intracranial EEG.

14.3.6 Propagation of Focal Seizures on fMRI

The propagation of epileptic seizures teaches us about the connectivity of intrinsic brain networks and provides an explanation for the evolving clinical features that occur as a seizure progresses. This typically occurs on a timescale of seconds, so fMRI is well suited to reveal seizure spread.

Two main types of fMRI seizure propagation have been highlighted (Tyvaert et al. 2009). The first is local extension of the primary activation within the same hemisphere. The second pattern is involvement of regions within the contralateral hemisphere, as the epileptic activity becomes bilateral. Other common regions of spread also included the thalamus (typically later in the seizure, more than 10 s after onset) and the anterior or posterior cingulate cortex (although default mode network involvement most often shows negative BOLD). In approximately half of patients (nine of 20 cases in one series), ictal propagation regions can be linked to symptomatic expression of the seizure, such as motor cortex involvement (with clonus), supplementary motor area (with "figure-of-4" posturing), middle frontal gyrus (eye deviation), or temporal lobe activity (oromanual automatisms) (Chaudhary et al. 2012).

From the classical epilepsy literature, there are several archetypal propagation patterns that are characteristic of particular brain regions or seizure types. A few of these have been shown on fMRI so far.

Demonstration of the "Jacksonian march" of focal motor seizures comes from a case of epilepsy due to a central cortex tumor. The first BOLD activation (signal more than 1.5% above baseline) was adjacent to the tumor. Nearly 1 min later, jerking of the foot began and fMRI activation was seen nearby, at the precentral gyrus foot motor area (Krings et al. 2000).

Occipital lobe seizures can have a characteristic pattern of posterior-to-bitemporal spread (Williamson et al. 1992). This is demonstrated by one fMRI case, where seizure activity is first seen in the occipital lobe and slowly spreads to the contralateral temporo-occipital region and then to the temporal lobes bilaterally, over the course of 2 min (Sonmezturk et al. 2011).

Propagation of one temporal lobe seizure has been demonstrated with concurrent intracranial EEG (Chaudhary et al. 2016). After early temporal lobe activity, later seizure phases showed involvement of default mode network regions and of the occipital lobe. An alternative analysis approach using EEG band-power regressors detected fMRI activation at the bilateral frontal lobes, which are also a common region of spread for temporal lobe seizures.

A surprising fMRI propagation pattern was seen in a seizure with insular onset. There was a long delay of more than 30 sec from the initial inferior insular involvement to the eventual seizure spread into the superior part of the insula (Auer et al. 2008). This suggests that either a functional blockage prevented local progression or that the seizure activity "jumped" to the superior insula via another region.

Effective connectivity analysis can give further insight into seizure propagation patterns, particularly when a lagged-regressor approach cannot differentiate the time of onset at each region. Dynamic causal modeling was used in a patient with a hypothalamic hamartoma to examine the influence of the hamartoma on distant regions of seizure activation (left frontal and left parietal in this case). The best fitting model had reciprocal connections from the hamartoma to the parietal region, which in turn connected to the frontal lobe region. Modulation of feed-forward connectivity was increased during the seizure, with a decrease of latent feedback (Murta et al. 2012).

Granger causality is another data-driven measure of directed influence between brain regions that has also been applied to seizure propagation. In four focal epilepsy cases with seizures arising from various lobes, the driving region was plausibly determined from the directed connectivity matrix (Tana et al. 2012). For example, a case of occipital lobe epilepsy showed propagation from the left to right occipital lobe and then into the temporal lobe. Another case arising from the parietal lobe showed that the postcentral gyrus was driving activity at the ipsilateral occipital lobe. However, the best approach for determining the nodes in this kind of analysis is unclear, and further technical development is needed before such findings can be considered robust.

14.3.7 Interpreting Decreased BOLD Signal in Focal Seizures

While some cases show only increased BOLD during focal seizures, there are many examples of decreased BOLD signal at variable locations remote from the seizure focus. This phenomenon is sometimes called "deactivation" or a "negative BOLD response." A relatively larger BOLD increase often precedes deactivation, for example one case series found activation at mean time +4.5 s versus later deactivation at +7 s (Tyvaert et al. 2009). Unlike for interictal discharges, there are no clear reports of purely decreased BOLD at the seizure focus.

Deactivation is sometimes seen immediately adjacent to the main area of activation, and "vascular steal" has been proposed as a possible explanation (Kobayashi et al. 2006). The idea is that vascular dilatation and increased perfusion at the focus cause diversion of perfusion from nearby tissue. Some evidence of this effect has been shown in animal models of focal epilepsy (seizures induced by localized microinjection of 4-aminopyridine), where optical imaging during acute seizures shows a large increase in blood flow (CBF) at the focus and a decrease at the surrounding neocortex by as much as 20% (Zhao et al. 2009). However, there is also a decrease in the metabolic rate of oxygen ($CMRO_2$) in the surround, so it remains possible that some of this effect is due to decreased neuronal activity as well.

Otherwise, negative BOLD can represent inhibition of cortical function distant from the seizure focus. This has been demonstrated by a case of frontal lobe epilepsy with seizures characterized by motor arrest and retained awareness. During the event, there was a BOLD decrease at the sensorimotor cortex bilaterally, along with the expected increase at the frontal lobe (Meletti et al. 2015). Another demonstration of seizure-related deactivation of motor cortex comes from a remarkable patient who had both focal (facial myoclonus) and generalized (absence) epileptic events (Chassagnon et al. 2009). The focal seizures showed much more localized deactivation at contralateral motor cortex only, compared to the absence seizures, where a typical widespread corticothalamic pattern of deactivation was seen. Here, the motor deactivation can be viewed as a physiological response related to inhibition of movement as the same effect can be seen between voluntary finger tapping in healthy controls.

Interictal deactivation is often associated with the EEG slow wave that follows an epileptic discharge, and which has been associated with prolonged hyperpolarization and functional inhibition (Pittau et al. 2013). It has been suggested that some seemingly negative-only interictal BOLD responses are due to the (low-amplitude) initial positive response being missed (Rathakrishnan et al. 2010), although this argument seems less applicable to seizures, where the events are longer and of more intense amplitude.

Ictal deactivation of regions corresponding to the default mode network (DMN) have been reported in focal events arising from the frontal lobe (Thornton et al. 2010), insula (Fahoum et al. 2013), and parietal lobe (Chaudhary et al. 2012). Compared to generalized absence seizures, the pattern of DMN deactivation in focal seizures is often less extensive and predominantly ipsilateral rather than engaging the whole network. As physiological DMN activity is associated with introspective thinking, it has been suggested that its involvement in seizures may be related to the impairment of awareness (Carney et al. 2010). In focal epilepsy, this is partly supported by an association between impaired awareness seizures and interictal discharges that show negative DMN

BOLD (Fahoum et al. 2012; Laufs et al. 2007). Furthermore, fMRI decreases at the DMN during focal seizures are more often (but not exclusively) observed during seizures where there is loss of consciousness (LOC) (in 64% with LOC versus 33% of cases without LOC) (Chaudhary et al. 2012). The electrographic correlate of decreased BOLD at the DMN is beta-frequency activity <30 Hz, with the suggestion that this may represent suspension of the normal function (Fahoum et al. 2013). However, the mechanism relating the seizure focus to DMN inhibition remains an open question. The "network inhibition hypothesis" of impaired consciousness during seizures proposes that the epileptic discharge is associated with inhibition of subcortical arousal systems, which normally maintain activities in cortical regions (including the DMN) that are important for consciousness (Blumenfeld 2012).

In the postictal phase, decreased BOLD at the seizure focus is the general rule, although the duration of this undershoot may be more sustained, which would be predicted by the usual canonical hemodynamic response function (Salek-Haddadi et al. 2002). This is related to hypoperfusion and can be exploited to identify the seizure onset zone using postictal arterial spin labeling MRI. This technique can be an effective approach, identifying a region concordant with the presumed seizure onset in 57% of patients studied (Gaxiola-Valdez et al. 2017).

14.3.8 The Preictal State in Focal Epilepsy

The preictal period represents a transition phase from near-normal baseline brain function to the acute pathological network dysfunction of a seizure. Examining the dynamic time course of BOLD changes over this period has yielded surprising results, given the conventional view that seizures begin abruptly at the onset of EEG and clinical signs.

The preictal period shows a relatively slow increase in BOLD at the seizure focus, which builds over several minutes or more, before the earliest clinical or EEG indication of the seizure onset (Fig. 14.2) (Auer et al. 2008; Donaire et al. 2009a; Federico et al. 2005). Although this pattern is not universally observed, for example, it was not seen in the seizure detected by intracranial EEG recording (Chaudhary et al. 2016), other case series have found preictal changes in

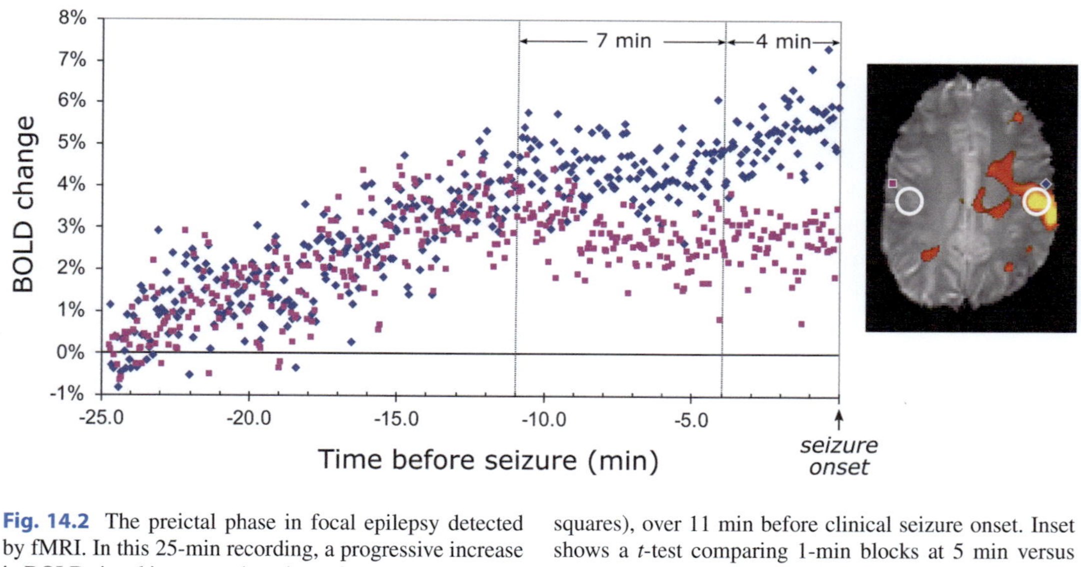

Fig. 14.2 The preictal phase in focal epilepsy detected by fMRI. In this 25-min recording, a progressive increase in BOLD signal is seen at the seizure focus in the left frontal lobe and postcentral gyrus (blue diamonds) compared to that at the homologous contralateral region (pink squares), over 11 min before clinical seizure onset. Inset shows a *t*-test comparing 1-min blocks at 5 min versus immediately prior to seizure activity. (Reproduced with permission from Federico et al. (2005))

nearly all focal seizures using a reduced statistical threshold (Chaudhary et al. 2012). Preictal BOLD increases are mostly congruent with the location of subsequent seizure activity but can also be seen at remote locations such as the frontal lobes (Federico et al. 2005). On some occasions, preictal fMRI activation can occur along with a buildup of irregular interictal epileptiform EEG discharges that precede the seizure (Storti et al. 2015). There is further support for these findings from optical imaging, where recordings of spontaneous seizures also demonstrate preictal changes in cerebral blood flow and oxygenation (Slone et al. 2012; Zhao et al. 2007).

Slowly increasing preictal fMRI signal may also be seen at homologous contralateral cortex to the focus. An interesting but speculative idea is that this represents an attempt to suppress pathological preseizure activity that is building up at the focus (Federico et al. 2005; Vinette et al. 2016). There is a physiological analog for such a phenomenon, specifically the interhemispheric inhibition that occurs between the left and right motor cortex in healthy brains during planned movements.

An alternative explanation is that increasing BOLD at the contralateral hemisphere represents excitatory pro-seizure activity, as part of a kindled mirror focus. This would fit with the additional observation that functional connectivity between the seizure focus and contralateral regions increases in the preictal period (Vinette et al. 2016).

14.3.9 Focal Reflex Seizures

In reflex epilepsies, seizures are provoked by stimuli that are specific for each patient. Triggers may include simple sensory or motor stimuli, such as a flash of light or a movement, or may be more elaborate cognitive tasks, such as listening to music, reading, or playing chess. Although quite uncommon, these cases are ideally suited to imaging with fMRI as clinical events can be induced during scanning. The following examples show how fMRI in reflex seizures has led to a new understanding of the seizure onset and mechanism.

Reading epilepsy is characterized by myoclonus of the mouth or jaw that is precipitated by reading, especially aloud, and may progress to a generalized tonic-clonic seizure (GTCS) if the patient continues. EEG during reading shows irregular sharp waves with a wide field, at times maximal at the left temporoparietal region. The fMRI correlate of these spikes is a positive BOLD signal at the left precentral gyrus, at the orbitofrontal region, and bilaterally in the central sulcus and basal ganglia (Archer et al. 2003; Salek-Haddadi et al. 2009). A block reading task in these patients shows a normal pattern of fMRI task activation in visual and language areas, which overlaps with the spike-related activity at the left middle frontal gyrus. The inference from this overlap is that seizure activity begins in the working memory areas of the left dorsolateral prefrontal cortex, with spread into the adjacent precentral gyrus to produce the typical symptoms (Archer et al. 2003). Alternatively, examination of the fMRI time course has been interpreted as showing the left premotor cortex as the primary source of epileptic activity, with effective connectivity analysis suggesting that the left piriform cortex may have a role in seizure initiation (Vaudano et al. 2012).

Writing-induced seizures occur with dystonia and myoclonic jerks of the writing hand. Most of these exceedingly rare cases have been associated with generalized epilepsy, in particular juvenile myoclonic epilepsy (Chifari et al. 2004), although one case that is due to focal cortical dysplasia at the right inferior parietal lobule has been reported (Racicot et al. 2016). Functional MRI during a right-handed writing task shows intense activation of the left frontal supplementary motor area (Abreu et al. 2005). The interpretation is that these seizures have a focal trigger zone in the language-dominant hemisphere that engages an apparently generalized epileptic network. Additional cases are needed to confirm this hypothesis.

Musicogenic epilepsy is another rare condition where seizures can be provoked by particular music. The triggering song is specific to each individual, and the experience often has an affective or emotional component. Seizures are focal, most often involving the right or left temporal lobe (Pittau et al. 2008). Several cases have now been studied with fMRI using block designs of listening to epileptogenic music versus neutral nonepileptogenic music. Prior to seizure onset, the trigger music generally induces more extensive BOLD increases than the neutral music, mostly in regions of the temporal and frontal lobes relevant to auditory and emotional processing, but with considerable individual variability (Diekmann and Hoppner 2014; Mórocz et al. 2003; Pittau et al. 2008). At the onset of the seizure, additional regions of fMRI activation are seen, particularly at the left or right anteromesial temporal lobe and at the orbitofrontal or frontopolar regions (Klamer et al. 2015; Marrosu et al. 2009; Mórocz et al. 2003). The main point of discussion is around which of these possible sites initiates the epileptic discharge. In one case, effective connectivity showed that temporal lobe activity drives the frontal lobe changes (Klamer et al. 2015). Hippocampal seizure onset was later confirmed on intracranial EEG recordings, and the patient had a good outcome after targeted temporal lobe resection, demonstrating the value of fMRI seizure localization for tailoring individual management. At a syndrome level, however, the fMRI findings are somewhat divergent, which adds support to other studies that have concluded that musicogenic epilepsy is a heterogenous condition that can arise from multiple different foci within the temporal lobe (Tayah et al. 2006).

14.4 Functional MRI of Generalized Seizures

14.4.1 Absence Seizures

Absences seizures (previously called *petit mal*) are the seizure type that has been most extensively studied with functional MRI because they are relatively common, occur frequently in affected patients, and are of short duration with minimal accompanying movement. Along with myoclonus and generalized tonic-clonic seizures, they are the main seizure type found in genetic (idiopathic) generalized epilepsies. They are recognized by a sudden halting of activity, blank stare, and unresponsiveness, lasting between a few and 30 sec. They occur spontaneously, sometimes many times per day in untreated patients, and can also be provoked by hyperventilation. The classical EEG correlate is 3–4-Hz generalized spike-wave (GSW) discharges, which are symmetrical, have high amplitude, and begin and end abruptly. These discharges last for the duration of the clinical event, but when the discharges are brief (lasting <3 s), there may be little or no obvious clinical expression (van Luijtelaar et al. 1991).

The underlying mechanisms of GSW are an ongoing topic of investigation and debate. The *corticoreticular hypothesis* (Gloor 1968) proposes that the basis of generalized spike-wave is the abnormal interaction between the cortex and projections of the thalamus and reticular system. This view attempts to reconcile earlier views that the cause was primarily based either within subcortical structures (centrencephalic epilepsy) or within the cortex.

Multiple human EEG–fMRI studies have demonstrated a characteristic BOLD pattern associated with GSW. There is an increase at the thalamus bilaterally, along with widespread symmetrical cortical decreases, especially at the frontal cortex, parietal cortex, and posterior cingulate (Bai et al. 2010; Hamandi et al. 2006). Additional deactivation has also been noted at the caudate and reticular nuclei (Fig. 14.3) (Carney et al. 2010). Some studies have also found variable positive BOLD activation in cortical regions, including at the mesial frontal cortex, bilateral insula, and cerebellum (Berman et al. 2010; Gotman et al. 2005). The magnitude of BOLD signal change is of the order of 3% increase at the thalamus versus 8% decrease at the cortex (Salek-Haddadi et al. 2003). Thalamic BOLD activation is a consistent finding across studies and has also been observed in animal models (Tenney et al. 2004), supporting the engagement of a thalamocortical network during absence seizures.

Network-based analysis of fMRI activity during absence seizures leads to a similar interpretation. Independent component analysis

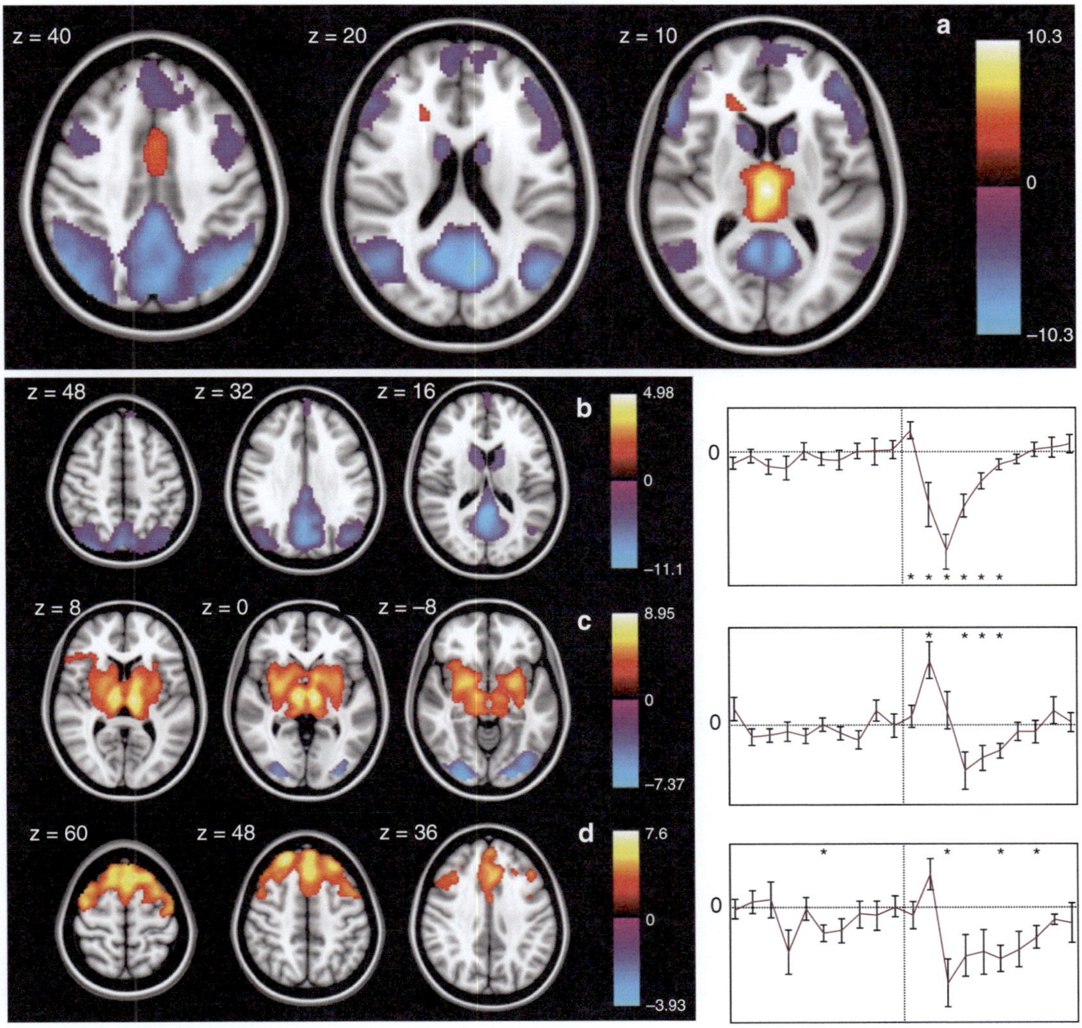

Fig. 14.3 Absence seizures. Functional MRI group analysis in childhood absence epilepsy (n = 8) with generalized spike-wave discharges. (**a**) Canonical hemodynamic response function model showing significant thalamic and anterior cingulate activation and widespread deactivation. (**b–d**) Selected components from an event-related independent component analysis (eICA) showing (**b**) default mode network deactivation, (**c**) thalamic and striatum activation, and (**d**) biphasic bifrontal changes with activation followed by rapid deactivation. Additional eICA components (not shown) demonstrate additional late salience and sensorimotor network changes. (Adapted from Masterton et al. (2013) with permission)

shows first an increase in thalamic intranetwork connectivity and then sequentially decreased intranetwork connectivity within the default mode, central executive, and dorsal attention networks. The extent of these changes has been correlated with the duration of GSW (Zhang et al. 2014b). Another analysis showed sequential involvement of default mode, task-positive, and then thalamic-sensorimotor networks (Guo et al. 2016). During seizures, strong anticorrelation between thalamocortical and default mode networks is seen, but in the postictal period, this anticorrelation decreases and dynamic network topology remains transiently perturbed (Liao et al. 2014).

Earlier observations had indicated that the general pattern of the BOLD response was independent of the duration of the GSW burst

(Aghakhani et al. 2004). However, in recent multicenter cohorts, increasing the duration of GSW has been shown to correspond to a linear increase in the BOLD signal amplitude at the thalamus and decrease at the posterior parts of the default mode network (Pugnaghi et al. 2014). No threshold effect for the duration of GSW was found, which can be interpreted mechanistically to indicate that there is no meaningful boundary between a burst of "interictal GSW" and an "absence seizure."

Patient age and the presence of antiepileptic medications do not substantially alter the BOLD pattern of absence seizures. This has been clearly demonstrated in children newly diagnosed with absence seizures who have not yet started on any antiepileptic treatment (Moeller et al. 2008).

Indeed, activation patterns are remarkably consistent for absence seizures in a given patient, with between-individual variability being much more significant (Moeller et al. 2010). Some patients show frontal lobe cortical activation and others deactivation, but the reason for this is not well understood. Comparison between these patients shows that positive BOLD at the dorsolateral prefrontal cortex is generally associated with greater activation amplitudes at other brain regions. This intrinsic difference may relate to different seizure mechanisms or genetic factors and provides an endophenotype for absence seizures (Carney et al. 2012).

Nevertheless, activation patterns for GSW are largely consistent across the various epilepsy syndromes. GSW in eyelid myoclonia with absences (EMA, Jeavon's syndrome) shows the same findings as in childhood absence epilepsy (CAE) (Labate et al. 2005; Liu et al. 2008). Comparison between CAE, juvenile absence epilepsy (JAE), and juvenile myoclonic epilepsy (JME) shows that cluster sizes of the BOLD response are largest in CAE and correspond to a longer mean duration of GSW (of 5.2 s, 2.3 s, and 1.8 s, respectively) (Pugnaghi et al. 2014). In myoclonic-astatic epilepsy (MAE, Doose syndrome), GSW shows the pattern described above but with some additional involvement of motor regions (Moeller et al. 2014). This activation occurs in the putamen and premotor cortex, which may account for the typical motor manifestations of this syndrome, where there is myoclonus, followed by a loss of muscle tone.

In contrast, atypical absence seizures show a notably different fMRI pattern (Pillay et al. 2013). These seizures differ from "typical" absences by their less abrupt onset, partially retained awareness, and they more often occur in patients with intellectual disability. Atypical absences also have a different EEG signature, showing irregular slow spike-and-wave (SSW) at 1.5–2.5 Hz. On fMRI, these discharges show extensive but variable BOLD decreases, often including the primary cortical regions. Thalamic activation is inconsistent and not always seen, and additional positive responses may sometimes be seen at the caudate and basal ganglia.

Why seizures end after a stereotyped duration is one of the least well understood aspects of epilepsy. Animal models of GSW have suggested that seizure termination may be related to full recruitment of all available neurons and metabolic changes, including tissue hypoxia, acidification, and potassium currents, which together lead to depressed synaptic responsiveness (Timofeev and Steriade 2004). The concluding phase of GSW shows a decrease of fMRI activity at the dorsolateral prefrontal cortex (below baseline) and an increase at the precuneus/posterior cingulate regions. These changes presumably reflect the recovery of function that was "suspended" during the seizure (Benuzzi et al. 2015).

14.4.2 Neurovascular Coupling and Negative BOLD Signal in Absence Seizures

Concurrent recordings of fMRI (BOLD) and arterial spin labeling (perfusion) show that the relationship between oxygen consumption and perfusion remains constant during absence seizures (Hamandi et al. 2008; Stefanovic et al. 2005). This has also been confirmed in animal models of GSW (Nersesyan et al. 2004). Preserved neurovascular coupling is also seen in areas of negative BOLD, further confirming that decreased fMRI signal during GSW corresponds to a decrease in cortical activity (Carmichael et al. 2008). Other methods, such as 133-xenon perfusion studies and near-infrared spectroscopy, also show decreased perfusion and increased deoxyhemoglobin supporting these conclusions (Buchheim et al. 2004; Sperling and Skolnick 1995).

Ideally, the meaning of decreased BOLD with GSW could be investigated in animals, but the rodent model of 7–8-Hz spike-wave discharges only shows positive BOLD responses (Tenney et al. 2004). A ferret absence-seizure model was developed as it replicates the human features of 3–4-Hz spike-wave and has a sulcated cortex, but this model did not show any negative BOLD responses either (Youngblood et al. 2015).

14.4.3 Impairment of Consciousness During Absence Seizures

How seizures cause loss of consciousness is a central question in the study of epilepsy. However, consciousness is not an "all-or-nothing" phenomenon, and the extent of impairment with absence seizures can be variable between patients and episodes, with differing involvement of cognitive functions (Blumenfeld 2005).

The default mode network consists of brain regions that are more metabolically active during the awake resting state while no specific cognitive task is being performed (Raichle et al. 2001). The BOLD signal decrease in these areas during absence seizures indicates a partial suspension of the baseline state of the brain, which may contribute to impaired awareness (Gotman et al. 2005; Laufs et al. 2006). While some studies report little change in BOLD signal when task performance is not impaired (Berman et al. 2010), others report typical BOLD decreases even when there is no clinical correlate of the GSW discharge (Li et al. 2009).

Comparing short (<4 s, no clinical correlate) and long GSW (>8 s, impaired awareness) shows that longer discharges have more widespread fMRI changes and greater statistical significance, particularly at the thalamus (Carney et al. 2010; Li et al. 2009). This has been replicated in a relatively large CAE cohort (more than 1000 seizures from 39 patients), showing that greater behavioral impairment corresponds to larger BOLD changes in each of the default mode, task-positive, and thalamic-sensorimotor networks (Guo et al. 2016).

Taken together, fMRI findings in absence seizures indicate that impaired awareness is linked to more intense epileptic engagement of these critical networks at (and before) seizure onset, accompanied by early and/or sustained thalamic activity, again supporting the central role of the thalamocortical circuit.

14.4.4 Preictal BOLD Changes in Absence Seizures

Prior to the onset of the scalp EEG spike-wave discharge in CAE, by 10 s or more, a gradual BOLD increase can be seen at several cortical regions. This occurs at the precuneus and lateral parietal cortex (Carney et al. 2010), as well as at the medial prefrontal, frontopolar, and lateral occipital cortex (Bai et al. 2010). Similar time course analysis in medication-resistant JME also shows the earliest positive changes at parietal and frontal cortex, with Granger causality analysis suggesting a directed influence from the frontal lobe to the thalamus during this period (Szaflarski et al. 2010). Dynamic network analysis indicates that persistently increased sensorimotor connectivity and decreased posterior-brain connectivity precede and may predispose to absence seizures (Tangwiriyasakul et al. 2018). Curiously, when events are separated into those with versus without impairment of consciousness, only the seizures leading to behavioral impairment show a preictal fMRI change (Guo et al. 2016), which may be related to the intensity of network activity as described above.

The meaning of these preictal BOLD changes is not yet well understood. They may represent early epileptic activity, which is not yet sufficiently synchronized to appear as a scalp discharge. Alternatively, it may correspond to physiological brain activity of a normal brain state (for example, normal engagement of the default mode network due to internally directed thinking), but which is permissive for seizures and has a higher probability that one will occur.

14.4.5 Photosensitive Epilepsy and the Photoparoxysmal Response

In photosensitive epilepsy, seizures can be triggered by visual stimuli such as viewing a visual pattern, eye closure, or watching television. It is the most common form of reflex epilepsy but is mostly found in association with generalized epilepsies (Martins da Silva and Leal 2017). These patients have a photoparoxysmal response (PPR) seen on EEG, where stimulation with a strobing light at frequencies between 1 Hz and 25 Hz induces a spike-wave discharge that can be either generalized or more limited to the occipital regions.

During fMRI, photic stimulation produces activation of the visual cortex in participants both with and without epilepsy. The area of visual cortex activation is greater in some epileptic patients (Hill et al. 1999), which has been interpreted as a marker of increased cortical excitability.

Surprisingly, the photoparoxysmal response itself does not show a consistent BOLD response with standard analysis. However, a novel approach detected increased fMRI signal at the intraparietal sulcus and the premotor cortex, 3 s earlier than would be predicted by the conventional hemodynamic response (Moeller et al. 2009a). This early BOLD activation may correspond to increased electrographic gamma synchrony, a phenomenon that has also been observed as a prelude to the spike-wave PPR discharge (Parra et al. 2003). Thus, initiation of PPR may be a relatively focal cortical event, driven out of frontoparietal cortex, before the "generalized" scalp EEG discharge is expressed.

A further case is reported where repeated photic stimulation triggered a tonic-clonic seizure (Moeller et al. 2009b). The PPR-related BOLD changes had a different pattern from preceding subclinical studies, showing additional activation at the thalamus and superior colliculi and deactivation of DMN frontoparietal regions, overall more akin to the fMRI pattern of GSW. At the visual cortex, BOLD amplitude progressively increased with each successive stimulus. In comparison, healthy controls have a stable nonincreasing visual cortex photic response (of around +2% baseline versus +6% baseline in the patient with epilepsy). The inference is that hyperexcitable visual cortex can initiate the PPR discharge from association cortex areas and that the subsequent development of a clinical seizure involves propagation into subcortical structures, including the thalamus.

14.4.6 Generalized Tonic-Clonic Seizures

Generalized tonic-clonic seizures (GTCS) are both a medical emergency and characterized by vigorous movement, making fMRI of human GTCS infeasible.

In animal models, GTCS can be induced by intravenous bicuculline (a $GABA_A$ antagonist), and high-field fMRI shows widespread symmetrical BOLD increases in both cortical and subcortical structures (Nersesyan et al. 2004). Typically, BOLD signal increase of 5–10% are seen, which is greater than the increase found in absence seizures (of 2–3%) in this model. The cortical activation of GTCS is very extensive, including primary regions such as visual and somatomotor cortex. Nevertheless, a few areas such as auditory cortex do remain relatively spared in GTCS, so even these seizures are not completely "generalized" in their cortical involvement. Once the GTCS ends, there is a widespread BOLD signal decrease and EEG slowing and attenuation, indicative of an extensive decrease in cortical neuronal activity.

Deactivation at the hippocampus may sometimes be seen later in the seizure (DeSalvo et al. 2010). This is surprising as local field power recordings from the hippocampus show dramatic increases in neural activity by as much as 30 times baseline, even exceeding the ictal activity recorded at the cortex (Schridde et al. 2008). The explanation is that local metabolic utilization of oxygen ($CMRO_2$) at the hippocampus exceeds the blood flow (CBF) that is required to maintain oxygenation. Even though CBF does increase at the hippocampus, the relative change of CBF/$CMRO_2$ is less than at the cortex. The result is a local hippocampal increase of deoxyhemoglobin and thus decreased BOLD in the presence of intense neural activity.

In contrast, postictal negative BOLD signal both at the hippocampus and across the cortex has a different explanation. This is caused by profound depression of neural activity and CBF and $CMRO_2$ return to baseline. This demonstrates how different mechanisms can produce negative BOLD (even during a single seizure) and that the interpretation of negative BOLD is different between GTCS and absence seizures.

In the preictal period for GTCS (in bicuculline-induced animal models), focal BOLD increases are observed more than 20 s before EEG onset (DeSalvo et al. 2010). This occurs in somatosensory cortex and then at the thalamus, with these areas remaining the most strongly activated throughout the seizure. Similarly in the pentylenetetrazol (PTZ) model of GTCS, early and intense activation of the thalamus, and retrosplenial cortex occur, with signal increases of more than 20% before clinical seizure activity (Brevard et al. 2006). Optical imaging in PTZ models supports this finding, with hemodynamic changes that parallel building electrographic gamma power in these regions (Zhang et al. 2014a). Together, these findings point to the role of a thalamocortical network in the generation of GTCS, possibly with preictal initiation in focal cortical regions.

The best gauge of whether these models are applicable to human GTCS is the findings from human cerebral perfusion studies using ictal SPECT. During spontaneous focal-to-bilateral TCS, with tracer injection after the seizure has begun, increased perfusion is seen at the thalamus, medial cerebellum, and basal ganglia and decreased perfusion at the regions of the default mode network (Blumenfeld et al. 2009). Likewise, in TCS induced by electroconvulsive shocks, early increased perfusion is seen at the thalamus and in the region of the bitemporal stimulating electrodes (Enev et al. 2007). These studies, while not directly comparable to animal models, also support the idea of a focal cortical onset that then engages a thalamic network and widespread cortical involvement.

14.4.7 Tonic Seizures

Tonic seizures are found in people with some of the severe developmental epilepsies, particularly Lennox–Gastaut syndrome, where it is one of the characteristic features. Tonic seizures consist of brief truncal stiffening with variable degrees of elevation of the arms, leg extension, and neck flexion, with a duration typically less than 10 s. EEG shows a high voltage slow wave, followed by diffuse low-voltage fast activity, which may reflect fast neuronal firing over a wide cortical area (Fig. 14.4) (Archer et al. 2014a).

The generalized paroxysmal fast activity (GPFA) of Lennox–Gastaut syndrome electrographically has a striking similarity to the signature of tonic seizures and has been studied in detail with fMRI. During GPFA, there is a uniform and widespread positive BOLD response involving cortical association areas, the thalamus, the brain stem, and the basal ganglia. Usually, no regions of BOLD decrease are seen (Pillay et al. 2013). Concurrent activation at the thalamus and pons appears to be an important mechanism of GPFA. Activation of this network has also been proposed as a common pathogenic mechanism in the development of Lennox–Gastaut syndrome (Siniatchkin et al. 2011).

Cerebral perfusion studies during tonic seizures reflect this fMRI pattern. In the early phase of seizure, there is hyperperfusion of the pons and cerebellar hemispheres and hypoperfusion at pericentral cortex. In a later phase, this develops into hyperperfusion of frontal and lateral parietal cortex (Intusoma et al. 2013).

Broad activation of frontal and parietal association cortex in tonic seizures (and in GPFA) as a single highly connected network is physi-

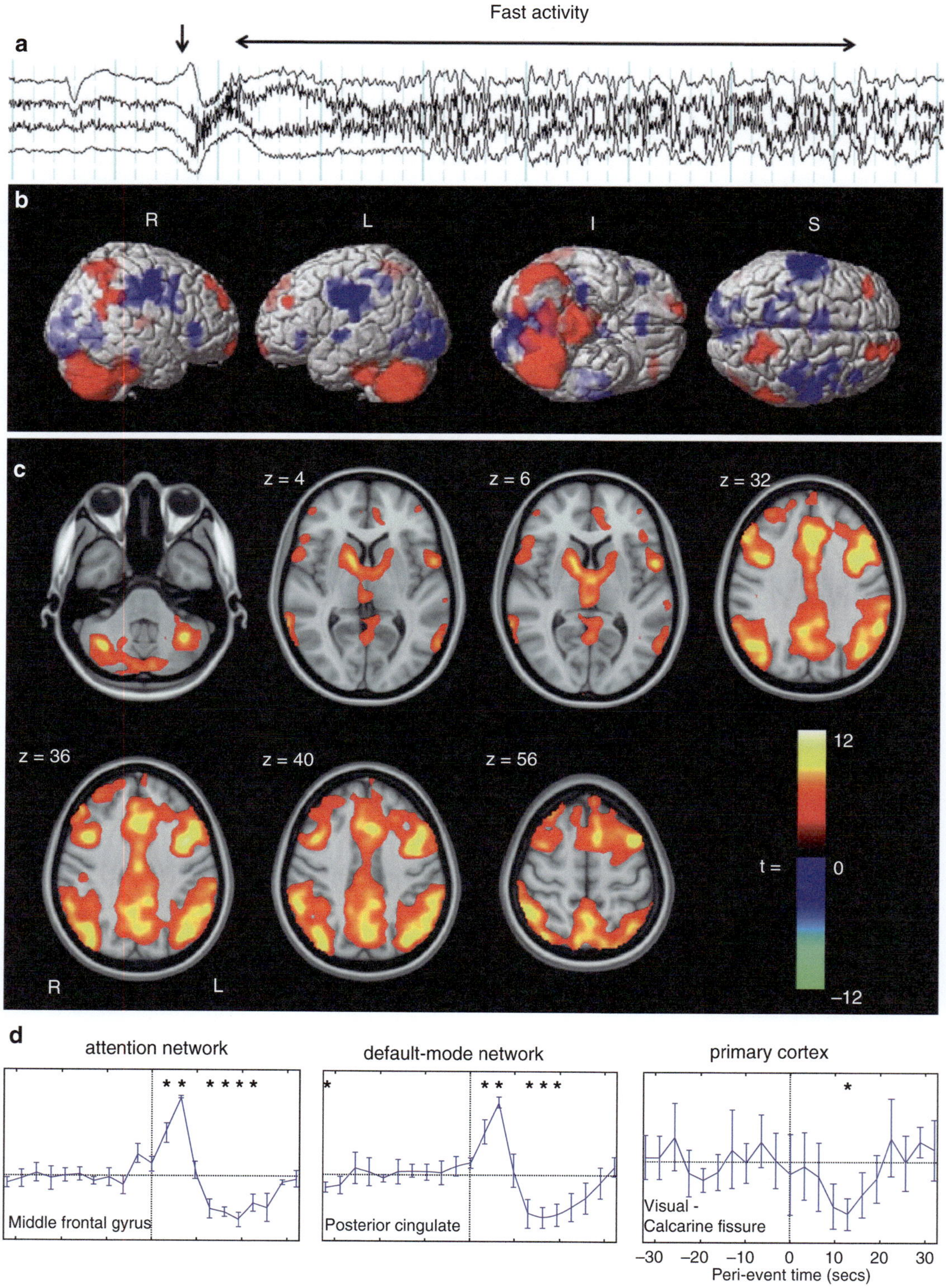

Fig. 14.4 Tonic seizures and the BOLD response to generalized paroxysmal fast activity. (**a**) EEG of a tonic seizure showing paroxysmal fast. (**b**) Early perfusion changes during tonic seizures measured by ictal SPECT. (**c**, **d**) fMRI shows increased BOLD throughout cortical and subcortical regions, with some deactivation of primary cortical regions. (Adapted from Intusoma et al. (2013) and Archer et al. (2014b) with permission)

ologically highly unusual as these regions corresponding to the attention network and default mode network respectively would be expected to counterfluctuate during normal physiological states (Fox et al. 2005). Consequently, Lennox–Gastaut syndrome has been described as a "secondary network epilepsy," indicating that the underlying cause (whether a genetic abnormality or a focal cortical lesion) produces seizures in this syndrome via abnormal and unstable interactions of large-scale brain networks (Archer et al. 2014b).

In summary, fMRI and perfusion data have led to the hypothesis that tonic seizures arise in frontal and/or parietal cortex, are amplified through the intrinsic attentional network, and project via the corticoreticular pathways to the pons leading to the characteristic motor expression (Intusoma et al. 2013).

14.5 Conclusions and Future Directions

In this chapter, we have reviewed the findings from fMRI performed during seizures. The development of fMRI acquisition and analysis methods has made this technically challenging task possible, so that the majority of seizure types have now been recorded in humans and/or in animal models. The data from these studies lead to the following observations:

1. The evolution of the BOLD signal during seizures is best understood from a network perspective, where epileptic activity engages and propagates through otherwise normal physiological networks. In focal seizures, there are many different patterns of network involvement with correspondingly diverse clinical signs, each related to the site of the epileptogenic focus. However, the common theme is of cortical onset with cortico-cortical propagation. The use of fMRI to elucidate the common archetypal network propagations has only just begun, but this is an approach that promises to greatly extend our understanding of clinical epileptology.
2. Generalized seizures show striking differences from focal seizures in their fMRI signature, beyond their (defined) early engagement of bilateral networks. Involvement of cortico-subcortical networks is the key feature, specifically of the thalamocortical circuit. The different generalized seizure types have dramatically varying clinical expressions, which makes sense when their specific network involvement is considered. Absence seizures, where thalamocortical activation leads to inhibition of the default mode network, are characterized by brief behavioral arrest and impaired awareness. Tonic seizures, which may arise in the frontoparietal attentional network and then drive pontine activation, are predominantly expressed by stereotyped brain stem posturing. Tonic-clonic seizures, whether evolving from a focal or generalized onset, show very widespread cortical activation, including of bilateral motor cortex, and in this phase are characterized by bilateral clonic jerking.
3. Preictal activation of specific networks, in the seconds or minutes before seizure onset, is an emerging, and now seemingly common, finding on fMRI. The location of these preictal signal changes is often limited to particular regions, suggesting the possibility that even generalized seizures have (in some sense) a focal basis. So far, this preictal phenomenon has not received a great deal of attention, perhaps because it is not apparent on conventional seizure EEG recordings. We predict that this will become an increasingly important area of research as any early marker of an impending seizure is of vital interest to the person experiencing it (as a warning would allow them to avoid injuries and to apply preventative treatment) and also provides a critical insight into the mechanisms of seizure generation.
4. Progress in defining the networks engaged by each seizure type is but the first step. The important future direction in seizure fMRI will be to examine how affected networks can be modulated to inhibit their recruitment by epileptic activity. Clearly, anti-epilepsy medi-

cations alter the function of brain networks, but so far we have limited ability to engineer specific network modulations for a particular patient or diagnosis. Other treatment approaches, such as deep brain stimulation, local ablation/resection, or targeted drug delivery also, have the ability to modulate specific networks via the connectivity of the intervention site. Thus, an important challenge will be to determine whether there are key "rich club" nodes where such strategies can be applied, in order to prevent the spread of local neighborhood epileptic activity into large-scale intrinsic networks. Such network hubs will be highly and flexibly connected into each of the critical large-scale intrinsic networks (for example, the thalamic nuclei and piriform cortex are possible candidates) and could therefore become common targets for effective intervention in refractory epilepsy.

5. Seizure-correlated head motion is the greatest technical barrier to future effective seizure fMRI data acquisition and analysis. The development of acquisition protocols that are resistant to motion effects, for example, by the inclusion of navigator sequences and/or recording multiple echo times, would be an important step forward. The increasing use of multiband fMRI with short repetition times will also advance the field by enabling dynamic imaging of seizures at much higher temporal resolutions.

In total, fMRI of seizures has already provided a proof of principle for the network basis of the epilepsies by revealing specific patterns of network engagement and propagation across various common seizure types. A broadening clinical spectrum where this technique can be feasibly applied, alongside emerging technical advances, will continue to provide important insights into onset mechanisms, clinical expression, and treatment targets for seizures, as well as further reveal the fundamental network organization of the human brain.

References

Abreu P, Ribeiro M, Forni A, Pires I, Sousa G (2005) Writing epilepsy: a neurophysiological, neuropsychological and neuroimaging study. Epilepsy Behav 6(3):463–466

Abreu R, Leal A, Figueiredo P (2018) EEG-informed fMRI: a review of data analysis methods. Front Hum Neurosci 12:29

Aghakhani Y, Bagshaw AP, Bénar CG, Hawco C, Andermann F, Dubeau F et al (2004) fMRI activation during spike and wave discharges in idiopathic generalized epilepsy. Brain 127(5):1127–1144

Archer JS, Briellmann RS, Syngeniotis A, Abbott DF, Jackson GD (2003) Spike-triggered fMRI in reading epilepsy: involvement of left frontal cortex working memory area. Neurology 60(3):415–421

Archer JS, Waites AB, Abbott DF, Federico P, Jackson GD (2006) Event-related fMRI of myoclonic jerks arising from dysplastic cortex. Epilepsia 47(9):1487–1492

Archer JS, Warren AEL, Jackson GD, Abbott DF (2014a) Conceptualizing Lennox–Gastaut syndrome as a secondary network epilepsy. Front Neurol 30:5

Archer JS, Warren AEL, Stagnitti MR, Masterton RAJ, Abbott DF, Jackson GD (2014b) Lennox-Gastaut syndrome and phenotype: secondary network epilepsies. Epilepsia 55(8):1245–1254

Auer T, Veto K, Dóczi T, Komoly S, Juhos V, Janszky J et al (2008) Identifying seizure-onset zone and visualizing seizure spread by fMRI: a case report. Epileptic Disord 10(2):93–100

Bai X, Vestal M, Berman R, Negishi M, Spann M, Vega C et al (2010) Dynamic time course of typical childhood absence seizures: EEG, Behavior, and functional magnetic resonance imaging. J Neurosci 30(17):5884–5893

Benuzzi F, Ballotta D, Mirandola L, Ruggieri A, Vaudano AE, Zucchelli M et al (2015) An EEG-fMRI study on the termination of generalized spike-and-wave discharges in absence epilepsy. PLoS One 10(7):e0130943

Berg AT, Berkovic SF, Brodie MJ, Buchhalter J, Cross JH, van Emde BW et al (2010) Revised terminology and concepts for organization of seizures and epilepsies: report of the ILAE Commission on Classification and Terminology, 2005–2009. Epilepsia 51(4):676–685

Berman R, Negishi M, Vestal M, Spann M, Chung MH, Bai X et al (2010) Simultaneous EEG, fMRI, and behavior in typical childhood absence seizures. Epilepsia 51(10):2011–2022

Blumenfeld H (2005) Consciousness and epilepsy: why are patients with absence seizures absent? In: Laureys S (ed) Progress in brain research. Elsevier, London, pp 271–603

Blumenfeld H (2012) Impaired consciousness in epilepsy. Lancet Neurol 11(9):814–826

Blumenfeld H, Varghese GI, Purcaro MJ, Motelow JE, Enev M, McNally KA et al (2009) Cortical and subcortical networks in human secondarily generalized tonic-clonic seizures. Brain 132(Pt 4):999–1012

Brevard ME, Kulkarni P, King JA, Ferris CF (2006) Imaging the neural substrates involved in the genesis of pentylenetetrazol-induced seizures. Epilepsia 47(4):745–754

Buchheim K, Obrig HV, Pannwitz W, Müller A, Heekeren H, Villringer A et al (2004) Decrease in haemoglobin oxygenation during absence seizures in adult humans. Neurosci Lett 354(2):119–122

Carmichael DW, Hamandi K, Laufs H, Duncan JS, Thomas DL, Lemieux L (2008) An investigation of the relationship between BOLD and perfusion signal changes during epileptic generalised spike wave activity. Magn Reson Imaging 26(7):870–873

Carney PW, Masterton RAJ, Harvey AS, Scheffer IE, Berkovic SF, Jackson GD (2010) The core network in absence epilepsy differences in cortical and thalamic BOLD response. Neurology 75(10):904–911

Carney PW, Masterton RAJ, Flanagan D, Berkovic SF, Jackson GD (2012) The frontal lobe in absence epilepsy: EEG-fMRI findings. Neurology 78(15):1157–1165

Chassagnon S, Hawko CS, Bernasconi A, Gotman J, Dubeau F (2009) Coexistence of symptomatic focal and absence seizures: video-EEG and EEG-fMRI evidence of overlapping but independent epileptogenic networks. Epilepsia 50(7):1821–1826

Chaudhary UJ, Carmichael DW, Rodionov R, Thornton RC, Bartlett P, Vulliemoz S et al (2012) Mapping preictal and ictal haemodynamic networks using video-electroencephalography and functional imaging. Brain 135(12):3645–3663

Chaudhary UJ, Duncan JS, Lemieux L (2013) Mapping hemodynamic correlates of seizures using fMRI: a review. Hum Brain Mapp 34(2):447–466

Chaudhary UJ, Centeno M, Thornton RC, Rodionov R, Vulliemoz S, McEvoy AW et al (2016) Mapping human preictal and ictal haemodynamic networks using simultaneous intracranial EEG-fMRI. NeuroImage: Clinical 11:486–493

Chifari R, Piazzini A, Turner K, Canger R, Canevini MP, Wolf P (2004) Reflex writing seizures in two siblings with juvenile myoclonic epilepsy. Acta Neurol Scand 109(3):232–235

DeSalvo MN, Schridde U, Mishra AM, Motelow JE, Purcaro MJ, Danielson N et al (2010) Focal BOLD fMRI changes in bicuculline-induced tonic–clonic seizures in the rat. NeuroImage 50(3):902–909

Detre JA, Sirven JI, Alsop DC, O'Connor MJ, French JA (1995) Localization of subclinical ictal activity by functional magnetic resonance imaging: Correlation with invasive monitoring. Ann Neurol 38(4):618–624

Diekmann V, Hoppner AC (2014) Cortical network dysfunction in musicogenic epilepsy reflecting the role of snowballing emotional processes in seizure generation: an fMRI-EEG study. Epileptic Disord 16(1):31–44

Donaire A, Bargallo N, Falcón C, Maestro I, Carreno M, Setoain J et al (2009a) Identifying the structures involved in seizure generation using sequential analysis of ictal-fMRI data. NeuroImage 47(1):173–183

Donaire A, Falcón C, Carreno M, Bargallo N, Rumià J, Setoain J et al (2009b) Sequential analysis of fMRI images: a new approach to study human epileptic networks. Epilepsia 50(12):2526–2537

Dymond AM, Crandall PH (1976) Oxygen availability and blood flow in the temporal lobes during spontaneous epileptic seizures in man. Brain Res 102(1):191–196

Enev M, McNally KA, Varghese G, Zubal IG, Ostroff RB, Blumenfeld H (2007) Imaging onset and propagation of ECT-induced seizures. Epilepsia 48(2):238–244

Fahoum F, Lopes R, Pittau F, Dubeau F, Gotman J (2012) Widespread epileptic networks in focal epilepsies: EEG-fMRI study. Epilepsia 53(9):1618–1627

Fahoum F, Zelmann R, Tyvaert L, Dubeau F, Gotman J (2013) Epileptic discharges affect the default mode network—fMRI and intracerebral EEG evidence. PLoS One 8(6):e68038

Federico P, Abbott DF, Briellmann RS, Harvey AS, Jackson GD (2005) Functional MRI of the pre-ictal state. Brain 128(Pt 8):1811–1817

Fisher RS, Cross JH, D'Souza C, French JA, Haut SR, Higurashi N et al (2017) Instruction manual for the ILAE 2017 operational classification of seizure types. Epilepsia 58(4):531–542

Flanagan D, Badawy RAB, Jackson GD (2014) EEG–fMRI in focal epilepsy: local activation and regional networks. Clin Neurophysiol 125(1):21–31

Fox MD, Snyder AZ, Vincent JL, Corbetta M, Van Essen DC, Raichle ME (2005) The human brain is intrinsically organized into dynamic, anticorrelated functional networks. Proc Natl Acad Sci U S A 102(27):9673–9678

Franck G, Sadzot B, Salmon E, Depresseux JC, Grisar T, Peters JM et al (1986) Regional cerebral blood flow and metabolic rates in human focal epilepsy and status epilepticus. Adv Neurol 44:935–948

Gaxiola-Valdez I, Singh S, Perera T, Sandy S, Li E, Federico P (2017) Seizure onset zone localization using postictal hypoperfusion detected by arterial spin labelling MRI. Brain 140(11):2895–2911

Gloor P (1968) Generalized cortico-reticular epilepsies some considerations on the pathophysiology of generalized bilaterally synchronous spike and wave discharge. Epilepsia 9(3):249–263

Goense J, Merkle H, Logothetis NK (2012) High-resolution fMRI reveals laminar differences in neurovascular coupling between positive and negative BOLD responses. Neuron 76(3):629–639

Gotman J, Pittau F (2011) Combining EEG and fMRI in the study of epileptic discharges. Epilepsia 52:38–42

Gotman J, Grova C, Bagshaw A, Kobayashi E, Aghakhani Y, Dubeau F (2005) Generalized epileptic discharges show thalamocortical activation and suspension of the default state of the brain. Proc Natl Acad Sci U S A 102(42):15236–15240

Guo JN, Kim R, Chen Y, Negishi M, Jhun S, Weiss S et al (2016) Impaired consciousness in patients with absence seizures investigated by functional MRI,

EEG, and behavioural measures: a cross-sectional study. Lancet Neurol 15(13):1336–1345

Hamandi K, Salek-Haddadi A, Laufs H, Liston A, Friston K, Fish DR et al (2006) EEG–fMRI of idiopathic and secondarily generalized epilepsies. NeuroImage 31(4):1700–1710

Hamandi K, Laufs H, Nöth U, Carmichael DW, Duncan JS, Lemieux L (2008) BOLD and perfusion changes during epileptic generalised spike wave activity. NeuroImage 39(2):608–618

Harris S, Boorman L, Bruyns-Haylett M, Kennerley A, Ma H, Zhao M et al (2014) Contralateral dissociation between neural activity and cerebral blood volume during recurrent acute focal neocortical seizures. Epilepsia 55(9):1423–1430

Harris SS, Boorman LW, Kennerley AJ, Sharp PS, Martin C, Redgrave P et al (2018) Seizure epicenter depth and translaminar field potential synchrony underlie complex variations in tissue oxygenation during ictal initiation. NeuroImage 171:165–175

Hill RA, Chiappa KH, Huang-Hellinger F, Jenkins BG (1999) Hemodynamic and metabolic aspects of photosensitive epilepsy revealed by functional magnetic resonance imaging and magnetic resonance spectroscopy. Epilepsia 40(7):912–920

Intusoma U, Abbott DF, Masterton RAJ, Stagnitti MR, Newton MR, Jackson GD et al (2013) Tonic seizures of Lennox-Gastaut syndrome: periictal single-photon emission computed tomography suggests a corticopontine network. Epilepsia 54(12):2151–2157

Jackson GD, Connelly A, Cross JH, Gordon I, Gadian DG (1994) Functional magnetic resonance imaging of focal seizures. Neurology 44(5):850

Klamer S, Rona S, Elshahabi A, Lerche H, Braun C, Honegger J et al (2015) Multimodal effective connectivity analysis reveals seizure focus and propagation in musicogenic epilepsy. NeuroImage 113:70–77

Kobayashi E, Hawco CS, Grova C, Dubeau F, Gotman J (2006) Widespread and intense BOLD changes during brief focal electrographic seizures. Neurology 66(7):1049–1055

Kokkinos V, Zountsas B, Kontogiannis K, Garganis K (2012) Epileptogenic networks in two patients with hypothalamic hamartoma. Brain Topogr 25(3):327–331

Kreisman NR, Magee JC, Brizzee BL (1991) Relative hypoperfusion in rat cerebral cortex during recurrent seizures. J Cereb Blood Flow Metab 11(1):77–87

Krings T, Töpper R, Reinges MHT, Foltys H, Spetzger U, Chiappa KH et al (2000) Hemodynamic changes in simple partial epilepsy: a functional MRI study. Neurology 54(2):524

Kubota F, Kikuchi S, Ito M, Shibata N, Akata T, Takahashi A et al (2000) Ictal brain hemodynamics in the epileptic focus caused by a brain tumor using functional magnetic resonance imaging (fMRI). Seizure 9(8):585–589

Labate A, Briellmann RS, Abbott DF, Waites AB, Jackson GD (2005) Typical childhood absence seizures are associated with thalamic activation. Epileptic Disord 7(4):373–377

Laufs H, Lengler U, Hamandi K, Kleinschmidt A, Krakow K (2006) Linking generalized spike-and-wave discharges and resting state brain activity by using EEG/fMRI in a patient with absence seizures. Epilepsia 47(2):444–448

Laufs H, Hamandi K, Salek-Haddadi A, Kleinschmidt AK, Duncan JS, Lemieux L (2007) Temporal lobe interictal epileptic discharges affect cerebral activity in "default mode" brain regions. Hum Brain Mapp 28(10):1023–1032

LeVan P, Tyvaert L, Moeller F, Gotman J (2010) Independent component analysis reveals dynamic ictal BOLD responses in EEG-fMRI data from focal epilepsy patients. NeuroImage 49(1):366–378

Li Q, Luo C, Yang T, Yao Z, He L, Liu L et al (2009) EEG–fMRI study on the interictal and ictal generalized spike-wave discharges in patients with childhood absence epilepsy. Epilepsy Res 87(2–3):160–168

Liao W, Zhang Z, Mantini D, Xu Q, Ji G-J, Zhang H et al (2014) Dynamical intrinsic functional architecture of the brain during absence seizures. Brain Struct Funct 219(6):2001–2015

Liu Y, Yang T, Liao W, Yang X, Liu I, Yan B et al (2008) EEG-fMRI study of the ictal and interictal epileptic activity in patients with eyelid myoclonia with absences. Epilepsia 49(12):2078–2086

Ma H, Zhao M, Schwartz TH (2013) Dynamic neurovascular coupling and uncoupling during ictal onset, propagation, and termination revealed by simultaneous in vivo optical imaging of neural activity and local blood volume. Cereb Cortex 23(4):885–899

Marrosu F, Barberini L, Puligheddu M, Bortolato M, Mascia M, Tuveri A et al (2009) Combined EEG/fMRI recording in musicogenic epilepsy. Epilepsy Res 84(1):77–81

Martins da Silva A, Leal B (2017) Photosensitivity and epilepsy: Current concepts and perspectives—a narrative review. Seizure 50:209–218

Masterton RAJ, Carney PW, Abbott DF, Jackson GD (2013) Absence epilepsy subnetworks revealed by event-related independent components analysis of functional magnetic resonance imaging. Epilepsia 54(5):801–808

Meletti S, Vaudano AE, Tassi L, Caruana F, Avanzini P (2015) Intracranial time–frequency correlates of seizure-related negative BOLD response in the sensory-motor network. Clin Neurophysiol 126(4):847–849

Moeller F, Siebner HR, Wolff S, Muhle H, Granert O, Jansen O et al (2008) Simultaneous EEG-fMRI in drug-naive children with newly diagnosed absence epilepsy. Epilepsia 49(9):1510–1519

Moeller F, Siebner HR, Ahlgrimm N, Wolff S, Muhle H, Granert O et al (2009a) fMRI activation during spike and wave discharges evoked by photic stimulation. NeuroImage 48(4):682–695

Moeller F, Siebner HR, Wolff S, Muhle H, Granert O, Jansen O et al (2009b) Mapping brain activity on the verge of a photically induced generalized tonic–clonic seizure. Epilepsia 50(6):1632–1637

Moeller F, LeVan P, Muhle H, Stephani U, Dubeau F, Siniatchkin M et al (2010) Absence seizures: individual patterns revealed by EEG-fMRI. Epilepsia 51(10):2000–2010

Moeller F, Groening K, Moehring J, Muhle H, Wolff S, Jansen O et al (2014) EEG-fMRI in myoclonic astatic epilepsy (Doose syndrome). Neurology 82(17):1508–1513

Mórocz IA, Karni A, Haut S, Lantos G, Liu G (2003) fMRI of triggerable aurae in musicogenic epilepsy. Neurology 60(4):705–709

Murta T, Leal A, Garrido MI, Figueiredo P (2012) Dynamic causal modelling of epileptic seizure propagation pathways: a combined EEG–fMRI study. NeuroImage 62(3):1634–1642

Murta T, Leite M, Carmichael DW, Figueiredo P, Lemieux L (2015) Electrophysiological correlates of the BOLD signal for EEG-informed fMRI: electrophysiological correlates of the BOLD signal. Hum Brain Mapp 36(1):391–414

Nersesyan H, Hyder F, Rothman DL, Blumenfeld H (2004) Dynamic fMRI and EEG recordings during spike-wave seizures and generalized tonic-clonic seizures in WAG/Rij Rats. J Cereb Blood Flow Metab 24(6):589–599

Parra J, Kalitzin SN, Iriarte J, Blanes W, Velis DN (2003) Lopes da Silva FH. Gamma-band phase clustering and photosensitivity: is there an underlying mechanism common to photosensitive epilepsy and visual perception? Brain 126(Pt 5):1164–1172

Penfield W (1933) The evidence for a cerebral vascular mechanism in epilepsy. Ann Intern Med 7(3):303

Pillay N, Archer JS, Badawy RAB, Flanagan DF, Berkovic SF, Jackson G (2013) Networks underlying paroxysmal fast activity and slow spike and wave in Lennox-Gastaut syndrome. Neurology 81(7):665–673

Pittau F, Tinuper P, Bisulli F, Naldi I, Cortelli P, Bisulli A et al (2008) Videopolygraphic and functional MRI study of musicogenic epilepsy. A case report and literature review. Epilepsy Behav 13(4):685–692

Pittau F, Fahoum F, Zelmann R, Dubeau F, Gotman J (2013) Negative BOLD response to interictal epileptic discharges in focal epilepsy. Brain Topogr 26(4):627–640

Pugnaghi M, Carmichael DW, Vaudano AE, Chaudhary UJ, Benuzzi F, Di Bonaventura C et al (2014) Generalized spike and waves: effect of discharge duration on brain networks as revealed by BOLD fMRI. Brain Topogr 27(1):123–137

Racicot F, Obaid S, Bouthillier A, Guillon-Létourneau L, Clément J-F, Nguyen DK (2016) Praxis-induced reflex seizures mainly precipitated by writing due to a parietal focal cortical dysplasia. Epilepsy Behav Case Rep 6:52–54

Raichle ME, MacLeod AM, Snyder AZ, Powers WJ, Gusnard DA, Shulman GL (2001) A default mode of brain function. Proc Natl Acad Sci U S A 98(2):676–682

Rathakrishnan R, Moeller F, Levan P, Dubeau F, Gotman J (2010) BOLD signal changes preceding negative responses in EEG-fMRI in patients with focal epilepsy. Epilepsia 51(9):1837–1845

Salek-Haddadi A, Merschhemke M, Lemieux L, Fish DR (2002) Simultaneous EEG-correlated ictal fMRI. NeuroImage 16(1):32–40

Salek-Haddadi A, Lemieux L, Merschhemke M, Friston KJ, Duncan JS, Fish DR (2003) Functional magnetic resonance imaging of human absence seizures. Ann Neurol 53(5):663–667

Salek-Haddadi A, Mayer T, Hamandi K, Symms M, Josephs O, Fluegel D et al (2009) Imaging seizure activity: a combined EEG/EMG-fMRI study in reading epilepsy. Epilepsia 50(2):256–264

Schridde U, Khubchandani M, Motelow JE, Sanganahalli BG, Hyder F, Blumenfeld H (2008) Negative BOLD with large increases in neuronal activity. Cereb Cortex 18(8):1814–1827

Shariff S, Suh M, Zhao M, Ma H, Schwartz TH (2006) Recent developments in oximetry and perfusion-based mapping techniques and their role in the surgical treatment of neocortical epilepsy. Epilepsy Behav 8(2):363–375

Siniatchkin M, Coropceanu D, Moeller F, Boor R, Stephani U (2011) EEG-fMRI reveals activation of brainstem and thalamus in patients with Lennox-Gastaut syndrome. Epilepsia 52(4):766–774

Slone E, Westwood E, Dhaliwal H, Federico P, Dunn JF (2012) Near-infrared spectroscopy shows preictal haemodynamic changes in temporal lobe epilepsy. Epileptic Disord 14(4):371–378

Song Y, Torres RA, Garcia S, Frometa Y, Bae J, Deshmukh A et al (2016) Dysfunction of neurovascular/metabolic coupling in chronic focal epilepsy. IEEE Trans Biomed Eng 63(1):97–110

Sonmezturk HH, Morgan V, Abou-Khalil B (2011) Focal seizure propagation illustrated by fMRI. Epileptic Disord 13(1):92–95

Sperling MR, Skolnick BE (1995) Cerebral blood flow during spike-wave discharges. Epilepsia 36(2):156–163

Stefanovic B, Warnking JM, Kobayashi E, Bagshaw AP, Hawco C, Dubeau F et al (2005) Hemodynamic and metabolic responses to activation, deactivation and epileptic discharges. NeuroImage 28(1):205–215

Storti SF, Del Felice A, Formaggio E, Boscolo Galazzo I, Bongiovanni LG, Cerini R et al (2015) Spatial and temporal EEG-fMRI changes during preictal and postictal phases in a patient with posttraumatic epilepsy. Clin EEG Neurosci 46(3):247–252

Szaflarski JP, DiFrancesco M, Hirschauer T, Banks C, Privitera MD, Gotman J et al (2010) Cortical and subcortical contributions to absence seizure onset examined with EEG/fMRI. Epilepsy Behav 18(4):404–413

Tana MG, Bianchi AM, Sclocco R, Franchin T, Cerutti S, Leal A (2012) Parcel-based connectivity analysis of fMRI data for the study of epileptic seizure propagation. Brain Topogr 25(4):345–361

Tangwiriyasakul C, Perani S, Centeno M, Yaakub SN, Abela E, Carmichael DW et al (2018) Dynamic brain network states in human generalized spike-wave discharges. Brain 141(10):2981–2994

Tayah TF, Abou-Khalil B, Gilliam FG, Knowlton RC, Wushensky CA, Gallagher MJ (2006) Musicogenic seizures can arise from multiple temporal lobe foci: intracranial EEG analyses of three patients. Epilepsia 47(8):1402–1406

Tenney JR, Duong TQ, King JA, Ferris CF (2004) fMRI of brain activation in a genetic rat model of absence seizures. Epilepsia 45(6):576–582

Thornton RC, Rodionov R, Laufs H, Vulliemoz S, Vaudano A, Carmichael D et al (2010) Imaging haemodynamic changes related to seizures: comparison of EEG-based general linear model, independent component analysis of fMRI and intracranial EEG. NeuroImage 53(1):196–205

Timofeev I, Steriade M (2004) Neocortical seizures: initiation, development and cessation. Neuroscience 123(2):299–336

Tousseyn S, Dupont P, Goffin K, Sunaert S, Paesschen WV (2015) Correspondence between large-scale ictal and interictal epileptic networks revealed by single photon emission computed tomography (SPECT) and electroencephalography (EEG)–functional magnetic resonance imaging (fMRI). Epilepsia 56(3):382–392

Tyvaert L, Hawco C, Kobayashi E, LeVan P, Dubeau F, Gotman J (2008) Different structures involved during ictal and interictal epileptic activity in malformations of cortical development: an EEG-fMRI study. Brain 131(8):2042–2060

Tyvaert L, LeVan P, Dubeau F, Gotman J (2009) Noninvasive dynamic imaging of seizures in epileptic patients. Hum Brain Mapp 30(12):3993–4011

van Luijtelaar EL, de Bruijn SF, Declerck AC, Renier WO, Vossen JM, Coenen AM (1991) Disturbances in time estimation during absence seizures in children. Epilepsy Res 9(2):148–153

Vaudano AE, Carmichael DW, Salek-Haddadi A, Rampp S, Stefan H, Lemieux L et al (2012) Networks involved in seizure initiation A reading epilepsy case studied with EEG-fMRI and MEG. Neurology 79(3):249–253

Vinette SA, Premji S, Beers CA, Gaxiola-Valdez I, Pittman DJ, Slone EG et al (2016) Pre-ictal BOLD alterations: two cases of patients with focal epilepsy. Epilepsy Res 127:207–220

Williamson PD, Thadani VM, Darcey TM, Spencer DD, Spencer SS, Mattson RH (1992) Occipital lobe epilepsy: clinical characteristics, seizure spread patterns, and results of surgery. Ann Neurol 31(1):3–13

Youngblood MW, Chen WC, Mishra AM, Enamandram S, Sanganahalli BG, Motelow JE et al (2015) Rhythmic 3–4 Hz discharge is insufficient to produce cortical BOLD fMRI decreases in generalized seizures. NeuroImage 109:368–377

Zhang T, Zhou J, Jiang R, Yang H, Carney PR, Jiang H (2014a) Pre-seizure state identified by diffuse optical tomography. Sci Rep 21:4

Zhang Z, Liao W, Wang Z, Xu Q, Yang F, Mantini D et al (2014b) Epileptic discharges specifically affect intrinsic connectivity networks during absence seizures. J Neurol Sci 336(1):138–145

Zhang C, Bélanger S, Pouliot P, Lesage F (2015) Measurement of local partial pressure of oxygen in the brain tissue under normoxia and epilepsy with phosphorescence lifetime microscopy. PLoS One 10(8):e0135536

Zhao M, Suh M, Ma H, Perry C, Geneslaw A, Schwartz TH (2007) Focal increases in perfusion and decreases in hemoglobin oxygenation precede seizure onset in spontaneous human epilepsy. Epilepsia 48(11):2059–2067

Zhao M, Ma H, Suh M, Schwartz TH (2009) Spatiotemporal dynamics of perfusion and oximetry during ictal discharges in the rat neocortex. J Neurosci 29(9):2814–2823

15 The Functional Anatomy of Speech Processing: From Auditory Cortex to Speech Recognition and Speech Production

Gregory Hickok

15.1 Introduction

Lesion-based research has been successful in providing a broad outline of the neuroanatomy of speech/language processes (Dronkers et al. 2000; Hillis 2007) and continues to play a crucial role in the development of functional anatomic models of cognitive processes (Fellows et al. 2005). However, lesion studies lack the spatial resolution to assess more detailed functional anatomical hypotheses. Functional imaging methods such as functional magnetic resonance imaging (fMRI), when appropriately guided and constrained by lesion and other methods, can provide much-needed information.

In this chapter, we will review evidence regarding the functional anatomy of the human auditory cortex as it relates to speech recognition and speech production. Figure 15.1 displays an organizational framework for this discussion.

15.2 Hierarchical Organization of Auditory Cortex

The monkey auditory cortex is organized hierarchically with a core region at the center, a belt region surrounding the core, and a parabelt region surrounding the belt area, each containing subdivisions. The core corresponds to the primary auditory cortex, showing a distinct primary-type cytoarchitecture and robust single-unit responses to pure tones, with sharp tuning curves relative to belt regions. Both the core and the belt areas receive inputs from the medial geniculate nucleus (MGN), although from different subregions, MGv and MGd, respectively. The parabelt also receives direct ascending auditory input from MGd but is distinguished from the belt area in that it does not receive direct input from the core. Instead, information reaching the parabelt from the core appears to be mediated by the belt region, which projects heavily to the parabelt (Kaas and Hackett 2000; Kaas et al. 1999).

The human auditory cortex appears to be similar in its hierarchical organization. Simple acoustic stimulation, such as noise bursts or tones, activates the auditory cortex in and around Heschl's gyrus. In addition, more complex stimuli, such as speech, activate a broader region, including the superior temporal sulcus (STS) (Binder et al. 2000).

In both human and nonhuman primates, there is evidence for two broad projection streams, sometimes referred to as the ventral and dorsal pathways (Hickok and Poeppel 2000, 2007; Rauschecker 1998; Romanski et al. 1999; Scott 2005). There is a general agreement that the ventral stream supports recognition of the content of auditory information (a "what" pathway), but there is disagreement regarding the nature of the

G. Hickok (✉)
Department of Cognitive Sciences, Center for Cognitive Neuroscience, University of California, Irvine, Irvine, CA, USA
e-mail: gshickok@uci.edu

S. Ulmer, O. Jansen (eds.), *fMRI*, https://doi.org/10.1007/978-3-030-41874-8_15

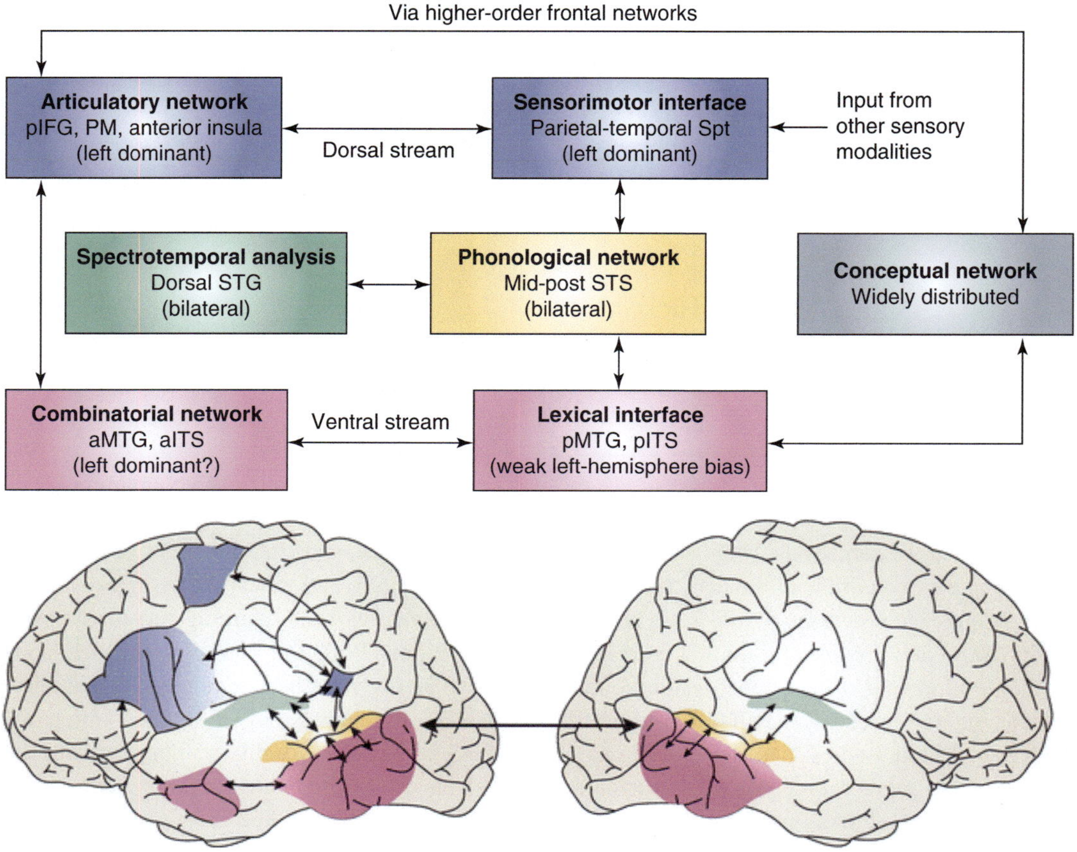

Fig. 15.1 The dual-stream model of the functional anatomy of language. (**a**) Schematic diagram of the dual-stream model. The earliest stage of cortical speech processing involves some form of spectrotemporal analysis, which is carried out in auditory cortices bilaterally in the supratemporal plane. These spectrotemporal computations appear to differ between the two hemispheres. Phonological-level processing and representation involves the middle to posterior portions of the superior temporal sulcus (STS) bilaterally, although there may be a weak left-hemisphere bias at this level of processing. Subsequently, the system diverges into two broad streams, a dorsal pathway (*blue*) that maps sensory or phonological representations onto articulatory motor representations and a ventral pathway (*pink*) that maps sensory or phonological representations onto lexical conceptual representations. (**b**) Approximate anatomical locations of the dual-stream model components, specified as precisely as available evidence allows. Regions shaded *green* depict areas on the dorsal surface of the superior temporal gyrus (STG) that are proposed to be involved in spectrotemporal analysis. Regions shaded *yellow* in the posterior half of the STS are implicated in phonological-level processes. Regions shaded *pink* represent the ventral stream, which is bilaterally organized with a weak left-hemisphere bias. The more posterior regions of the ventral stream, posterior middle, and inferior portions of the temporal lobes correspond to the lexical interface, which links phonological and semantic information, whereas the more anterior locations correspond to the proposed combinatorial network. Regions shaded *blue* represent the dorsal stream, which is strongly left dominant. The posterior region of the dorsal stream corresponds to an area in the Sylvian fissure at the parietotemporal boundary (area Spt), which is proposed to be a sensorimotor interface, whereas the more anterior locations in the frontal lobe, probably involving Broca's region and a more dorsal premotor site, correspond to portions of the articulatory network. Arrows indicate reciprocal connections. *aITS* anterior inferior temporal sulcus, *aMTG* anterior middle temporal gyrus, *pIFG* posterior inferior frontal gyrus, *PM* premotor cortex. (Reprinted with permission from Hickok and Poeppel (2007))

dorsal stream, with some authors promoting a location-based function ("where" pathway) (Rauschecker 1998) and others an auditory-motor integration function (Hickok et al. 2003; Hickok and Poeppel 2000, 2007; Warren et al. 2005). These hypotheses are not necessarily incompatible.

15.3 STS Supports Phonological Aspects of Speech Recognition

A number of studies have found that portions of the STS are important for representing and/or processing phonological information (Fig. 15.1, yellow; Binder et al. 2000; Hickok and Poeppel 2004, 2007; Indefrey and Levelt 2004; Liebenthal et al. 2005; Price et al. 1996). The STS is activated by several tasks that tap phonological information such as speech perception, speech production (Indefrey and Levelt 2004), and the active short-term maintenance of phonemic information (Buchsbaum et al. 2001; Hickok et al. 2003). Functional activation studies that have used subtraction methodologies to isolate phonological processes have found activation along the STS (Liebenthal et al. 2005; Narain et al. 2003; Obleser et al. 2006; Scott et al. 2000; Spitsyna et al. 2006; Vouloumanos et al. 2001), as have studies that manipulate psycholinguistic variables that tap phonological networks (Okada and Hickok 2006). Although a common view is that the phonological system is strongly left dominant, both lesion and imaging evidence (Hickok and Poeppel 2007) suggest a bilateral organization.

One currently unresolved question is the relative contribution of anterior vs. posterior STS regions in phonological processing. A majority of functional imaging studies targeting phonological processing in perception have highlighted regions in the posterior half of the STS (Hickok and Poeppel 2007). Other studies, however, have reported *anterior* STS activation in perceptual speech tasks (Mazoyer et al. 1993; Narain et al. 2003; Scott et al. 2000; Spitsyna et al. 2006). These studies involved sentence-level stimuli, raising the possibility that anterior STS regions may be responding to some other aspect of the stimuli such as its syntactic or prosodic organization (Friederici et al. 2000; Humphries et al. 2001, 2005, 2006; Vandenberghe et al. 2002). Lesion evidence indicates that damage to posterior temporal lobe areas is most predictive of auditory comprehension deficits (Bates et al. 2003). The weight of the available evidence, therefore, suggests that the critical portion of the STS that is involved in phonological-level processes is bounded anteriorly by the anterolateral-most aspect of Heschl's gyrus and posteriorly by the posterior-most extent of the Sylvian fissure (Hickok and Poeppel 2007).

15.4 Access to Conceptual-Semantic Information May Involve Middle Temporal Regions

Comprehension of speech involves more than just processing and recognizing phonological information in speech. It crucially involves using speech sound information to access conceptual-semantic representations. Although the organization of semantic knowledge in the brain is far from understood, a common view is that conceptual-semantic information is widely distributed throughout the cortex (Damasio and Damasio 1994; Gage and Hickok 2005; Hickok and Poeppel 2000, 2004, 2007; Martin 1998; Martin and Chao 2001; Mesulam 1998; Squire 1986). Access to this system via auditory-linguistic channels, however, may be more focal. The posterior, middle, and ventral temporal lobe (~BA 37) appears to be an important node in the interface between auditory/speech systems and conceptual-semantic knowledge (Fig. 15.1, posterior pink-shaded area). This conclusion is supported by lesion evidence showing that damage to this region results in semantic-level deficits in both comprehension and production (Chertkow et al. 1997; Hart and Gordon 1990; Hickok and Poeppel 2004, 2007).

Functional imaging studies have implicated these same regions in lexical-semantic processing. For example, Binder and colleagues asked subjects to make semantic decisions about auditorily presented words (Binder et al. 1997). In comparison to a tone-decision control task, semantic decisions strongly activated portions of the STS and middle temporal and inferior temporal gyri (in additional to frontal and parietal regions), but did not activate the superior temporal gyrus (STG). In the context of studies on phonological-level processes discussed above, a reasonable interpretation is that the STS activation reflects phonological aspects of word processing, whereas the more ventral activations, which do not show up reliably in studies of phonological processing, reflect postphonemic mechanisms involved in processing or accessing lexical-semantic information.

Similar conclusions are derived from studies of lexical-semantic processing that use different approaches. Some studies have found greater activation in inferior posterior temporal regions for words compared to nonwords (Binder et al. 2005; Rissman et al. 2003). This contrast should emphasize lexical-semantic processes as nonwords have minimal lexical-semantic associations. Posterior middle temporal regions have also been implicated in processing semantically ambiguous words. Rodd et al. found that listening to sentences that contained high levels of lexical ambiguity produced more activation in the left posterior MTG (Rodd et al. 2005).

Imaging studies of semantic priming, which also should highlight regions involved in lexical-semantic processing, have, however, led to a different conclusion. These studies (Copland et al. 2003; Rissman et al. 2003) have found a more anterior middle temporal site that shows a reduction in activation for semantically related, compared to semantically unrelated, word pairs (priming is typically reflected as a reduction of brain activity; Henson 2003). The implication of anterior temporal regions is not consistent with stroke-based lesion studies, as noted above. However, it is consistent with recent claims derived from studies of semantic dementia that the anterior temporal lobes play a critical role in the representation of conceptual knowledge (Hodges and Patterson 2007; Patterson et al. 2007).

Much work remains to be done in understanding the functional anatomy of semantic-related processes, particularly the relation between the posterior and anterior regions which have been implicated. It is possible to make the generalization that while phonemic-level processes involve auditory-responsive regions in the STS, higher-level lexical- and conceptual-semantic processes involve regions surrounding the STS, both ventrally and posteriorly.

15.5 Sensory Systems Participate in Speech Production

There is unequivocal evidence that posterior sensory-related cortex in the left, but not right, hemisphere participates in speech production. For example, damage to the left posterior temporal lobe often results not only in comprehension deficits but also in speech *production* deficits (Damasio 1991, 1992; Geschwind 1971; Goodglass 1993; Goodglass et al. 2001). Disruption to phonological systems appears to account for some of these production deficits. Damage to the left dorsal STG and/or the supramarginal gyrus/temporal-parietal junction is associated with conduction aphasia, a syndrome that is characterized by good comprehension but with frequent phonemic errors in speech production, naming difficulties that often involve tip-of-the-tongue states (implicating a breakdown in phonological encoding), and difficulty with verbatim repetition (Damasio and Damasio 1980; Goodglass 1992).[1] Conduction aphasia has classically been considered a disconnection syndrome involving damage to the arcuate fasciculus (Geschwind 1965). However, there is now good evidence that this syndrome results from cortical

[1]Although conduction aphasia is often characterized as a disorder of repetition, it is clear that the deficit extends well beyond this one task (Hickok et al. 2000). In fact, Wernicke first identified conduction aphasia as a disorder of speech production in the face of preserved comprehension (Wernicke 1874/1969). It was only later that Lichtheim introduced repetition as a convenient diagnostic tool for assessing the integrity of the link between sensory and motor-speech systems (Lichtheim 1885).

dysfunction (Anderson et al. 1999; Hickok et al. 2000). Thus, conduction aphasia provides evidence for the involvement of left posterior auditory-related brain regions in phonological aspects of speech production (Hickok 2000; Hickok et al. 2000).

Functional imaging evidence also implicates left superior posterior temporal regions in speech production generally (Hickok et al. 2000; Price et al. 1996) and phonological stages of the process in particular (Indefrey and Levelt 2000, 2004). With respect to the latter, the posterior portion of the left planum temporale region, which is within the distribution of lesions associated with conduction aphasia, activates during picture naming, exhibits length effects (Okada et al. 2003) and frequency effects (Graves et al. 2007), and has a time course of activation, measured electromagnetically, that is consistent with the phonological encoding stage of naming (Levelt et al. 1998).

Taken together, the lesion and physiological evidence reviewed in this section make a compelling argument for the involvement of left posterior superior temporal regions in phonological aspects of speech production.

15.6 The Posterior Planum Temporale Supports Sensorimotor Integration

If left posterior superior temporal regions are involved in phonological aspects of speech *production*, there must be a mechanism for interfacing posterior and anterior brain regions. The need for such a mechanism has long been acknowledged and, in classical models, was instantiated as a simple white-matter pathway, the arcuate fasciculus (Geschwind 1971). More recent proposals have argued, instead, for a *cortical* system that serves to integrate sensory and motor aspects of speech (Hickok et al. 2000, 2003; Hickok and Poeppel 2000, 2004, 2007; Warren et al. 2005), which is consistent with much research on sensorimotor integration systems studied in the context of the monkey visual system (Andersen 1997; Colby and Goldberg 1999; Milner and Goodale 1995).

A series of studies over the last several years have identified a cortical network for speech and related abilities (e.g., music), which has many of the properties exhibited by sensorimotor networks studied in other domains. These properties include sensorimotor responses, connectivity with frontal motor systems, motor effector specificity, and multisensory responses (Andersen 1997; Colby and Goldberg 1999). The speech-related network with these response properties includes an area (termed Spt) in the left posterior planum temporal (Okada and Hickok 2009) region (Fig. 15.1, posterior blue-shaded region) that has been argued to support sensorimotor integration for speech (Hickok et al. 2003). We will review the evidence for this claim below.

15.6.1 Spt Exhibits Sensorimotor Response Properties

A number of studies have demonstrated the existence of an area in the left posterior planum temporale that responds both during the perception and production of speech, even when speech is produced covertly (subvocally) so that there is no overt auditory feedback (Buchsbaum et al. 2001, 2005a, b; Hickok et al. 2003). Spt is not speech-specific, however. It responds equally well to the perception and (covert) production via humming of melodic stimuli (Hickok et al. 2003; Pa and Hickok 2008).

15.6.2 Spt Is Functionally Connected to Motor Speech Areas

Spt activity is tightly correlated with activity in frontal speech production-related areas, such as the pars opercularis (BA 44; Buchsbaum et al. 2001), suggesting that the two regions are functionally connected. Furthermore, cortex in the posterior portion of the planum temporale (area Tpt) has a cytoarchitectonic structure that is similar to BA44. Galaburda writes, "area Tpt ... exhibits a degree of specialization like that of Area 44 in Broca's region. It contains prominent pyramids in layer IIIc and a broad lamina IV....

the intimate relationship and similar evolutionary status of Areas 44 and Tpt allows for a certain functional overlap" (Galaburda 1982).

15.6.3 Spt Activity Is Modulated by Motor Effector Manipulations

In monkey, parietal cortex sensorimotor integration areas are organized around motor effector systems (e.g., ocular vs. manual actions in LIP and AIP; Andersen 1997; Colby and Goldberg 1999). Recent evidence suggests that Spt may be organized around the vocal tract effector system: Spt was less active when skilled pianists listened to and then imagined playing a novel melody than when they listened to and covertly hummed the same melody (Pa and Hickok 2008).

15.6.4 Spt Is Sensitive to Speech-Related Visual Stimuli

Many neurons in sensorimotor integration areas of the monkey parietal cortex are sensitive to inputs from more than one sensory modality (Andersen 1997). The planum temporale, while often thought to be an auditory area, also activates in response to sensory input from other modalities. For example, silent lip-reading has been shown to activate auditory cortex in the vicinity of the planum temporale (Calvert et al. 1997; Calvert and Campbell 2003). Although these studies typically report the location as "auditory cortex" including primary regions, group-based localizations in this region can be unreliable. Indeed, a recent fMRI study using individual subject analyses has found that activation to visual speech and activation using the standard Spt-defining auditory-motor task (listen then covertly produce) are found in the same regions of the left posterior planum temporale. Thus, Spt appears to be sensitive also to visual input that is relevant to vocal tract actions.

In summary, Spt exhibits all the features of sensorimotor integration areas as identified in the parietal cortex of the monkey. This suggests that Spt is a sensorimotor integration area for vocal tract actions (Pa and Hickok 2008), placing it in the context of a network of sensorimotor integration areas in the posterior parietal and temporal/parietal cortex, which receive multisensory input and are organized around motor effector systems (Andersen 1997). Although area Spt is not language specific, it counts sensorimotor integration for phonological information as a prominent function.

15.7 Summary

Data from functional imaging studies has augmented a long history of language-brain research based on traditional neuropsychological methods. This work converges on several broad conclusions that are particularly relevant to an understanding of the neural organization of speech processing. Human auditory cortex is hierarchically organized, with early areas primarily involved in the spectrotemporal analysis of acoustic signals. Higher-order representations/processes, such as those involved in the analysis of phonological information, involve auditory-related regions in the STS, which are probably several steps downstream from primary auditory cortex. Beyond these high-level auditory-related systems in the STS, portions of the middle and inferior temporal gyri are important for mapping auditory-related representations onto conceptual-semantic systems. These systems, involved in mapping acoustic input onto conceptual-semantic representations, comprise the ventral stream and are bilaterally organized in their early stages, becoming somewhat left dominant at the level of conceptual-semantic access. A dorsal stream connects portions of the auditory system to articulatory motor systems, thus enabling speech production and related functions. This circuit involves the posterior planum temporale (area Spt), which may function as a sensorimotor interface system for the vocal tract.

References

Andersen R (1997) Multimodal integration for the representation of space in the posterior parietal cortex. Philos Trans R Soc Lond Ser B Biol Sci 352:1421–1428

Anderson JM, Gilmore R et al (1999) Conduction aphasia and the arcuate fasciculus: a reexamination of the Wernicke-Geschwind model. Brain Lang 70:1–12

Bates E, Wilson SM et al (2003) Voxel-based lesion-symptom mapping. Nat Neurosci 6(5):448–450

Binder JR, Frost JA et al (1997) Human brain language areas identified by functional magnetic resonance imaging. J Neurosci 17:353–362

Binder JR, Frost JA et al (2000) Human temporal lobe activation by speech and nonspeech sounds. Cereb Cortex 10:512–528

Binder JR, Westbury CF et al (2005) Distinct brain systems for processing concrete and abstract concepts. J Cogn Neurosci 17(6):905–917

Buchsbaum B, Hickok G et al (2001) Role of left posterior superior temporal gyrus in phonological processing for speech perception and production. Cogn Sci 25:663–678

Buchsbaum BR, Olsen RK et al (2005a) Human dorsal and ventral auditory streams subserve rehearsal-based and echoic processes during verbal working memory. Neuron 48(4):687–697

Buchsbaum BR, Olsen RK et al (2005b) Reading, hearing, and the planum temporale. Neuroimage 24(2):444–454

Calvert GA, Campbell R (2003) Reading speech from still and moving faces: the neural substrates of visible speech. J Cogn Neurosci 15:57–70

Calvert GA, Bullmore ET et al (1997) Activation of auditory cortex during silent lipreading. Science 276:593–596

Chertkow H, Bub D et al (1997) On the status of object concepts in aphasia. Brain Lang 58(2):203–232

Colby CL, Goldberg ME (1999) Space and attention in parietal cortex. Annu Rev Neurosci 22:319–349

Copland DA, de Zubicaray GI et al (2003) Brain activity during automatic semantic priming revealed by event-related functional magnetic resonance imaging. Neuroimage 20(1):302–310

Damasio H (1991) Neuroanatomical correlates of the aphasias. In: Sarno M (ed) Acquired aphasia, 2nd edn. Academic, San Diego, pp 45–71

Damasio AR (1992) Aphasia. N Engl J Med 326:531–539

Damasio H, Damasio AR (1980) The anatomical basis of conduction aphasia. Brain 103:337–350

Damasio AR, Damasio H (1994) Cortical systems for retrieval of concrete knowledge: the convergence zone framework. In: Koch C, Davis JL (eds) Large-scale neuronal theories of the brain. MIT Press, Cambridge, pp 61–74

Dronkers NF, Redfern BB et al (2000) The neural architecture of language disorders. In: Gazzaniga MS (ed) The new cognitive neurosciences. MIT Press, Cambridge, pp 949–958

Fellows LK, Heberlein AS et al (2005) Method matters: an empirical study of impact in cognitive neuroscience. J Cogn Neurosci 17(6):850–858

Friederici AD, Meyer M et al (2000) Auditory language comprehension: an event-related fMRI study on the processing of syntactic and lexical information. Brain Lang 74:289–300

Gage N, Hickok G (2005) Multiregional cell assemblies, temporal binding, and the representation of conceptual knowledge in cortex: a modern theory by a "classical" neurologist, Carl Wernicke. Cortex 41:823–832

Galaburda AM (1982) Histology, architectonics, and asymmetry of language areas. In: Arbib MA, Caplan D, Marshall JC (eds) Neural models of language processes. Academic, San Diego, pp 435–445

Geschwind N (1965) Disconnexion syndromes in animals and man. Brain 88(237–294):585–644

Geschwind N (1971) Aphasia. N Engl J Med 284:654–656

Goodglass H (1992) Diagnosis of conduction aphasia. In: Kohn SE (ed) Conduction aphasia. Lawrence Erlbaum, Hillsdale, pp 39–49

Goodglass H (1993) Understanding aphasia. Academic, San Diego

Goodglass H, Kaplan E et al (2001) The assessment of aphasia and related disorders, 3rd edn. Lippincott Williams and Wilkins, Philadelphia

Graves WW, Grabowski TJ et al (2007) A neural signature of phonological access: distinguishing the effects of word frequency from familiarity and length in overt picture naming. J Cogn Neurosci 19:617–631

Hart JJ, Gordon B (1990) Delineation of single-word semantic comprehension deficits in aphasia, with anatomical correlation. Ann Neurol 27:226–231

Henson RNA (2003) Neuroimaging studies of priming. Prog Neurobiol 70:53–81

Hickok G (2000) Speech perception, conduction aphasia, and the functional neuroanatomy of language. In: Grodzinsky Y, Shapiro L, Swinney D (eds) Language and the brain. Academic, San Diego, pp 87–104

Hickok G, Poeppel D (2000) Towards a functional neuroanatomy of speech perception. Trends Cogn Sci 4:131–138

Hickok G, Poeppel D (2004) Dorsal and ventral streams: a framework for understanding aspects of the functional anatomy of language. Cognition 92:67–99

Hickok G, Poeppel D (2007) The cortical organization of speech processing. Nat Rev Neurosci 8(5): 393–402

Hickok G, Erhard P et al (2000) A functional magnetic resonance imaging study of the role of left posterior superior temporal gyrus in speech production: implications for the explanation of conduction aphasia. Neurosci Lett 287:156–160

Hickok G, Buchsbaum B et al (2003) Auditory-motor interaction revealed by fMRI: speech, music, and working memory in area Spt. J Cogn Neurosci 15:673–682

Hillis AE (2007) Aphasia: progress in the last quarter of a century. Neurology 69(2):200–213

Hodges JR, Patterson K (2007) Semantic dementia: a unique clinicopathological syndrome. Lancet Neurol 6(11):1004–1014

Humphries C, Willard K et al (2001) Role of anterior temporal cortex in auditory sentence comprehension: an fMRI study. Neuroreport 12:1749–1752

Humphries C, Love T et al (2005) Response of anterior temporal cortex to syntactic and prosodic manipulations during sentence processing. Hum Brain Mapp 26:128–138

Humphries C, Binder JR et al (2006) Syntactic and semantic modulation of neural activity during auditory sentence comprehension. J Cogn Neurosci 18(4):665–679

Indefrey P, Levelt WJM (2000) The neural correlates of language production. In: Gazzaniga MS (ed) The new cognitive neurosciences. MIT Press, Cambridge, pp 845–865

Indefrey P, Levelt WJ (2004) The spatial and temporal signatures of word production components. Cognition 92(1–2):101–144

Kaas JH, Hackett TA (2000) Subdivisions of auditory cortex and processing streams in primates. Proc Natl Acad Sci U S A 97(22):11793–11799

Kaas JH, Hackett TA et al (1999) Auditory processing in primate cerebral cortex. Curr Opin Neurobiol 9(2):164–170

Levelt WJM, Praamstra P et al (1998) An MEG study of picture naming. J Cogn Neurosci 10:553–567

Lichtheim L (1885) On aphasia. Brain 7:433–484

Liebenthal E, Binder JR et al (2005) Neural substrates of phonemic perception. Cereb Cortex 15(10):1621–1631

Martin A (1998) The organization of semantic knowledge and the origin of words in the brain. In: Jablonski NG, Aiello LC (eds) The origins and diversification of language. California Academy of Sciences, San Francisco, pp 69–88

Martin A, Chao LL (2001) Semantic memory and the brain: structure and processes. Curr Opin Neurobiol 11(2):194–201

Mazoyer BM, Tzourio N et al (1993) The cortical representation of speech. J Cogn Neurosci 5:467–479

Mesulam M-M (1998) From sensation to cognition. Brain 121:1013–1052

Milner AD, Goodale MA (1995) The visual brain in action. Oxford University Press, Oxford

Narain C, Scott SK et al (2003) Defining a left-lateralized response specific to intelligible speech using fMRI. Cereb Cortex 13(12):1362–1368

Obleser J, Zimmermann J et al (2006) Multiple stages of auditory speech perception reflected in event-related fMRI. Cereb Cortex 17:2251–2257

Okada K, Hickok G (2006) Identification of lexical-phonological networks in the superior temporal sulcus using fMRI. Neuroreport 17:1293–1296

Okada K, Hickok G (2009) Two cortical mechanisms support the integration of visual and auditory speech: a hypothesis and preliminary data. Neurosci Lett 452(3):219–223

Okada K, Smith KR et al (2003) Word length modulates neural activity in auditory cortex during covert object naming. Neuroreport 14:2323–2326

Pa J, Hickok G (2008) A parietal-temporal sensory-motor integration area for the human vocal tract: evidence from an fMRI study of skilled musicians. Neuropsychologia 46:362–368

Patterson K, Nestor PJ et al (2007) Where do you know what you know? The representation of semantic knowledge in the human brain. Nat Rev Neurosci 8(12):976–987

Price CJ, Wise RJS et al (1996) Hearing and saying: the functional neuro-anatomy of auditory word processing. Brain 119:919–931

Rauschecker JP (1998) Cortical processing of complex sounds. Curr Opin Neurobiol 8(4):516–521

Rissman J, Eliassen JC et al (2003) An event-related FMRI investigation of implicit semantic priming. J Cogn Neurosci 15(8):1160–1175

Rodd JM, Davis MH et al (2005) The neural mechanisms of speech comprehension: fMRI studies of semantic ambiguity. Cereb Cortex 15:1261–1269

Romanski LM, Tian B et al (1999) Dual streams of auditory afferents target multiple domains in the primate prefrontal cortex. Nat Neurosci 2:1131–1136

Scott SK (2005) Auditory processing - speech, space and auditory objects. Curr Opin Neurobiol 15(2):197–201

Scott SK, Blank CC et al (2000) Identification of a pathway for intelligible speech in the left temporal lobe. Brain 123:2400–2406

Spitsyna G, Warren JE et al (2006) Converging language streams in the human temporal lobe. J Neurosci 26(28):7328–7336

Squire LR (1986) Mechanisms of memory. Science 232:1612–1619

Vandenberghe R, Nobre AC et al (2002) The response of left temporal cortex to sentences. J Cogn Neurosci 14(4):550–560

Vouloumanos A, Kiehl KA et al (2001) Detection of sounds in the auditory stream: event-related fMRI evidence for differential activation to speech and non-speech. J Cogn Neurosci 13(7):994–1005

Warren JE, Wise RJ et al (2005) Sounds do-able: auditory-motor transformations and the posterior temporal plane. Trends Neurosci 28(12):636–643

Wernicke C (1874/1969) The symptom complex of aphasia: a psychological study on an anatomical basis. In: Cohen RS, Wartofsky MW (eds) Boston studies in the philosophy of science. D. Reidel, Dordrecht, pp 34–97

16

Mapping of Recovery from Poststroke Aphasia: Comparison of PET and fMRI

Wolf-Dieter Heiss

16.1 The Principle of Activation Studies

The energy demand of the brain is very high and relies almost entirely on the oxidative metabolism of glucose. Glucose metabolized in neuronal cell bodies mainly supports cellular, vegetative, and housekeeping functions, for example, axonal transport, biosynthesis of nucleic acids, proteins, and lipids, as well as other energy-consuming processes not related directly to action potentials. Therefore, the energy demand of neuronal cell bodies is relatively low and essentially unaffected by neuronal functional activation (Sokoloff 1999). A larger portion of energy consumption is required for signaling, mainly action potential propagation and postsynaptic ion fluxes; this might account for up to 87% of the total energy consumed, with only 13% expended in maintaining membrane resting potential (Attwell and Laughlin 2001). As a consequence, the rate of glucose consumption of neuronal cell bodies is essentially unaffected by functional activation, whereas increases in metabolism (and in the coupled regional blood flow) evoked by functional activation are confined to synapse-rich regions, that is, the neutrophil that contains axonal terminals, dendritic processes, and the astrocytic processes that envelop the synapses (Magistretti 2004). The magnitudes of these increases are linearly related to the frequency of action potentials in the afferent pathways, and increases of metabolism and blood flow in the projection zones occur regardless of whether the pathway is excitatory or inhibitory. Only at the next downstream projection zones, glucose utilization (and, as a consequence, blood supply) is depressed in inhibited neurons and increased in excited neurons.

Mapping of neuronal activity in the brain can be primarily achieved by quantitation of the regional cerebral metabolic rate for glucose (rCMRGlc), as introduced for autoradiographic experimental studies by Sokoloff (Sokoloff 1999) and adapted for positron emission tomography (PET) in humans (Reivich et al. 1979). Functional mapping, as it is widely used now, relies primarily on the hemodynamic response assuming a close association between energy metabolism and blood flow. While it is well documented that increases in blood flow and glucose consumption are closely coupled during neuronal activation, the increase in oxygen consumption is considerably delayed, leading to a decreased oxygen extraction fraction (OEF) during activation (Mintun et al. 2001). PET detects and, if required, can quantify changes in CBF and CMRGlc accompanying different activation states of the brain tissue. The regional values of CBF or CMRGlc represent the brain activity due to a specific state, task, or stimulus, in comparison to the

W.-D. Heiss (✉)
Max Planck Institute for Metabolism Research, Cologne, Germany
e-mail: wdh@nf.mpg.de

S. Ulmer, O. Jansen (eds.), *fMRI*, https://doi.org/10.1007/978-3-030-41874-8_16

resting condition, and color-coded maps can be analyzed or coregistered to morphologic images. Due to the radioactivity of the necessary tracers, activation studies with PET are limited to a maximum of 12 doses of ^{15}O-labeled tracers, for example, 12 flow scans, or two doses of ^{18}F-labeled tracers, for example, two metabolic scans. Especially for studies of glucose consumption, the time to metabolic equilibrium (20–40 min), as well as the time interval between measurements required for isotope decay (HT for ^{18}F 108 min, for ^{15}O 2 min), must be taken into consideration.

Functional magnetic resonance imaging (fMRI) measures signals that depend on the differential magnetic properties of oxygenated and deoxygenated hemoglobin, termed the blood-oxygen-level-dependent (BOLD) signal, which gives an estimate of changes in oxygen availability (Ogawa et al. 1990). This means that mainly the amount of deoxyhemoglobin in small blood vessels is recorded, which depends on the flow of well-oxygenated arterial blood (CBF), on the outflow of O_2 to the tissue ($CMRO_2$) and on the cerebral blood volume (CBV) (Turner et al. 1997). The magnitude of these changes in signal intensity relative to the resting conditions are color coded to produce fMRI images that map changes in brain function, which can be superimposed on the anatomical image. This results in a spatial resolution of fMRI of 1–3 mm with a temporal resolution of approximately 10 s. As fMRI does not involve ionizing radiation and, thus, is also used without limitations in healthy subjects, allowing more rapid signal acquisition and more flexible experimental setups, it has become the dominant technique for functional imaging. Therefore, fMRI has become the most used method to demonstrate changes in activation patterns during recovery from aphasia (Hartwigsen and Saur 2019; Price 2012). There are some advantages of PET, however—physiologically specific measures, better quantitation, better signal-to-noise ratio, fewer artifacts, and actual activated and reference values—which support its continued use especially in complex clinical situations and in combination with special stimulating techniques, such as transcranial magnetic stimulation (TMS).

16.2 Language Activation in Healthy Subjects

The capacity to understand and to speak language is strictly lateralized in most subjects to the dominant hemisphere. With a few exceptions, this is the left hemisphere in right-handers, whereas in left-handers, language may be represented in either hemisphere or even bilaterally (Knecht et al. 2002; Thiel et al. 1998). In addition to language dominance, details of the anatomical localization of sensory and motor language areas (Wernicke's and Broca's region) may vary considerably even in normal individuals. A considerable variety of language activation paradigms have been applied for localization of language functions by PET and fMRI (Hickok and Poeppel 2007; Petersen et al. 1988; Price 2000; Wise 2003), producing a vast amount of partly contradictory data (Demonet et al. 1996). For the analysis of aphasia after stroke or due to brain tumors, the application of a simplified scheme may be justified (Fig. 16.1; Price 2000).

The processing of hearing words activates bilaterally the upper temporal gyrus, and the semantic attribution to a meaningful content is achieved in left posterior temporal, temporo-parietal, and anterior lower cortical areas. For the production of speech, the activity in the posterior upper temporal sulcus and in the left posterior lower temporal cortex is increased. The activity in the posterior upper temporal sulci is further increased, if words or sequences are repeated or read. In contrast, the left posterior lower temporal cortex in the neighborhood of the middle fusiform semantic area is activated by word fluency. This area is participating in lexical speech production. Independently, planning of articulation activates the left anterior insula and the bordering frontal operculum. Phonologic word retrieval requires the integration of the anterior insula/operculum and the posterior upper temporal sulcus or left posterior lower temporal gyrus. Finally, the bilateral sensomotoric cortex is activated for the motoric control of speech production, and the hearing of the spoken response augments the activation in the upper temporal gyrus.

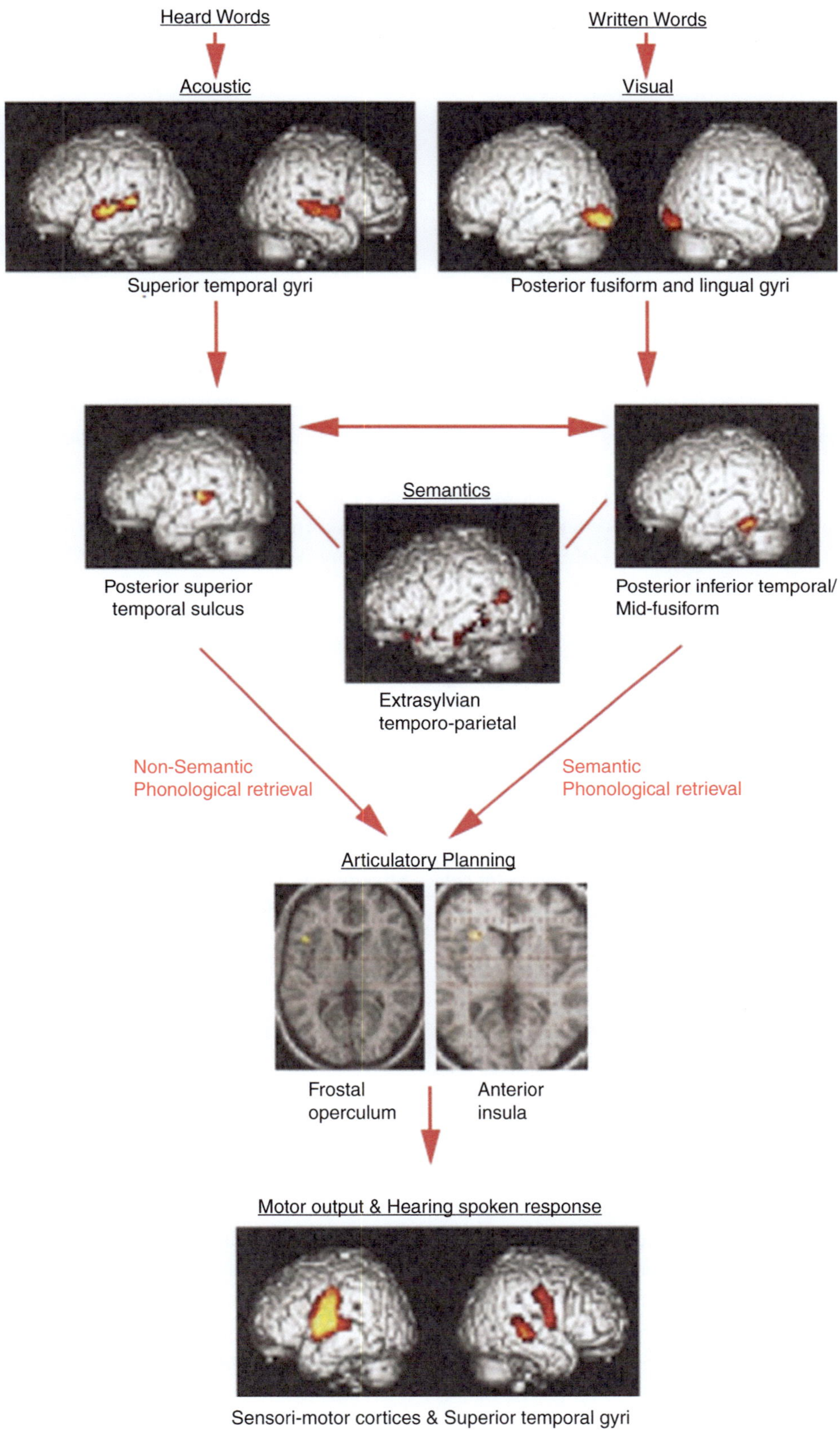

Fig. 16.1 Proposed neurological and cognitive model of language with brain areas activated by different tasks. (From Price (2000))

In the processing of written words, the same areas are involved. Reading selectively activates the posterior fusiform and lingual gyrus, which are also involved in picture naming. For reading, the visual cortex and the posterior upper temporal sulci are activated, which contribute to the functional integration of the language network. According to this model, the function of the Wernicke region is represented in the upper part of the sulcus temporalis, the sulcus temporalis posterior superior; the anterior insula and not the Broca's area is responsible for planning articulation; the gyrus angularis is involved in semantic connection and not specific for visualization of words; the meaning of words is located in the left lower and middle temporal gyrus; reading and retrieval of names activate the posterior lower temporal lobe. For these functions—and also for the severity of functional damage—the hierarchy of individual areas within the network and the dominance of left cortical regions are of utmost importance (Heiss and Thiel 2006), which are induced and manifested by collateral and transcallosal inhibition (Karbe et al. 1998; Nudo et al. 1996).

It has to be kept in mind that all usual language functions, which are complex and require integration of several partial functions, activate larger parts of the bilateral network. For instance, the retrieval of substantives and verbs activates large areas in the left dorsomedial prefrontal cortex and the anterior cingulum as well as the supplementary motor area. The processing of meaningful connections activates the left middle temporal gyrus, the left and right temporal pole, as well as the left prefrontal area. Hearing and processing of nouns and generating verbs in relation to nouns involve a network consisting of pars opercularis and triangularis of the left lower frontal gyrus, the posterior part of the temporal sulcus up to the planum temporale, and the anterior part of the left lower temporal gyrus. In this network, even some parts of the cerebellum and of the basal ganglia are integrated (Booth et al. 2007). These complex activation patterns involving widely distributed areas impair the prediction of severity and recovery of speech disturbances caused by infarcts or other localized brain damage.

16.3 Poststroke Aphasia

Aphasia is a severely incapacitating symptom of stroke and is a main cause of functional disturbance. Estimates suggest that more than 20% of patients suffering a stroke develop aphasia and 10–18% of survivors are left with a persistent speech deficit (Wade et al. 1986). Most patients with aphasia due to acute nonprogressive brain damage, such as in the case of stroke or head injury, show some degree of recovery of language function during the days, months, or even years following the initial insult. The recuperation is variable, ranging from the hardly noticeable improvement of auditory comprehension of the global aphasia to the apparently complete recovery of the patient with mild fluent aphasia due to small subcortical stroke. It is also well known that improvement can be observed not only in patients submitted to language rehabilitation but also in cases that have not undergone any specific treatment.

16.4 Disturbance of Regional Metabolism and Flow Versus Severity and Persistence of Language Deficit

Studies of glucose metabolism after stroke (Cappa et al. 1997) have shown metabolic disturbances in the ipsilateral hemisphere caused by the lesion and contralateral hemisphere caused by functional deactivation (diaschisis; Feeney and Baron 1986). Most studies have been performed in right-handed individuals with language dominance in the left hemisphere. The left temporo-parietal region, in particular, the angular gyrus, the supramarginal gyrus, and the lateral and transverse superior temporal gyrus (STG), is most frequently and consistently impaired, and the degree of impairment is related to the severity of aphasia (Karbe et al. 1989; Metter et al. 1990). In contrast, metabolic impairment in subcortical structures is related mainly to language fluency and other behavioral aspects, but not to aphasia severity (Metter et al. 1988). In patients with aphasia attributable to purely subcortical strokes, deactivation of temporo-parietal cortex is regularly found, which is probably responsible for the aphasic symptoms (Kumar et al. 1996).

The recovery of metabolism in both the hemispheres was correlated with the recovery of aphasia. One specific region crucial for the recovery of language perception has been found in the left temporo-parietal cortex (Karbe et al. 1989; Metter et al. 1987) and metabolic disturbance in these areas is related to outcome (Heiss et al. 1993). Investigations in the subacute state after stroke showed a highly significant correlation with language performance assessed at follow-up after 2 years (Karbe et al. 1995). The receptive language disorder is correlated with rCMRGlc in the left temporal cortex, and word fluency is correlated with rCMRGlc in the left prefrontal cortex. These results indicate that the functional disturbance as measured by rCMRGlc in speech-relevant brain regions early after stroke is predictive of the eventual outcome of aphasia. However, not only functional deactivation (diaschisis) but also neuronal loss may contribute to metabolic and perfusional changes in the neighborhood of the infarct, and the condition of the surrounding tissue may affect the recovery of individual patients. In this context, it is important to note that early reperfusion to specific areas is able to restore disturbed function, as demonstrated for the recovery of naming by reperfusion to the key areas BA37, BA 44/45 (Broca), and BA 22 (Wernicke; Hillis et al. 2006).

16.5 Changes in Activation Patterns Versus Recovery of Language Function

On this basis, it is not surprising that in patients with a poor outcome of poststroke aphasia, metabolism in the hemisphere outside the infarct was significantly less than in those with good language recovery, indicating significant cell loss caused by the ischemic episode outside the ischemic core (Heiss et al. 1993). In addition, the functionality of the network was reduced in patients with an eventual poor outcome; during task performance, patients with an eventual good recovery predominantly activated structures in the ipsilateral hemisphere. It must be kept in mind that aphasia symptoms—and consequently also activation patterns—improve with the restoration of regional blood flow (Jordan and Hillis 2006).

One of the central issues of aphasia research is the question why recovery from aphasia is taking place and what the responsible mechanisms for this recovery are. Converging evidence from clinical studies and neural imaging studies of aphasic patients suggests that primary candidates for recovery in right-handed, left-hemisphere language-dominant patients include undamaged portions of the language network in the left hemisphere and—to a lesser extent—homologous right-hemisphere areas (Rosen et al. 2000). Since the language network is not confined to the dominant hemisphere, the role of the right hemisphere after infarcts in the left hemisphere has been addressed in several studies. Generally, more right-hemispheric activations were seen in the subacute phase of an infarct with language activation than in normals with the same tasks (Ohyama et al. 1996; Price and Crinion 2005; Saur et al. 2006; Weiller et al. 1995). Despite such responses in the right superior temporal gyrus, especially in fluent Wernicke's patients (Musso et al. 1999; Weiller et al. 1995) and in the inferior frontal gyrus (Ohyama et al. 1996), efficient restoration of language is usually achieved only if left temporal areas are preserved and can be reintegrated into the functional network (Gainotti 1993; Basso et al. 1989). Only the basic function of mere word repetition appears to be sufficiently supported by sole right-hemisphere activation (Berthier et al. 1991). Based on their study in chronic nonfluent aphasia patients, Belin et al. (1996) suggested that the increased activation within the right hemisphere may be a marker of failed or faulty recovery attempts in the sense of maladaptive plasticity or the breakdown of normal interhemispheric control within the distributed neural network. Language recovery in the months immediately after aphasia onset was associated with regression of functional depression (diaschisis) in structurally unaffected regions, in particular in the right hemisphere (Cappa et al. 1997; Saur et al. 2006).

Right-hemispheric activations after left frontal or temporal-parietal damage are not related to the level of recovery (Fernandez et al. 2004), but may reflect transcallosal inhibition as a maladaptive neuronal reorganization rather than functional compensation (Price and Crinion 2005). Although the brain recruits right-hemispheric regions for speech processing when the left-hemispheric centers are impaired (Raboyeau et al. 2008), outcome studies reveal that this strategy is significantly less effective than repair of the speech-relevant network in adults (Karbe et al. 1998). The effectiveness of right-hemispheric compensation appears to be higher in childhood than later (Muller et al. 1998). In studies of reorganization of the functional network in the course of aphasia, it is important to take into consideration the specificity of the tasks, the influence of site and extent of lesion, and the effect of treatment focused on a particular language domain on the recruitment of different aspects of the language network, especially if compensatory treatment to access limited functional responses would stimulate only required pathways and would do little to stimulate reorganization of the language system (Thompson 2000).

Changes in the activation pattern induced by repeating words in the course after ischemic stroke were related to recovery from poststroke aphasia (Heiss et al. 1999). Repeating words activated blood flow in ten normal controls by more than 10% relative to resting condition in both upper temporal gyri, by 5–10% in planum temporale and Heschl gyrus of both sides and in the lower part of the central gyrus of the left side, and by less than 5% in the left Broca's area. This test procedure was applied to 23 patients with aphasia of different types. Morphological defects were defined on MRI/CT, and the patients were grouped according to the site of the lesion. Activation PET studies were performed in the subacute stage approximately 2 weeks after the stroke and repeated 6 weeks later. On matched MRIs, regions of interest were defined in 14 identified structures of the bilateral language-related network.

The three groups of aphasic patients showed different patterns of activation in the acute and chronic phase, and their improvement was different: Although subcortical and frontal infarcts improved considerably in several tests, temporal infarcts showed only little improvement. These differences in improvement of speech deficits were reflected in different patterns of activation in the course after stroke (Fig. 16.2). The subcortical and frontal groups improved substantially and activated the right inferior frontal gyrus and the right superior temporal gyrus (STG) at baseline and regained regional left STG activation at follow-up. The temporal group improved only in word comprehension; it activated the left Broca's area and supplementary motor areas at baseline and the precentral gyrus bilaterally as well as the right STG at follow-up, but could not reactivate the left STG. These differential activation patterns were also obvious when subcortical and frontal infarcts were grouped together according to the extent of improvement: Those with a decrease in Token test errors by more than 50% could activate the left STG; those with a more unfavorable and unsatisfactory outcome were not able to do this. Similar reactivation patterns were observed in smaller groups of patients (Cao et al. 1999; Warburton et al. 1999). A recent study with repeated fMRI and parallel language testing from the acute to the chronic stage after stroke demonstrated a similar pattern (Saur et al. 2006). All 14 patients recovered clinically as shown by a set of aphasia tests. In the acute phase (mean, 1.8 days poststroke), group analysis showed little early activation of noninfarcted left-hemispheric language structures, while in the subacute phase (12.1 days poststroke), a large increase of activation in the bilateral language network, with a peak in the right Broca homologue, was observed. In the chronic phase (1321 days poststroke), a normalization of activation with a reshift to left-hemispheric areas was observed. This reorganization with recruitment of homologue language zones correlated with improvement, the normalization possibly reflected recovery and consolidation of the language system.

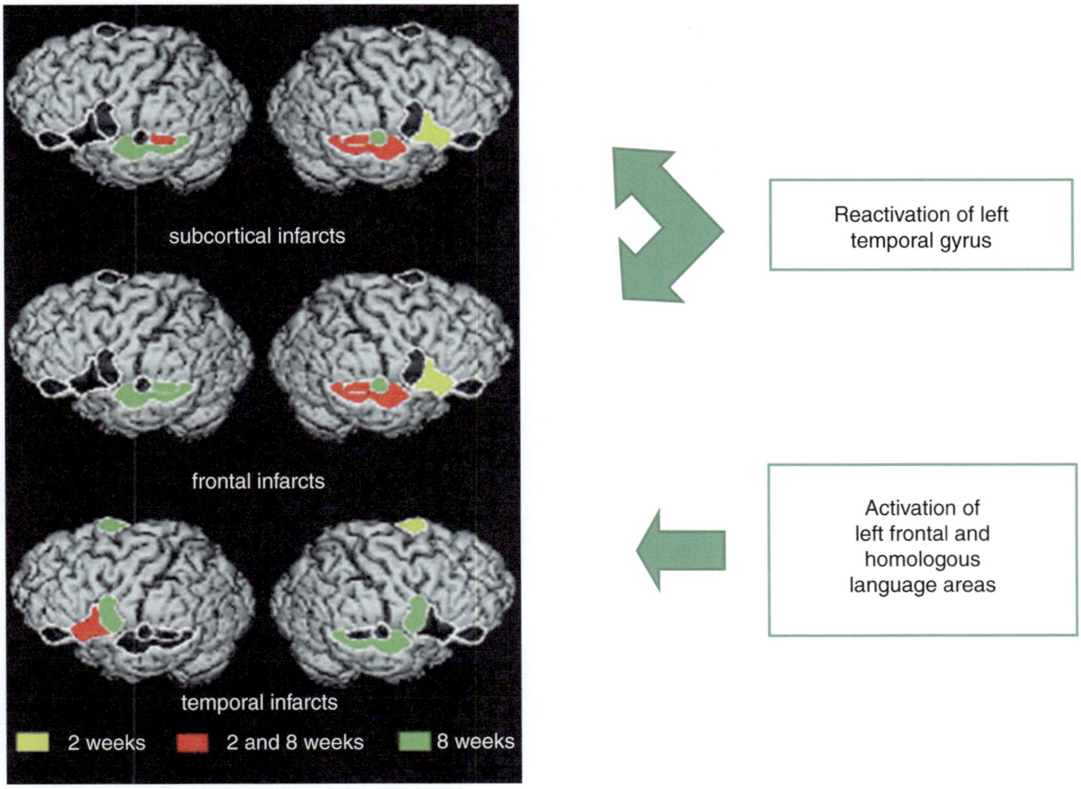

Fig. 16.2 Activation patterns in patients with left-hemispheric stroke 2 and 8 weeks after stroke. In the case of subcortical and frontal infarction, the left temporal areas are reactivated, correlating to better recovery of language function. (From Heiss et al. (1999))

16.6 Effect of Treatment in Poststroke Aphasia

Although the effect of physiotherapy on the improvement of sensorimotor deficits is unchallenged, the efficiency of speech therapy is still controversial, with several randomized controlled trials yielding no difference in outcome between treated and untreated groups (Ferro et al. 1999; Greener et al. 2001a). Many trials were undertaken to enhance the recovery from aphasia with adjuvant pharmacotherapy, but again, only a few studies demonstrated efficacy: In a double-blind placebo-controlled study, Walker-Batson et al. (2001) observed a significantly increased gain in score in patients treated with dextroamphetamine before speech therapy sessions compared to the placebo group, but the difference was not significant at 6 months' follow-up. Similarly, donepezil improved the effect of speech therapy only temporarily (Berthier et al. 2006). A large Cochrane Review (Greener et al. 2001b) identified piracetam as the only drug with a significant effect on recovery of language, which was also observed in a large multicenter trial (Orgogozo 1998). In order to investigate the question if the effect of piracetam is reflected in altered activation patterns, we performed a study in 24 patients with aphasia after stroke (Kessler et al. 2000). All these patients had speech therapy and were randomly assigned to placebo or 2 × 2.4 g piracetam. With respect to performance in the aphasia tests, the piracetam group did significantly better especially in subtests reflecting the ability for spontaneous speech, whereas the placebo experienced—as the verum group—improvements in Token test, reading and writing, and comprehension. It was impressive to see that these differences in improvement were also reflected in differences in the achieved activation patterns: In the piracetam group, the increase in activation was significantly higher in the left transverse temporal gyrus, the left triangular part of the inferior frontal gyrus, and the left posterior temporal gyrus after the treatment period compared with the initial measures. In the right inferior frontal gyrus, a trend toward a decrease in activation was observed. The placebo group showed an increase in the activation effect only in the left vocalization area, which is the inferior part of the precentral gyrus where the primary motor area of mouth, tongue, and larynx is localized. It might be concluded from the controlled clinical trials and our study of activation patterns that piracetam as an adjuvant to speech therapy improves recovery of various language functions and that this effect is accompanied by task-related flow activation in eloquent areas of the left hemisphere. This again points to the important role of (re)activated areas in the left hemisphere in the recovery of language function. Other imaging studies with individualized aphasia treatment in small numbers of patients did not show conclusive changes in fMRI activation patterns (review in Crinion and Leff 2007).

16.7 Combination of Repetitive Transcranial Magnetic Stimulation (rTMS) with Activated Imaging

rTMS is a noninvasive procedure to create electric currents in discrete brain areas (Pascual-Leone et al. 2002), which, depending on frequency, intensity, and duration, can lead to transient increases and decreases in the excitability of the affected cortex. Low frequencies of rTMS (below 5 Hz) can suppress the excitability of the cortex, while higher-frequency stimulation (5–20 Hz) leads to an increase in cortical excitability (Kobayashi and Pascual-Leone 2003). As in the motor system (Chen et al. 1997), it can also be applied to identify the various areas involved in language processing and production by a selective disturbance of partial function with low-frequency rTMS (Kapoor 2017; Leon Ruiz et al. 2018; Norise and Hamilton 2016). Most frequently, rTMS is used in the so-called lesion mode to interfere with normal brain function. In our studies cited below, rTMS was applied with 4 Hz at resting motor threshold for 10–30 s. These parameter settings were chosen because Wassermann et al. (2002) has shown that 4 Hz is the lowest frequency that consistently interferes with language function and simultaneously minimizes the risk of inducing seizures.

Increases in relative cerebral blood volume (CBV) in contralateral homologous language regions during overt propositional speech fMRI in chronic, nonfluent aphasia patients indicated overactivation of right language homologues (Naeser et al. 2004). This right-hemisphere overactivation may represent a maladaptive strategy, as suggested previously by Belin et al. (1996) and Rosen et al. (2000) in their studies with chronic, nonfluent aphasia patients. This overactivation in the right-hemisphere homologous language areas during overt propositional speech can be interpreted as a result of decreased transcallosal inhibition due to damage of the specialized and lateralized speech areas (Karbe et al. 1998). TMS studies by Martin et al. (2004) and Naeser et al. (2005a) have reported improved picture-naming ability in chronic nonfluent aphasia patients following a series of ten 20-min 1 Hz rTMS sessions to suppress a portion of the right pars triangularis area in the right Broca's area. Picture-naming ability was significantly improved at 2 months following ten 20-min rTMS sessions (90% of motor threshold). The authors hypothesized that suppression of the right pars triangularis modulated the bihemispheric neural network for naming, resulting in improved picture naming after the rTMS treatment series.

Both types of inhibition—collateral ipsilateral and transcallosal contralateral—can be demonstrated by simultaneous rTMS and PET activation studies (Thiel et al. 2006). In six normal male volunteers, the Broca's area, as defined by maximal activation during verb generation in the left inferior frontal gyrus, was stimulated by rTMS (4 Hz at resting motor threshold for 30 s) to interfere with normal language function.

Interference with language function (positive TMS effect) is usually classified into three types on the behavioral level: (1) no response to the stimulus (e.g., no verb generated to a presented noun), (2) wrong response to the stimulus (e.g., a verb is generated which is not semantically related to the presented noun), and (3) the reaction time latency to the stimulus is changed (e.g., faster response means facilitation, slower response means inhibition). At rest, rTMS decreased blood flow ipsilaterally and contralaterally. During verb generation, rCBF was decreased during rTMS ipsilateral under the coil, but increased ipsilateral outside the coil and in the contralateral homologous area (Fig. 16.3). The effect of rTMS was accompanied by a prolongation of reaction time latencies to verbal stimuli.

The role of activation in the right hemisphere for residual language performance can be investigated by combining rTMS with functional imaging, for example, PET (Siebner et al. 2001). Such an approach was used in 11 patients with predominantly nonfluent aphasia 2 weeks after left-sided middle cerebral artery infarction (Winhuisen et al. 2005). rTMS stimulation sites were selected according to maximum flow activation within left and right inferior frontal gyrus (IFG). Of these patients, three activated the left and eight the bilateral IFG. rTMS (4 Hz, as described above) resulted in increased reaction time latency or error rate in the word-generation task in five patients with right IFG activation, indicating essential language function. In a verbal fluency task, these patients had a lower performance than patients with effects of rTMS only over the left IFG, suggesting a less effective compensatory potential of right-sided network areas. These results were supported by studies in tumor patients.

As suggested previously (Belin et al. 1996; Rosen et al. 2000), the overactivation of the right-hemisphere homologous areas might represent a maladaptive strategy, and the activated right-hemisphere centers might actually hinder the recovery of the primary centers in the left hemisphere. Several case reports indicate persistent positive effects of repeatedly administered inhibitory rTMS to the right-hemispheric Broca homologue in patients with chronic aphasia (Naeser et al. 2005a, b), but a favorable response was not

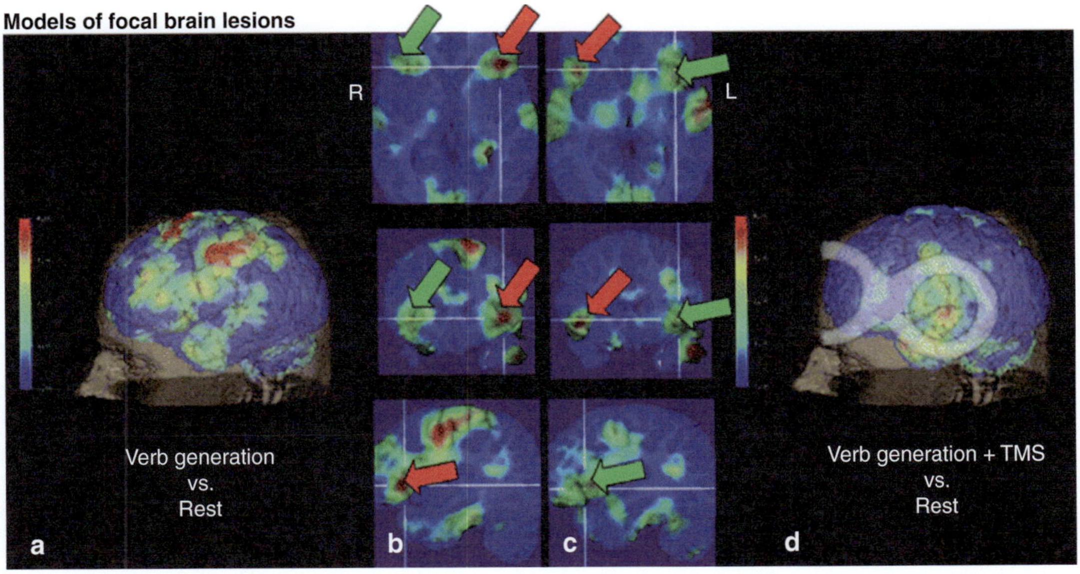

Fig. 16.3 Effect of repetitive transcranial magnetic stimulation on activation pattern by verb generation. Activation pattern (**a**) and coil position (**d**) shown in 3D rendering. Images in 3D (**b**) show activation of left inferior frontal gyrus during verb generation (*red arrows*); images (**c**) clearly show the decreased activation on the left (*green arrow*) and increased activity on the right side (*red arrows*) during rTMS interference. (Modified from Thiel et al. (2006))

obtained in all patients (Martin et al. 2009). Low-frequency rTMS over the area that was homologous to the most activated one during word repetition improved performance in another case series (Kakuda et al. 2010), suggesting that transcallosal inhibition of the compensating region should be suppressed irrespective of the hemisphere. As all of these studies lack a control group, a conclusion on the efficacy of this treatment strategy cannot be drawn.

Most non-invasive brain stimulation (NIBS) studies in poststroke aphasia employed inhibitory low-frequency rTMS for stimulation of the contralesional pars triangularis of the right inferior frontal gyrus (BA 45) in order to reduce right hemisphere hyperactivity and transcallosal inhibition on the left Broca's area and a meta-analysis of seven studies involving 160 stroke patients showed a positive effect on language recovery (Ren et al. 2014). Several studies attempted to restore perilesional activity in the left inferior frontal gyrus by applying excitatory (high-frequency) rTMS (Szaflarski et al. 2011). In one small study, a single session of excitatory rTMS over the right inferior frontal gyrus was more effective than inhibitory stimulation of this region (Chieffo et al. 2014). Combined bihemispheric stimulation with excitatory rTMS over the left and inhibitory rTMS over the right inferior frontal gyrus and language training significantly improved aphasia scores (Khedr et al. 2014).

In a randomized controlled study, the effect of inhibitory rTMS on pars triangularis of the right inferior frontal gyrus (IFG) in comparison to rTMS vertex stimulation in combination to speech and language therapy (SLT) on the pattern of brain activation and on the recovery of poststroke aphasia in the subacute stage was investigated. Twenty-nine right-handed patients with left-hemispheric infarcts were included, 15 received right inferior frontal gyrus stimulation, 14 were sham stimulated over the vertex and served as controls (Thiel et al. 2013). The change in global AAT test scores between initial and follow-up assessment was significantly higher ($P = 0.002$, t-test for independent samples) in rTMS-treated right-handed patients (22.4 ± 11.77) than in sham-treated patients (8.6 ± 10.06). There was no significant interaction between treatment effect and AAT-subtests, indicating that all subtests contribute equally to the observed treatment effect, with the largest difference in picture-naming performance (6.1 ± 3.35).

During verb stimulation before the initiation of treatment, all patients showed an abnormal activation pattern involving large parts of the language network in the non-dominant right hemisphere. In this study, PET could be applied during NIBS to demonstrate the immediate modulation of network activity as well as longer-lasting alterations related to recovery, thus lending direct support to the hypothesis of the relationship between activation shift and improvement of subacute poststroke aphasia ("proof-of-principle"). The clinical results have been confirmed in a large controlled multicenter study (Thiel et al. 2015).

Several studies were performed with excitatory transcranial direct current stimulation (tDCS) of the left frontal cortex to improve speech production in aphasics (Darkow et al. 2017; Holland et al. 2016; Marangolo et al. 2013; Zheng et al. 2016) and demonstrated positive effects in small groups of patients. Simultaneous tDCS and fMRI allowed identification of widespread changes in whole-brain functional connectivity (Meinzer et al. 2014). However, larger control studies were not performed yet.

16.8 Language Function in Brain Tumors

The speed of the development of a brain lesion may have an effect on the functional impairment and on the mechanisms of compensation and reorganization of the involved networks. In a study on 61 patients with tumors in the dominant left hemisphere (Thiel et al. 2001), a verb-generation paradigm not only increased flow in the left IFG (Brodman 44 and 55), both superior temporal gyri and the cerebellum (the pattern observed in the control group), but additionally in the left frontal medial gyrus (BA 46) and the orbital part of the IFG (BA 47), the anterior insula and the left cerebellum. Contrary to the healthy volunteers, two-thirds of the right-handed patients showed also an activation of the right IFG, that is, the area homologous to the Broca's area. In 18% of the patients, a reversed dominance was indicated by a negative laterality index. It was interesting to note that successful resection of a left fronto-temporal tumor improved aphasia and restored left-hemispheric dominance, suggesting the reversibility of the effect of disinhibition by removal of the cause of primary functional damage. In a further study (Thiel et al. 2005), the role of involvement of the right IFG in speech performance was tested by disturbing the IFG function with rTMS. In all patients, rTMS over the left IFG prolonged word-generation latencies, indicating that the left IFG is still essential for the performance of this task, as it is in normals. However, in patients but not in controls, significantly longer latencies were also observed during rTMS over the right IFG corresponding to higher right IFG activation. The right IFG, therefore, can be regarded as essential for language performance because patients and controls activate the IFG only during word generation, for example, retrieval of verbs and nouns contrasted with a number of control states (Warburton et al. 1996) and TMS over the right interfered with this task in patients as over the left in controls. The lateralization indices, as determined by PET, were significantly lower in patients with right-sided TMS effect than in those without. As described in the article by Thiel et al. (2006), there was a significant correlation between the laterality index and the performance in a verbal fluency test (FAS, Lezak et al. 2004) in patients without right-positive TMS effect (4 Hz for 20 s, as described above), whereas in patients with a predominant right-positive TMS effect, the performance in the verbal fluency test was comparable with that in controls. This result may indicate that in a few patients with left-hemispheric brain tumors, the slow progression of damage leads to a shift in language function to the right hemisphere, which can compensate for the defect on the left side.

16.9 Hierarchical Organization for Recovery?

The different dynamics of recovery of language function observed in patients after stroke and with tumors in the left hemisphere suggest various mechanisms for compensation of the lesion within the functional network. Despite the limited number of longitudinal studies, the heterogeneity with respect to the type of aphasia in the patients included, and the differences among the activation and stimulation paradigms (Zahn et al. 2006), a hierarchy for effective recovery might be deduced from these data (Fig. 16.4; Heiss and Thiel 2006):

- Best, even complete recovery of function can usually be achieved only by the restoration of the original activation pattern within the network of the dominant hemisphere; this is only feasible after small brain damage, probably only affecting an area of minor importance, permitting functional restitution of the main interconnected components.
- If primary functional centers are damaged, the reduction in collateral inhibition leads to activation of areas around the lesion; this intrahemispheric compensation involving secondary centers of the ipsilateral network is the basis for incomplete but often satisfactory improvement of language function.
- If ipsilateral network components are severely damaged, the reduction in transcallosal inhibition causes activation of contralateral homotopic areas; this interhemispheric compensation involving homotopic contralesional areas contributes to some improvement in function, which is dependent on the extent of the functional shift between the hemispheres, but usually is not as efficient as intrahemispheric compensation. However, in some patients with slowly developing brain damage—and perhaps also an a priori not highly lateralized functional network—the language function can be completely shifted to the right hemisphere, and in these cases, speech performance can be preserved or completely

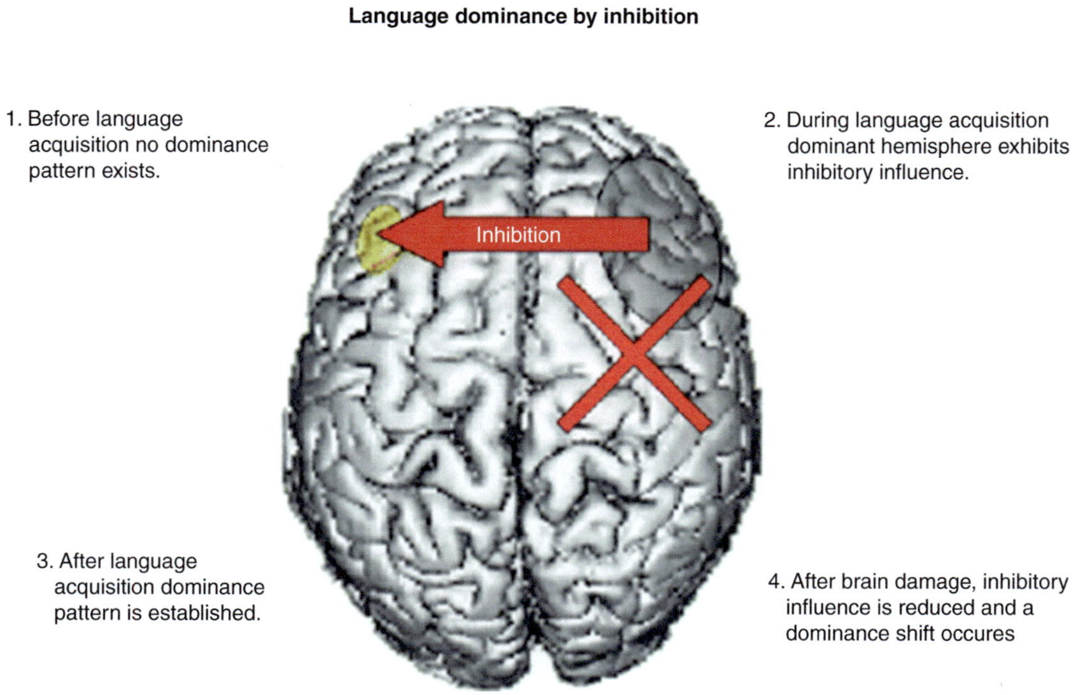

Fig. 16.4 Development of language dominance and changes in hierarchy of areas by lesions. (*1*) before language acquisition, no dominance pattern exists; (*2*) during language acquisition, dominant hemisphere exhibits inhibitory influence; (*3*) after language acquisition, dominance pattern is established; (*4*) after brain damage, inhibitory influence is reduced and a dominance shift occurs. (Courtesy of Thiel)

recovered despite the damage in the left (previously dominant) hemisphere.

The concept of the difference between the effectiveness of intrahemispheric compensation and interhemispheric compensation may be taken one step further. The blockade of the contralateral intact area by rTMS can be utilized to modulate the inhibitory interactions. In a controlled feasibility study, prevention of right-hemispheric overactivation by rTMS over the Broca's homologous area of the right hemisphere was related to improved language performance (Weiduschat et al. 2011). The authors postulated that rTMS decreased excitation in right BA 45, which in turn modulated activity in the distributed, bihemispheric language network. This result suggests that in aphasia patients, contralateral overactivation (likely due to transcallosal disinhibition secondary to dominant, left-hemisphere lesion) may be tempered or suppressed, following a series of slow, 1 Hz rTMS treatments to a posterior portion of the right pars triangularis. The clinical and long-term efficacy of this novel complementary treatment for aphasia was proven in larger clinical trials (Thiel et al. 2015).

16.10 Conclusions

Specific brain functions, such as language, can be localized by comparing CBF or CMRGlc during the performance of a select task with a "resting" condition. This was originally made possible by PET using FDG. With ^{15}O-water or other ultrashort-lived CBF tracers, multiple replications of conditions in the same subject could be performed. This technique was widely used, especially for the study of higher brain function (cognitive neuroscience) and for evaluating disturbed activation patterns in disease, as in poststroke aphasia. In recent years, fMRI has become the dominating imaging technique in this field because it does not involve ionizing radiation and, therefore, is easily used in normal controls, allowing more rapid signal acquisition and more complex experimental designs. However, PET provides a more physiologically specific signal, a better signal-to-noise ratio, and fewer artifacts in individual acquisitions. PET also provides actual activated and reference regional values, which may show a better correlation with task performance than the difference signal provided by fMRI. Additionally, magnetic stimulations can be performed during PET examinations. These advantages support its continued use in pathophysiologically complex clinical situations such as stroke and brain tumors, where CBF responses to activation may be altered and may involve unexpected components of a functional network.

References

Attwell D, Laughlin SB (2001) An energy budget for signaling in the grey matter of the brain. J Cereb Blood Flow Metab 21(10):1133–1145

Basso A, Gardelli M et al (1989) The role of the right hemisphere in recovery from aphasia. Two case studies. Cortex 25:555–566

Belin P, van Eeckhout P et al (1996) Recovery from nonfluent aphasia after melodic intonation therapy: a PET study. Neurology 47(6):1504–1511

Berthier ML, Green C et al (2006) A randomized, placebo-controlled study of donepezil in poststroke aphasia. Neurology 67:1687–1689

Berthier ML, Starkstein SE et al (1991) Transcortical aphasia. Importance of the nonspeech dominant hemisphere in language repetition. Brain 114(Pt 3):1409–1427

Booth JR, Wood L et al (2007) The role of the basal ganglia and cerebellum in language processing. Brain Res 1133:136–144

Cao Y, Vikingstad EM et al (1999) Cortical language activation in stroke patients recovering from aphasia with functional MRI. Stroke 30:2331–2340

Cappa SF, Perani D et al (1997) A PET follow-up study of recovery after stroke in acute aphasics. Brain Lang 56:55–67

Chen R, Classen J et al (1997) Depression of motor cortex excitability by low-frequency transcranial magnetic stimulation. Neurology 48:1398–1403

Chieffo R, Ferrari F, Battista P, Houdayer E, Nuara A et al (2014) Excitatory deep transcranial magnetic stimulation with H-coil over the right homologous Broca's region improves naming in chronic post-stroke aphasia. Neurorehabil Neural Repair 28:291–298

Crinion JT, Leff AP (2007) Recovery and treatment of aphasia after stroke: functional imaging studies. Curr Opin Neurol 20:667–673

Darkow R, Martin A, Wurtz A, Floel A, Meinzer M (2017) Transcranial direct current stimulation effects on neural processing in post-stroke aphasia. Hum Brain Mapp 38:1518–1531

Demonet JF, Fiez JA et al (1996) PET studies of phonological processing: a critical reply to Poeppel. Brain Lang 55:352–379

Feeney DM, Baron JC (1986) Diaschisis. Stroke 17:817–830

Fernandez B, Cardebat D et al (2004) Functional MRI follow-up study of language processes in healthy subjects and during recovery in a case of aphasia. Stroke 35:2171–2176

Ferro JM, Mariano G et al (1999) Recovery from aphasia and neglect. Cerebrovasc Dis 9(Suppl 5):6–22

Gainotti G (1993) The riddle of the right hemisphere's contribution to the recovery of language. Eur J Disord Commun 28:227–246

Greener J, Enderby P et al (2001a) Speech and language therapy for aphasia following stroke (Cochrane Review). The Cochrane Library 3 Oxford: update software

Greener J, Enderby P et al (2001b) Pharmacological treatment for aphasia following stroke. Cochrane Database Syst Rev 2001(4):CD000424. Review

Hartwigsen G, Saur D (2019) Neuroimaging of stroke recovery from aphasia – insights into plasticity of the human language network. Neuroimage 190:14–31

Heiss WD, Emunds HG et al (1993) Cerebral glucose metabolism as a predictor of rehabilitation after ischemic stroke. Stroke 24:1784–1788

Heiss WD, Kessler J et al (1993) Cerebral glucose metabolism as a predictor of recovery from aphasia in ischemic stroke. Arch Neurol 50:958–964

Heiss WD, Kessler J et al (1999) Differential capacity of left and right hemispheric areas for compensation of poststroke aphasia. Ann Neurol 45:430–438

Heiss WD, Thiel A (2006) A proposed regional hierarchy in recovery of post-stroke aphasia. Brain Lang 98:118–123

Hickok G, Poeppel D (2007) The cortical organization of speech processing. Nat Rev Neurosci 8:393–402

Hillis AE, Kleinman JT et al (2006) Restoring cerebral blood flow reveals neural regions critical for naming. J Neurosci 26:8069–8073

Holland R, Leff AP, Penny WD, Rothwell JC, Crinion J (2016) Modulation of frontal effective connectivity during speech. Neuroimage 140:126–133

Jordan LC, Hillis AE (2006) Disorders of speech and language: aphasia, apraxia and dysarthria. Curr Opin Neurol 19:580–585

Kakuda W, Abo M et al (2010) Functional MRI-based therapeutic rTMS strategy for aphasic stroke patients: a case series pilot study. Int J Neurosci 120(1):60–66

Kapoor A (2017) Repetitive transcranial magnetic stimulation therapy for post-stroke non-fluent aphasia: a critical review. Top Stroke Rehabil 24:547–553

Karbe H, Herholz K et al (1989) Regional metabolic correlates of token test results in cortical and subcortical left hemispheric infarction. Neurology 39:1083–1088

Karbe H, Kessler J et al (1995) Long-term prognosis of poststroke aphasia studied with positron emission tomography. Arch Neurol 52:186–190

Karbe H, Thiel A et al (1998) Brain plasticity in poststroke aphasia: what is the contribution of the right hemisphere? Brain Lang 64:215–230

Kessler J, Thiel A et al (2000) Piracetam improves activated blood flow and facilitates rehabilitation of poststroke aphasic patients. Stroke 31:2112–2116

Khedr EM, Abo El-Fetoh N, Ali AM, El-Hammady DH, Khalifa H et al (2014) Dual-hemisphere repetitive transcranial magnetic stimulation for rehabilitation of poststroke aphasia: a randomized, double-blind clinical trial. Neurorehabil Neural Repair 28:740–750

Knecht S, Floel A et al (2002) Degree of language lateralization determines susceptibility to unilateral brain lesions. Nat Neurosci 5:695–699

Kobayashi M, Pascual-Leone A (2003) Transcranial magnetic stimulation in neurology. Lancet Neurol 2:145–156

Kumar R, Masih AK et al (1996) Global aphasia due to thalamic hemorrhage: a case report and review of the literature. Arch Phys Med Rehabil 77:1312–1315

Leon Ruiz M, Rodriguez Sarasa ML, Sanjuan Rodriguez L, Benito-Leon J, Garcia-Albea Ristol E, Arce Arce S (2018) Current evidence on transcranial magnetic stimulation and its potential usefulness in poststroke neurorehabilitation: opening new doors to the treatment of cerebrovascular disease. Neurologia 33:459–472

Lezak M, Howieson D et al (2004) Neuropsycho-logical assessment. Oxford University Press, Oxford

Magistretti PJ (2004) Brain energy metabolism. In: Byrne JH, Roberts JL (eds) From molecules to networks. Elsevier, Amsterdam, pp 67–90

Marangolo P, Fiori V, Calpagnano MA, Campana S, Razzano C et al (2013) tDCS over the left inferior frontal cortex improves speech production in aphasia. Front Hum Neurosci 7:539

Martin PI, Naeser MA et al (2004) Transcranial magnetic stimulation as a complementary treatment for aphasia. Semin Speech Lang 25:181–191

Martin PI, Naeser MA et al (2009) Overt naming fMRI pre- and post-TMS: two nonfluent aphasia patients, with and without improved naming post-TMS. Brain Lang 111(1):20–35

Meinzer M, Lindenberg R, Darkow R, Ulm L, Copland D, Floel A (2014) Transcranial direct current stimulation and simultaneous functional magnetic resonance imaging. J Vis Exp (86). https://doi.org/10.3791/51730

Metter EJ, Hanson WR et al (1990) Temporoparietal cortex in aphasia. Evidence from positron emission tomography. Arch Neurol 47:1235–1238

Metter EJ, Kempler D et al (1987) Cerebellar glucose metabolism in chronic aphasia. Neurology 37:1599–1606

Metter EJ, Riege WH et al (1988) Subcortical structures in aphasia. An analysis based on (18 F)-fluorodeoxyglucose, positron emission tomography, and computed tomography. Arch Neurol 45:1229–1234

Mintun MA, Lundstrom BN et al (2001) Blood flow and oxygen delivery to human brain during functional activity: theoretical modeling and experimental data. Proc Natl Acad Sci U S A 98:6859–6864

Muller RA, Rothermel RD et al (1998) Brain organization of language after early unilateral lesion: a PET study. Brain Lang 62:422–451

Musso M, Weiller C et al (1999) Training-induced brain plasticity in aphasia. Brain 122(Pt 9):1781–1790

Naeser MA, Martin PI et al (2004) Overt propositional speech in chronic nonfluent aphasia studied with the dynamic susceptibility contrast fMRI method. Neuroimage 22:29–41

Naeser MA, Martin PI et al (2005a) Improved picture naming in chronic aphasia after TMS to part of right Broca's area: an open-protocol study. Brain Lang 93:95–105

Naeser MA, Martin PI et al (2005b) Improved naming after TMS treatments in a chronic, global aphasia patient–case report. Neurocase 11(3):182–193

Norise C, Hamilton RH (2016) Non-invasive brain stimulation in the treatment of post-stroke and neurodegenerative aphasia: parallels, differences, and lessons learned. Front Hum Neurosci 10:675

Nudo RJ, Wise BM et al (1996) Neural substrates for the effects of rehabilitative training on motor recovery after ischemic infarct. Science 272:1791–1794

Ogawa S, Lee TM et al (1990) Brain magnetic resonance imaging with contrast dependent on blood oxygenation. Proc Natl Acad Sci U S A 87:9868–9872

Ohyama M, Senda M et al (1996) Role of the nondominant hemisphere and undamaged area during word repetition in poststroke aphasics – a PET activation study. Stroke 27:897–903

Orgogozo JM (1998) Piracetam in the treatment of acute stroke. CNS Drugs 9:41–49

Pascual-Leone A, Davey N et al (2002) Handbook of transcranial magnetic stimula tion. Arnold Press, London

Petersen SE, Fox PT et al (1988) Positron emission tomographic studies of the cortical anatomy of single-word processing. Nature 331:585–589

Price CJ (2000) The anatomy of language: contributions from functional neuroimaging. J Anat 197(Pt 3):335–359

Price CJ (2012) A review and synthesis of the first 20 years of PET and fMRI studies of heard speech, spoken language and reading. Neuroimage 62:816–847

Price CJ, Crinion J (2005) The latest on functional imaging studies of aphasic stroke. Curr Opin Neurol 18:429–434

Raboyeau G, De Boissezon X et al (2008) Right hemisphere activation in recovery from aphasia: lesion effect or function recruitment? Neurology 70:290–298

Reivich M, Kuhl D et al (1979) The (18 F)fluorodeoxyglucose method for the measurement of local cerebral glucose utilization in man. Circ Res 44:127–137

Ren CL, Zhang GF, Xia N, Jin CH, Zhang XH et al (2014) Effect of low-frequency rTMS on aphasia in stroke

patients: a meta-analysis of randomized controlled trials. PLoS One 9:e102557
Rosen HJ, Petersen SE et al (2000) Neural correlates of recovery from aphasia after damage to left inferior frontal cortex. Neurology 55:1883–1894
Saur D, Lange R et al (2006) Dynamics of language reorganization after stroke. Brain 129:1371–1384
Siebner HR, Takano B et al (2001) Continuous transcranial magnetic stimulation during positron emission tomography: a suitable tool for imaging regional excitability of the human cortex. Neuroimage 14:883–890
Sokoloff L (1999) Energetics of functional activation in neural tissues. Neurochem Res 24:321–329
Szaflarski JP, Vannest J, Wu SW, DiFrancesco MW, Banks C, Gilbert DL (2011) Excitatory repetitive transcranial magnetic stimulation induces improvements in chronic post-stroke aphasia. Med Sci Monit 17:CR132–CR139
Thiel A, Black SE, Rochon EA, Lanthier S, Hartmann A et al (2015) Non-invasive repeated therapeutic stimulation for aphasia recovery: a multilingual, multicenter aphasia trial. J Stroke Cerebrovasc Dis 24: 751–758
Thiel A, Habedank B et al (2005) Essential language function of the right hemisphere in brain tumor patients. Ann Neurol 57:128–131
Thiel A, Habedank B et al (2006) From the left to the right: how the brain compensates progressive loss of language function. Brain Lang 98:57–65
Thiel A, Hartmann A, Rubi-Fessen I, Anglade C, Kracht L et al (2013) Effects of noninvasive brain stimulation on language networks and recovery in early poststroke aphasia. Stroke 44:2240–2246
Thiel A, Herholz K et al (1998) Localization of language-related cortex with 15O-labeled water PET in patients with gliomas. Neuroimage 7:284–295
Thiel A, Herholz K et al (2001) Plasticity of language networks in patients with brain tumors: a PET activation study. Ann Neurol 50:620–629
Thiel A, Schumacher B et al (2006) Direct demonstration of transcallosal disinhibition in language networks. J Cereb Blood Flow Metab 26:1122–1127
Thompson CK (2000) The neurobiology of language recovery in aphasia. Brain Lang 71:245–248
Turner R, Howseman A et al (1997) Functional imaging with magnetic resonance. In: Frackowiak RSJ, Friston KJ, Frith CD, Dolan RJ, Mazziotta JC (eds) Human brain function. Academic, San Diego, pp 467–486
Wade DT, Hewer RL et al (1986) Aphasia after stroke: natural history and associated deficits. J Neurol Neurosurg Psychiatry 49:11–16
Walker-Batson D, Curtis S et al (2001) A double-blind, placebo-controlled study of the use of amphetamine in the treatment of aphasia. Stroke 32:2093–2098
Warburton E, Price CJ et al (1999) Mechanisms of recovery from aphasia: evidence from positron emission tomography studies. J Neurol Neurosurg Psychiatry 66:155–161
Warburton E, Wise RJS et al (1996) Noun and verb retrieval by normal subjects studies with PET. Brain 119:159–179
Wassermann EM, Pascual-Leone A et al (2002) Safety and side-effects of transcranial magnetic stimulation and repetitive transcranialmagnetic stimulation. In: Handbook of transcranial magnetic stimulation. Arnold Press, London, pp 39–49
Weiduschat N, Thiel A et al (2011) Effects of repetitive transcranial magnetic stimulation in aphasic stroke: a randomized controlled pilot study. Stroke 42(2):409–415
Weiller C, Isensee C et al (1995) Recovery from Wernicke's aphasia: a positron emission tomographic study. Ann Neurol 37:723–732
Winhuisen L, Thiel A et al (2005) Role of the contralateral inferior frontal gyrus in recovery of language function in poststroke aphasia: a combined repetitive transcranial magnetic stimulation and positron emission tomography study. Stroke 36:1759–1763
Wise RJ (2003) Language systems in normal and aphasic human subjects: functional imaging studies and inferences from animal studies. Br Med Bull 65:95–119
Zahn R, Schwarz M et al (2006) Functional activation studies of word processing in the recovery from aphasia. J Physiol Paris 99:370–385
Zheng X, Dai W, Alsop DC, Schlaug G (2016) Modulating transcallosal and intra-hemispheric brain connectivity with tDCS: implications for interventions in aphasia. Restor Neurol Neurosci 34:519–530

17 Use of fMRI Language Lateralization for Quantitative Prediction of Naming and Verbal Memory Outcome in Left Temporal Lobe Epilepsy Surgery

Jeffrey R. Binder

Partial removal of the anterior temporal lobe (ATL) is the most commonly performed surgical procedure for intractable epilepsy. ATL resection is highly effective for seizure control in patients with temporal lobe epilepsy (TLE), resulting in long-term cure rates of 60–80% (Jeong et al. 2005; McIntosh et al. 2001; Tellez-Zenteno et al. 2005). The undeniable benefit of ATL surgery is partially offset by the occurrence of neuropsychological morbidity in some patients receiving this treatment. Evidence suggests a 30–60% incidence of significant naming decline (Bell et al. 2000b; Busch et al. 2016; Hermann et al. 1999a, b, 1994; Langfitt and Rausch 1996; Sabsevitz et al. 2003) and a similar risk for decline in verbal memory ability (Baxendale et al. 2006; Binder et al. 2008a; Chelune et al. 1993; Gleissner et al. 2004; Helmstaedter and Elger 1996; Lineweaver et al. 2006; Martin et al. 1998; Sabsevitz et al. 2001; Stroup et al. 2003) after left ATL surgery. Patients are generally aware of these deficits, which adversely affect quality of life and employability (Helmstaedter et al. 2003; Langfitt et al. 2007; Lineweaver et al. 2004; Perrine et al. 1995; Stroup et al. 2003). Cognitive deficits from right ATL resection have been much less consistently observed (Binder et al. 2008a; Busch et al. 2016; Lee et al. 2002; Loring et al. 1990a, 1995b; Pigot and Milner 1993; Pillon et al. 1999). Although the first priority in treating intractable epilepsy is seizure control, the importance of cognitive side effects for some patients undergoing left ATL surgery should not be underestimated or denied. Indeed, considerable resources have been devoted to developing methods for predicting and preventing cognitive morbidity, and many such methods are used routinely in the evaluation of surgical candidates despite ongoing controversy regarding their effectiveness.

This chapter focuses on recent advances in the prediction of postoperative language and verbal memory deficits using preoperative functional magnetic resonance imaging (fMRI). The value of such risk assessment is that it provides the patient and the physician with additional information that can be useful in deciding whether to proceed with treatment in elective situations. The use of fMRI activation maps intraoperatively for defining surgical resection boundaries is a separate issue that will not be addressed in detail here.

17.1 Use of fMRI for Predicting Naming Outcome

17.1.1 Measuring Language Lateralization

The intracarotid amobarbital (Wada) test was developed to assess the risk of language decline in patients undergoing resective brain surgery

J. R. Binder (✉)
Department of Neurology, Medical College of Wisconsin, Milwaukee, WI, USA
e-mail: JBinder@mcw.edu

S. Ulmer, O. Jansen (eds.), *fMRI*, https://doi.org/10.1007/978-3-030-41874-8_17

(Wada and Rasmussen 1960), under the assumption that operating on the language-dominant hemisphere entailed increased risk. Although the Wada test has been in use for more than 60 years, until recently the relationship between Wada language asymmetry and postoperative language outcome had never been quantified. The historical reasons for this relate to the fact that language lateralization was traditionally viewed as dichotomous (left or right) or trichotomous (left, right, or "bilateral"). Under this schema, it seemed obvious that operating on a nondominant hemisphere would be safer than operating on a language-dominant hemisphere. Several aspects of this formulation have changed in recent decades. First, language lateralization has come to be seen as a continuously graded rather than an all-or-none phenomenon, with relative *degrees* of dominance rather than distinct categories (Binder et al. 1996; Chlebus et al. 2007; Knecht et al. 2000b, 2002; Loring et al. 1990b; Seghier 2008; Springer et al. 1999). Thus, while the vast majority (~80%) of patients who undergo left hemisphere surgery for epilepsy are left dominant for language, there is variation within this group in terms of the degree of left dominance. This variability raises the question of whether graded degrees of language dominance are reflected in graded levels of risk. Second, neuropsychological methods for identifying postoperative language deficits have steadily improved and become more widespread, resulting in a shift of the clinical focus, particularly in left ATL cases, away from prediction of severe aphasia (which is very rare after standard left ATL resection) and toward prediction of more moderate degrees of language decline.

The effort to develop fMRI methods for predicting language outcome in ATL epilepsy surgery is therefore motivated by two critical assumptions. First, it is assumed that patients show varying degrees of language (mainly naming) deficit after surgery and that it is desirable to know before surgery what degree of decline can be expected. Second, it is assumed that the degree of decline will be related, at least in part, to the degree of language lateralization toward the surgical hemisphere. The goal of fMRI in this context is thus to provide a reliable and valid measure of language lateralization. A variety of fMRI language activation paradigms have been described, differing in the type of language stimuli, stimulus modality, language task, control stimuli, and control task used, raising the question of which of these paradigms, if any, is optimal. Although different paradigms have seldom been compared quantitatively, a survey of extant studies shows that they can produce very different, in some cases entirely nonoverlapping, activation patterns. This variation is related primarily to the cognitive, sensory, and motor processes engaged by the tasks, and the degree to which the language and control conditions differ in engaging these specific processes (Binder 2016; Binder et al. 2008b).

Several simple criteria can be applied in assessing the usefulness of different language paradigms. First, the pattern of activation obtained in healthy, right-handed adults should be lateralized strongly to the left hemisphere, given that almost all such individuals are left-hemisphere dominant for language (Knecht et al. 2000a; Loring et al. 1990b; Springer et al. 1999). Second, the activation should be robust; that is, it should be reliably obtained across individuals and in the same general brain regions from person to person. Third, there should be concordance between language lateralization measured with the fMRI paradigm and lateralization measured with other techniques, such as the Wada test, in the same individuals. Finally, in some cases it may be desirable that the paradigm produces activation in particular target brain regions. In the case of ATL surgery, for example, activation asymmetry in the temporal lobe might be more predictive of outcome than activation in the frontal lobe; thus, a paradigm that activates the temporal lobe would have advantages over one that does not.

Figure 17.1 illustrates some of these issues. The figure shows average fMRI (i.e., blood oxygenation-level dependent, or BOLD) activations obtained from 26 healthy right-handed participants while they listened to spoken words and performed a semantic decision task (Binder et al. 1997, 2008b). In the top panel, BOLD signal during this task is compared to a "resting" base-

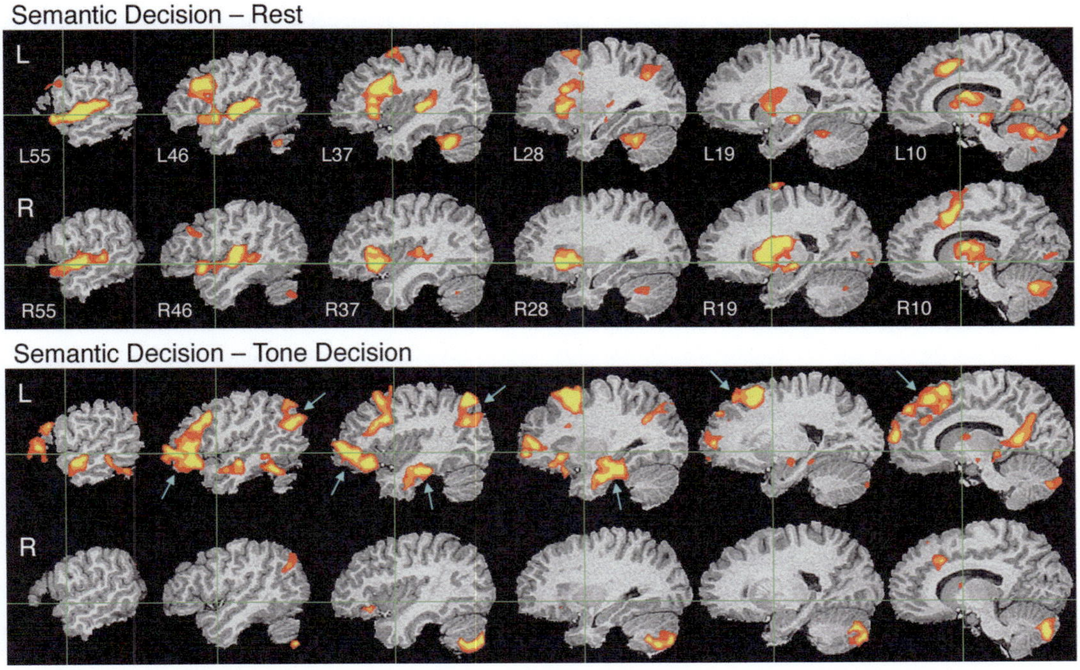

Fig. 17.1 Group fMRI activation maps from two auditory word comprehension experiments in the same 26 participants. *Top*: semantic decision relative to resting. *Bottom*: semantic decision relative to tone decision. Data are displayed as serial sagittal sections through the brain at 9-mm intervals. *X*-axis locations for each slice are given in the *top panel*. Both maps are thresholded at a whole-brain corrected $p<0.05$ using voxel-wise $p<0.0001$ and cluster extent>200 mm^3. The three steps in each color continuum represent voxel-wise p thresholds of 10^{-4}, 10^{-5}, and 10^{-6}. *Blue arrows* in the lower image indicate left-hemisphere language areas that are active during the resting state and thus visible only when an active nonlinguistic task is used as the baseline (adapted from Binder et al. 2008b)

line. The activated regions are largely bilateral, including bilateral auditory (superior temporal), working memory (dorsolateral prefrontal), and attention (cingulo-opercular-insular) networks. In the lower panel of the figure, the semantic decision task is compared to a nonlinguistic auditory control task that requires attention and working memory processes. In this case, the activated regions are strongly left-lateralized, including several left temporal, parietal, and prefrontal regions (indicated by blue arrows) that were not observed when the resting baseline was used. These data illustrate in a dramatic fashion how activation patterns depend on the choice of control condition. In the lower panel, the use of an active nonlinguistic control task "subtracts out" bilateral activation in early auditory, general executive, and attention networks, leaving activation in left-lateralized language networks. These results also demonstrate that certain high-level language processing regions are active during the "resting" state and can only be observed when an active nonlinguistic control condition is employed (Binder et al. 1999, 2008b).

Many fMRI language paradigms have been compared to Wada language testing (Adcock et al. 2003; Baciu et al. 2001; Bahn et al. 1997; Benke et al. 2006; Benson et al. 1999; Binder et al. 1996; Carpentier et al. 2001; Chlebus et al. 2007; Deblaere et al. 2004; Desmond et al. 1995; Gaillard et al. 2004; Hertz-Pannier et al. 1997; Janecek et al. 2013b; Lehéricy et al. 2000; Rutten et al. 2002; Sabbah et al. 2003; Spreer et al. 2002; Woermann et al. 2003; Worthington et al. 1997; Yetkin et al. 1998). A sample-size-weighted average across 23 such studies showed an overall concordance rate of 85%, a value that agrees closely with the rate observed in the largest study, which showed concordance of 86% in a sample of 229 patients (Janecek et al. 2013b). In assessing the rate of concordance, patients are usually assigned to categories such as "left dominant," "right dominant," or "mixed" on each test. The proportion of concordant cases depends on how these arbitrary categories are defined as well as other factors. Another method for comparing fMRI and Wada results is to calculate the correlation between continuous measures of lateralization on both tests. In the case of fMRI, a standard approach is to calculate a laterality index (LI) expressing the asymmetry of activation in numerical form. The first such LI was based on a simple count of the voxels that survived thresholding in each hemisphere (Binder et al. 1996). The formula $(L - R)/(L+R)$, where L and R refer to the voxel counts in each hemisphere, yields a number that varies from +1 when all activated voxels are on the left side to −1 when all activated voxels are on the right side. LI values obtained with this method vary as a function of the threshold used for defining activated voxels; thus, several authors have explored alternative asymmetry measures that do not require thresholding (Adcock et al. 2003; Chlebus et al. 2007; Nagata et al. 2001; Seghier 2008; Wilke and Schmithorst 2006). No consensus regarding the optimal method for calculating activation asymmetry has yet emerged from these studies.

17.1.2 Predicting Naming Outcome

With so many studies focusing on fMRI/Wada correlations, it is easy to forget that the actual aim of measuring language lateralization prior to brain surgery is prediction of language outcome. In the case of left ATL resection, an fMRI procedure that reliably identifies patients at risk for postoperative naming deficits would be a valuable clinical tool, especially if the fMRI results added information over and above other available sources. Previous behavioral studies have identified demographic and behavioral variables that may predict outcome. For example, left ATL patients who develop seizures at an earlier age generally have a lower risk for postoperative language decline (Busch et al. 2016; Hermann et al. 1999b; Saykin et al. 1995; Stafiniak et al. 1990), presumably because earlier age at onset is associated with a higher probability of language shift to the right hemisphere (Springer et al. 1999). Age at surgery was shown to be an important independent predictor in a recent large study, with older patients showing more decline (Busch et al. 2016). Better preoperative naming performance is associated with a higher risk for decline (Busch et al. 2016; Hermann et al. 1994). As noted earlier, although Wada language testing has been assumed to predict language outcome, apart from a few case reports of patients with right language dominance who did not decline (Langfitt and Rausch 1996; Wada and Rasmussen 1960), this assumption went untested for many years.

In the first study to examine fMRI language lateralization as a predictor of naming outcome, Sabsevitz et al. (Sabsevitz et al. 2003) studied 24 consecutively encountered patients undergoing left ATL resection. The fMRI paradigm used a contrast between an auditory semantic decision task and a nonlinguistic tone decision task (Fig. 17.1, lower panel). Asymmetry of activation with this task paradigm is generally concordant with language lateralization on the Wada test (Binder et al. 1996; Janecek et al. 2013b). Sabsevitz et al. computed separate LIs for the whole hemisphere, frontal lobe, temporal lobe, and angular gyrus. All patients also underwent Wada testing and preoperative assessment of confrontation naming using the 60-item Boston Naming Test (BNT). The BNT was administered again at 6 months after surgery, and a change score was calculated as the difference between postoperative and preoperative BNT scores. Surgeries were performed blind to the fMRI data.

Compared to a control group of 32 right ATL patients, the left ATL group declined postoperatively on the BNT ($p<0.001$), with an average raw change score of −9. Within the left ATL group, however, there was considerable variability, with 13 patients (54%) showing variable degrees of decline relative to the control group, and others showing minimal or no decline. The temporal lobe fMRI LI was the strongest predictor of outcome ($r=-0.64$, $p<0.001$), indicating that stronger language lateralization toward the left (surgical) temporal lobe was related to poorer naming outcome, whereas lateralization toward the right temporal lobe was associated with little or no decline. This fMRI measure showed 100% sensitivity, 73% specificity, and a positive predictive value of 81% in predicting significant decline. By comparison, the Wada language LI showed a somewhat weaker correlation with outcome ($r = -0.50$, $p < 0.05$), 92% sensitivity, 43% specificity, and a positive predictive value of 67%.

Sabsevitz et al. also created multivariate models to determine the contribution of fMRI relative to other noninvasive predictors. Both age at epilepsy onset ($r = -0.35$, $p = 0.09$) and preoperative performance ($r = -0.39$, $p = 0.06$) showed strong trends toward a correlation with outcome, and together these variables predicted about 27% of the variance in outcome. Adding the temporal lobe fMRI LI to this model accounted for an additional 23% of the variance ($p < 0.01$), indicating a significant increase in predictive power. Addition of the Wada language asymmetry score did not improve the model (R^2 change $= 0.01$, $p > 0.1$).

In a more recent study from the same research group, Janecek et al. updated this fMRI prediction model, using data from 55 left ATL surgery patients (Janecek et al. 2013a). Similar to the results of Sabsevitz et al., fMRI LI accounted for an additional 19% of the variance in outcome relative to a model using preoperative BNT score alone ($p = 0.01$).

Three other studies have examined correlations between preoperative language fMRI LI and postoperative naming decline after left ATL surgery. Bonelli et al. (2012) found that greater leftward activation asymmetry in the middle frontal gyrus during a verbal fluency task was correlated with greater decline on a picture naming task ($r = -0.46$, $p = 0.03$) in 24 patients. The fMRI measure showed 100% sensitivity, 33% specificity, and a PPV of 60% for predicting significant decline. These more modest prediction results may reflect the fact that the authors excluded patients who were not left dominant by fMRI, thereby limiting the range of the predictor variable. Very similar results ($r = -0.50$, $p = 0.04$) were reported by Rosazza et al. in a sample of 17 left ATL patients (Rosazza et al. 2013). In contrast, Audrain et al. found no correlation between fMRI LI, based on a combination of word production activation tasks, and BNT change in 20 left ATL patients (Audrain et al. 2018). The explanation for this divergence from the previous studies is unclear.

Though still somewhat preliminary, the results overall suggest that language lateralization measured with preoperative fMRI may be an effective aid in predicting risk of naming decline after left ATL resection (Szaflarski et al. 2017). One study suggested a somewhat stronger predictive power for fMRI compared to the Wada language test (Sabsevitz et al. 2003). Although preoperative naming score and age at the onset of epilepsy are both useful predictors (Busch et al. 2016; Ives-Deliperi and Butler 2012), initial results suggest that fMRI adds predictive power compared to prediction based on preoperative naming score alone (Janecek et al. 2013a; Rosazza et al. 2013; Sabsevitz et al. 2003).

Additional evidence on the relative predictive power of fMRI and Wada testing comes from a study that examined naming outcome in 10 left ATL patients who had discordant fMRI and Wada language results preoperatively (Janecek et al. 2013a). Such patients are rare because the baseline rate of discordance is only ~15%, less than half of these discordant cases are likely to have left ATL surgery, and not all treated patients are available for postoperative testing. Predicted change scores were computed using either the fMRI LI or the Wada language asymmetry index in optimized multivariate prediction models for each method. Of the ten cases, naming outcomes were more accurately predicted by the fMRI model in seven, more accurately by the Wada model in two, and equally well by both tests in the remaining case.

17.1.3 "Resting-State Language Network" Mapping

Low-frequency temporal fluctuations in the "resting" fMRI BOLD signal show correlations across brain regions, a phenomenon believed to reflect neural connectivity (Biswal et al. 1995). Numerous studies have shown that these connections are organized into large-scale networks (e.g., Fox et al. 2005; Smith et al. 2009; Vincent et al. 2008; Yeo et al. 2011), including some identified as resting-state "language networks" (Smith et al. 2009; Tomasi and Volkow 2012). Preliminary studies have identified relationships between the strength of functional connectivity in particular regions and language lateralization derived with standard task fMRI methods (Doucet et al. 2015; Smitha et al. 2017; Wang et al. 2014). This technique might therefore provide an important alternative method for language mapping, especially in children and cognitively impaired individuals who have difficulty performing tasks. At present, the specific methods used for identifying network components and computing lateralization indexes have varied substantially and are still being investigated. No studies have yet validated these asymmetry measures against Wada testing or clinical outcomes.

Audrain et al. examined a novel metric using preoperative resting-state fMRI connectivity as a predictor of naming outcome after ATL resection (Audrain et al. 2018). A connectivity matrix was created from the fMRI data in each participant by measuring connectivity between all possible pairs in a set of 66 regions putatively involved in language. These matrices were then averaged across 19 healthy control participants to create a "normative template." A "matrix similarity" metric was then computed for each of 20 left ATL surgery patients by correlating the patient's connectivity matrix with the normative template. One way to conceptualize this metric is that it quantifies the global degree of deviation of each patient's connectome from the "normal" pattern. Interestingly, patients with a more "normal" connectome (i.e., stronger correlation with the normative template) showed less postoperative naming decline ($R^2 = 0.4$, $p = 0.003$). The results suggest that resting fMRI connectivity may provide a unique measure of "functional reserve" that predicts resilience of the naming network to ATL resection.

17.2 "Tailoring" Temporal Lobe Resections

It remains to be seen how useful fMRI language activation maps will be for planning resection boundaries in temporal lobe surgery. At least three significant problems complicate progress: (1) variation in language maps produced by different activation protocols; (2) generally poor activation of the ATL, where the majority of temporal lobe surgeries are performed; and (3) an inadequate understanding of the specificity of fMRI activations.

As indicated earlier, different fMRI language activation protocols in current clinical use produce markedly different patterns of activation (Binder 2016). These findings suggest that activation maps are strongly dependent on the specific composition of cognitive processes engaged during the scan, and how these differ between the language and control tasks used (see discussion earlier). Most language activation protocols currently used in clinical studies do not elicit robust ATL activation, especially in inferior portions of the ATL. Because the dominant ATL is known to contribute to language processing (Damasio et al. 1996; Hamberger et al. 2001; Humphries et al. 2006; Rogers et al. 2006), and left ATL resection not infrequently results in language decline (Bell et al. 2000b; Davies et al. 1998a; Hermann et al. 1999b; Langfitt and Rausch 1996; Sabsevitz et al. 2003), it follows that these protocols are not detecting crucial language areas.

Considerable evidence suggests that the ATL plays a role in semantic processing, that is, storage and retrieval of conceptual knowledge that underlies word and sentence meaning (Binder et al. 2009; Patterson et al. 2007; Visser et al. 2010). Damage to this semantic system has been proposed as a major cause of the naming deficits observed in patients with ATL lesions (Bell et al. 2001; Lambon Ralph et al. 2001). Several methodological factors appear to influence the sensitivity of fMRI in detecting these ATL semantic networks. First, the ATL is more strongly activated by sentences than by single words or strings of unrelated words (Friederici et al. 2000; Humphries et al. 2006, 2005; Mazoyer et al. 1993;

Vandenberghe et al. 2002; Xu et al. 2005). This observation suggests that the ATL is particularly necessary for integrating meaning across multiple words. Other studies have implicated the ATL specifically in processing semantic knowledge related to social interactions, as in stories depicting agents, actions, emotional states, motives, and so on (Olson et al. 2013; Ross and Olson 2010; Zahn et al. 2007). Finally, ATL activation is more likely to be observed when an active control task is used as a baseline, rather than a "resting" state (Binder et al. 2008b; Spitsyna et al. 2006; Stark and Squire 2001; Visser et al. 2010). For example, Stark and Squire (2001) observed activation in medial ATL regions during a picture-encoding task when an active decision task was used as a baseline but not when a "rest" baseline was used. Similarly, Spitsyna et al. (2006) observed activation in the anterior fusiform and inferior temporal gyri during a story comprehension task when an active decision task was used as a baseline but not when a "passive" baseline was used. These observations suggest that semantic processes carried out by the ATL occur even during resting or passive states, perhaps comprising a component of normal consciousness that supports planning, problem solving, daydreaming, and other high-level integrative processes that depend on semantic knowledge (Binder et al. 1999, 2009). Active, attentionally demanding control tasks disrupt these ongoing "default" processes, which would otherwise mask ATL activation.

On the basis of these considerations, Binder et al. designed an fMRI protocol aimed specifically at eliciting reliable ATL activation (Binder et al. 2011). An auditory story comprehension task ("Story") was selected to engage rapid integration of semantic information, including social concepts. This task was contrasted with an active, attentionally demanding arithmetic task ("Math") involving auditorily presented addition and subtraction problems. Prior evidence indicates that arithmetic, particularly addition and subtraction operations, does not engage the temporal lobe (Baldo and Dronkers 2007; Cappelletti et al. 2001; Crutch and Warrington 2002; Diesfeldt 1993); thus, this task was expected to interrupt ongoing "default mode" processing in the ATL and to cause minimal ATL activation. An additional feature of the arithmetic task is that it used verbal, sentence-like stimuli that could be matched to the stories on low-level features like auditory and phonological input. A second aim of this study was to test whether comparable results could be achieved across different centers using a variety of imaging hardware and software platforms.

The Story > Math contrast elicited strong activation throughout the ATL, lateral temporal lobe, and medial temporal lobe bilaterally in an initial cohort of 18 healthy participants (Fig. 17.2). The task protocol was then implemented at six other imaging centers using identical methods. Data from a second cohort of participants scanned at these centers closely replicated the results from the initial cohort. The results have since been replicated further by the Human Connectome Project (Barch et al. 2013). Compared to other fMRI protocols commonly used to elicit temporal lobe activation, the Story-Math protocol activates a much larger extent of the region typically removed in a standard ATL resection (Fig. 17.3).

In addition to these problems concerning sensitivity of the activation protocol, the problem of activation specificity is critical to address before language fMRI maps are used to tailor temporal

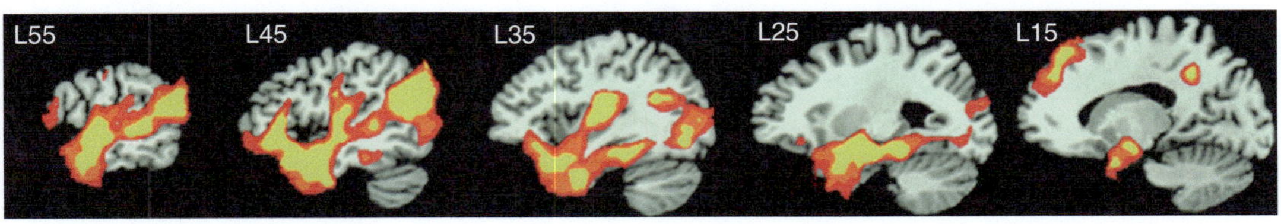

Fig. 17.2 Areas of greater activation for the Story condition relative to the Math condition (thresholded at whole-brain corrected $p < 0.05$), shown in serial sagittal sections through the left hemisphere. Stereotaxic locations are given in the *upper left corner* of each slice (adapted from Binder et al. 2011)

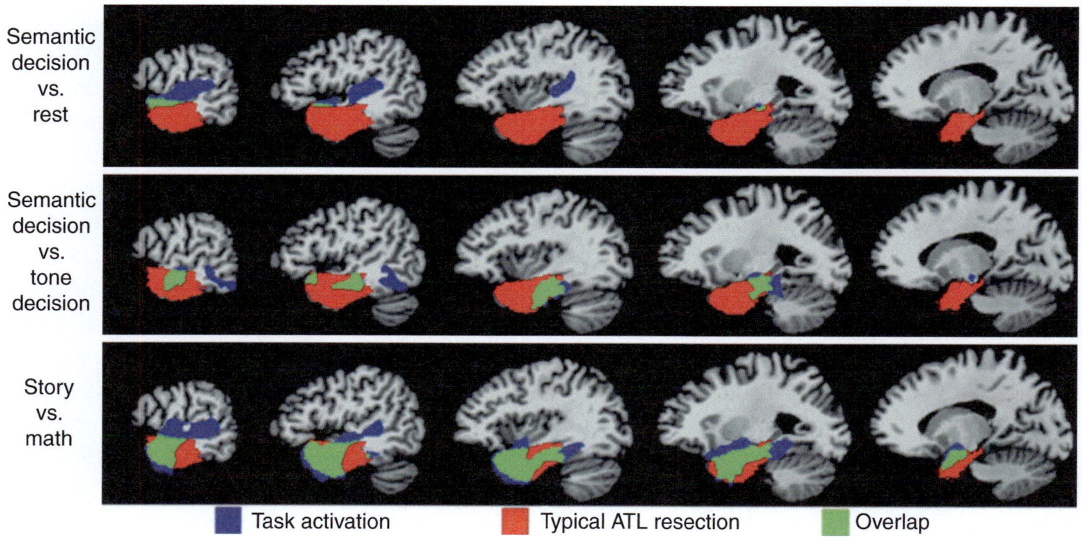

Fig. 17.3 Overlap between activated areas in three fMRI language comprehension paradigms and regions typically resected in left ATL surgery. *Red* indicates areas of lesion overlap in 23 left ATL surgery patients, based on spatially normalized postoperative MRI scans. *Blue* indicates temporal lobe regions activated with each paradigm (all thresholded at whole-brain corrected $p<0.05$) that do not fall within this typical resection zone (see Fig. 17.1. and Binder et al. (2008a) for details regarding the semantic decision vs. rest and the semantic decision vs. tone decision paradigms). *Green* indicates activated regions that overlap with the typical resection zone. Overlap with the targeted surgical zone differs markedly between the language paradigms and is greatest for the Story-Math contrast (adapted from Binder et al. 2011)

lobe resections. Some regions activated during fMRI tasks may play a minor or nonspecific role rather than a critical role in language. Resection of these "active" foci may not necessarily produce clinically relevant or persisting deficits. Thus, using fMRI activation maps to decide which brain regions can be resected involves two potential risks: (1) resection of critical language zones that are "not activated" because of insensitivity of the particular language activation protocol employed, resulting in postoperative language decline, and (2) sparing of "activated" regions that are in fact not critical for language, resulting in suboptimal seizure control. Only through very carefully designed studies—in which resections are performed blind to the fMRI data, standardized procedures are used for assessing outcome, and quantitative measures are made of the anatomical and functional lesion—will the usefulness of fMRI language maps for "tailoring" surgical resections be determined. One such study, the FMRI in Anterior Temporal Epilepsy Surgery (FATES) study, is currently underway. This prospective, multicenter study will evaluate whether language outcome after left ATL resection is related to the amount of "activated" brain tissue removed, as defined by preoperative fMRI.

17.3 Prediction of Verbal Memory Outcome

ATL resection typically involves removal of much of the anterior medial temporal lobe (MTL), including portions of the hippocampus and parahippocampus, which are known to be critical for encoding and retrieval of long-term episodic memories (Squire 1992). Verbal memory decline after left ATL resection is a consistent finding in group studies and is observed in 30–60% of such patients (Baxendale et al. 2006; Binder et al. 2008a; Chelune et al. 1991, 1993; Chiaravalloti and Glosser 2001; Gleissner et al. 2004; Helmstaedter and Elger 1996; Hermann et al. 1995; Kneebone et al. 1995; Lee et al. 2002; Lineweaver et al. 2006; Loring et al. 1995b; Martin et al. 1998; Sabsevitz et al. 2001; Stroup et al. 2003). In contrast, nonverbal memory decline after right ATL resection is less consistently observed in groups and individuals (Lee et al. 2002; Stroup et al. 2003; Lineweaver et al. 2006; Binder et al. 2008a, b). A main focus of the preoperative evaluation in ATL surgery candidates is, therefore, to estimate the risk of verbal memory decline in patients undergoing left ATL resection.

The Wada memory test was originally developed for the purpose of predicting global amnesia after ATL resection (Milner et al. 1962 #1496). Studies of its ability to predict relative verbal memory decline have been inconsistent, with several studies suggesting good predictive value (Bell et al. 2000a; Chiaravalloti and Glosser 2001; Kneebone et al. 1995; Loring et al. 1995b; Sabsevitz et al. 2001) and others showing little or none, particularly when used in combination with noninvasive tests (Binder et al. 2008a; Chelune and Najm 2000; Kirsch et al. 2005; Lacruz et al. 2004; Lineweaver et al. 2006; Stroup et al. 2003). Some authors have questioned the general validity and reliability of Wada memory results (Kubu et al. 2000; Lee et al. 1995; Loddenkemper et al. 2007; Loring et al. 1990a; Martin and Grote 2002; Novelly and Williamson 1989; Simkins-Bullock 2000). Others have emphasized the sensitivity of the test to certain details of the stimulus presentation, procedures used for recall, and other methodological factors (Alpherts et al. 2000; Carpenter et al. 1996; Loring et al. 1995a, 1994). Other presurgical tests of MTL functional or anatomical asymmetry are also modestly predictive of memory outcome, including structural MRI of the hippocampus (Cohen-Gadol et al. 2004; Lineweaver et al. 2006; Stroup et al. 2003; Trenerry et al. 1993; Wendel et al. 2001) and interictal positron emission tomography (Griffith et al. 2000). Preoperative neuropsychological testing also has predictive value, in that patients with good memory abilities prior to surgery are more likely to decline than patients with poor preoperative memory (Baxendale et al. 2006, 2007; Binder et al. 2008a; Chelune et al. 1991; Davies et al. 1998b; Gleissner et al. 2004; Helmstaedter and Elger 1996; Hermann et al. 1995; Jokeit et al. 1997; Lineweaver et al. 2006; Stroup et al. 2003).

17.3.1 fMRI of the Medial Temporal Lobe

MTL activation during memory encoding and retrieval tasks has been a subject of intense research with fMRI (for reviews, see Gabrieli 2001; Hwang and Golby 2006; Paller and Wagner 2002; Rugg et al. 2002; Schacter and Addis 2007; Schacter and Wagner 1999; Vilberg and Rugg 2008). Hippocampal activation has been demonstrated using a variety of task paradigms (e.g., Binder et al. 2005; Binder et al. 1997; Constable et al. 2000; Davachi and Wagner 2002; Eldridge et al. 2000; Fernandez et al. 1998; Greene et al. 2006; Hassabis et al. 2007; Henke et al. 1997; Kensinger et al. 2003; Killgore et al. 2002; Martin 1999; Otten et al. 2001; Parsons et al. 2006; Prince et al. 2007; Small et al. 2001; Sperling et al. 2001; Stark and Squire 2001; Vincent et al. 2006; Weis et al. 2004; Zeinah et al. 2003), although fMRI of this region is not without technical challenges. The hippocampal formation is small relative to typical voxel sizes used in fMRI. Within-voxel averaging of signals from active and inactive structures may thus impair detection of hippocampal activity. Loss of MRI signal in the medial ATL due to macroscopic field inhomogeneity can affect the amygdala and occasionally the anterior hippocampus (Constable et al. 2000; Fransson et al. 2001; Morawetz et al. 2008). Finally, the "baseline" state employed in subtraction analyses is probably of critical importance. Hippocampal encoding processes probably continue beyond the duration of the stimulus or event (Alvarez and Squire 1994), and human imaging evidence suggests that the hippocampus is relatively activated in the "resting" state (Andreasen et al. 1995; Binder et al. 1999; Martin 1999; Stark and Squire 2001).

Hippocampal activation paradigms generally employ one of three approaches. The first, based on electrophysiological studies showing that the hippocampus responds more strongly to novel than to repeated stimuli (Grunwald et al. 1998;

Knight 1996; Li et al. 1993; Riches et al. 1991), involves a contrast between encoding novel and repeated stimuli. The encoding task might involve explicit memorization for later retrieval testing or a decision task designed to produce implicit encoding. Such novelty contrasts mainly activate the posterior parahippocampus and adjacent fusiform gyrus, with involvement of the posterior hippocampus in some but not all studies (Binder et al. 2005; Fransson et al. 2001; Gabrieli et al. 1997; Hunkin et al. 2002; Kirchhoff et al. 2000; Stern et al. 1996; Tulving et al. 1996). The second approach involves manipulating the degree of associative/semantic processing that occurs during encoding. Hippocampal encoding is thought to involve the creation of "relational" representations that tie together sensory, semantic, affective, and other codes activated by an event (Cohen and Eichenbaum 1993; McClelland et al. 1995; O'Reilly and Rudy 2001). External events that are meaningful and activate semantic and emotional associations engage the hippocampus more robustly and are thus more effectively recorded (Craik and Lockhart 1972). Thus many fMRI studies have demonstrated hippocampal activation using contrasts between a stimulus (e.g., a word or picture) or task that engages associative/semantic processing and a stimulus (e.g., a nonword or unrecognizable visual form) or task that engages only sensory processing (Bartha et al. 2003; Binder et al. 1997, 2005; Davachi and Wagner 2002; Henke et al. 1997, 1999; Kensinger et al. 2003; Killgore et al. 2002; Martin 1999; Otten et al. 2001; Small et al. 2001; Sperling et al. 2001; Wagner et al. 1998; Zeinah et al. 2003). Finally, a third approach uses subsequent recognition performance as a direct index of MTL activity during encoding. Items encoded during the fMRI scan are sorted according to whether they were later remembered during postscan testing, and a contrast is made between successfully and unsuccessfully encoded items. These studies consistently show greater MTL activation during subsequently remembered compared to subsequently forgotten stimuli, although the precise MTL regions showing this effect have varied considerably (Brewer et al. 1998; Buckner et al. 2001; Constable et al. 2000; Davachi and Wagner 2002; Fernandez et al. 1998; Kirchhoff et al. 2000; Otten et al. 2001; Prince et al. 2005, 2007; Uncapher and Rugg 2005; Wagner et al. 1998; Weis et al. 2004).

Finally, the lateralization of MTL activation detected by fMRI depends on the type of stimulus material encoded. MTL activation is left-lateralized for verbal stimuli and generally symmetric for pictorial stimuli (Binder et al. 1997, 2005; Golby et al. 2001; Kelley et al. 1998; Martin 1999; Otten et al. 2001; Powell et al. 2005; Reber et al. 2002).

17.3.2 Medial Temporal Lobe fMRI as a Predictor of Memory Outcome

Several fMRI studies have examined the relationship between preoperative MTL activation and memory outcome after ATL surgery (Table 17.1). Rabin et al. (2004) studied 23 patients undergoing ATL resection (10 left and 13 right) using a scene encoding task that activates the posterior MTL bilaterally (Detre et al. 1998). Patients were tested for delayed recognition of the same pictures immediately after scanning. Delayed picture recognition was then tested again after surgery, and the change on this recognition task was used as the primary memory outcome variable. About half of the patients in both left and right surgery groups declined on this measure. Preoperative fMRI activation lateralization toward the side of surgery was correlated with decline, as was the extent of activation on the side of surgery. These results were the first to demonstrate a relationship between preoperative fMRI activation asymmetry and outcome, yet they are of limited relevance to the problem of predicting verbal memory outcome. In the left ATL patients studied by Rabin et al., neither Wada memory nor fMRI activation asymmetry predicted verbal memory decline as measured by standard psychometric tests.

Richardson, Powell, and colleagues studied correlations between hippocampal activation and verbal memory outcome in three small studies (Powell et al. 2008; Richardson et al. 2004, 2006). Patients performed a semantic decision task with words during the fMRI scan and then took a recognition test after scanning. Words that were subsequently recognized were contrasted with words

Table 17.1 fMRI studies of verbal memory outcome prediction in ATL surgery

Author	Year	*N*	fMRI contrast	Memory measure	Summary
Rabin et al.	2004	10 L 13 R	Indoor/outdoor decision on visual scenes vs. passive viewing of scrambled scenes	Recognition of scenes encoded during fMRI	MTL LI predicts outcome on scene recognition task in both surgery groups
Richardson et al.	2004	10 L	Subsequently recognized vs. familiar but not recognized words encoded during a semantic decision task	Word-list learning and story recall (Adult Memory and Information Processing Battery)	Activation asymmetry in a hippocampus region of interest (ROI) predicts verbal memory outcome
Richardson et al.	2006	12 L	Same as Richardson et al. (2004)	Same as Richardson et al. (2004)	Unilateral activation in ether left or right hippocampus ROI predicts verbal memory outcome
Binder et al.	2008a	60 L	Semantic decision on auditory words vs. sensory decision on tones	Word-list learning and delayed recall (Selective Reminding Test)	LI predicts verbal memory outcome, adds value beyond other predictors
Frings et al.	2008	9 L 10 R 12 R	Memorizing and recognizing object locations vs. comparing size of two objects	Word-list learning (Verbaler Lern- and Merkfaehigkeitstest)	Hippocampal LI predicts verbal memory outcome, mainly in left group
Köylü et al.	2008	14 L 12 R	Semantic decision on auditory words vs. sensory decision on tones	Word-list learning and delayed recall (Münchner Gedächtnistest)	MTL activation correlates with pre- and postoperative memory
Powell et al.	2008	7 L 8 R	Subsequently recognized vs. forgotten words and faces encoded during a semantic decision task	Word-list learning and visual design learning	Unilateral activation in dominant-side hippocampus ROI predicts verbal memory outcome in dominant resection
Binder et al.	2010	30 L 37 R	Indoor/outdoor decision on visual scenes vs. perceptual matching of scrambled scenes	Word-list learning and delayed recall (Selective Reminding Test)	Hippocampal LI for scenes does not predict verbal memory outcome
Bonelli et al.	2010	29 L 25 R	Same paradigm as in Powell et al. (2008)	Same as Powell et al. (2008)	Anterior and posterior MTL LIs from the word-encoding condition predict verbal memory outcome
Sidhu et al.	2015	23 L 27 R	Semantic decision on visual words vs. resting baseline	Word-list learning (Brain Injury Rehabilitation Trust Memory and Information Processing Battery)	Frontotemporal LI predicts verbal memory outcome in the left surgery group

that were judged to be familiar but not recognized. In the first of these studies (Richardson et al. 2004), the authors observed a focus in the anterior hippocampus where *asymmetry* of activation (i.e., left-right) predicted verbal memory outcome on a standardized word-list learning test after left ATL resection. Greater activation in this region on the left side relative to the right side predicted greater decline. The second study by the same authors, however, showed correlations between outcome and hippocampal activation on either side (Richardson et al. 2006). That is, greater activation unilaterally on the left or the right was associated with poorer outcome. The correlation between verbal memory decline after *left* ATL resection and activation in the *right* hippocampus is difficult to explain, as patients with greater activation in the right hippocampus preoperatively would be expected to have a better outcome, not a worse outcome (Chelune 1995). This finding was not replicated in the third study (Powell et al. 2008), which reported a correlation between left hippocampus activation and poor outcome but no correlation between right hippocampus activation and outcome. A methodological limitation in all of these studies is that they are based on fMRI activation values extracted from a small region of interest defined by searching the volume for voxels that show a correlation with outcome across a group of patients. As the coordinates of these correlated voxels have varied across the studies, it is not clear how this method of extracting activation values would be applied to a newly encountered patient.

Frings et al. studied the relationship between preoperative hippocampal activation asymmetry and verbal memory outcome in a small sample of patients undergoing left or right ATL resection (Frings et al. 2008). The fMRI protocol used a task in which patients viewed a virtual-reality environment containing colored geometric shapes and either memorized the location of these objects or performed a recognition decision following memorization. These "memory" tasks were contrasted with a control task in which patients saw two versions of a geometric object and indicated which one was larger. This fMRI contrast had been shown previously to activate posterior MTL regions (mainly posterior parahippocampus) bilaterally. An LI was computed over the entire hippocampus, defined using a stereotaxic atlas. Verbal memory change was marginally correlated (1-tailed, $p=0.077$) with preoperative LI in the left ATL surgery group, but not in the right surgery group. A significant correlation (1-tailed, $p<0.05$) was obtained when the groups were combined, indicating greater verbal memory decline when preoperative hippocampal activation was lateralized more toward the side of surgery.

Binder et al. (2010) measured hippocampal activation asymmetry in 30 left and 37 right ATL surgery patients using a scene-encoding task. An anterior hippocampal ROI was defined using a probabilistic atlas in standard stereotaxic space. When contrasted with a perceptual matching task, this paradigm activates the anterior hippocampus bilaterally (Binder et al. 2005). Activation asymmetry was correlated with side of seizure focus ($p=0.004$) and with Wada memory testing performed in the same patients ($p=0.009$). This activation asymmetry, however, did not predict verbal memory outcome.

In the most significant study on this topic to date, Bonelli et al. (2010) examined verbal and nonverbal memory outcome in 54 patients undergoing left or right ATL surgery. The fMRI paradigm used the subsequent recognition contrast with words and faces developed by Powell et al. (2005, 2008). The authors operationally defined ROIs in each individual as the location where activation asymmetry was highest. An "asymmetry image" was created in each individual by contrasting activation levels in mirror-symmetric voxels in the left and right temporal lobes. A small sphere around the voxel with the highest asymmetry value was used as the ROI. Two such ROIs were created in each patient, one in the anterior MTL and one in the posterior MTL. The main finding was a strong correlation ($R^2=0.23$, $p=0.008$) between anterior MTL ROI asymmetry during word encoding and verbal memory change scores in the left ATL surgery group, such that the greater the asymmetry toward the left, the greater the decline in verbal memory. Interestingly, there was a significant correlation ($R^2=0.14$, $p=0.04$) in the opposite direction for the posterior MTL ROI, such that greater asymmetry toward the left was associated with *less* verbal memory decline. Given that the posterior hippocampus is typically spared in ATL resections, the authors interpreted the latter finding as evidence that intrahemispheric recruitment of the posterior left hippocampus in left TLE is important for preservation of verbal memory processes.

These studies are informative in several ways. Three studies (Binder et al. 2010; Frings et al. 2008; Rabin et al. 2004) used scene-encoding tasks that activate the MTL bilaterally on fMRI, a pattern that suggests activation of both verbal and nonverbal memory encoding systems. Prediction of verbal memory outcome using these paradigms appears to be weak at best (see Mechanic-Hamilton et al. 2009, for further evidence). In contrast, the verbal memory fMRI paradigms used by Richardson, Powell, and Bonelli et al. provide better predictive information regarding verbal memory outcome. These results provide further support for the long-standing concept of material-specific encoding in the episodic memory system. The results of Bonelli et al., though based on a relatively small sample of 29 left ATL surgery patients, are particularly promising and should be confirmed prospectively in a larger group of patients.

17.3.3 Language Lateralization as a Predictor of Verbal Memory Outcome

Binder et al. studied the relationship between preoperative language lateralization and verbal memory outcome (Binder et al. 2008a). The premise underlying this approach is that the verbal episodic memory encoding system is likely to be colateralized with language. More generally, the authors proposed that the type of material preferentially encoded by the left or right episodic memory system depends on the type of information it receives from the ipsilateral neocortex. If this model is correct, then the MTL in the language-dominant hemisphere is likely to be more critical for supporting verbal episodic memory, and language lateralization should be a reliable indicator of verbal memory lateralization.

The study included 60 patients who underwent left ATL resection and a control group of 63 patients who underwent right ATL resection. The fMRI paradigm used a contrast between an auditory semantic decision task and a nonlinguistic tone decision task (Fig. 17.1, lower panel). Verbal memory was measured preoperatively and 6 months after surgery using the Selective Reminding Test, a word-list learning and retention test (Buschke and Fuld 1974). Other neuropsychological testing included the story recall and visual reproduction subtests from Wechsler Memory Scale (Wechsler 1997). Language LIs were computed from the fMRI data using a large region of interest covering the lateral two-thirds of each hemisphere (Springer et al. 1999). All patients also underwent preoperative Wada language and object memory testing.

The left ATL surgery group showed substantial changes in verbal memory, with an average raw score decline of 43% on word-list learning and 45% on delayed recall of the word list. Of the individual patients in this group, 33% declined significantly on the learning measure and 55% on the delayed recall measure. In contrast, the right ATL surgery group improved slightly on both measures. Neither groups showed significant changes on any nonverbal memory tests. Preoperative measures that predicted verbal memory decline in the left surgery group included the preoperative score, the fMRI language LI, the Wada language asymmetry score, the age at onset of epilepsy, and the Wada memory asymmetry score (Table 17.2, Fig. 17.4).

Table 17.2 Preoperative predictors of verbal memory outcome in 60 left ATL surgery patients

Predictor variable	List learning	*p*	Delayed recall	*p*
Preoperative score	−0.662	<0.0001	−0.654	<0.0001
fMRI language LI	−0.432	<0.001	−0.316	<0.05
Wada language asymmetry	−0.398	<0.01	−0.363	<0.01
Age at epilepsy onset	−0.341	<0.01	−0.390	<0.01
Wada memory asymmetry	−0.331	<0.05	−0.135	ns

List learning and delayed recall refer to the consistent long-term recall and delayed recall subtests of the selective reminding test. Simple correlation values and *p* values for each correlation are shown

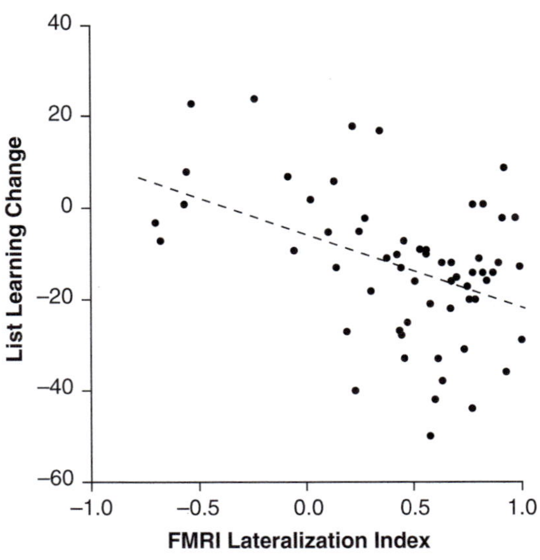

Fig. 17.4 Relationship between fMRI lateralization indexes and individual change scores on a word-list learning verbal memory test (Continuous Long-Term Recall from the Selective Reminding Test) in 60 left ATL surgery patients ($r = -0.432$, $p < 0.001$) (adapted from Binder et al. 2008a)

Similar results were reported by Sidhu et al. in a study of 23 patients with left ATL resection (Sidhu et al. 2015). During fMRI, the patients performed a semantic decision ("is it pleasant or unpleasant?") on visually presented concrete words. Delayed recognition of the words was tested after scanning, and the activation associated with correctly recognized words was then computed. Although the authors refer to this as a memory paradigm, this analysis differs from the standard subsequent memory paradigm (used by Powell, Richardson, and other authors) in that remembered words were compared with a resting baseline rather than with nonremembered words. Rather than specifically identifying activation from episodic memory encoding processes, this contrast would capture all of the linguistic, attention, and even motor response processes that accompany the semantic decision task. Activations were accordingly widespread, including in right-hand motor regions. An ROI covering frontal and temporal regions included many typical language regions. Leftward activation asymmetry in this ROI was correlated with pre- to postoperative decline on a word-list learning test ($r = -0.66$, $p = 0.001$). Somewhat surprisingly, memory change was not related to preoperative score, age at onset of epilepsy, or hippocampal volumes. No preoperative variables were related to memory change in a group of 27 right ATL surgery patients.

In applying these results to real clinical situations, the main questions to resolve are the following: which tests make a significant independent contribution to predicting outcome and how should results from these tests be optimally combined? Binder et al. (2008a) addressed these questions in a series of stepwise multiple regression analyses. The first variables entered in all analyses were preoperative test performance and age at the onset of epilepsy. The rationale for including these variables first is that they can be obtained with relatively little expense and at no risk to the patient. Next, the fMRI language LI was added, followed by simultaneous addition of both the Wada memory and Wada language asymmetry scores. The rationale for adding fMRI in the second step is that fMRI is noninvasive and carries less risk than the Wada test. The two Wada scores were added together in the final step because these measures are typically obtained together.

Preoperative score and age at the onset of epilepsy together accounted for 49% of the variance in List Learning outcome and 54% of the variance in Delayed Recall outcome. The fMRI LI accounted for an additional 10% of the variance in List Learning outcome ($p=0.001$) and 7% of the variance in Delayed Recall outcome ($p=0.003$). Addition of the Wada language and memory data did not significantly improve the predictive power of either model (R^2 change for List Learning=0.025, R^2 change for Delayed Recall=0.017, both $p>0.1$). When patients were categorized as showing decline or no decline based on a negative change score 1.5 standard deviations or more from the mean change score in the right ATL surgery group, the List Learning outcome model showed sensitivity of 90% and specificity of 80% for predicting decline on List Learning. The delayed recall outcome model showed sensitivity of 81% and specificity of 100% for predicting decline on Delayed Recall.

These results are interesting for several reasons. Most intriguing is the finding that *language* lateralization, whether measured by fMRI or the Wada test, was a better predictor of verbal *memory* outcome than Wada memory testing. The explanation for this paradox rests on two hypotheses. One, mentioned earlier, is that verbal memory encoding processes tend to colateralize with language processes. The second hypothesis is that many tests of memory lateralization do not specifically assess verbal memory encoding. That is, visual stimuli such as objects and pictures can be dually encoded using both verbal and visual codes. Wada memory procedures that use such stimuli (including the Wada test used by Binder et al.) therefore do not provide a measure of verbal memory lateralization but rather a measure of overall memory lateralization that includes both verbal and nonverbal encoding processes. Together, these two hypotheses suggest that lan-

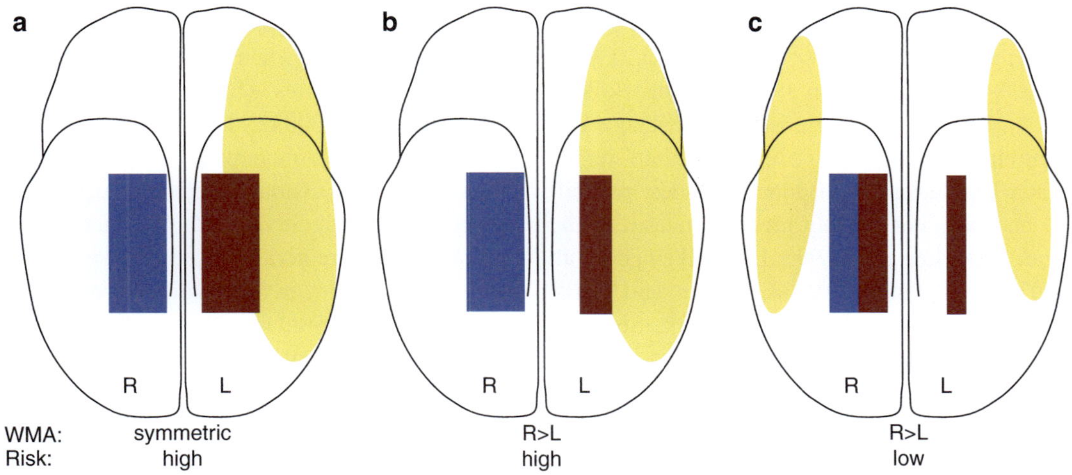

Fig. 17.5 Schematic diagram of a hypothetical model of memory and language representation in temporal lobe epilepsy (TLE). The *yellow* ovals represent language systems, *red* rectangles represent verbal episodic memory encoding systems in the MTL, and *blue* rectangles represent nonverbal episodic memory encoding systems in the MTL. (**a**) Typical state in healthy subjects and patients with late-onset epilepsy. Language and verbal memory processes are strongly left-lateralized, placing the patient at high risk for verbal memory decline. (**b**) Chronic left TLE without shift. The left MTL is dysfunctional, causing Wada memory asymmetry (WMA) to the right, but verbal memory has not shifted, leaving the patient at high risk for verbal memory decline. (**c**) Chronic left TLE with shift. Both language and verbal memory functions have shifted partially to the right, lowering the risk for verbal memory decline. Note the partial lack of correspondence, across patient types, between Wada memory asymmetry and level of risk (adapted from Binder et al. 2008a)

guage asymmetry may be more closely correlated than Wada memory asymmetry with verbal memory lateralization (Fig. 17.5). In particular, some patients with left temporal seizures show right-lateralized memory on the Wada test due to a strong nonverbal memory component in the right hemisphere but are nevertheless at high risk for verbal memory decline because their *verbal* memory remains strongly lateralized to the left (Fig. 17.5b).

These data also have direct implications for clinical practice. First, they confirm the utility of fMRI for predicting verbal memory outcome in patients undergoing left ATL resection. The fMRI language LI is a safe, noninvasive measure that improves prediction accuracy relative to other noninvasive measures. The finding that Wada memory lateralization is not a strong predictor of verbal memory outcome and adds no predictive value beyond these noninvasive measures confirms several previous studies that also examined multivariate prediction models (Chelune and Najm 2000; Kirsch et al. 2005; Lacruz et al. 2004; Lineweaver et al. 2006; Stroup et al. 2003). Although Binder et al. found that Wada language asymmetry is a stronger predictor of verbal memory outcome than Wada memory lateralization, even the addition of both Wada tests together did not contribute additional predictive power after inclusion of available noninvasive data (including fMRI). These results call into question the routine use of the Wada test for predicting material-specific verbal memory outcome, particularly if a validated fMRI measure of language lateralization is available. Some practitioners continue to value the Wada test as a means of predicting more severe "global" amnesia, such is known to occur after bilateral MTL damage (Di Gennaro et al. 2006; Guerreiro et al. 2001; Milner et al. 1962; Scoville and Milner 1957). According to this theory, anesthetization of the to-be-resected MTL is necessary to discover whether the contralateral hemisphere is healthy enough to support memory on its own. Empirical observations, however, provide little support for such an approach. Cases of global amnesia following unilateral temporal lobe resection—especially modern, well-documented cases—appear to be rare in the extreme (Baxendale 1998; Kapur and Prevett 2003; Kubu et al. 2000; Loring et al. 1990a; Novelly and Williamson 1989; Simkins-Bullock 2000). Furthermore, there is ample evidence that contralateral hemisphere "memory failure" on the Wada test suffers from poor test–retest reliability and does not reliably predict amnesia (Kubu et al. 2000; Lee et al. 1995; Loddenkemper et al. 2007; Loring et al. 1990a; Martin and Grote 2002; Novelly and Williamson 1989; Simkins-Bullock 2000). Given the availability of fMRI for predicting material-specific verbal memory outcome, perhaps the use of the Wada test should be reserved only for those patients at greatest risk for global amnesia, that is, patients undergoing unilateral ATL resection who have structural or functional evidence of damage to the contralateral MTL. Because it is noninvasive and requires fewer personnel, fMRI is also likely to be considerably less costly than Wada testing.

17.4 Conclusions

Recent studies demonstrate that preoperative fMRI can be used to predict postoperative naming and verbal memory changes in patients undergoing left ATL resection. Most importantly, two studies showed that fMRI significantly improves prediction accuracy when combined with other noninvasive measures (Binder et al. 2008a; Sabsevitz et al. 2003). Thus, fMRI provides patients and practitioners with a tool for making better informed decisions based on a quantitative assessment of cognitive risk. The quantitative nature of these predictions represents something of a paradigm shift, in that traditional predictive models using the Wada test tended to be implemented as a dichotomous "pass or fail" judgment. The alternative approach followed in many recent studies involves the development of multivariable formulas that compute predicted change scores (Fig. 17.6). These quantitative predictions provide a much more realistic picture of the actual outcomes, which are not dichotomous but instead vary smoothly along a continuum. Ultimately, of course, the decision whether to undergo surgery is a categorical one, but the categorical nature of the decision does not obviate the need for precision regarding the factors that enter into the decision. An unemployed patient with frequent seizures may be willing to tolerate a substantial decline in naming or verbal memory, whereas a patient who depends on such cognitive abilities for his livelihood may be willing to risk a small decline but not a large one.

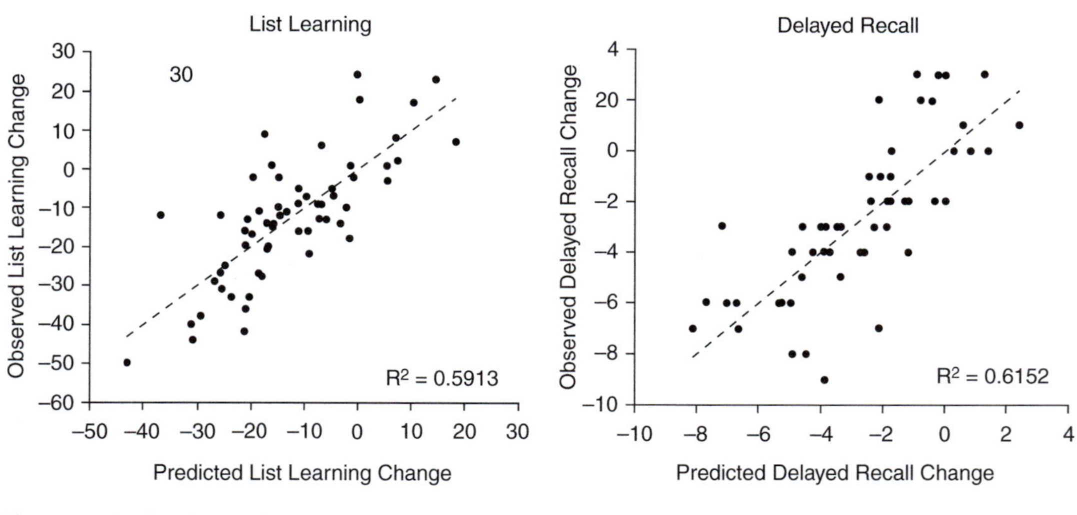

Fig. 17.6 Predicted vs. observed individual memory change scores in 60 left ATL surgery patients on tests of List Learning and Delayed Recall. Predicted list learning change scores were computed from the formula 17.67 − 0.704 (preoperative score) − 0.280 (age at onset) − 12.19 (fMRI LI). Predicted delayed recall change scores were computed from the formula 0.76 − 0.688 (preoperative score) − 0.093 (age at onset) − 2.14 (fMRI LI) (adapted from Binder et al. 2008a)

In practice, the use of fMRI for predicting outcome in epilepsy surgery depends critically on the validity of the fMRI protocol and the involvement of clinicians with the necessary clinical expertise. Language fMRI is a complex test of higher brain function, which will produce high-quality results only if high-quality methods are used. Unlike a structural imaging study, the patient is required to perform a specific mental task or tasks during fMRI, must understand fully what to do, and must be monitored for compliance during the study. The task conditions must be designed to reliably and specifically identify the mental processes of interest, based on modern scientific knowledge about these processes rather than on folk psychology or nineteenth-century neurology. These challenges can best be met through close involvement of cognitive scientists in the design of task protocols and by direct involvement of clinicians with expertise in cognitive testing to provide patient instruction and performance assessment during scanning.

Acknowledgments Thanks to Linda Allen, Christopher Anderson, Chad Carlson, Lisa Conant, Bill Gross, Thomas Hammeke, Yu Liu, Wade Mueller, Thomas Prieto, Manoj Raghavan, Megan Rozman, David Sabsevitz, Sara Swanson, Laura Umfleet, and other personnel at the Froedtert-MCW Comprehensive Epilepsy Center for assistance with this research, which was also supported by National Institute of Neurological Diseases and Stroke grant R01 NS35929, National Institutes of Health General Clinical Research Center grant M01 RR00058, and the Charles A. Dana Foundation.

References

Adcock JE, Wise RG, Oxbury JM, Oxbury SM, Matthews PM (2003) Quantitative fMRI assessment of the differences in lateralization of language-related brain activation in patients with temporal lobe epilepsy. NeuroImage 18:423–438

Alpherts WC, Vermeulen J, van Veelen CW (2000) The Wada test: prediction of focus lateralization by asymmetric and symmetric recall. Epilepsy Res 39(3):239–249

Alvarez P, Squire LR (1994) Memory consolidation and the medial temporal lobe: a simple network model. Proc Natl Acad Sci U S A 91:7041–7045

Andreasen NC, O'Leary DS, Cizadlo T, Arndt S, Rezai K, Watkins GL et al (1995) Remembering the past: two facets of episodic memory explored with positron emission tomography. Am J Psychiatr 152:1576–1585

Audrain S, Barnett AJ, McAndrews MP (2018) Language network measures at rest indicate individual differences in naming decline after anterior temporal lobe resection. Hum Brain Mapp 39:4404–4419

Baciu M, Kahane P, Minotti L, Charnallet A, David D, Le Bas JF et al (2001) Functional MRI assessment of the hemispheric predominance for language in epileptic patients using a simple rhyme detection task. Epileptic Disord 3(3):117–124

Bahn MM, Lin W, Silbergeld DL, Miller JW, Kuppusamy K, Cook RJ et al (1997) Localization of language cortices by functional MR imaging compared with intracarotid amobarbital hemispheric sedation. Am J Radiol 169:575–579

Baldo JV, Dronkers NF (2007) Neural correlates of arithmetic and language comprehension: a common substrate? Neuropsychologia 45:229–235

Barch DM, Burgess GC, Harms MP, Petersen SE, Schlaggar BL, Corbetta M et al (2013) Function in the human connectome: task-fMRI and individual differences in behavior. NeuroImage 80:169–189

Bartha L, Brenneis C, Schocke M, Trinka E, Koylu B, Trieb T et al (2003) Medial temporal lobe activation during semantic language processing: fMRI findings in healthy left- and right-handers. Cogn Brain Res 17:339–346

Baxendale S (1998) Amnesia in temporal lobectomy patients: historical perspective and review. Seizure 7(1):15–24

Baxendale S, Thompson P, Harkness W, Duncan J (2006) Predicting memory decline following epilepsy surgery: a multivariate approach. Epilepsia 47(11):1887–1894

Baxendale S, Thompson P, Harkness W, Duncan J (2007) The role of the intracarotid amobarbital procedure in predicting verbal memory decline after temporal lobe resection. Epilepsia 48(3):546–552

Bell BD, Davies KG, Haltiner AM, Walters GL (2000a) Intracarotid amobarbital procedure and prediction of postoperative memory in patients with left temporal lobe epilepsy and hippocampal sclerosis. Epilepsia 41:992–997

Bell BD, Davies KG, Hermann BP, Walters G (2000b) Confrontation naming after anterior temporal lobectomy is related to age of acquisition of the object names. Neuropsychologia 38:83–92

Bell BD, Hermann BP, Woodard AR, Jones JE, Rutecki PA, Sheth R et al (2001) Object naming and semantic knowledge in temporal lobe epilepsy. Neuropsychology 15(4):434–443

Benke T, Koylu B, Visani P, Karner E, Brenneis C, Bartha L et al (2006) Language lateralization in temporal lobe epilepsy: a comparison between fMRI and the Wada Test. Epilepsia 47(8):1308–1319

Benson RR, FitzGerald DB, LeSeuer LL, Kennedy DN, Kwong KK, Buchbinder BR et al (1999) Language dominance determined by whole brain functional MRI in patients with brain lesions. Neurology 52:798–809

Binder JR (2016) fMRI of language systems. In: Filippi M (ed) fMRI techniques and protocols, 2nd edn. Humana Press, New York, pp 355–386

Binder JR, Swanson SJ, Hammeke TA, Morris GL, Mueller WM, Fischer M et al (1996) Determination of language dominance using functional MRI: a comparison with the Wada test. Neurology 46: 978–984

Binder JR, Frost JA, Hammeke TA, Cox RW, Rao SM, Prieto T (1997) Human brain language areas identified by functional MRI. J Neurosci 17(1):353–362

Binder JR, Frost JA, Hammeke TA, Bellgowan PSF, Rao SM, Cox RW (1999) Conceptual processing during the conscious resting state: a functional MRI study. J Cogn Neurosci 11(1):80–93

Binder JR, Bellgowan PSF, Hammeke TA, Possing ET, Frost JA (2005) A comparison of two fMRI protocols for eliciting hippocampal activation. Epilepsia 46(7):1061–1070

Binder JR, Sabsevitz DS, Swanson SJ, Hammeke TA, Raghavan M, Mueller WM (2008a) Use of preoperative functional MRI to predict verbal memory decline after temporal lobe epilepsy surgery. Epilepsia 49:1377–1394

Binder JR, Swanson SJ, Hammeke TA, Sabsevitz DS (2008b) A comparison of five fMRI protocols for mapping speech comprehension systems. Epilepsia 49(12):1980–1997

Binder JR, Desai R, Conant LL, Graves WW (2009) Where is the semantic system? A critical review and meta-analysis of 120 functional neuroimaging studies. Cereb Cortex 19:2767–2796

Binder JR, Swanson SJ, Sabsevitz DS, Hammeke TA, Raghavan M, Mueller WM (2010) A comparison of two fMRI methods for predicting verbal memory decline after left temporal lobectomy: language lateralization vs. hippocampal activation asymmetry. Epilepsia 51(4):618–626

Binder JR, Gross W, Allendorfer JB, Bonilha L, Chapin J, Edwards JC et al (2011) Mapping anterior temporal language areas with fMRI: a multi-center normative study. NeuroImage 54(2):1465–1475

Biswal BB, Yetkin FZ, Haughton VM, Hyde JS (1995) Functional connectivity in the motor cortex of resting human brain using echo-planar MRI. Magn Reson Med 34:537–541

Bonelli SB, Powell RHW, Yogarajah M, Samson RS, Symms MR, Thompson PJ et al (2010) Imaging memory in temporal lobe epilepsy: predicting the effects of temporal lobe resection. Brain 133:1186–1199

Bonelli SB, Thompson PJ, Yogarajah M, Vollmar C, Powell RHW, Symms MR et al (2012) Imaging language networks before and after anterior temporal lobe resection: results of a longitudinal fMRI study. Epilepsia 53(4):639–650

Brewer JB, Zhao Z, Desmond JE, Glover GH, Gabrieli JDE (1998) Making memories: brain activity that predicts how well visual experience will be remembered. Science 281:1185–1188

Buckner RL, Wheeler ME, Sheridan MA (2001) Encoding processes during retrieval tasks. J Cogn Neurosci 13(3):406–415

Busch RM, Floden DP, Prayson B, Chapin JS, Kim KH, Ferguson L et al (2016) Estimating risk of word-finding problems in adults undergoing epilepsy surgery. Neurology 87:2363–2369

Buschke H, Fuld PA (1974) Evaluating storage, retention, and retrieval in disordered memory and learning. Neurology 24:1019–1025

Cappelletti M, Butterworth B, Kopelman M (2001) Spared numerical abilities in a case of semantic dementia. Neuropsychologia 39(11):1224–1239

Carpenter K, Oxbury JM, Oxbury S, Wright GD (1996) Memory for objects presented after intracarotid sodium amytal: a sensitive clinical neuropsychological indicator of temporal lobe pathology. Seizure 5:103–108

Carpentier A, Pugh KR, Westerveld M, Studholme C, Skrinjar O, Thompson JL et al (2001) Functional MRI of language processing: dependence on input modality and temporal lobe epilepsy. Epilepsia 42:1241–1254

Chelune GC (1995) Hippocampal adequacy versus functional reserve: predicting memory functions following temporal lobectomy. Arch Clin Neuropsychol 10:413–432

Chelune GJ, Najm IM (2000) Risk factors associated with postsurgical decrements in memory. In: Luders HO, Comair Y (eds) Epilepsy surgery, 2nd edn. Lippincott, Philadelphia, pp 497–504

Chelune GJ, Naugle RI, Lüders H, Awad IA (1991) Prediction of cognitive change as a function of preoperative ability level among temporal lobectomy patients at six months follow-up. Neurology 41:399–404

Chelune GJ, Naugle RI, Lüders H, Sedlak J, Awad IA (1993) Individual change after epilepsy surgery: Practice effects and base-rate information. Neuropsychology 7:41–52

Chiaravalloti ND, Glosser G (2001) Material-specific memory changes after anterior temporal lobectomy as predicted by the intracarotid amobarbital test. Epilepsia 42:902–911

Chlebus P, Mikl M, Brazdil M, Pazourkova M, Krupa P, Rektor I (2007) fMRI evaluation of hemispheric language dominance using various methods of laterality index calculation. Exp Brain Res 179:365–374

Cohen NJ, Eichenbaum H (1993) Memory, amnesia, and the hippocampal system. MIT Press, Cambridge, MA

Cohen-Gadol AA, Westerveld M, Alvarez-Carilles J, Spencer DD (2004) Intracarotid amytal memory test and hippocampal magnetic resonance imaging volumetry: validity of the Wada test as an indicator of hippocampal integrity among candidates for epilepsy surgery. J Neurosurg 101:926–931

Constable RT, Carpentier A, Pugh K, Westerveld M, Oszunar Y, Spencer DD (2000) Investigation of the hippocampal formation using a randomized event-related paradigm and z-shimmed functional MRI. NeuroImage 12:55–62

Craik FIM, Lockhart RS (1972) Levels of processing: a framework for memory research. J Verbal Learn Verbal Behav 11:671–684

Crutch SJ, Warrington EK (2002) Preserved calculation skills in a case of semantic dementia. Cortex 38:389–399

Damasio H, Grabowski TJ, Tranel D, Hichwa RD, Damasio AR (1996) A neural basis for lexical retrieval. Nature 380:499–505

Davachi L, Wagner AD (2002) Hippocampal contributions to episodic memory: insights from relational and item-based learning. J Neurophysiol 88:982–990

Davies KG, Bell BD, Bush AJ, Hermann BP, Dohan FC, Jaap AS (1998a) Naming decline after left anterior temporal lobectomy correlates with pathological status of resected hippocampus. Epilepsia 39:407–419

Davies KG, Bell BD, Bush AJ, Wyler AR (1998b) Prediction of verbal memory loss in individuals after anterior temporal lobectomy. Epilepsia 39:820–828

Deblaere K, Boon PA, Vandemaele P, Tieleman A, Vonck K, Vingerhoets G et al (2004) MRI language dominance assessment in epilepsy patients at 1.0 T: region of interest analysis and comparison with intracarotid amytal testing. Neuroradiology 46(6):413–420

Desmond JE, Sum JM, Wagner AD, Demb JB, Shear PK, Glover GH et al (1995) Functional MRI measurement of language lateralization in Wada-tested patients. Brain 118:1411–1419

Detre JA, Maccotta L, King D, Alsop DC, D'Esposito M, Zarahn E et al (1998) Functional MRI lateralization of memory in temporal lobe epilepsy. Neurology 50:926–932

Di Gennaro G, Grammaldo LG, Quarato PP, Esposito V, Mascia A, Sparano A et al (2006) Severe amnesia following bilateral medial temporal lobe damage occurring on two distinct occasions. Neurol Sci 27(2):129–133

Diesfeldt HFA (1993) Progressive decline of semantic memory with preservation of number processing and calculation. Behav Neurol 6:239–242

Doucet G, Pustina D, Skidmore C, Sharan A, Sperling M, Tracy J (2015) Resting-state functional connectivity predicts the strength of hemispheric lateralization for language processing in temporal lobe epilepsy and normals. Hum Brain Mapp 36:288–303

Eldridge LL, Knowlton BJ, Furmanski CS, Bookheimer SY, Engel SA (2000) Remembering episodes: a selective role for the hippocampus during retrieval. Nat Neurosci 3(11):1149–1152

Fernandez G, Weyerts H, Schrader-Bölsche M, Tendolkar I, Smid HG, Tempelmann C et al (1998) Successful verbal encoding into episodic memory engages the posterior hippocampus: a parametrically analyzed functional magnetic resonance imaging study. J Neurosci 18:1841–1847

Fox MD, Snyder AZ, Vincent JL, Corbetta M, Van Essen DC, Raichle ME (2005) The human brain is intrinsically organized into dynamic, anticorrelated functional networks. Proc Natl Acad Sci U S A 102:9673–9678

Fransson P, Merboldt KD, Ingvar M, Petersson KM, Frahm J (2001) Functional MRI with reduced susceptibility artifact: high-resolution mapping of episodic memory encoding. Neuroreport 12(7):1415–1420

Friederici AD, Meyer M, von Cramon DY (2000) Auditory language comprehension: an event-related fMRI study on the processing of syntactic and lexical information. Brain Lang 74:289–300

Frings L, Wagner K, Halsband U, Schwarzwald R, Zentner J, Schulze-Bonhage A (2008) Lateralization of hippocampal activation differs between left and right temporal lobe epilepsy patients and correlates with postsurgical verbal learning decrement. Epilepsy Res 78(2–3):161–170

Gabrieli JDE (2001) Functional imaging of episodic memory. In: Cabeza R, Kingstone A (eds) Handbook of functional neuroimaging of cognition. MIT Press, Cambridge, MA, pp 253–291

Gabrieli JDE, Brewer JB, Desmond JE, Glover GH (1997) Separate neural bases of two fundamental memory processes in human medial temporal lobe. Science 276:264–266

Gaillard WD, Balsamo L, Xu B, McKinney C, Papero PH, Weinstein S et al (2004) fMRI language task panel improves determination of language dominance. Neurology 63(8):1403–1408

Gleissner U, Helmstaedter C, Schramm J, Elger CE (2004) Memory outcome after selective amygdalohippocampectomy in patients with temporal lobe epilepsy: one-year follow-up. Epilepsia 45(8):960–962

Golby AJ, Poldrack RA, Brewer JB, Spencer D, Desmond JE, Aron AP et al (2001) Material-specific lateralization in the medial temporal lobe and prefrontal cortex during memory encoding. Brain 124(Pt 9):1841–1854

Greene AJ, Gross WL, Elsinger CL, Rao SM (2006) An fMRI analysis of the human hippocampus: inference, context, and task awareness. J Cogn Neurosci 18(7):1156–1173

Griffith HR, Perlman SB, Woodard AR, Rutecki PA, Jones JC, Ramirez LF et al (2000) Preoperative FDG-PET temporal lobe hypometabolism and verbal memory after temporal lobectomy. Neurology 54:1161–1165

Grunwald T, Lehnertz K, Heinze HJ, Helmstaedter C, Elger CE (1998) Verbal novelty detection within the human hippocampus proper. Proc Natl Acad Sci U S A 95:3193–3197

Guerreiro CAM, Jones-Gotman M, Andermann F, Cendes F (2001) Severe amnesia in epilepsy: causes, anatomopsychological considerations, and treatment. Epilepsy Behav 2:224–246

Hamberger MJ, Goodman RR, Perrine K, Tamny TR (2001) Anatomic dissociation of auditory and visual naming in the lateral temporal cortex. Neurology 56:56–61

Hassabis D, Kumaran D, Maguire EA (2007) Using imagination to understand the neural basis of episodic memory. J Neurosci 27(52):14365–14374

Helmstaedter C, Elger CE (1996) Cognitive consequences of two-thirds anterior temporal lobectomy on verbal memory in 144 patients: a three-month follow-up study. Epilepsia 37:171–180

Helmstaedter C, Kurthen M, Lux S, Reuber M, Elger CE (2003) Chronic epilepsy and cognition: a longitudinal study in temporal lobe epilepsy. Ann Neurol 54:425–432

Henke K, Buck A, Weber B, Wieser HG (1997) Human hippocampus establishes associations in memory. Hippocampus 7:249–256

Henke K, Weber B, Kneifel S, Wieser HG, Buck A (1999) Human hippocampus associates information in memory. Proc Natl Acad Sci U S A 96:5884–5889

Hermann BP, Wyler AR, Somes G, Clement L (1994) Dysnomia after left anterior temporal lobectomy without functional mapping: frequency and correlates. Neurosurgery 35:52–57

Hermann BP, Seidenberg M, Haltiner A, Wyler AR (1995) Relationship of age at onset, chronologic age, and adequacy of preoperative performance to verbal memory change after anterior temporal lobectomy. Epilepsia 36(2):137–145

Hermann B, Davies K, Foley K, Bell B (1999a) Visual confrontation naming outcome after standard left anterior temporal lobectomy with sparing versus resection of the superior temporal gyrus: a randomized prospective clinical trial. Epilepsia 40(8):1070–1076

Hermann BP, Perrine K, Chelune GJ, Barr W, Loring DW, Strauss E et al (1999b) Visual confrontation naming following left anterior temporal lobectomy: a comparison of surgical approaches. Neuropsychology 13(1):3–9

Hertz-Pannier L, Gaillard WD, Mott S, Cuenod CA, Bookheimer S, Weinstein S et al (1997) Noninvasive assessment of language dominance in children and adolescents with functional MRI: a preliminary study. Neurology 48:1003–1012

Humphries C, Swinney D, Love T, Hickok G (2005) Response of anterior temporal cortex to syntactic and prosodic manipulations during sentence processing. Hum Brain Mapp 26:128–138

Humphries C, Binder JR, Medler DA, Liebenthal E (2006) Syntactic and semantic modulation of neural activity during auditory sentence comprehension. J Cogn Neurosci 18:665–679

Hunkin NM, Mayes AR, Gregory LJ, Nicholas AK, Nunn JA, Brammer MJ et al (2002) Novelty-related activation within the medial temporal lobes. Neuropsychologia 40(8):1456–1464

Hwang DY, Golby AJ (2006) The brain basis for episodic memory: insights from functional MRI, intracranial EEG, and patients with epilepsy. Epilepsy Behav 8(1):115–126

Ives-Deliperi VL, Butler JT (2012) Naming outcomes after temporal lobectomy in epilepsy patients: a systematic review of the literature. Epilepsy Behav 24:194–198

Janecek JK, Swanson SJ, Sabsevitz DS, Hammeke TA, Raghavan M, Binder JR (2013a) Naming outcome prediction in patients with discordant Wada and fMRI language lateralization. Epilepsy Behav 27:399–403

Janecek JK, Swanson SJ, Sabsevitz DS, Hammeke TA, Raghavan M, Rozman ME et al (2013b) Language lateralization by fMRI and Wada testing in 229 patients with epilepsy: rates and predictors of discordance. Epilepsia 54(2):314–322

Jeong S-W, Lee SK, Hong K-S, Kinm K-K, Chung C-K, Kim H (2005) Prognostic factors for the surgery for mesial temporal lobe epilepsy: longitudinal analysis. Epilepsia 46(8):1273–1279

Jokeit H, Ebner A, Holthausen H, Markowitsch HJ, Moch A, Pannek H et al (1997) Individual prediction of change in delayed recall of prose passages after left-sided anterior temporal lobectomy. Neurology 49:481–487

Kapur N, Prevett M (2003) Unexpected amnesia: are there lessons to be learned from cases of amnesia following unilateral temporal lobe surgery? Brain 126(12):2573–2585

Kelley WM, Miezin FM, McDermott KB, Buckner RL, Raichle ME, Cohen NJ et al (1998) Hemispheric specialization in human dorsal frontal cortex and medial temporal lobe for verbal and nonverbal memory encoding. Neuron 20:927–936

Kensinger EA, Clarke RJ, Corkin S (2003) What neural correlates underlie successful encoding and retrieval? A functional magnetic resonance imaging study using a divided attention paradigm. J Neurosci 23(6):2407–2415

Killgore WD, Casasanto DJ, Yurgelun-Todd DA, Maldjian JA, Detre JA (2002) Functional activation of the left amygdala and hippocampus during associative encoding. Neuroreport 11:2259–2263

Kirchhoff BA, Wagner AD, Maril A, Stern CE (2000) Prefrontal-temporal circuitry for episodic encoding and subsequent memory. J Neurosci 20(16):6173–6180

Kirsch HE, Walker JA, Winstanley FS, Hendrickson R, Wong ST, Barbaro NM et al (2005) Limitations of Wada memory asymmetry as a predictor of outcomes after temporal lobectomy. Neurology 65:676–680

Knecht S, Deppe M, Dräger B, Bobe L, Lohmann H, Ringelstein EB et al (2000a) Language lateralization in healthy right-handers. Brain 123:74–81

Knecht S, Dräger B, Deppe M, Bobe L, Lohmann H, Flöel A et al (2000b) Handedness and hemispheric language dominance in healthy humans. Brain 123:2512–2518

Knecht S, Floel A, Drager B, Breitenstein C, Sommer J, Henningsen H et al (2002) Degree of language lateralization determines susceptibility to unilateral brain lesions. Nat Neurosci 5(7):695–699

Kneebone AC, Chelune GJ, Dinner DS, Naugle RI, Awad IA (1995) Intracarotid amobarbital procedure as a predictor of material-specific memory change after anterior temporal lobectomy. Epilepsia 36:857–865

Knight RT (1996) Contribution of the human hippocampal region to novelty detection. Nature 383:256–259

Kubu CS, Girvin JP, McLachlan RS, Pavol M, Harnadek MC (2000) Does the intracarotid amobarbital procedure predict global amnesia after temporal lobectomy? Epilepsia 41:1321–1329

Lacruz ME, Alarcon G, Akanuma N, Lum FC, Kissani N, Koutroumanidis M et al (2004) Neuropsychological effects associated with temporal lobectomy and amygdalohippocampectomy depending on Wada test failure. J Neurol Neurosurg Psychiatry 75:600–607

Lambon Ralph MA, McClelland J, Patterson K, Galton CJ, Hodges JR (2001) No right to speak? The relationship between object naming and semantic impairment: neuropsychological evidence and a computational model. J Cogn Neurosci 13:341–356

Langfitt JT, Rausch R (1996) Word-finding deficits persist after left anterotemporal lobectomy. Arch Neurol 53:72–76

Langfitt JT, Westerveld M, Hamberger MJ, Walczak TS, Cicchetti DV, Berg AT et al (2007) Worsening of quality of life after epilepsy surgery: effect of seizures and memory decline. Neurology 68(23):1988–1994

Lee GP, Loring DW, Smith JR, Flanigin HF (1995) Intraoperative hippocampal cooling and Wada memory testing in the evaluation of amnesia risk following anterior temporal lobectomy. Arch Neurol 52:857–861

Lee TMC, Yip JTH, Jones-Gotman M (2002) Memory deficits after resection of left or right anterior temporal lobe in humans: a meta-analytic review. Epilepsia 43:283–291

Lehéricy S, Cohen L, Bazin B, Samson S, Giacomini E, Rougetet R et al (2000) Functional MR evaluation of temporal and frontal language dominance compared with the Wada test. Neurology 54:1625–1633

Li L, Miller EK, Desimone R (1993) The representation of stimulus familiarity in anterior inferior temporal cortex. J Neurophysiol 69:1918–1929

Lineweaver TT, Naugle RI, Cafaro AM, Bingaman W, Luders HO (2004) Patients' perceptions of memory functioning before and after surgical intervention to treat medically refractory epilepsy. Epilepsia 45:1604–1612

Lineweaver TT, Morris HH, Naugle RI, Najm IM, Diehl B, Bingaman W (2006) Evaluating the contributions of state-of-the-art assessment techniques to predicting memory outcome after unilateral anterior temporal lobectomy. Epilepsia 47(11):1895–1903

Loddenkemper T, Morris HH, Lineweaver TT, Kellinghaus C (2007) Repeated intracarotid amobarbital tests. Epilepsia 48(3):553–558

Loring DW, Lee GP, Meador KJ, Flanigin HF, Figueroa RE, Martin RC (1990a) The intracarotid amobarbital procedure as a predictor of memory failure following unilateral temporal lobectomy. Neurology 40:605–610

Loring DW, Meador KJ, Lee GP, Murro AM, Smith JR, Flanigin HF et al (1990b) Cerebral language lateralization: evidence from intracarotid amobarbital testing. Neuropsychologia 28(8):831–838

Loring DW, Meador KJ, Lee GP, King DW, Gallagher BB, Murro AM et al (1994) Stimulus timing effects on Wada memory testing. Arch Neurol 51:806–810

Loring DW, Hermann BP, Perrine K, Plenger PM, Lee GP, Nichols ME et al (1995a) Memory for real objects is superior to line drawing recognition in discrimination of lateralized temporal lobe impairment during the Wada test. J Int Neuropsychol Soc 1:134

Loring DW, Meador KJ, Lee GP, King DW, Nichols ME, Park YD et al (1995b) Wada memory asymmetries predict verbal memory decline after anterior temporal lobectomy. Neurology 45:1329–1333

Martin A (1999) Automatic activation of the medial temporal lobe during encoding: lateralized influences of meaning and novelty. Hippocampus 9:62–70

Martin RC, Grote CL (2002) Does the Wada test predict memory decline following epilepsy surgery. Epilepsy Behav 3(1):4–15

Martin RC, Sawrie SM, Roth DL, Giliam FG, Faught E, Morawetz RB et al (1998) Individual memory change after anterior temporal lobectomy: a base rate analysis using regression-based outcome methodology. Epilepsia 39:1075–1082

Mazoyer BM, Tzourio N, Frak V, Syrota A, Murayama N, Levrier O et al (1993) The cortical representation of speech. J Cogn Neurosci 5(4):467–479

McClelland JL, McNaughton BL, O'Reilly RC (1995) Why are there complementary learning systems in the hippocampus and neocortex: insights from the success and failures of connectionist models of learning and memory. Psychol Rev 102:409–457

McIntosh AM, Wilson SJ, Berkovic SF (2001) Seizure outcome after temporal lobectomy: current research practice and findings. Epilepsia 42(10):1288–1307

Mechanic-Hamilton D, Korczykowski M, Yushkevich PA, Lawler K, Pluta J, Glynn S et al (2009) Hippocampal volumetry and functional MRI of memory in temporal lobe epilepsy. Epilepsy Behav 16(1):128–138

Milner B, Branch C, Rasmussen T (1962) Study of short-term memory after intracarotid injection of sodium amytal. Trans Am Neurol Assoc 87:224–226

Morawetz C, Holz P, Lange C, Baudewig J, Weniger G, Irle E et al (2008) Improved functional mapping of the human amygdala using a standard functional magnetic resonance imaging sequence with simple modifications. Magn Reson Imaging 26:45–53

Nagata S, Uchimura K, Hirakawa W, Kuratsu J (2001) Method for quantitatively evaluating the lateralization of linguistic function using functional MR imaging. Am J Neuroradiol 22:985–991

Novelly RA, Williamson PD (1989) Incidence of false-positive memory impairment in the intracarotid Amytal procedure. Epilepsia 30:711

Olson IR, McCoy D, Klobusicky E, Ross LA (2013) Social cognition and the anterior temporal lobes: a review and theoretical framework. Soc Cogn Affect Neurosci 8(2):123–133

O'Reilly RC, Rudy JW (2001) Conjunctive representations in learning and memory: principles of cortical and hippocampal function. Psychol Rev 108: 311–345

Otten LJ, Henson RNA, Rugg MD (2001) Depth of processing effects on neural correlates of memory encoding. Relationship between findings from across- and within-task comparisons. Brain 124(2):399–412

Paller KA, Wagner AD (2002) Observing the transformation of experience into memory. Trends Cogn Sci 6:93–102

Parsons MW, Haut MW, Lemieux SK, Moran MT, Leach SG (2006) Anterior medial temporal lobe activation during encoding of words: FMRI methods to optimize sensitivity. Brain Cogn 60(3):253–261

Patterson K, Nestor PJ, Rogers TT (2007) Where do you know what you know? The representation of semantic knowledge in the human brain. Nat Rev Neurosci 8:976–987

Perrine K, Hermann BP, Meador KJ, Vickrey BG, Cramer JA, Hays RD et al (1995) The relationship of neuropsychological functioning to quality of life in epilepsy. Arch Neurol 52(10):997–1003

Pigot S, Milner B (1993) Memory for different aspects of complex visual scenes after unilateral-temporal or frontal-lobe resection. Neuropsychologia 13: 1–15

Pillon B, Bazin B, Deweer B, Ehrle N, Baulac M, Dubois B (1999) Specificity of memory deficits after right or left temporal lobectomy. Cortex 35:561–571

Powell HW, Koepp MJ, Symms MR, Boulby PA, Salek-Haddadi A, Thompson PJ et al (2005) Material-specific lateralization of memory encoding in the medial temporal lobe: blocked versus event-related design. NeuroImage 48:1512–1525

Powell HWR, Richardson MP, Symms MR, Boulby PA, Thompson PJ, Duncan JS et al (2008) Preoperative fMRI predicts memory decline following anterior temporal lobe resection. J Neurol Neurosurg Psychiatry 79:686–693

Prince SE, Daselaar SM, Cabeza R (2005) Neural correlates of relational memory: successful encoding and retrieval of semantic and perceptual associations. J Neurosci 25(5):1203–1210

Prince SE, Tsukiura T, Cabeza R (2007) Distinguishing the neural correlates of episodic memory encoding and semantic memory retrieval. Psychol Sci 18(2):144–151

Rabin ML, Narayan VM, Kimberg DY, Casasanto DJ, Glosser G, Tracy JI et al (2004) Functional MRI predicts post-surgical memory following temporal lobectomy. Brain 127(10):2286–2298

Reber PJ, Wong EC, Buxton RB (2002) Encoding activity in the medial temporal lobe examined with anatomically constrained fMRI analysis. Hippocampus 12(3):363–376

Richardson MP, Strange BA, Thompson PJ, Baxendale SA, Duncan JS, Dolan RJ (2004) Pre-operative verbal memory fMRI predicts post-operative memory decline after left anterior temporal lobe resection. Brain 127:2419–2426

Richardson MP, Strange BA, Duncan JS, Dolan RJ (2006) Memory fMRI in left hippocampal sclerosis. Optimizing the approach to predicting postsurgical memory. Neurology 66:699–705

Riches IP, Wilson FAW, Brown MW (1991) The effects of visual stimulation and memory on neurones of the hippocampal formation and neighboring parahippocampal gyrus and inferior temporal cortex of the primate. J Neurosci 11:1763–1779

Rogers TT, Hocking J, Noppeney U, Mechelli A, Gorno-Tempini ML, Patterson K et al (2006) Anterior temporal cortex and semantic memory: reconciling findings from neuropsychology and functional imaging. Cogn Affect Behav Neurosci 6(3):201–213

Rosazza C, Ghielmetti F, Minati L, Vitali P, Giovagnoli AR, Deleo F et al (2013) Preoperative language lateralization in temporal lobe epilepsy (TLE) predicts peri-ictal, pre- and post-operative language performance: an fMRI study. NeuroImage: Clinical 3:73–83

Ross LA, Olson IR (2010) Social cognition and the anterior temporal lobes. NeuroImage 49:3452–3462

Rugg MD, Otten LJ, Henson RNA (2002) The neural basis of episodic memory: evidence from functional neuroimaging. Philos Trans Royal Soc Lond Ser B 357:1097–1110

Rutten G-J, Ramsey N, van Rijen P, Alpherts W, van Veelen C (2002) fMRI-determined language lateralization in patients with unilateral or mixed language dominance according to the Wada test. NeuroImage 17:447–460

Sabbah P, Chassoux F, Leveque C, Landre E, Baudoin-Chial S, Devaux B et al (2003) Functional MR imaging in assessment of language dominance in epileptic patients. NeuroImage 18:460–467

Sabsevitz DS, Swanson SJ, Morris GL, Mueller WM, Seidenberg M (2001) Memory outcome after left anterior temporal lobectomy in patients with expected and reversed Wada memory asymmetry scores. Epilepsia 42:1408–1415

Sabsevitz DS, Swanson SJ, Hammeke TA, Spanaki MV, Possing ET, Morris GL et al (2003) Use of preoperative functional neuroimaging to predict language deficits from epilepsy surgery. Neurology 60:1788–1792

Saykin AJ, Stafiniak P, Robinson LJ, Flannery K, Gur R, O'Connor MJ et al (1995) Language before and after temporal lobectomy: specificity of acute changes and relation to early risk factors. Epilepsia 36:1071–1077

Schacter DL, Addis DR (2007) The cognitive neuroscience of constructive memory: remembering the past and imagining the future. Philos Trans Royal Soc Lond: Ser B 362(1481):773–786

Schacter DL, Wagner AD (1999) Medial temporal lobe activations in fMRI and PET studies of episodic encoding and retrieval. Hippocampus 9:7–24

Scoville WB, Milner B (1957) Loss of recent memory after bilateral hippocampal lesions. J Neurol Neurosurg Psychiatry 20:11–21

Seghier ML (2008) Laterality index in functional MRI: methodological issues. Magn Reson Imaging 26(5):594–601

Sidhu MK, Stretton J, Winston GP, Symms M, Thompson PJ, Koepp MJ et al (2015) Memory fMRI predicts verbal memory decline after anterior temporal lobe resection. Neurology 84:1512–1519

Simkins-Bullock J (2000) Beyond speech lateralization: a review of the variability, reliability, and validity of the intracarotid amobarbital procedure and its nonlanguage uses in epilepsy surgery candidates. Neuropsychol Rev 10:41–74

Small SA, Nava AS, Perera GM, DeLaPaz R, Mayeux R, Stern Y (2001) Circuit mechanisms underlying memory encoding and retrieval in the long axis of the hippocampal formation. Nat Neurosci 4(4):442–449

Smith SM, Fox PT, Miller KL, Glahn DC, Fox PM, Mackay CE et al (2009) Correspondence of the brain's functional architecture during activation and rest. Proc Natl Acad Sci U S A 106(31):13040–13045

Smitha XKA, Arun XKM, Rajesh XPG, Thomas XB, Kesavadas XC (2017) Resting-state seed-based analysis: an alternative to task-based language fMRI and its laterality index. Am J Neuroradiol 38:1187–1192

Sperling RA, Bates JF, Cocchiarella AJ, Schacter DL, Rosen BR, Albert MS (2001) Encoding novel face-name associations: a functional MRI study. Hum Brain Mapp 14(3):129–139

Spitsyna G, Warren JE, Scott SK, Turkheimer FE, Wise RJS (2006) Converging language streams in the human temporal lobe. J Neurosci 26(28):7328–7336

Spreer J, Arnold S, Quiske A, Ziyeh S, Altenmüller DM, Herpers M et al (2002) Determination of hemisphere dominance for language: comparison of frontal and temporal fMRI activation with intracarotid amytal testing. Neuroradiology 44:467–474

Springer JA, Binder JR, Hammeke TA, Swanson SJ, Frost JA, Bellgowan PSF et al (1999) Language dominance in neurologically normal and epilepsy subjects: a functional MRI study. Brain 122:2033–2045

Squire LR (1992) Memory and the hippocampus: a synthesis from findings with rats, monkeys, and humans. Psychol Rev 99:195–231

Stafiniak P, Saykin AJ, Sperling MR, Kester DB, Robinson LJ, O'Connor MJ et al (1990) Acute naming deficits following dominant temporal lobectomy: prediction by age at first risk for seizures. Neurology 40:1509–1512

Stark CE, Squire LR (2001) When zero is not zero: the problem of ambiguous baseline conditions in fMRI. Proc Natl Acad Sci U S A 98(22):12760–12766

Stern CE, Corkin S, González RG, Guimaraes AR, Baker JA, Jennings PJ et al (1996) The hippocampal formation participates in novel picture encoding: evidence from functional magnetic resonance imaging. Proc Natl Acad Sci U S A 93:8660–8665

Stroup E, Langfitt JT, Berg M, McDrmott M, Pilcher W, Como P (2003) Predicting verbal memory decline following anterior temporal lobectomy (ATL). Neurology 60:1266–1273

Szaflarski JP, Gloss D, Binder JR, Gaillard WD, Golby AJ, Holland SK et al (2017) Practice guideline summary: Use of fMRI in the presurgical evaluation of patients with epilepsy. Report of the Guideline Development, Dissemination, and Implementation Subcommittee of the American Academy of Neurology. Neurology 88(4):395–402

Tellez-Zenteno JF, Dhar R, Wiebe S (2005) Long-term seizure outcomes following epilepsy surgery: a systematic review and meta-analysis. Brain 128:1188–1198

Tomasi D, Volkow ND (2012) Resting functional connectivity of language networks: characterization and reproducibility. Mol Psychiatry 17(8):841–854

Trenerry MR, Jack CRJ, Ivnik RJ, Sharbrough FW, Cascino GD, Hirschorn KA et al (1993) MRI hippocampal volumes and memory function before and after temporal lobectomy. Neurology 43(9):1800–1805

Tulving E, Markowitsch HJ, Crail FIM, Habib R, Houle S (1996) Novelty and familiarity activations in PET studies of memory encoding and retrieval. Cereb Cortex 6:71–79

Uncapher MR, Rugg MD (2005) Encoding and durability of episodic memory: a functional magnetic resonance imaging study. J Neurosci 25(31):7260–7267

Vandenberghe R, Nobre AC, Price CJ (2002) The response of left temporal cortex to sentences. J Cogn Neurosci 14(4):550–560

Vilberg KL, Rugg MD (2008) Memory retrieval and the parietal cortex: a review of evidence from a dual-process perspective. Neuropsychologia 46(7):1787–1799

Vincent JL, Snyder AZ, Fox MD, Shannon BJ, Andrews JR, Raichle ME et al (2006) Coherent spontaneous activity identifies a hippocampal-parietal memory network. J Neurophysiol 96(6):3517–3531

Vincent JL, Kahn I, Snyder AZ, Raichle ME, Buckner RL (2008) Evidence for a frontoparietal control system revealed by intrinsic functional connectivity. J Neurophysiol 100(6):3328–3342

Visser M, Jefferies E, Lambon Ralph MA (2010) Semantic processing in the anterior temporal lobes: a meta-analysis of the functional neuroimaging literature. J Cogn Neurosci 22(6):1083–1094

Wada J, Rasmussen T (1960) Intracarotid injection of sodium amytal for the lateralization of cerebral speech dominance. J Neurosurg 17:266–282

Wagner AD, Schacter DL, Rotte M, Koutstaal W, Maril A, Dale AM et al (1998) Building memories: remembering and forgetting of verbal experiences as predicted by brain activity. Science 281:1188–1191

Wang D, Buckner RL, Liu H (2014) Functional specialization in the human brain estimated by intrinsic hemispheric interaction. J Neurosci 34:12341–12352

Wechsler D (1997) Wechsler memory scale—Third Edition. WMS-III Administration and scoring manual. Psychological Corporation, San Antonio, TX

Weis S, Klaver P, Reul J, Elger CE, Fernández G (2004) Temporal and cerebellar brain regions that support both declarative memory formation and retrieval. Cereb Cortex 14:256–267

Wendel JD, Trenerry MR, Xu YC, Sencakova D, Cascino GD, Britton JW et al (2001) The relationship between quantitative T2 relaxometry and memory in nonlesional temporal lobe epilepsy. Epilepsia 42:863–869

Wilke M, Schmithorst VJ (2006) A combined bootstrap/histogram analysis approach for computing a lateralization index from neuroimaging data. NeuroImage 33:522–530

Woermann FG, Jokeit H, Luerding R, Freitag H, Schulz R, Guertler S et al (2003) Language lateralization by

Wada test and fMRI in 100 patients with epilepsy. Neurology 61(5):699–701

Worthington C, Vincent DJ, Bryant AE, Roberts DR, Vera CL, Ross DA et al (1997) Comparison of functional magnetic resonance imaging for language localization and intracarotid speech amytal testing in presurgical evaluation for intractable epilepsy. Stereotact Funct Neurosurg 69:197–201

Xu J, Kemeny S, Park G, Frattali C, Braun A (2005) Language in context: emergent features of word, sentence, and narrative comprehension. NeuroImage 25:1002–1015

Yeo BT, Krienen FM, Sepulcre J, Sabuncu MR, Lashkari D, Hollinshead M et al (2011) The organization of the human cerebral cortex estimated by intrinsic functional connectivity. J Neurophysiol 106:1125–1165

Yetkin FZ, Swanson S, Fischer M, Akansel G, Morris G, Mueller W et al (1998) Functional MR of frontal lobe activation: Comparison with Wada language results. Am J Neuroradiol 19:1095–1098

Zahn R, Moll J, Krueger F, Huey ED, Garrido G, Grafman J (2007) Social concepts are represented in the superior anterior temporal cortex. Proc Natl Acad Sci U S A 104:6430–6435

Zeinah MM, Engel SA, Thompson PM, Bookheimer SY (2003) Dynamics of the hippocampus during encoding and retrieval of face-name pairs. Science 299: 577–580

18 Preoperative Blood Oxygen Level-Dependent (BOLD) Functional Magnetic Resonance Imaging (fMRI) of Motor and Somatosensory Function

Christoph Stippich and Anthony Tyndall

18.1 Rationale for fMRI in Rolandic Neurosurgery

Surgery in or around the "central region" entails a high risk for intraprocedural damage of the precentral and postcentral gyrus with consecutive motor and sensory deficits that can impact the patient's quality of life considerably. By non-invasively providing a precise localization of the different representations of the human body in relation to the surgical target, blood oxygen level-dependent (BOLD) functional magnetic resonance imaging (fMRI) facilitates the selection of candidates for surgery as well as the planning and performance of more aggressive but safe and function-preserving resections (Petrella et al. 2006). This also implies that fMRI plays a role in identifying those patients who are not the ideal candidates for surgery and who may profit more from less invasive therapeutic options like radiation or chemotherapy. Such patients often present with diffusely infiltrating or recurrent malignancies of the brain, where a complete resection and a surgical cure cannot be achieved. In this situation, deficits associated with the treatment should be kept to a minimum. Prior to treatment, fMRI provides important diagnostic information to evaluate the risks and chances on an individual basis and to optimize the therapeutic strategy accordingly. fMRI brain mapping is not generalizable and must be done in a patient-specific fashion, as each patient's brain anatomy is unique and the functional anatomy may demonstrate pathology-induced atypical organization or reorganization (Bates et al. 2003; Duffau 2005). In addition, functional landmarks are helpful to plan partial resections or biopsies. This also applies for awake craniotomies or epilepsy surgery. Hence, the majority of preoperative fMRI studies are performed in patients with brain tumors and epilepsies to preserve the adjacent eloquent brain areas. In nonresective neurosurgery also, fMRI can be applied, for example, in patients with medically intractable chronic pain. Here, it has been demonstrated that fMRI facilitates the placement of stimulation electrodes over the motor cortex (Pirotte et al. 2005a, b). Ideally, preoperative fMRI studies are conducted for functional neuronavigation and in combination with diffusion tensor imaging (DTI), to also visualize important fiber bundles during surgery, for example, the pyramidal tract (Nimsky et al. 2006).

It is important to note that the central region can be localized easily and reliably on the basis of morphological images of the brain using different anatomical structures as landmarks (for details, see Chap. 2; Fig. 18.1). The most robust anatomical landmark is the "hand knob" of the precentral gyrus, representing the structural correlate of the motor hand area on transverse

C. Stippich (✉) · A. Tyndall
Department of Neuroradiology, University Hospital Zürich, Zürich, Switzerland
e-mail: christoph.stippich@usz.ch; anthony.devere-tyndall@usz.ch

S. Ulmer, O. Jansen (eds.), *fMRI*, https://doi.org/10.1007/978-3-030-41874-8_18

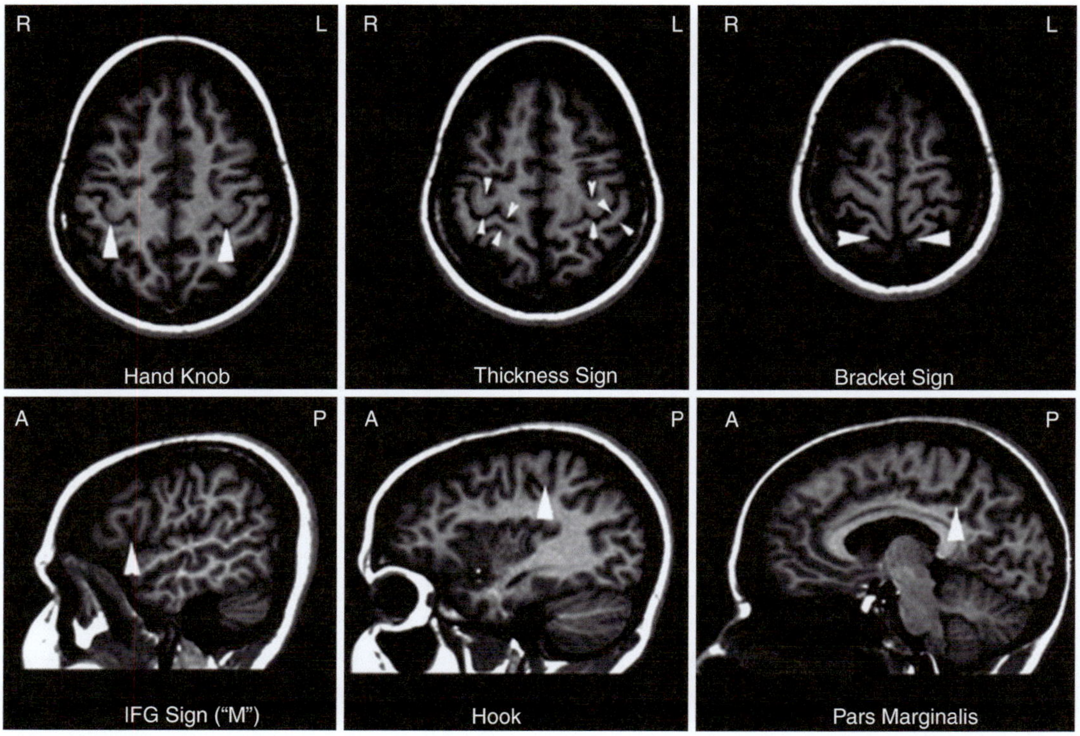

Fig. 18.1 Anatomical landmarks on morphological MRI according to Naidich and Yousry in transverse (*upper row*) and sagittal (*lower row*) views. *White arrowheads* indicate the relevant anatomical structures. The "hand knob" and "hook" are synonyms for the "precentral knob" (Reprinted from Stippich 2007, p. 90, with permission)

cross-sectional images (Yousry et al. 1997), which also corresponds to the "precentral hook" on sagittal images. The existence of these morphological landmarks substantiates the controversy whether functional imaging is necessary at all for rolandic neurosurgery. This view, however, does not account for the important limitations of morphological brain imaging in the presence of anatomical variants or under pathological conditions (e.g., mass effects, infiltration, destruction, postoperative state in recurrent malignancies), both precluding proper identification of the different gyri and sulci. More importantly, the motor hand area is the only functional area that can be identified reliably using anatomical criteria alone. All other representations of the human body can be identified only by using functional neuroimaging (Fesl et al. 2003), both in the primary motor cortex (M1) and in the primary somatosensory cortex (S1). A substantial body of research supports the role of fMRI as a valid and valuable preoperative imaging modality (Stippich et al. 2007). Hence, the rationale for preoperative fMRI results largely from the limitations of structural brain imaging (Rolls et al. 2007). Furthermore, neuroplasticity and functional reorganization induced by the lesion or by the treatment can be assessed using fMRI (Shinoura et al. 2006), for example, in patients with motor and somatosensory deficits that are not explained conclusively by anatomical consideration and in patients who are candidates for repeated neurosurgery because of recurrent malignancies.

Taken together, the rationale for carrying out presurgical fMRI is often based on the limitations of imaging morphology, clinical and electrophysiological diagnostics, and the need to include data on physiological and neuroplastic changes or pathologic (e.g., epileptic) activation of the brain in treatment planning. This diagnostic information may be generated by fMRI in a single investigation before treatment by means of a

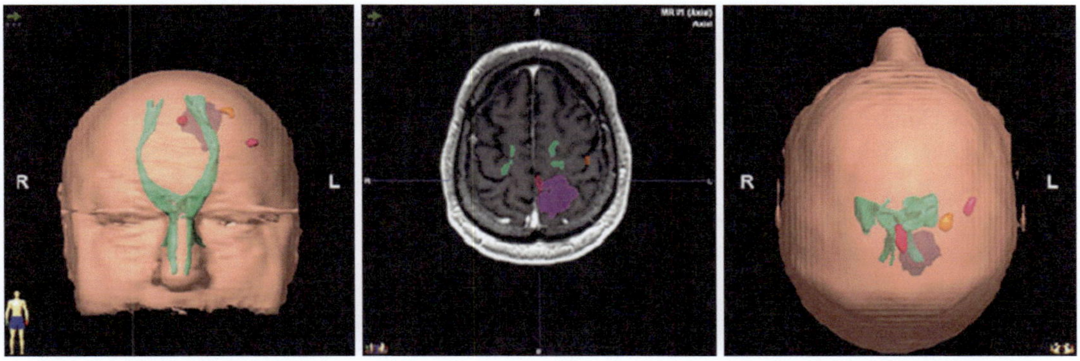

Fig. 18.2 Integration of BOLD-fMRI and DTI-tractography for functional neuronavigation. Three-dimensional (3D)-surface projections (*left*: anterior–posterior; *right*: top–down) and two-dimensional (2D)-navigation view (*middle*). The spatial relationship of the cortical toe (*red*), finger (*orange*), and tongue (*pink*) motor representations and of the pyramidal tract (*green*) to the segmented brain tumor (*purple*) is clearly depicted. The tumor affects the superior parietal lobule and invades the postcentral gyrus extending toward the cortical motor representation of the lower extremity

combined visualization of anatomy, pathology, and function. Combination of other modern methods of magnetic resonance imaging (MRI), for example, by mapping fractional anisotropy (FA) or DTI, may be helpful in depicting important fiber pathways such as the pyramidal tract (Schonberg et al. 2006; Fig. 18.2).

18.2 Review of Literature

fMRI is currently the most frequently used noninvasive neuroimaging modality for presurgical planning and proven useful in guiding tumor and epilepsy surgery involving primary motor areas (Hirsch et al. 2000; Bartsch et al. 2006; Petrella et al. 2006; Sunaert 2006; Rosen and Savoy 2012; Pillai 2010, Orringer et al. 2012; Silva et al. 2018). Mapping the primary motor cortex in patients with rolandic brain tumors has been the first clinical application of fMRI (Jack et al. 1994). Shortly after the first reports on BOLD-fMRI in healthy subjects (Belliveau et al. 1991; Bandettini et al. 1992; Kwong et al. 1992; Ogawa et al. 1993), the potential usefulness of functional imaging techniques in clinical context and particularly in presurgical identification of motor and somatosensory cortices was postulated. The first description of presurgical fMRI as a clinically useful application dates back to 1994, when Jack et al. provided proof of principle in two patients with brain tumors in the sensorimotor cortex, validating their preliminary results with established electrophysiological techniques (Jack et al. 1994). Soon after, several case studies (Baumann et al. 1995; Cosgrove et al. 1996) and reports with small number of patients (Puce et al. 1995; Pujol et al. 1996; Mueller et al. 1996; Krings et al. 1998), harboring glial tumors or arteriovenous malformations (AVM), confirmed technical and practical feasibility of fMRI using motor and sensory tasks in the clinical context and stressed the high potential value of this new upcoming technique for preoperative risk assessment, therapeutic decision-making, and surgical planning.

During the following years, investigations with larger number of tumor patients (up to 50) were carried out, claiming their results to represent an important factor for surgical decision (Schlosser et al. 1997; Pujol et al. 1998). Comparisons of presurgical fMRI data with the established reference procedure intracortical stimulation (ICS) were numerous, and only those specifically dealing with brain tumor patients will be mentioned here, since a detailed description of validation studies is offered in Chaps. 11–13, 21, and 22. Virtually all studies report highly concordant data of presurgical fMRI and ICS in patients with lesions around the central sulcus (Dymarkowski et al. 1998; Achten et al. 1999; Roux et al. 1999a, b), with agreement between fMRI and ICS data ranging from 83% in 33 patients (Majos et al. 2005) to 92% in 60 patients (Lehericy et al. 2000). Motor mapping with fMRI has consistently shown a reasonable correlation with electrocortical stimulation, higher than for language mapping, but may yet be too disconcordant to replace it (Bizzi et al. 2008; Kapsalakis et al. 2012). Task sensitivity for identification of the sensorimotor region with fMRI estimated in large groups of tumor patients was 85% in 103 patients (Krings et al. 2001), 97% in 125 patients (Hirsch et al. 2000), and 96% in 268 patients (Tyndall et al. 2017). Furthermore, it should be briefly noted that various groups focused on the correlation of fMRI results in patients with central lesions with those of other functional imaging procedures, for example, positron-emission tomography (PET; Bittar et al. 1999).

One of the first attempts to evaluate the impact of fMRI on neurosurgical planning was published by Lee et al. The authors applied preoperative fMRI sensorimotor mapping in 32 tumor patients and reported that the results were used to determine feasibility of surgical resection in 55%, to aid in surgical planning in 22%, and to select patients for invasive surgical functional mapping in 78%. Overall, the fMRI results were useful in one or more of these surgical decision-making categories in 89% of all examined tumor patients (Lee et al. 1999). A similar range was documented by Ternovoi et al., who found that presurgical fMRI results had an influence on therapeutic tactics in 69% of 16 tumor patients (Ternovoi et al. 2004). Other investigators tried to establish a functional risk predictor for postoperative clinical outcome. Haberg et al. examined 25 patients with primary brain tumors near sensorimotor regions. In 80% of the patients, successful fMRI measurements were obtained, out of which 75% were used in preoperative planning. The risk of postoperative loss of function was significantly lower, when the distance between tumor periphery and BOLD activation was 10 mm or more (Haberg et al. 2004). Similarly, Krishnan et al., who evaluated BOLD activation in 54 patients, found that a lesion-to-activation distance of less than 5 mm and incomplete resection were predictors of new postoperative neurological deficits and recommended cortical stimulation within a 10-mm range (Krishnan et al. 2004). In patients with medial frontal lesions, preoperative fMRI was used to establish the area at risk for resection of specific parts of the supplementary motor area (SMA), associated with transient postoperative motor deficits and speech disorders (Krainik et al. 2001, 2003, 2004). In one study, the authors used fMRI-guided resection in 16 patients with low-grade gliomas. Since these tumors are generally not contrast enhancing, resection borders are particularly difficult to establish based on morphological imaging alone. Using fMRI for the determination of resection borders, no permanent neurological deficits and no radiographic tumor progression, within a median follow-up time of 25 months, were observed (Hall et al. 2005). However, the data available to quantify a safe distance between functional activation and resection borders with respect to surgically induced neurological deficits are still very limited and do not justify any general conclusion or recommendation.

Overall, although the abovementioned studies clearly demonstrated feasibility of presurgical fMRI in clinical environment and postulated a contribution of the obtained additional clinical information to pretherapeutic decision-making, an effect on the decrease in posttherapeutic morbidity was not corroborated. In order to achieve this, controlled clinical trials using optimized and standardized protocols would be required. Although most investigators agree on the necessity of a standardized routine, and several methodological studies presenting optimized protocols for clinical use were published (Hirsch et al. 2000; Ramsey et al. 2001; Rutten et al. 2002; Stippich et al. 1999, 2000, 2002a, b, 2004; Stippich 2005), no large-scale randomized clinical trials addressing actual benefit for the patient, in terms of decrease in morbidity, have been undertaken so far (Sunaert 2006).

Although sensorimotor areas are identified with high success rates using fMRI in patients with central lesions by most investigators, a frequently encountered phenomenon is an altered pattern of activation as compared to the normal brain function, currently denominated as lesion-induced reorganization or plasticity. In an early study in seven patients with intracerebral gliomas of the primary sensorimotor cortex, activation was found to be displaced or reduced (Atlas et al. 1996). Roux et al. correlated the type of activation with histologic tumor characteristics in 17 patients. In infiltrating tumors, intratumoral activation was detected, which was displaced and scattered correlated with the degree of infiltration, whereas in noninfiltrating tumors, activation showed extra-tumoral shift. In tumors at a distance from the motor cortex, no intratumoral activation was measured (Roux et al. 1997). Likewise, a PET study with 51 patients describes that central lesions are more frequently associated with altered patterns of activation than lesions in noncentral locations (Bittar et al. 2000). Other studies found significant BOLD-signal decrease in areas adjacent to tumor tissue in motor and sensory cortices as compared to the contralateral side. This effect was present in glial tumors, most pronounced in glioblastoma, and presumably related to tumor-induced changes in local cerebral hemodynamics (Holodny et al. 1999, 2000; Krings et al. 2002a, b), while in nonglial tumors (metastasis, cavernoma, abscess, AVM, meningioma), no BOLD-signal decrease was found (Schreiber et al. 2000).

A report on 33 patients, with different intra- and extra-axial tumors, established the influence of tumor type and distance from eloquent cortex on activation volumes in fMRI (Liu et al. 2005). In addition to displacement or reduction of activation in the primary sensorimotor cortex harboring the tumor, other patterns of lesion-induced reorganization encompass activation of solely the contralesional cortex or an enhanced activation of nonprimary sensorimotor areas with increasing degree of paresis (Alkadhi et al. 2000; Carpentier et al. 2001; Krings et al. 2002a, b). Also in patients with prior surgery (Kim et al. 2005) or newly acquired central paresis after resection (Reinges et al. 2005), significant decreases in BOLD activation are observed. One possible explanation for this tumor-induced BOLD-signal loss was lately proposed by an fMRI study where tumor blood volume and perfusion were measured. The authors concluded that the BOLD amplitude correlates with total intratumoral blood volume and, thus, reduced peritumoral perfusion due to a tumor-aspirating perfusion (steal phenomenon) goes along with reduced BOLD activation (Ludemann et al. 2006). Of note is, however, that resection of glioma with preoperative edema may cause transient increase in BOLD activation ipsilateral to the tumor, presumably by a decrease in pressure on the brain (Kokkonen et al. 2005). Lesion-induced functional reorganization may reflect the recruitment of plastic neuronal networks to compensate for sensory or motor impairment. On the level of a functional diagnosis in presurgical fMRI, these reorganization phenomena are of major clinical significance for the planning of resections, since they can potentially cause false-negative results.

During the past years, the use of combined presurgical fMRI and DTI techniques for tractography was suggested to provide a better estimate of proximity of tumor borders to eloquent cortex than fMRI measurements alone. In particular, for space-occupying lesions affecting the central region, visualization of the origin, direction, and functionality of large white matter tracts, allowing imaging of functional connectivity, was put forward to improve surgical outcome and to promise a decrease in patient morbidity (Krings et al. 2001; Parmar et al. 2004; Ulmer et al. 2004; Shinoura et al. 2005; Stippich et al. 2003; Holodny et al. 2001).

The application of real-time fMRI in clinical environment enables quick preliminary online analysis of fMRI data, which is particularly useful in surgical diagnostics, considering that fMRI data acquisition and processing are very time consuming. Möller et al. demonstrated the technical feasibility of presurgical real-time fMRI examination in ten patients with central area tumors immediately prior to surgery (Moller et al. 2005). In another study, motor and language tasks were used for real-time fMRI in 11 tumor patients. The authors reported satisfactory activation for hand motor tasks, weaker activation for foot motor tasks, and no useful activation for language tasks at the chosen threshold, concluding that the procedure needed to be optimized but was generally feasible in clinical routine (Schwindack et al. 2005). Furthermore, Gasser et al. achieved the recording of intraoperative fMRI in four anesthetized patients with lesions in the vicinity of the central region. Using a passive stimulation paradigm and analyzing the data during acquisition by online statistical evaluation, they obtained intraoperative identification of eloquent brain areas taking brain shift into account (Gasser et al. 2005).

Finally, with the introduction of higher magnetic field scanners to clinical diagnostics, practicability of presurgical fMRI at 3 Tesla (T) was established in patients with brain tumors (Roessler et al. 2005; Van Westen et al. 2005; Feigl et al. 2008). Today the clinical implementation of preoperative fMRI is possible also in regional hospitals (Geerts et al. 2007). For a general review on the role of imaging in disease management and the development of improved image-guided therapies in neurooncology, see also the article by Jacobs et al. (2005) and Pillai (2010).

Note: Very recently the American Medical Association (www.ama-assn.org) has released CPT-codes (Current Procedural Terminology) for clinical fMRI applications. General instructions for clinical fMRI can be found in the Current Protocols for Magnetic Resonance Imaging (Thulborn 2006).

18.3 General Considerations

Motor cortex mapping is the predominant preoperative application of fMRI because of its easy implementation in a clinical setting and the robust and valid functional localizations. Blocked-design fMRI is currently more widely implemented than event-related fMRI for motor cortex mapping, probably due to its high detection power, relatively easy design, and better patient participation (Tie et al. 2009). Typically, a simple block design consisting of three to five stimulation-baseline cycles is applied while the patients perform self-paced movements with the tongue or lips, hand or fingers, and foot or toes to investigate the motor cortex somatotopy.

Essentials for the success of clinical fMRI examinations are (1) motor tasks that are feasible also in patients with paresis, (2) reduction of motion to a minimum, and (3) short scanning times. Under these conditions, BOLD activations in the primary motor cortex are generally very reliable. This can be achieved when the "most feasible" motor tasks have been selected from clinical testing, when patient positioning and head fixation is optimal during the fMRI scans, when appropriate motion correction is applied for data processing, and when the fMRI scanning protocols have been evaluated in volunteers for robust functional localization, high BOLD-signal yield, and low scanning time. For the diagnostic interpretation of clinical fMRI data, it is indispensable that the whole fMRI procedure is fully standardized (scanning, data processing, and evaluation) and that normative data are available for all applied fMRI scanning protocols (ideally including data for important influencing factors like handedness) as well as a precise assessment of each patient's neurological deficits at the time of the preoperative fMRI measurement. For the latter, the importance of the individual training of the investigator with each patient before the actual fMRI measurement cannot be overestimated. To control for incorrect task performance, a video monitoring during the fMRI measurements is highly recommended. In uncooperative patients, it may even be necessary that the investigator is inside the scanner room to give instructions directly (e.g., by tapping the hand when the movement is started and stopped). All erroneous measurements must be excluded from evaluation and repeat measurements must be performed.

The investigation of patients with pareses can be challenging, however. Dedicated paradigms based on somatosensory stimulation (Stippich et al. 1999, 2004; Stippich 2005) or complex finger movements of the unimpaired hand (Stippich et al. 2000) may help to overcome the problem. A somatosensory stimulation can also be useful in uncooperative or sedated patients and in children. Automated devices deliver reproducible stimuli and are ideal for follow-up measurements under standardized conditions (Golaszewski et al. 2002; Kurth et al. 1998; Stippich et al. 1999). For more details, see paragraphs in Sects. 18.6 and 18.7. A review of literature regarding the various fMRI paradigms for motor and somatosensory function is beyond the scope of this chapter. We refer the reader to the extensive database available. It is of note that most manufacturers offer online data-processing software for functional BOLD imaging with their magnetic resonance (MR) imagers today, providing easy access to the method.

18.4 Diagnostic Aims

The primary diagnostic aim of preoperative fMRI is to localize the primary motor cortex and/or the primary somatosensory cortex in relation to the surgical target and the different cortical representations of the human body of the precentral gyrus and/or postcentral gyrus. The secondary aims include the detection of neuroplastic changes and functional reorganization prior to treatment in patients with neurological deficits and in patients scheduled for repeated neurosurgery, investigating the natural course of brain activation in patients with rolandic pathologies, or investigating the effects of a specific (surgical or alternative) treatment on brain function, which may represent further diagnostic aims of follow-up measurements.

18.5 Selection of Candidates for Preoperative fMRI

Most patients referred to preoperative motor and somatosensory fMRI present with rolandic brain tumors, metastases, AVMs, and epileptogenic lesions. In general, patients with meningiomas and other (noninfiltrative) extra-axial masses should not be considered for fMRI, except for difficult cases on request of the surgeon. fMRI is also not necessary for patients with frontal or parietal pathologies that do not involve the central region directly.

As a basic principle, candidates for preoperative fMRI should be selected by anatomical consideration first using morphological MR images and on the basis of clinical findings (motor and/or sensory deficit), both clearly indicating an involvement of the primary motor and/or somatosensory cortex. The appropriate examination protocol should be selected accordingly. Depending on the site and extent of the lesion, a single fMRI reading can suffice; however, it is often necessary to examine the entire motor and, where appropriate, somatosensory somatotopy.

Preoperative fMRI studies are justified when the following anatomical criteria apply: (1) complete destruction of the rolandic anatomy precluding identification of the precentral gyrus, central sulcus, and postcentral gyrus; (2) compression or displacement of the precentral gyrus precluding reliable localization of the hand knob and the MR—morphologic reference of the motor hand area is absent as an orientation point for the somatotopic organization of the precentral gyrus respectively; (3) the surgical target lies below or above the hand knob and a precise localization of the cortical face or lower-extremity representations is warranted; (4) the surgical target is postcentral—a somatosensory stimulation may be applied; other (nonanatomical) criteria include (5) suspected neuroplastic changes/functional reorganization with respect to neurological signs and symptoms; and (6) repeated neurosurgery.

Note: The size of the BOLD clusters and the center of gravity varies with the statistical threshold applied for data evaluation. As a consequence, fMRI studies should not be performed to determine resection borders or a "safe" distance between lesion and functional area. In a strict sense, this is not possible to date on the basis of fMRI data as the material published on that topic is very limited (Haberg et al. 2004; Krishnan et al. 2004; Hall et al. 2005). Furthermore, non-standardized measurements in "interesting cases" are not feasible for clinical decision-making and should be avoided. However, such patients may be enrolled in research trials.

18.6 Paradigms for Clinical Motor and Somatosensory fMRI

When designing motor paradigms in a block design, it is of principal importance to establish whether only the primary motor cortex activation needs to be measured or secondary areas should also be considered. In the case where only the primary motor cortex is the target, paradigms can also include movements in both sides of the body (e.g., right hand vs. left hand). Since unilateral movements lead to activation of secondary areas in both hemispheres, secondary areas are active during alternating movements of the right and left body sides throughout the entire measurement, but continuous activation is not shown in the statistical evaluation of fMRI data, acquired using conventional block designs, due to the lack of "contrast" between the various stimulation blocks. If information needs to be obtained regarding secondary motor activation, paradigms with strictly unilateral movements of a single body part should be applied, with "resting" as the control condition. Alternatively, three different stimulation conditions could be integrated in the paradigm, that is, right movement, rest, and left movement. However, the number of blocks per paradigm is then increased and, consequently, the examination time and susceptibility to motion artifacts also increases. In addition, it should be borne in mind that information on brain activation in the tumor-unaffected hemisphere is largely insignificant for treatment. Also, paradigms enabling the examination of several cortical body representations are problematic in brain tumor patients (e.g., foot, hand, face). Although scan time could be reduced compared to three individual measurements, the time needed is still substantially longer than for each individual measurement alone. Particularly in the case of agitated patients or patients with paresis, the likelihood of motion artifacts increases, subsequently affecting all functional localizations (Seto et al. 2001, Bullmore et al. 1999). Only secondary functional areas that are exclusive to the respective movement can be localized. All jointly recruited areas escape detection on diagnostic fMRI. In conclusion, paradigms with movements of a single part of the body alternating with true rest that provide short scan times are most appropriate for preoperative fMRI (Fig. 18.3).

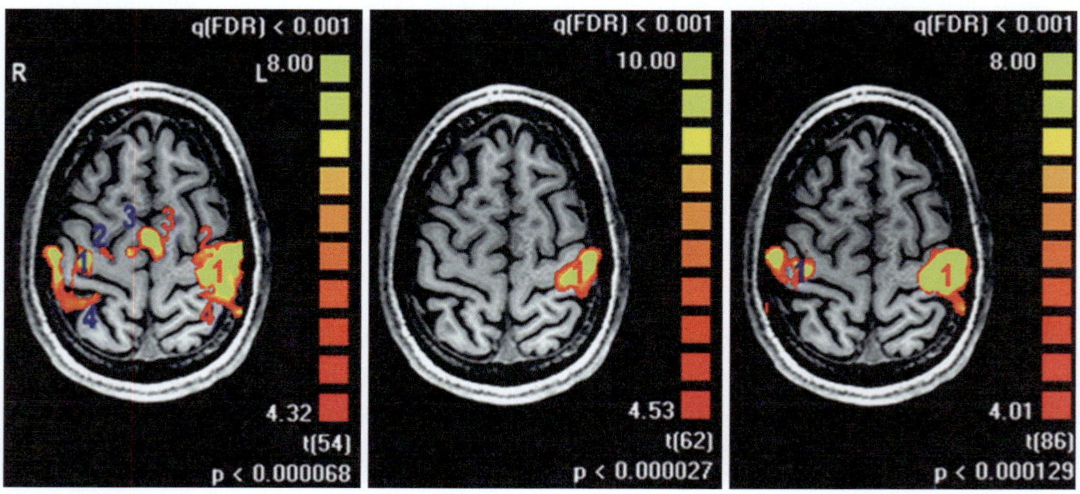

Fig. 18.3 Variation of paradigms to localize the motor hand area results in different activation patterns. *Left*: complex finger opposition of the right hand vs. rest; strong activation of cortical motor network in both hemispheres. The large contralateral cluster (*left*) covers the primary sensorimotor cortex (*1*), premotor cortex (*2*), and parietal cortex (*4*). Bilateral supplementary motor activation (*3*, *3*) is displayed in the midline as well as ipsilateral (*right*) premotor activation (*2*), primary sensorimotor coactivation (*1*), and parietal activation (*4*). *Middle*: complex finger opposition of the right vs. left hand; strong contralateral (*left*) primary sensorimotor activation (*1*), but no activation of secondary areas. *Right*: complex finger opposition of the right hand vs. right toe movements and tongue movements; strong contralateral (*left*) primary sensorimotor activation (*1*) and ipsilateral primary sensorimotor coactivation (*1*), but no activation of secondary areas (Reprinted from Stippich 2007, p. 106, with permission)

Clinical feasibility tests, carried out on neurosurgical patients with and without tumor-related pareses or sensory disturbances, showed that self-triggered movement tasks are better suited to preoperative fMRI than controlled paradigms, since only in this way each patient can perform within his or her ability. To keep the likelihood of motion artifacts to a minimum (Hoeller et al. 2002; Krings et al. 2001), the following movement tasks were chosen each with "rest" as control condition: repetitive tongue movements with the mouth closed, opposition of fingers D2–D5 to D1 with free choice of sequence, and repetitive flexion and extension of all five toes without moving the ankle (Stippich et al. 2002a, b; Fig. 18.4). Alternatively, in the case of mild paresis of the upper extremity, fist clenching/releasing can be tested. Face, arm, and leg movements, or movement of the feet, can often lead to poor diagnostic evaluation of data due to strong motion artifacts; therefore, they are not recommended for clinical fMRI. A paradigm with a block duration of 20 s and three repeat cycles (four rest conditions alternating with three stimulation conditions), adding to an examination time of 140 s, is a suitable compromise between robust functional localization of the primary motor cortex, high BOLD signals, and short scan time (Fig. 18.5).

Determination of motor function with preoperative fMRI is limited in patients with high-grade paresis (Pujol et al. 1998; Krings et al. 2002a, b). BOLD-signal changes are known to be less reliable for motor tasks involving paretic body parts (Mazzetto-Betti et al. 2010). In the case where the fMRI protocol is based solely on self-triggered movements contralateral to the tumor, a reliable preoperative fMRI diagnosis is not guaranteed—the pareses are results of

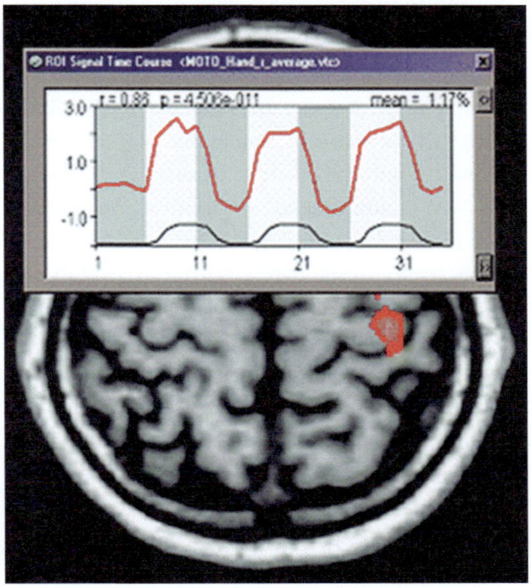

Fig. 18.5 Clinical standard protocol for motor paradigms. The block-designed paradigm consists of four rest periods (*light gray*) alternating with three stimulation periods (*white*), each 20 s in duration. The BOLD-signal time course of the motor hand area activation (*red line*) shows task-related increases in regional hemodynamics. The *black line* indicates the hemodynamic reference function (hrf) (Reprinted from Stippich 2007, p. 107, with permission)

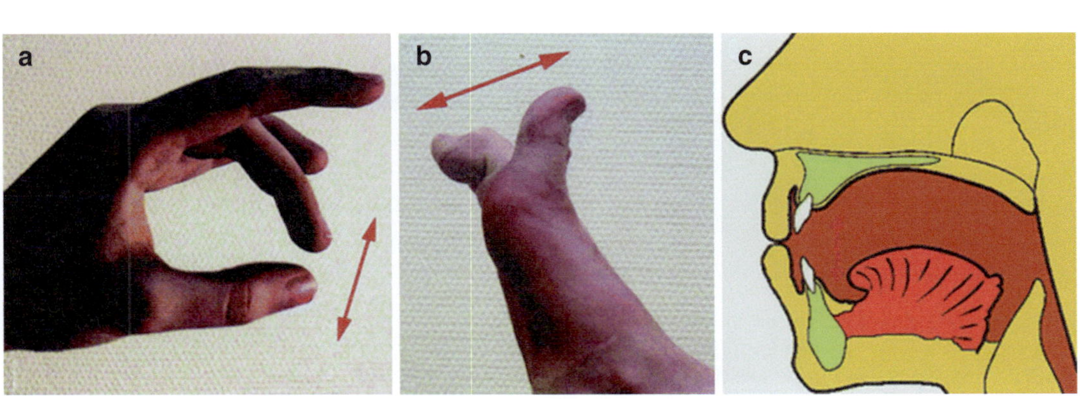

Fig. 18.4 (**a**–**c**) Recommended self-paced movements to investigate sensorimotor somatotopy in clinical fMRI. (**a**) Complex finger opposition of digits 2–5 against the thumb in a random order. Movement frequency ~3 Hz. (**b**) Toe up and down movements, frequency > 1 Hz. (**c**) Tongue up and down movements with the mouth closed. Movement frequency ~3 Hz (Reprinted from Stippich 2007, p. 106, with permission)

insufficient residual function of the primary motor cortex, which can lead to weak, or even absent, BOLD signals. Nevertheless, many patients with tumor-related paresis can be successfully examined by activating the primary somatosensory lip, finger, and toe representations of the postcentral gyrus (Stippich et al. 1999). Assisted motor tasks or substitution of imagined tasks may activate the primary motor area (M1) and supplementary motor area (SMA; Mizuguchi et al. 2013). While most investigators apply somatosensory stimuli manually (e.g., brushing the palm), automated devices provide reproducible and standardized stimulation conditions. Such manipulandum devices have shown to reliably activate motor cortex with less motion artifacts when compared to healthy controls (Shriver et al. 2013). Stimulators in use include electric (Kurth et al. 1998; Kampe et al. 2000; Golaszewski et al. 2004), tactile (Stippich et al. 1999; Wienbruch et al. 2006), or vibrotactile (Golaszewski et al. 2002, 2006). The fully automatic pneumatically driven 24-channel tactile stimulation used in our institution works artifact-free and produces reproducible stimuli and consistent examination conditions for comparative and outcome studies. The whole unit can be set up and removed within 5 min (Fig. 18.6). Scan

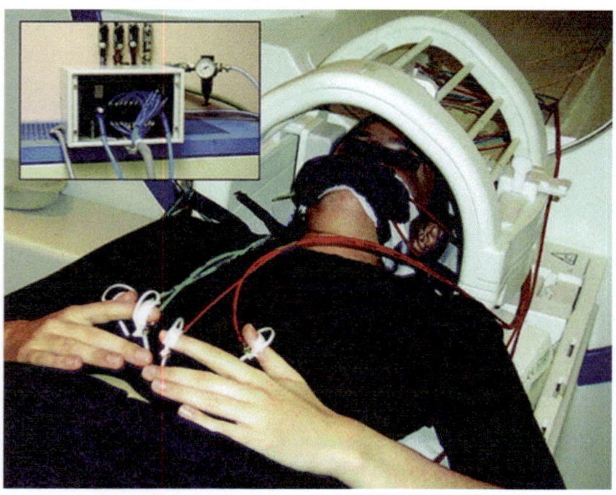

Fig. 18.6 Fully automated pneumatically driven tactile stimulation. Flexible membranes (4D Neuroimaging, Aachen, Germany) connected to pressure-resistant pneumatic tubes transmit the stimuli to the lips, fingers, or toes (not shown). *Upper left*: the 24-channel high-precision electromagnetic valve system was designed to investigate somatosensory somatotopy (Reprinted from Stippich 2007, p. 94, with permission)

times per measurement are 66 s for S1 (Stippich et al. 2004) or 105 s for S2 (Stippich 2005). The S1-paradigm consists of five repeat cycles (six rest conditions alternating with five stimulation conditions, duration 6 s each), the S2-paradigm of three repeat cycles (four rest conditions alternating with three stimulation conditions, duration 15 s each). For the latter paradigm, S1 activation is also robust.

As a further adjunct to investigate paretic patients, complex finger opposition of the nonparetic hand (ipsilateral to the pathology) can be used for the standard motor paradigm (140 s) to elicit robust premotor activation as an additional functional landmark for the precentral gyrus on the lesion side (Stippich et al. 2000; Fig. 18.7).

18.7 Preoperative fMRI in Patients With Rolandic Brain Tumors

18.7.1 Somatotopic Mapping of the Primary Motor Cortex (Standard Protocol)

Somatotopic mapping of the motor cortex is the most frequently used preoperative fMRI protocol in patients with rolandic lesions (Stippich et al. 2002a, b). The protocol contains three different fMRI measurements with a scanning time of 140 s each. Typical paradigms include tongue movements and finger and toe movements contralateral to the lesion to localize the motor homunculus in relation to the surgical target (Fig. 18.8). Even in case of complete destruction of the rolandic anatomy, fMRI provides three functional landmarks for different body representations (face, upper, and lower extremities). This diagnostic information is relevant to confirm the indication to operate and to plan and implement safer surgery. The same holds true for lesions that preclude proper identification of the hand knob as the anatomical reference for the motor hand area by compression or displacement (Fig. 18.9). In patients with small lesions that are—by anatomical consideration—not critical for all body representations, it seems appropriate to shorten the protocol by leaving the least relevant body representations unexamined

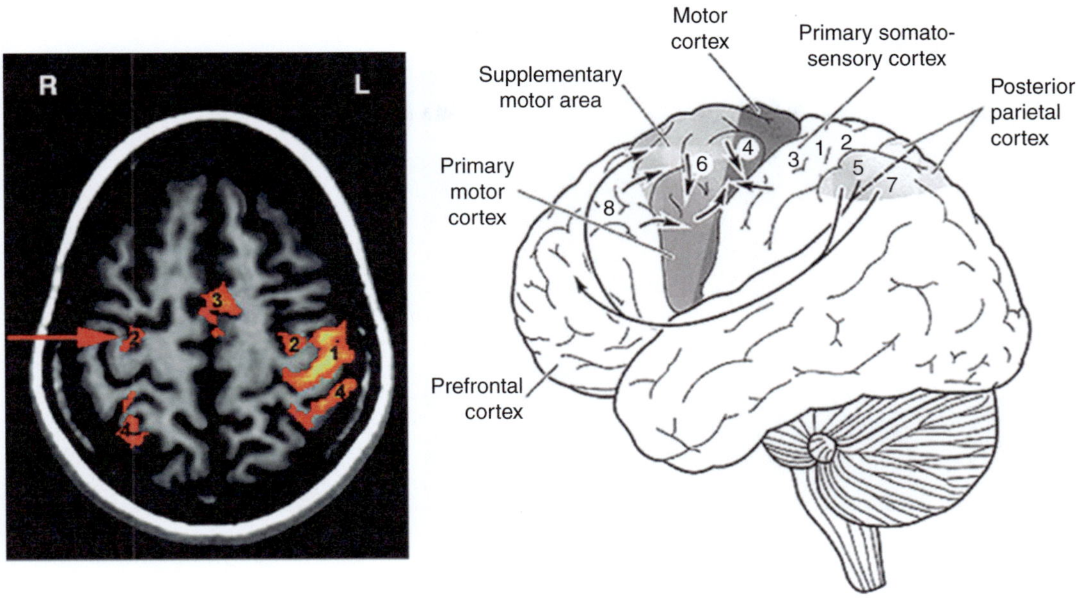

Fig. 18.7 Typical cortical activation pattern of complex finger opposition (right hand). Premotor activation ipsilateral to the moving hand (*red arrow*) serves as a functional landmark for the precentral gyrus in hemiparetic patients (a clinical case is presented in Fig. 18.13). Premotor activation is typically localized at the anterior wall of the precentral gyrus directly adjacent to the junction of the precentral sulcus with the superior frontal sulcus. It is important to note that this functional landmark does not localize the motor hand area! In the drawing of the cortical motor and somatosensory network (*right*), numbers indicate Brodmann areas (Reprinted from Stippich 2007, p. 113, with permission)

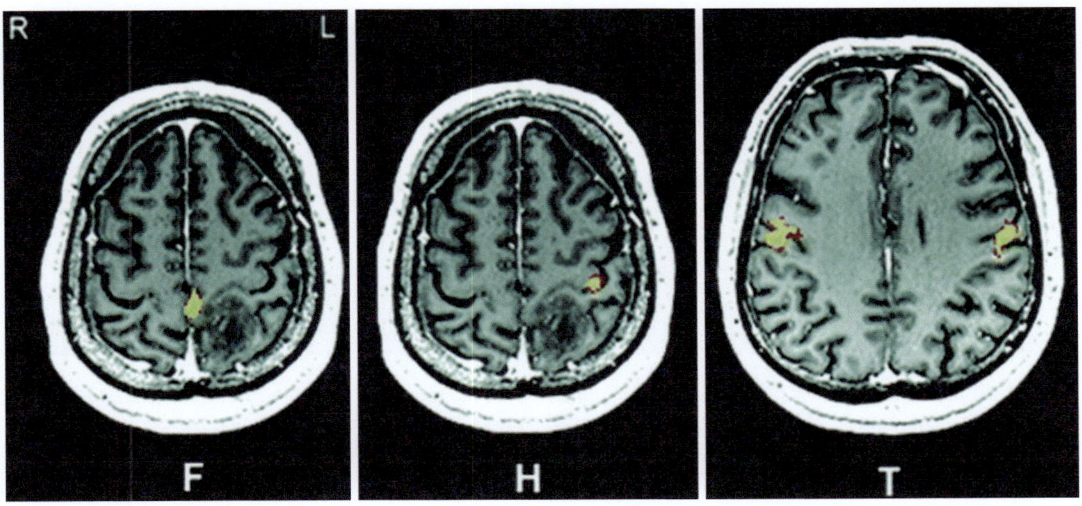

Fig. 18.8 Standard presurgical fMRI protocol: Somatotopic mapping of the motor cortex (same patient as in Fig. 18.2). The cortical foot representation (*F*) is closely related to the left parieto-postcentral anaplastic glioma. BOLD activation of the motor hand area (*H*) is localized at the hand knob and the bilateral tongue representations (*T*) at the level of the ventricular roof

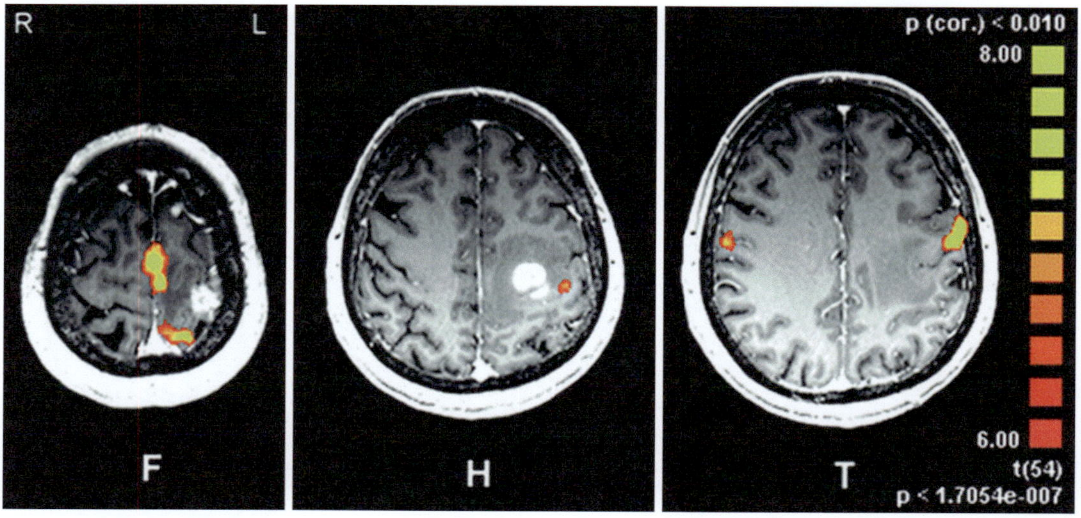

Fig. 18.9 Somatotopic fMRI mapping of the motor cortex in a patient with a left precentral glioblastoma precluding identification of the motor hand area using morphological landmarks. fMRI clearly indicates the position of the motor hand area during contralateral hand movements (*H*) as well as the cortical foot (*F*) and tongue representations (*T*)

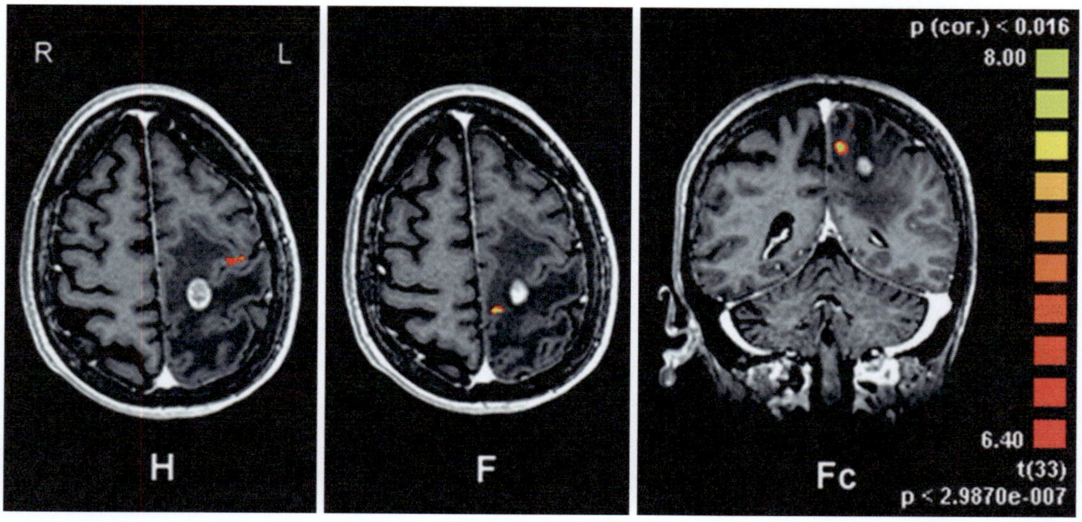

Fig. 18.10 Somatotopic fMRI mapping of the upper motor cortex in a patient with a left central metastasis indicating the spatial relationship to the cortical hand (*H*) and foot (*F*) representation. The latter is also displayed in coronal view (*Fc*). Additional fMRI localization of the motor tongue representations was not necessary by anatomical consideration

(Fig. 18.10). However, the examination of a single body representation alone, for example, the motor hand representation, is often not sufficient to provide the required diagnostic information. Somatotopic mapping enables also to assess plastic changes in cortical motor activation, for example, in patients with recurrent malignancies prior to repeated surgical treatment (Fig. 18.11). The abovementioned protocol has proven robust over a time period of 13 years over multiple MRI scanners, as demonstrated in a series of 268 presurgical patients with successful M1 activation

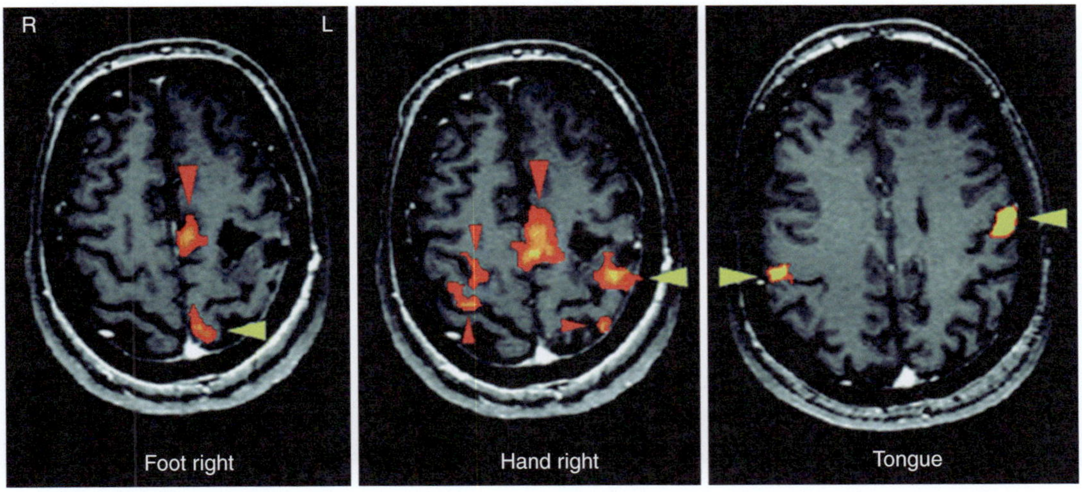

Fig. 18.11 Presurgical fMRI somatotopic mapping of the motor cortex in a hemiparetic patient with a recurrent left rolandic astrocytoma prior to repeated surgery. Foot, hand, and tongue movements revealed robust fMRI activation of the respective primary motor cortex body representations (*yellow arrowheads*). Note the increased activation in secondary areas (*red arrowheads*): in the supplementary motor area during toe and finger movements and in the whole cortical motor network in both hemispheres during finger movements (Reprinted from Stippich 2007, p. 111, with permission)

in 98.6% (hand: 95.4%; foot: 94.4%; tongue: 98.1%), with no statistically significant difference between 3 T and 1.5 T scanners (Tyndall et al. 2017).

18.7.2 Somatotopic Mapping of the Primary Somatosensory Cortex

This fMRI protocol was designed to localize the different somatosensory was designed to localize the different somatosensory body representations of the postcentral gyrus (Stippich et al. 1999). The somatosensory stimuli are transmitted to the lips, fingers, and toes contralateral to the brain lesion. In presurgical fMRI, somatotopic somatosensory mapping is mostly used as diagnostic adjunct, when motor paradigms are difficult to apply—for example, in uncooperative, sedated, or hemiparetic patients or in children—but there is also potential for standardized follow-up measurements on neuroplastic changes in the somatosensory system. This presurgical fMRI protocol enables a fully automated assessment of the spatial relationship between brain tumors and the postcentral gyrus, facilitating the estimation of possible postoperative sensory deficits (Fig. 18.12). Diagnostic information about the spatial relationship between the central sulcus or precentral gyrus and precentral or frontal brain tumors can be obtained rather indirectly as both anatomical structures are directly adjacent to the postcentral gyrus in the anterior direction. In the abovementioned study over 13 years, a somatosensory success rate of 82% was demonstrated for localizing S1 in 31 patients (Tyndall et al. 2017).

18.7.3 Localization of the Precentral Gyrus in Patients With Paresis

This special protocol was designed in volunteers to help localize the precentral gyrus in patients with contralateral paresis (Stippich et al. 2000). The clinical application is still experimental and requires own validation. In these patients, the primary motor cortex is commonly infiltrated by the tumor or severely compressed precluding both reliable identification of the rolandic anatomy on morphological images and proper performance

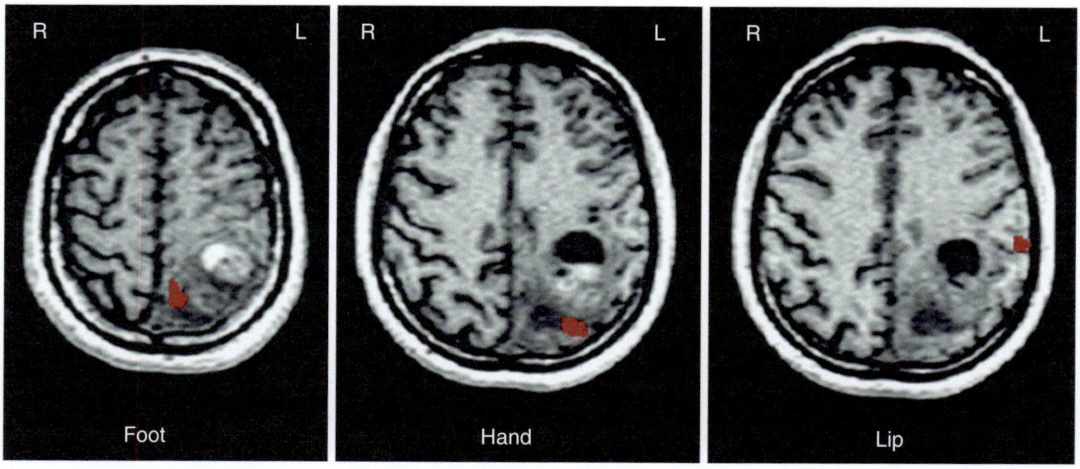

Fig. 18.12 Presurgical fMRI somatotopic mapping of the primary somatosensory cortex (S1) in a left parietal malignant glioma indicated compression of the upper postcentral gyrus at the level of the foot representation and tumor growth into the lower postcentral gyrus with dorsal displacement of the S1 hand representation (Reprinted from Stippich 2007, p. 112, with permission)

of contralateral movements for presurgical fMRI. However, as a basic principle, residual contralateral motor function and passive somatosensory stimulation should be used first for the functional localization of the pre- and postcentral gyrus. As a further adjunct, complex finger opposition of the nonparetic hand ipsilateral to the brain tumor can be used to activate the whole cortical motor network in both hemispheres. The premotor activation on the tumor side may serve as an additional functional landmark for the precentral gyrus, by localizing the anterior wall of the precentral gyrus near the junction of the precentral sulcus with the posterior part of the superior frontal sulcus (Fig. 18.13). It is important to note that the risk of surgery-related motor deficits cannot be estimated using premotor activation as a functional landmark! However, in healthy volunteers, primary motor coactivation can be observed frequently localizing the motor hand area ipsilateral to the moving hand (Stippich et al. 2007). Our initial clinical experience indicates that ipsilateral primary motor coactivation may be supportive to localize the motor hand area on the tumor side in hemiparetic patients.

Note: For all preoperative fMRI protocols presented here, the combination with anisotropic diffusion-weighted MRI or DTI (FA-mapping, DTI-tractography) is highly recommended to also delineate the effects of the rolandic pathologies on the pyramidal tract (Stippich et al. 2003).

18.8 Limitations, Pitfalls, and Outlook

Traditionally, functional areas are electrophysiologically mapped intraoperatively to reliably assess the spatial relationship between brain tumor and functional cortex (Ojemann et al. 1989; Duffau et al. 1999). Intraoperative electrocorticography (EcoG) is considered very reliable, but the sensitivity to detect motor function in the proximity of rolandic brain tumors can be low (Shinoura et al. 2005) and the method comprises several disadvantages. Surgery time can be substantially prolonged or patients need to be subjected to awake craniotomy. Furthermore, it is possible to derive activations only from the brain surface, while the by far larger portion of the cortex deep in the cerebral convolutions remains inaccessible (Cosgrove et al. 1996). Another significant disadvantage of EcoG is that the information is not available preoperatively and cannot be implemented in the assessment of the indication to operate and the planning of function-

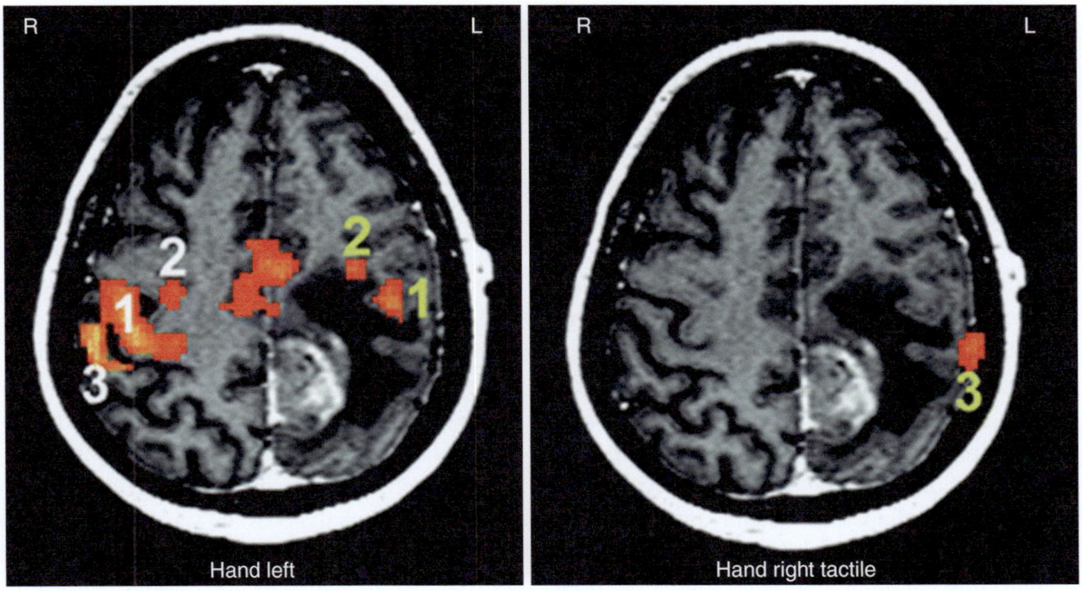

Fig. 18.13 Presurgical fMRI protocol for patients with preexisting paresis. This protocol may serve as an adjunct to the standard protocol using movements contralateral to the brain tumor. The application is still experimental and requires own validation. In this hemiparetic patient (grade 3/5) with a left malignant glioma, only weak BOLD activation was available from contralateral (*right*) hand movements precluding reliable localization of the motor hand area (not shown). By using complex finger opposition of the unimpaired hand ipsilateral to the tumor (*left*) and fully automated tactile stimulation of the right digits, BOLD activation is achievable in the motor hand area (*1*), premotor cortex (*2*), and primary somatosensory cortex (*3*) on the tumor side. Note the corresponding activations in the unimpaired hemisphere (*right*) associated with the left finger movements (*white numbers*). Bilateral supplementary motor activation is in the midline

preserving surgery. After all, morphological imaging provides very detailed information about intracranial pathologies (Osborn 2004), but not about brain function. fMRI is capable of overcoming these disadvantages of the "traditional diagnostic procedures" by visualizing anatomy, pathology, and function noninvasively in a single examination even prior to surgery.

When carried out in a standard way, fMRI is basically capable of providing a clinical "functional diagnosis" for individual patients (Thulborn 2006). Functional landmarks help to estimate possible therapy-related deficits and are thus particularly useful in providing patient information, verifying the indication, and selecting a sparing therapeutic procedure. Once the operation has been decided upon, careful planning and appropriate selection of incision, trepanation, surgical access, and resection margins are essential to function-preserving surgery. Intraoperatively, functional localizations facilitate surgical orientation, although inaccuracies resulting from displaced brain tissue need to be taken into consideration (Stippich et al. 2002a, b, 2003). All these factors increase patient safety and reduce the risk of postoperative deficits that additionally reduce quality of life.

According to current knowledge, one can assume that presurgical fMRI is able to contribute to a reduction in invasive diagnostic procedures both before and during neurosurgical interventions in patients with brain tumors. Whether fMRI can have a positive effect on surgery-related morbidity and disease-related mortality remains to be determined in prospective randomized studies. Prerequisites for this include a consensus on performance, analysis, and medical appraisal of presurgical fMRI, as well as the delineation of recommendations and guidelines by the assigned medical societies.

Preoperative fMRI has limitations imposed by patient-specific and methodological factors.

Cognitive tasks can coactivate other functions; thus, interpreting fMRI results by dividing the task into components may be challenging. As normal motor function depends on sensory feedback (proprioreceptive, haptic, visual information), this sensory feedback can augment activation in the motor task region as well as in confounding sensory regions, which are difficult to control for (Noble et al. 2013). Despite intensive patient training, optimized examination protocols, and appropriate head fixation, some patients cannot be examined due to poor cooperation or marked restlessness. When motor paradigms are used, undesirable continuation of movement during resting periods, mostly uncontrolled and interspersed accompanying movements in other parts of the body, can significantly compromise the quality of the examination, even if individually adjusted evaluation is used to register the error precisely. In the end, after this time-consuming process, examination results often need to be discarded. The same holds true for strong motion artifacts that cannot be corrected at later data-processing stages. Stimulus-related motion artifacts can simulate activations, leading to false high BOLD signals or even to incorrect localization (Hajnal et al. 1994; Krings et al. 2001; Hoeller et al. 2002; Steger and Jackson 2004). With regard to the appearance of motion artifacts, tongue and toe movements as well as finger opposition tasks are less critical than hand, foot, and lip movements. It is worth noting that despite the abovementioned pitfalls the necessity for repetition runs is usually low (2.4% for motor paradigms in one study), which more often than not achieve a sufficient BOLD activation (Tyndall et al. 2017).

The problems associated with investigating motor function in patients with tumor-related hemipareses have already been addressed (see Sect. 4.4). In most cases, functional localization of the pre- and postcentral gyrus can be achieved by using residual motor function in the affected extremities and applying special paradigms (Stippich et al. 2003). Compared to motor fMRI, BOLD signals are significantly weaker on tactile stimulation. Particularly in the lower extremities, tactile stimulation does not always achieve sufficient activation. This is accounted for by the lower number of receptors in toe tips, the comparatively small cortical toe representation, and ill-defined compressed air pulses when long pneumatic tubes are used.

The BOLD signals based on fMRI originate mainly in the capillary bed of the activated brain area and downstream veins (Frahm et al. 1994; Menon et al. 1995). Thus, fMRI measures a hemodynamic secondary phenomenon and not neuronal activity directly. Possible localization errors due to BOLD signals from draining veins can be identified by superimposing functional image data onto contrast-enhanced anatomical T1-weighted image sequences (Krings et al. 1999). Careful analysis of the signal–time curves of functional raw data helps to distinguish between parenchymatous and venous activation, since these rise at different rates (Krings et al. 2001). By causing vessel compression and pathological changes in vascular autoregulation, brain tumors can affect the localization and intensity of the BOLD signals measured (Holodny et al. 1999, 2000; Krings et al. 2002a, b; Ulmer et al. 2003, 2004; Kim et al. 2005; Liu et al. 2005; Hou et al. 2006; Ludemann et al. 2006). Whether artificial activations can occur due to their neovascularization remains to be clarified. For this reason, activations within contrast-enhanced tumor portions should be assessed as artifacts until reliable study results are available. Such activations should not be used for risk assessment, surgery planning, or functional neuronavigation. The same is true for BOLD signals in strongly vascularized cerebral metastases AVM (Lazar et al. 1997; Alkadhi et al. 2000; Lehericy et al. 2002; Ozdoba et al. 2002).

Investigator-dependent inaccuracies occur in manual superposition of echo-planar imaging (EPI) data, distorted by the method, onto anatomical three-dimensional (3D) data sets. As a precaution, a possible localization error of approximately 0.5 cm should always be assumed (Stippich et al. 2003). Improvements are expected in the future when distortion corrections for EPI data sets are available for clinical application (Weiskopf et al. 2005; Liu and Ogawa 2006; Priest et al. 2006), enabling superposition routines to be automated. We consider defining resection margins in presurgical diagnostics on the basis of fMRI data as unreliable, since the spatial extent of activated areas depends on the evaluation parameters chosen and can therefore vary. In addition, the position of brain structures can change intraoperatively ("brain shift"), with the result that data obtained preoperatively no longer accurately reflect the intraoperative situation (Wirtz et al. 1997; Wittek et al. 2005; Nimsky et al. 2006). Effluent cerebrospinal fluid alone can lead to shifts of several millimeters after opening of the dura. Moreover, there is often a sharp shift in the position of the brain due to tissue resection. For these reasons, preoperative fMRI cannot replace intraoperative mapping of brain function completely. Irrespective of functional imaging, additional technical inaccuracies must be taken into consideration in neuronavigation and referencing. Proposed computational models have shown to predict brain shift and adjust preoperative imaging for intraoperative guidance, yet must be validated in the clinical practice (Kyriacou et al. 2002; Onofrey et al. 2013). Alternatively, one can correlate intraoperative structural MRI images with preoperative fMRI to measure and compensate for brain shift (Archip et al. 2007).

Magnetic field strength does correlate with higher functional sensitivity, such as for primary hand motor area localization in a 7 T system, however at the cost of increased ghosting and head motion artifacts (Beisteiner et al. 2011). Whether this is relevant in the clinical context remains unclear. Even when comparing the more ubiquitous field strengths of 3 T and 1.5 T, motor mapping appears almost equally feasible at both field strengths (Tyndall et al. 2017).

More recently, resting-state fMRI (rs-fMRI), which detects spontaneous brain activity in a resting-state task-free environment, has shown promising results for motor mapping, including for presurgical planning, although still rarely applied in clinical practice (Rosazza et al. 2014; Schneider et al. 2016; Dierker et al. 2017). Demonstrated advantages over task-based fMRI include acceleration of the acquisition process, minimum paradigm design requirements, reduced reliance on patient cooperation (more relevant in patients with neurological deficits), and simultaneous mapping of multiple regions (Lee et al. 2013; Lang et al. 2014; Mitchell et al. 2013). However, rs-fMRI may be more prone to head motion artifact than task-based fMRI (Huijbers et al. 2017). Susceptibility artifact and neurovascular uncoupling have been shown to affect rs-fMRI similarly to task-based fMRI (Agarwal et al. 2017). rs-fMRI has also been implemented intraoperatively for motor mapping, with a sensitivity of 61.7% and specificity of 93.7% (Qiu et al. 2017). The robustness and potential of rs-fMRI as a valid method to guide clinical decision-making requires further investigation.

Acknowledgments Text and figures have been reproduced in part from Stippich (2007) with permission.

References

Achten E, Jackson GD et al (1999) Presurgical evaluation of the motor hand area with functional MR imaging in patients with tumors and dysplastic lesions. Radiology 210(2):529–538

Agarwal S, Sair HI et al (2017) Limitations of resting-state functional MR imaging in the setting of focal brain lesions. Neuroimaging Clin N Am 27(4):645–661

Alkadhi H, Kollias SS et al (2000) Plasticity of the human motor cortex in patients with arteriovenous malformations: a functional MR imaging study. AJNR Am J Neuroradiol 21(8):1423–1433

Archip N, Clatz O et al (2007) Non-rigid alignment of pre-operative MRI, fMRI, and DT-MRI with intra-operative MRI for enhanced visualization and navigation in image-guided neurosurgery. NeuroImage 35(2):609–624

Atlas SW, Howard RS II et al (1996) Functional magnetic resonance imaging of regional brain activity in patients with intracerebral gliomas: findings and implications for clinical management. Neurosurgery 38(2):329–338

Bandettini PA, Wong EC et al (1992) Time course EPI of human brain function during task activation. Magn Reson Med 25(2):390–397

Baumann SB, Noll DC et al (1995) Comparison of functional magnetic resonance imaging with positron emission tomography and magnetoencephalography to identify the motor cortex in a patient with an arteriovenous malformation. J Image Guid Surg 1(4):191–197

Bartsch AJ, Homola G et al (2006) Diagnostic functional MRI: illustrated clinical applications and decision-making. J Magn Reson Imaging 23(6):921–932
Bates E, Wilson SM et al (2003) Voxel-based lesion-symptom mapping. Nat Neurosci 6(5):448–450
Beisteiner R, Robinson S et al (2011) Clinical fMRI: evidence for a 7T benefit over 3T. Neuroimage 57(3):1015–1021
Belliveau JW, Kennedy DN et al (1991) Functional mapping of the human visual cortex by magnetic resonance imaging. Science 254(5032):716–719
Bittar RG, Olivier A et al (1999) Presurgical motor and somatosensory cortex mapping with functional magnetic resonance imaging and positron emission tomography. J Neurosurg 91(6):915–921
Bittar RG, Olivier A et al (2000) Cortical motor and somatosensory representation: effect of cerebral lesions. J Neurosurg 92(2):242–248
Bizzi A, Blasi V et al (2008) Presurgical functional MR imaging of language and motor functions: validation with intraoperative electrocortical mapping. Radiology 248(2):579–589
Bullmore ET, Brammer MJ et al (1999) Methods for diagnosis and treatment of stimulus-correlated motion in generic brain activation studies using fMRI. Hum Brain Mapp 7(1):38–48
Carpentier AC, Constable RT et al (2001) Patterns of functional magnetic resonance imaging activation in association with structural lesions in the rolandic region: a classification system. J Neurosurg 94(6):946–954
Cosgrove GR, Buchbinder BR et al (1996) Functional magnetic resonance imaging for intracranial navigation. Neurosurg Clin N Am 7(2):313–322
Dierker D, Roland J et al (2017) Resting-state functional magnetic resonance imaging in Presurgical functional mapping: sensorimotor localization. Neuroimaging Clin N Am 27(4):621–633
Duffau H, Capelle L et al (1999) Intra-operative direct electrical stimulations of the central nervous system: the Salpetriere experience with 60 patients. Acta Neurochir 141(11):1157–1167
Duffau H (2005) Lessons from brain mapping in surgery for low-grade glioma: insights into associations between tumour and brain plasticity. Lancet Neurol 4(8):476–486
Dymarkowski S, Sunaert S et al (1998) Functional MRI of the brain: localisation of eloquent cortex in focal brain lesion therapy. Eur Radiol 8(9):1573–1580
Feigl GC, Safavi-Abbasi S et al (2008) Real-time 3 T fMRI data of brain tumour patients for intra-operative localization of primary motor areas. Eur J Surg Oncol 34(6):708–715
Fesl G, Moriggl B et al (2003) Inferior central sulcus: variations of anatomy and function on the example of the motor tongue area. NeuroImage 20(1):601–610
Frahm J, Merboldt KD et al (1994) Brain or vein—oxygenation or flow? On signal physiology in functional MRI of human brain activation. NMR Biomed 7(1–2):45–53
Gasser T, Ganslandt O et al (2005) Intraoperative functional MRI: implementation and preliminary experience. NeuroImage 26(3):685–693
Geerts J, Martens M et al (2007) Functional magnetic resonance imaging for preoperative localisation of eloquent brain areas relative to brain tumours: clinical implementation in a regional hospital. JBR-BTR 90(4):258–263
Golaszewski SM, Zschiegner F et al (2002) A new pneumatic vibrator for functional magnetic resonance imaging of the human sensorimotor cortex. Neurosci Lett 324(2):125–128
Golaszewski SM, Siedentopf CM et al (2004) Modulatory effects on human sensorimotor cortex by whole-hand afferent electrical stimulation. Neurology 62(12):2262–2269
Golaszewski SM, Siedentopf CM et al (2006) Human brain structures related to plantar vibrotactile stimulation: a functional magnetic resonance imaging study. NeuroImage 29(3):923–929
Haberg A, Kvistad KA et al (2004) Preoperative blood oxygen level-dependent functional magnetic resonance imaging in patients with primary brain tumors: clinical application and outcome. Neurosurgery 54(4):902–914. discussion 914–915
Hajnal JV, Myers R et al (1994) Artifacts due to stimulus correlated motion in functional imaging of the brain. Magn Reson Med 31(3):283–291
Hall WA, Liu H et al (2005) Functional magnetic resonance imaging-guided resection of low-grade gliomas. Surg Neurol 64(1):20–27. discussion 27
Hirsch J, Ruge MI et al (2000) An integrated functional magnetic resonance imaging procedure for preoperative mapping of cortical areas associated with tactile, motor, language, and visual functions. Neurosurgery 47(3):711–721. discussion 721–722
Hoeller M, Krings T et al (2002) Movement artefacts and MR BOLD signal increase during different paradigms for mapping the sensorimotor cortex. Acta Neurochir 144(3):279–284. discussion 284
Holodny AI, Schulder M et al (1999) Decreased BOLD functional MR activation of the motor and sensory cortices adjacent to a glioblastoma multiforme: implications for image-guided neurosurgery. AJNR Am J Neuroradiol 20(4):609–612
Holodny AI, Schulder M et al (2000) The effect of brain tumors on BOLD functional MR imaging activation in the adjacent motor cortex: implications for image-guided neurosurgery. AJNR Am J Neuroradiol 21(8):1415–1422
Holodny AI, Schwartz TH et al (2001) Tumor involvement of the corticospinal tract: diffusion magnetic resonance tractography with intraoperative correlation. J Neurosurg 95(6):1082
Hou BL, Bradbury M et al (2006) Effect of brain tumor neovasculature defined by rCBV on BOLD fMRI activation volume in the primary motor cortex. NeuroImage 32(2):489–497
Huijbers W, Van Dijk KR et al (2017) Less head motion during MRI under task than resting-state conditions. NeuroImage 147:111–120

Jack CR, Thompson PM et al (1994) Sensory motor cortex: correlation of presurgical mapping with functional MR imaging and invasive cortical mapping. Radiology 190(1):85–92

Jacobs AH, Kracht LW et al (2005) Imaging in neurooncology. NeuroRx 2(2):333–347

Kampe KK, Jones RA et al (2000) Frequency dependence of the functional MRI response after electrical median nerve stimulation. Hum Brain Mapp 9(2):106–114

Kapsalakis IZ, Kapsalaki EZ et al (2012) Preoperative evaluation with FMRI of patients with intracranial gliomas. Radiol Res Pract 2012:727810

Kim MJ, Holodny AI et al (2005) The effect of prior surgery on blood oxygen level-dependent functional MR imaging in the preoperative assessment of brain tumors. AJNR Am J Neuroradiol 26(8):1980–1985

Kokkonen SM, Kiviniemi V et al (2005) Effect of brain surgery on auditory and motor cortex activation: a preliminary functional magnetic resonance imaging study. Neurosurgery 57(2):249–256. discussion 249–256

Krainik A, Lehericy S et al (2001) Role of the supplementary motor area in motor deficit following medial frontal lobe surgery. Neurology 57(5):871–878

Krainik A, Lehericy S et al (2003) Postoperative speech disorder after medial frontal surgery: role of the supplementary motor area. Neurology 60(4):587–594

Krainik A, Duffau H et al (2004) Role of the healthy hemisphere in recovery after resection of the supplementary motor area. Neurology 62(8):1323–1332

Krings T, Reul J et al (1998) Functional magnetic resonance mapping of sensory motor cortex for image-guided neurosurgical intervention. Acta Neurochir 140(3):215–222

Krings T, Erberich SG et al (1999) MR blood oxygenation level-dependent signal differences in parenchymal and large draining vessels: implications for functional MR imaging. AJNR Am J Neuroradiol 20(10):1907–1914

Krings T, Reinges MH et al (2001) Functional MRI for presurgical planning: problems, artefacts, and solution strategies. J Neurol Neurosurg Psychiatry 70(6):749–760

Krings T, Reinges MH et al (2002a) Factors related to the magnitude of T2* MR signal changes during functional imaging. Neuroradiology 44(6):459–466

Krings T, Topper R et al (2002b) Activation in primary and secondary motor areas in patients with CNS neoplasms and weakness. Neurology 58(3):381–390

Krishnan R, Raabe A et al (2004) Functional magnetic resonance imaging-integrated neuronavigation: correlation between lesion-to-motor cortex distance and outcome. Neurosurgery 55(4):904–914. discussion 914–915

Kurth R, Villringer K et al (1998) FMRI assessment of somatotopy in human Brodmann area 3b by electrical finger stimulation. Neuroreport 9(2):207–212

Kwong KK, Belliveau JW et al (1992) Dynamic magnetic resonance imaging of human brain activity during primary sensory stimulation. Proc Natl Acad Sci U S A 89(12):5675–5679

Kyriacou SK, Mohamed A et al (2002) Brain mechanics for neurosurgery: modeling issues. Biomech Model Mechanobiol 1(2):151–164

Lazar RM, Marshall RS et al (1997) Anterior translocation of language in patients with left cerebral arteriovenous malformation. Neurology 49(3):802–808

Lang S, Duncan N et al (2014) Resting state fMRI: review of neurosurgical applications. Neurosurgery 74(5):453–464

Lee CC, Ward HA et al (1999) Assessment of functional MR imaging in neurosurgical planning. AJNR Am J Neuroradiol 20(8):1511–1519

Lee MH, Smyser CD et al (2013) Resting-state fMRI: a review of methods and clinical applications. AJNR Am J Neuroradiol 34(10):1866–1872

Lehericy S, Duffau H et al (2000) Correspondence between functional magnetic resonance imaging somatotopy and individual brain anatomy of the central region: comparison with intraoperative stimulation in patients with brain tumors. J Neurosurg 92(4):589–598

Lehericy S, Biondi A et al (2002) Arteriovenous brain malformations: is functional MR imaging reliable for studying language reorganization in patients? Initial observations. Radiology 223(3):672–682

Liu G, Ogawa S (2006) EPI image reconstruction with correction of distortion and signal losses. J Magn Reson Imaging 24(3):683–689

Liu WC, Feldman SC et al (2005) The effect of tumour type and distance on activation in the motor cortex. Neuroradiology 47(11):813–819

Ludemann L, Forschler A et al (2006) BOLD signal in the motor cortex shows a correlation with the blood volume of brain tumors. J Magn Reson Imaging 23(4):435–443

Majos A, Tybor K et al (2005) Cortical mapping by functional magnetic resonance imaging in patients with brain tumors. Eur Radiol 15(6):1148–1158

Mazzetto-Betti KC, Leoni RF et al (2010) The stability of the blood oxygenation level-dependent functional MRI response to motor tasks is altered in patients with chronic ischemic stroke. Stroke 41(9):1921–1926

Menon RS, Ogawa S et al (1995) BOLD based functional MRI at 4 Tesla includes a capillary bed contribution: echo-planar imaging correlates with previous optical imaging using intrinsic signals. Magn Reson Med 33(3):453–459

Mitchell TJ, Hacker CD et al (2013) A novel data-driven approach to preoperative mapping of functional cortex using resting-state functional magnetic resonance imaging. Neurosurgery 73(6):969–982

Mizuguchi N, Nakata H et al (2013) Brain activity during motor imagery of an action with an object: a functional magnetic resonance imaging study. Neurosci Res 76(3):150–155

Moller M, Freund M et al (2005) Real time fMRI: a tool for the routine presurgical localisation of the motor cortex. Eur Radiol 15(2):292–295

Mueller WM, Yetkin FZ et al (1996) Functional magnetic resonance imaging mapping of the motor cortex in patients with cerebral tumors. Neurosurgery 39(3):515–520. discussion 520–521

Nimsky C, Ganslandt O et al (2006) Intraoperative visualization for resection of gliomas: the role of functional neuronavigation and intraoperative 1.5 T MRI. Neurol Res 28(5):482–487

Noble JW, Eng JJ et al (2013) Effect of visual feedback on brain activation during motor tasks: an FMRI study. Mot Control 17(3):298–312

Ogawa S, Menon RS et al (1993) Functional brain mapping by blood oxygenation level-dependent contrast magnetic resonance imaging. A comparison of signal characteristics with a biophysical model. Biophys J 64(3):803–812

Ojemann G, Ojemann J et al (1989) Cortical language localization in left, dominant hemisphere. An electrical stimulation mapping investigation in 117 patients. J Neurosurg 71(3):316–326

Onofrey JA, Staib LH et al (2013) Learning nonrigid deformations for constrained multi-modal image registration. Med. Image Comput Assist Interv 16(Pt 3):171–178

Orringer DA, Vago DR et al (2012) Clinical applications and future directions of functional MRI. Semin Neurol 32(4):466–475

Osborn A (2004) Diagnostic imaging: brain. Amirsys, Salt Lake City

Ozdoba C, Nirkko AC et al (2002) Whole-brain functional magnetic resonance imaging of cerebral arteriovenous malformations involving the motor pathways. Neuroradiology 44(1):1–10

Parmar H, Sitoh YY et al (2004) Combined magnetic resonance tractography and functional magnetic resonance imaging in evaluation of brain tumors involving the motor system. J Comput Assist Tomogr 28(4):551–556

Petrella JR, Shah LM et al (2006) Preoperative functional MR imaging localization of language and motor areas: effect on therapeutic decision making in patients with potentially resectable brain tumors. Radiology 240(3):793–802

Pillai JJ (2010) The evolution of clinical functional imaging during the past 2 decades and its current impact on neurosurgical planning. AJNR Am J Neuroradiol 31(2):219–225

Pirotte B, Goldman S et al (2005a) Integration of [11C] methionine-positron emission tomographic and magnetic resonance imaging for image-guided surgical resection of infiltrative low-grade brain tumors in children. Neurosurgery 57(Suppl. 1):128–139

Pirotte B, Voordecker P et al (2005b) Combination of functional magnetic resonance imaging-guided neuronavigation and intraoperative cortical brain mapping improves targeting of motor cortex stimulation in neuropathic pain. Neurosurgery 56(Suppl. 2):344–359. discussion 344–359

Priest AN, De Vita E et al (2006) EPI distortion correction from a simultaneously acquired distortion map using TRAIL. J Magn Reson Imaging 23(4):597–603

Puce A, Constable RT et al (1995) Functional magnetic resonance imaging of sensory and motor cortex: comparison with electrophysiological localization. J Neurosurg 83(2):262–270

Pujol J, Conesa G et al (1996) Presurgical identification of the primary sensorimotor cortex by functional magnetic resonance imaging. J Neurosurg 84(1):7–13

Pujol J, Conesa G et al (1998) Clinical application of functional magnetic resonance imaging in presurgical identification of the central sulcus. J Neurosurg 88(5):863–869

Qiu TM, Gong FY et al (2017) Real-time motor cortex mapping for the safe resection of glioma: an intraoperative resting-state fMRI study. AJNR Am J Neuroradiol 38(11):2146–2152

Ramsey NF, Sommer IE et al (2001) Combined analysis of language tasks in fMRI improves assessment of hemispheric dominance for language functions in individual subjects. NeuroImage 13(4):719–733

Reinges MH, Krings T et al (2005) Prospective demonstration of short-term motor plasticity following acquired central pareses. NeuroImage 24(4):1248–1255

Roessler K, Donat M et al (2005) Evaluation of preoperative high magnetic field motor functional MRI (3 Tesla) in glioma patients by navigated electrocortical stimulation and postoperative outcome. J Neurol Neurosurg Psychiatry 76(8):1152–1157

Rolls HK, Yoo SS et al (2007) Rater-dependent accuracy in predicting the spatial location of functional centers on anatomical MR images. Clin Neurol Neurosurg 109(3):225–235

Roux FE, Ranjeva JP et al (1997) Motor functional MRI for presurgical evaluation of cerebral tumors. Stereotact Funct Neurosurg 68(1–4 Pt 1):106–111

Roux FE, Boulanouar K et al (1999a) Cortical intraoperative stimulation in brain tumors as a tool to evaluate spatial data from motor functional MRI. Investig Radiol 34(3):225–229

Roux FE, Boulanouar K et al (1999b) Usefulness of motor functional MRI correlated to cortical mapping in rolandic low grade astrocytomas. Acta Neurochir 141(1):71–79

Rosazza C, Aquino D et al (2014) Preoperative mapping of the sensorimotor cortex: comparative assessment of task-based and resting-state FMRI. PLoS One 9(6):e98860

Rosen BR, Savoy RL (2012) fMRI at 20: has it changed the world? NeuroImage 62(2):1316–1324

Rutten GJ, Ramsey NF et al (2002) Interhemispheric reorganization of motor hand function to the primary motor cortex predicted with functional magnetic resonance imaging and transcranial magnetic stimulation. J Child Neurol 17(4):292–297

Schlosser MJ, McCarthy G et al (1997) Cerebral vascular malformations adjacent to sensorimotor and visual cortex. Functional magnetic resonance imaging studies before and after therapeutic intervention. Stroke 28(6):1130–1137

Schonberg T, Pianka P et al (2006) Characterization of displaced white matter by brain tumors using combined DTI and fMRI. NeuroImage 30(4):1100–1111

Schneider FC, Pailler M et al (2016) Presurgical assessment of the sensorimotor cortex using resting-state fMRI. AJNR Am J Neuroradiol 37(1):101–107

Schreiber A, Hubbe U et al (2000) The influence of gliomas and nonglial space-occupying lesions on blood-oxygen-level-dependent contrast enhancement. AJNR Am J Neuroradiol 21(6):1055–1063

Schwindack C, Siminotto E et al (2005) Real-time functional magnetic resonance imaging (rt-fMRI) in patients with brain tumours: preliminary findings using motor and language paradigms. Br J Neurosurg 19(1):25–32

Seto E, Sela G et al (2001) Quantifying head motion associated with motor tasks used in fMRI. NeuroImage 14(2):284–297

Shinoura N, Yamada R et al (2005) Preoperative fMRI, tractography and continuous task during awake surgery for maintenance of motor function following surgical resection of metastatic tumor spread to the primary motor area. Minim Invasive Neurosurg 48(2):85–90

Shinoura N, Suzuki Y et al (2006) Restored activation of primary motor area from motor reorganization and improved motor function after brain tumor resection. AJNR Am J Neuroradiol 27(6):1275–1282

Shriver S, Knierim KE et al (2013) Pneumatically driven finger movement: a novel passive functional MR imaging technique for presurgical motor and sensory mapping. AJNR Am J Neuroradiol 34(1):E5–E7

Silva M, See A et al (2018) Challenges and techniques for presurgical brain mapping with functional MRI. NeuroImage: Clin 14:794–803

Steger TR, Jackson EF (2004) Real-time motion detection of functional MRI data. J Appl Clin Med Phys 5(2):64–70

Stippich C (2005) Clinical functional magnetic resonance imaging: basic principles and clinical applications. Radiol up2date 5:317–336

Stippich C (ed) (2007) Clinical functional MRI: presurgical functional neuroimaging. Springer, New York. isbn:978-3-540-24469-1

Stippich C, Hofmann R et al (1999) Somatotopic mapping of the human primary somatosensory cortex by fully automated tactile stimulation using functional magnetic resonance imaging. Neurosci Lett 277(1):25–28

Stippich C, Kapfer D et al (2000) Robust localization of the contralateral precentral gyrus in hemiparetic patients using the unimpaired ipsilateral hand: a clinical functional magnetic resonance imaging protocol. Neurosci Lett 285(2):155–159

Stippich C, Heiland S et al (2002a) Functional magnetic resonance imaging: physiological background, technical aspects and prerequisites for clinical use. Rofo 174(1):43

Stippich C, Ochmann H et al (2002b) Somatotopic mapping of the human primary sensorimotor cortex during motor imagery and motor execution by functional magnetic resonance imaging. Neurosci Lett 331(1):50–54

Stippich C, Kress B et al (2003) Preoperative functional magnetic resonance tomography (FMRI) in patients with rolandic brain tumors: indication, investigation strategy, possibilities and limitations of clinical application. Rofo 175(8):1042–1050

Stippich C, Romanowski A et al (2004) Fully automated localization of the human primary somatosensory cortex in one minute by functional magnetic resonance imaging. Neurosci Lett 364(2):90–93

Stippich C, Blatow M et al (2007) Global activation of primary motor cortex during voluntary movements in man. NeuroImage 34:1227–1237

Sunaert S (2006) Presurgical planning for tumor resectioning. J Magn Reson Imaging 23(6):887–905

Ternovoi SK, Sinitsyn VE et al (2004) Localization of the motor and speech zones of the cerebral cortex by functional magnetic resonance tomography. Neurosci Behav Physiol 34(5):431–437

Thulborn K (2006) Clinical functional magnetic resonance imaging. In: Haacke EM et al (eds) Current protocols in magnetic resonance imaging. Wiley, New York

Tie Y, Suarez RO et al (2009) Comparison of blocked and event-related fMRI designs for pre-surgical language mapping. NeuroImage 47(Suppl. 2):T107–T115

Tyndall AJ, Stippich C et al (2017) Presurgical motor, somatosensory and language fMRI: Technical feasibility and limitations in 491 patients over 13 years. Eur Radiol 27:267–278

Ulmer JL, Krouwer HG et al (2003) Pseudo-reorganization of language cortical function at fMR imaging: a consequence of tumor-induced neurovascular uncoupling. AJNR Am J Neuroradiol 24(2):213–217

Ulmer JL, Salvan CV et al (2004) The role of diffusion tensor imaging in establishing the proximity of tumor borders to functional brain systems: implications for preoperative risk assessments and postoperative outcomes. Technol Cancer Res Treat 3(6):567–576

Van Westen D, Skagerberg G et al (2005) Functional magnetic resonance imaging at 3 T as a clinical tool in patients with intracranial tumors. Acta Radiol 46(6):599–609

Weiskopf N, Klose U et al (2005) Single-shot compensation of image distortions and BOLD contrast optimization using multi-echo EPI for real-time fMRI. NeuroImage 24(4):1068–1079

Wienbruch C, Candia V et al (2006) A portable and low-cost fMRI compatible pneumatic system for the investigation of the somatosensory system in clinical and research environments. Neurosci Lett 398(3):183–188

Wirtz CR, Tronnier VM et al (1997) Image-guided neurosurgery with intraoperative MRI: update of frameless stereotaxy and radicality control. Stereotact Funct Neurosurg 68(1–4 Pt 1):39–43

Wittek A, Kikinis R et al (2005) Brain shift computation using a fully nonlinear biomechanical model. Med Image Comput Comput Assist Interv 8(Pt 2):583–590

Yousry TA, Schmid UD et al (1997) Localization of the motor hand area to a knob on the precentral gyrus. A new landmark. Brain 120(Pt 1):141–157

Resting State Functional MRI for Presurgical Planning

19

Joshua S. Shimony, Eric C. Leuthardt, Donna Dierker, Ki-Yun Park, Carl D. Hacker, and Abraham Z. Snyder

19.1 Introduction

19.1.1 Background

In order to optimize outcomes for brain tumor patients, the neurosurgeon faces a common dilemma between maximal tumor resection and minimizing functional loss. These two factors are often cited in the surgical literature as predictors of long-term survival (Gulati et al. 2011; Lacroix et al. 2001; McGirt et al. 2009), and have been recognized as such from the early days of neurosurgery (Dandy 1921). The gold standard for intraoperative functional localization is electrical cortical stimulation mapping (Ojemann 1993); however, functional magnetic resonance imaging (fMRI) has been used as an important adjunct measure for presurgical mapping of eloquent cortex and for intraoperative navigation (Petrella et al. 2006).

fMRI detects changes in the blood oxygen level dependent (BOLD) signal that reflect the neurovascular response to neural activity. Traditionally, localization of function in the brain using fMRI has been performed by presenting stimuli or imposing tasks (e.g., finger tapping or object naming) to elicit a neuronal response (Spitzer et al. 1995). More recently there has been growing appreciation for the use of resting state spontaneous BOLD fluctuations, also called intrinsic brain activity, or resting state fMRI (rsfMRI) as a tool to elucidate the brain's functional organization. That intrinsic brain activity could be utilized for functional localization was first suggested by Biswal and colleagues who demonstrated that BOLD fluctuations observed in the resting state are correlated within the somatomotor system (Biswal et al. 1995). The development of these methods has opened up many new options for neurocognitive research as well as clinical applications, such as presurgical planning (Kokkonen et al. 2009; Liu et al. 2009; Shimony et al. 2009).

19.1.2 Resting State Networks

Areas of the brain that demonstrate synchronous BOLD activity are defined as resting state networks (RSN) (Seeley et al. 2007). Figure 19.1 demonstrates an example of positive correlations between seed regions within the default mode network (DMN) and anticorrelations with respect to a different RSN. The most widely used measure of synchronous activity between seed regions is the Pearson product moment. The topography of RSNs closely corresponds to responses elicited by a wide variety of sensory, motor, and cognitive tasks (Smith et al. 2009).

J. S. Shimony (✉) · E. C. Leuthardt · D. Dierker
K.-Y. Park · C. D. Hacker · A. Z. Snyder
Washington University School of Medicine, Saint Louis, MO, USA
e-mail: shimonyj@wustl.edu; leuthardte@wustl.edu; donna@wustl.edu; k.park@wustl.edu; hackerc@wustl.edu; azsnyder@wustl.edu

S. Ulmer, O. Jansen (eds.), *fMRI*, https://doi.org/10.1007/978-3-030-41874-8_19

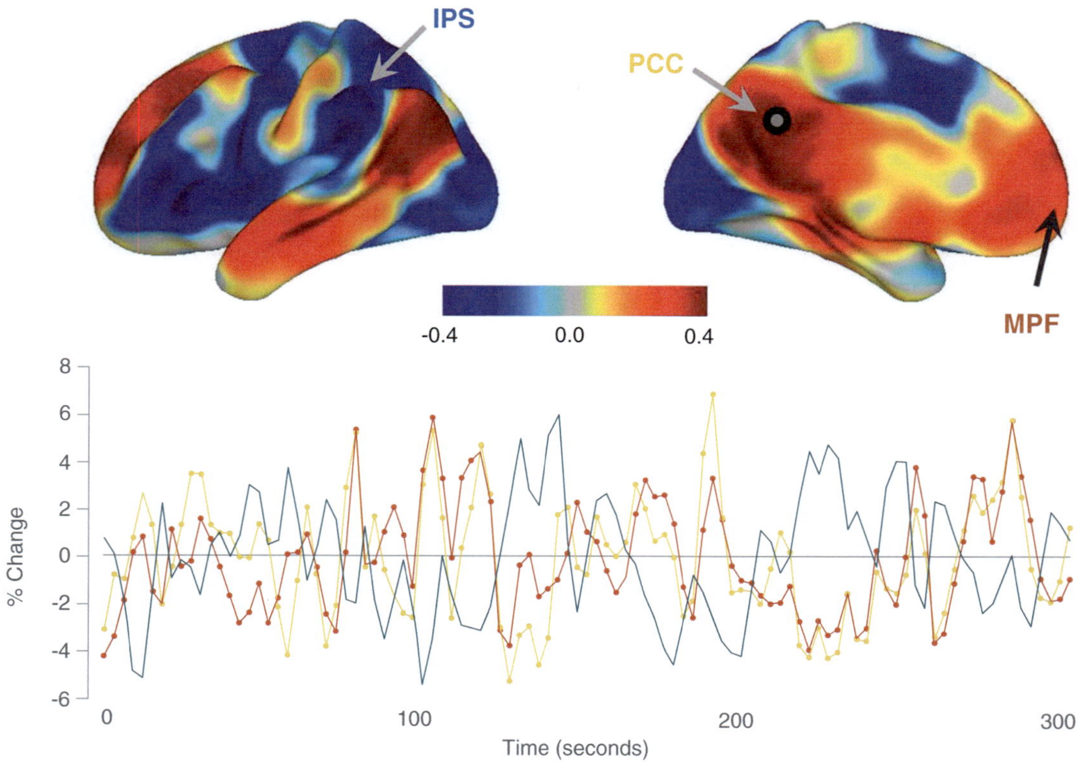

Fig. 19.1 Correlations between a seed region in the posterior cingulate cortex (PCC, part of the DMN) and all other voxels in the brain for a single subject during resting fixation. Positive correlations are denoted in warm colors and negative correlations are denoted in cold colors. The time course for a BOLD run is shown for the seed regions (PCC in yellow), the positively correlated medial prefrontal region (MPF, orange), and negatively correlated inferior parietal sulcus (IPS, blue)

Figure 19.2 demonstrates a collection of commonly identified RSN topographies. It has been established that intrinsic activity persists in a modified form during sleep (Larson-Prior et al. 2009; Samann et al. 2010) and under certain types of sedation (Mhuircheartaigh et al. 2010). RSNs have been identified in all mammalian species investigated to date (Hutchison et al. 2012; Nasrallah et al. 2013; Schwarz et al. 2013). This phylogenetic conservation implies that coherent intrinsic activity must be physiologically important despite its high metabolic cost (Raichle 2009, 2010).

The physiological function(s) of intrinsic neural activity remains an active area of research. One clue in this regard comes from studies of brain development. Thus, for example, retinal ganglion cell activity is required for proper development of synaptic connectivity within the lateral geniculate body during early brain development (Shatz 1990). This landmark result exemplifies *activity dependent synaptic plasticity*. Postnatally, young animals pass through a sequence of developmental critical periods during which brain structure is modified by *experience-dependent synaptic plasticity*. Examples of experience dependent plasticity include the classic experiments of Hubel and Wiesel in kittens (Hubel et al. 1977) and more recent experiments in rodents (Ackman and Crair 2014). Persistence of experience-dependent synaptic plasticity into adulthood provides the basis for *learning and memory*. Acquisition of new memories and motor skills necessarily unbalances synaptic weights (Tononi and Cirelli 2014). Thus, one primary function of intrinsic neural activity is thought to be rebalancing of synaptic weights (synaptic homeostasis) (Maffei and Fontanini 2009; Turrigiano 2011; Vitureira

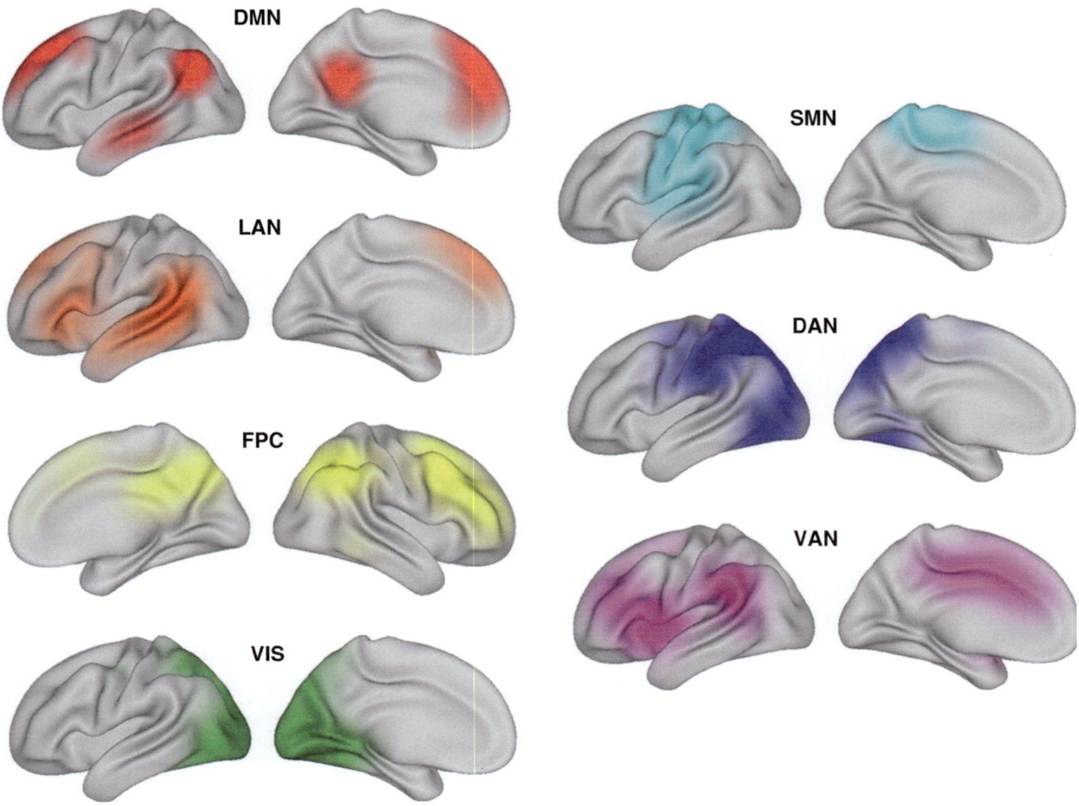

Fig. 19.2 Seven commonly identified RSNs, default mode network (DMN), frontoparietal control network (FPC), language network (LAN), ventral attention network (VAN), somatomotor network (SMN), vision network (VIS), and dorsal attention network (DAN). The right hemisphere is displayed for the ventral attention network because it was right lateralized

et al. 2012). The persistence of spontaneous fluctuations during states of reduced awareness suggests that intrinsic neuronal activity plays a role in the maintenance of the brain's functional integrity (Pizoli et al. 2011).

The spectral content of intrinsic BOLD signal fluctuations is approximately "1/f-like," or, "scale-free" (He 2011). The "1/f-like" spectral feature of BOLD fluctuations implies that these intrinsic signal fluctuations are aperiodic with the greatest fraction of power occurring at the lowest temporal frequencies. BOLD signal fluctuations are additionally confined to frequencies below ~0.2 Hz owing to the kinetics of the hemodynamic transduction, that is, the mechanisms regulating blood flow and metabolism in relation to neural activity. Direct measurements of the hemodynamic transduction transfer function using periodic stimuli show that the BOLD response is greatly attenuated at frequencies above ~0.2 Hz (Anderson 2008). It is likely that the same transduction mechanism underlies resting state BOLD fluctuations. This spectral feature carries important implications for the design of resting state fMRI artifact reduction strategies described below. Characteristics of BOLD fMRI spectral profiles are illustrated in multiple papers, for example (Larson-Prior et al. 2009; He 2011; Bianciardi et al. 2009; Fransson 2006).

Resting state networks are hierarchically organized (Cordes and Nandy 2006; Doucet et al. 2011; Lee et al. 2012). At the top of the hierarchy is a dichotomous distinction between the default mode network (DMN) and the rest of the brain (Fox et al. 2005; Hacker et al. 2013). Progressively finer distinctions between RSNs can be made at successively lower levels of the hierarchy. A consequence of this hierarchical organization is that unsupervised classification strategies may find any number of RSNs, depending on how many networks are requested (Lee et al. 2012). Another consequence of hierarchical organization is that RSN membership generally is not all-or-none. In other words, any part of the brain may belong to multiple RSNs, albeit unequally (Lee et al. 2012), although this point frequently is suppressed in winner-take-all representations of RSNs, for example, as in (Power et al. 2011). Second, the notion that RSN boundaries are well demarcated is variable across the brain. On the one hand, there exist contours on the cortical surface at which RSN membership changes abruptly as the boundary is crossed (Cohen et al. 2008; Wig et al. 2014). On the other hand, very few regions are completely enclosed by such contours. The neurobiological significance of this topological finding is unknown.

Several paradigmatic maneuvers are known to systematically change the statistics of intrinsic activity. One of the more interesting reported findings is that concurrent performance of a demanding working memory task reduces the amplitude of intrinsic activity throughout the DMN and markedly reduces measured functional connectivity between nodes of the DMN (Fransson 2006). In this experiment, the task was run at a pace faster than the hemodynamic response, thereby ensuring that task-induced responses did not contaminate the functional connectivity measures. Another frequently used maneuver is opening versus closing the eyes. Eye opening *suppresses* intrinsic activity within primary and higher order visual cortices (McAvoy et al. 2008). Moreover, presentation of a small visual stimulus in the eyes open state elicits a localized fMRI response in the retinotopically appropriate part of visual cortex but does not alter the ongoing activity (Bianciardi et al. 2009). In this last-mentioned experiment, the evoked response and the ongoing activity were separated in the temporal frequency domain by the use of a periodic stimulation paradigm. More generally, the available evidence suggests that task engagement tends to *suppress* intrinsic fluctuations in parts of the brain showing positive BOLD responses (He 2013). This principle constitutes one more indication that the primary function of intrinsic activity is not on-line processing. However, contrary evidence has been reported. Specifically, unilateral self-paced finger movement was observed to *increase* functional connectivity between sensorimotor and premotor cortices in the contralateral hemisphere (Marrelec et al. 2006).

Additional evidence for the role of rsfMRI correlations in the maintenance of long-term stability of the brain's functional organization was provided by Laumann et al. (2017). In this study, the authors investigated the stability of rsfMRI over time to evaluate for dynamic changes in the BOLD correlations that could reflect moment to moment changes in cognitive content of the brain. The authors concluded that changes in BOLD correlations over time are largely explained by a combination of sampling variability, head motion, and fluctuations in the sleep state during scanning. The authors concluded that a single correlation structure adequately describes the resting state structure of the brain as measured with BOLD fMRI.

The importance of RSNs to the mapping of brain function lies in the fact that their topography corresponds to activation maps elicited in task-based fMRI paradigms (Smith et al. 2009). These networks include the somatosensory, language, and visual networks, which can provide valuable information for the neurosurgeon in the preoperative setting. Other RSNs that are easily identified and are currently of research interest include the DMN, control, and attention networks (Fig. 19.2). Over the last decade we have been using resting state methods to provide presurgical planning information to the neurosurgeons at our hospital with very positive results. Over time these techniques have evolved and are now currently used routinely for patients with brain tumors or epilepsy, often combined with task fMRI and diffusion tensor imaging (DTI) in the intraoperative navigation system. In the rest of this chapter, we will discuss our clinical methods, analysis techniques, comparisons with task-based fMRI, and future prospects.

19.2 Methods

19.2.1 MRI and Clinical Protocols

Patients with newly diagnosed brain tumors are scanned using a 3 T scanner. The resting state data are acquired using a T2∗ echo plane imaging (EPI) sequence (3 × 3 × 3 mm cubic voxels; 128 volumes/run; TE = 27 ms; TR = 2.8 s; field of view = 256 mm; flip angle = 90°), while the patients are instructed to remain still and fixate on a visual crosshair without falling asleep (2 runs of 6 min each for a total time of 12 min). Tumor protocol anatomic imaging also includes T1-weighted magnetization prepared rapid acquisition gradient echo (MP-PAGE), T2-weighted fast spin echo, susceptibility-weighted imaging (SWI), diffusion-weighted imaging (DWI), and pre and postgadolinium contrast T1-weigted fast spin echo in multiple projections. All anatomic and functional magnetic resonance data are acquired in within 60 min.

The processing of the rsfMRI data is performed using a locally developed set of algorithms (Smyser et al. 2010) with details provided in http://4dfp.readthedocs.io. This processing, with its respective quality control (QC) measures, is implemented within the translational imaging platform (TIP), a custom XNAT-based informatics system (Marcus et al. 2007). The TIP includes an interface to query for and retrieve patient studies from the clinical picture archiving and communication system (PACS) and pipelines to fully automate the rsfMRI processing. The pipelines generate digital imaging and communications in medicine (DICOM)-formatted images of the resting state networks and a web-based QC report. Trained technicians manage the overall workflow and for studies that pass QC review, the generated DICOM images are pushed back to the PACS for use by clinicians. Studies that fail QC are reprocessed with adjusted parameters. In rare cases, the study is unable to be processed, typically due to severe subject motion, image artifacts, or poor spatial alignment with anatomic scans. Once the generated images are available on the clinical PACS, a neuroradiology fellow integrates them with the task fMRI, tractography, and anatomic images on a surgical planning station. The entire examination is reviewed by a neuroradiology attending, a report is dictated, and the intraoperative navigation-compatible fused imaging is transmitted to the operating room. If the quality of the rsfMRI data is determined to be suboptimal (either by the automatic QC measures or during the review by the neuroradiology fellow and attending) this will be included in the written report and the neurosurgery service will be notified. This set of procedures was refined over time in response to feedback from the personnel that implement the process and from the neurosurgeons who are the end users of this information. The service is frequently used by the neurosurgeons who perform tumor surgery at our institution.

From the neurosurgical point of view, the use of rsfMRI has been implemented to complement and enhance the currently established methods of task fMRI and DTI tractography. The rsfMRI information is especially valuable if the task fMRI is of poor quality or is nonexistent, such as can occur when patients are not able to cooperate with the task fMRI requirements. The rsfMRI data arrive in a format that is similar to that used for the task fMRI, that is, the rsfMRI data are provided as a graphical overlay of the location of the motor or language networks mapped on the brain. This is typically provided in several versions that are distinguished from each other by different threshold values that adjust the relative sensitivity and specificity of the maps. As part of the presurgical planning phase the neurosurgeon will review the rsfMRI maps in addition to the more traditional task fMRI and DTI tractography data (Fig. 19.3). During this phase the neurosurgeon will use these data (and their assessment of its quality) to help inform various decisions in regard to the surgery itself. These decisions may include some or all of the following items: (1) the location and size of the craniotomy; (2) the direction and path of approach to the tumor; (3) the need for a ventriculostomy catheter and where to place it; (4) the need for electrocortical stimulation equipment to confirm the MRI findings; (5) the need for an intraoperative MRI scan; and (6) the need to vary the type of anesthesia depending

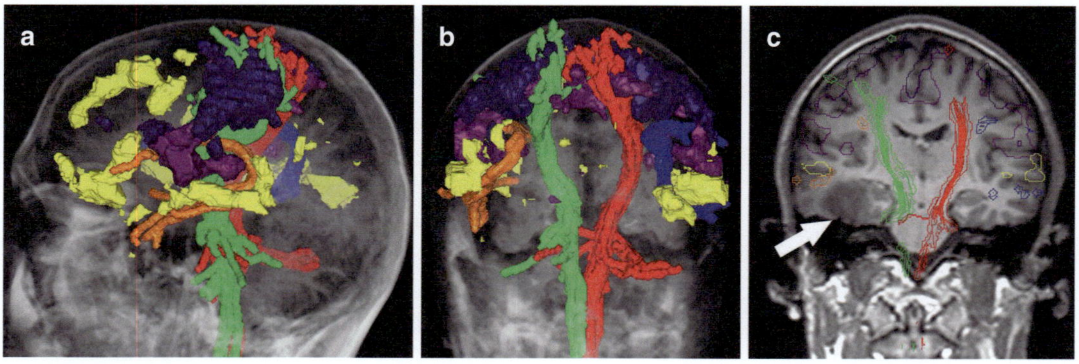

Fig. 19.3 Example of presurgical planning images from the intraoperative navigation system. (**a**) 3D left lateral view, (**b**) 3D coronal view, (**c**) 2D coronal view with regions and tracks superposed on a T1-weighted image. The white arrow points to the location of the tumor. Colored objects represent: Left corticospinal track (green), right corticospinal track (red), left arcuate fasciculus (orange), right arcuate fasciculus (blue), language RSN (yellow), somatomotor regions from both task and resting state (two shades of purple)

on the type of anticipated stimulation mapping. Every case is different, and the MRI information can provide valuable help in decreasing morbidity and optimizing the tumor resection.

19.2.2 Overview of Processing Methods for rsfMRI

Investigators interested in pursuing rsfMRI experiments need to be aware of certain practical considerations. A new investigator may wish to use one of the freely available software packages to help process their data. The following three packages include all the basic operations needed to analyze rsfMRI data: FSL (Jenkinson et al. 2012), AFNI (Cox 2012), SPM (www.fil.ion.ucl.ac.uk/spm/). Each package is downloadable at no cost, is documented in an easily accessible web site, provides on-line support, and is associated with regularly scheduled training workshops. FSL and AFNI are the most modular. Modular organization requires the user to understand the sequence of analysis operations and discourages "push-button" or rote analyses.

Basic preprocessing common to both task-based and rsfMRI must precede all subsequent analyses (detailed below). Once basic fMRI preprocessing is complete, the investigator must choose between two principal modes of rsfMRI analysis: (1) seed-based correlation (SBC) mapping and (2) spatial independent component analysis (sICA). SBC mapping is well suited to investigations of the functional connectivity of *a priori* targeted regions of interest but requires extensive preprocessing to reduce the impact of artifact (see below). sICA provides a direct means of separating artifact from neural signals (McKeown et al. 2003) but is less well suited to investigating targeted regions of interest. Both SBC and sICA yield highly reproducible results at the group level (Damoiseaux et al. 2006). RSNs near the top of the hierarchy, especially, the DMN, appear very much the same whether mapped by SBC or sICA; at lower levels of the hierarchy, RSN topography derived by the two methods systematically differs. Some networks are lateralized using sICA analysis, whereas SBC mapping generally yields highly symmetric maps (Fox et al. 2006; Salvador et al. 2005). Modest asymmetry can be observed with SBC if seeds are placed in homotopic parts of the brain instantiating language (left hemisphere) and orienting (external capture of attention; right hemisphere) (Fox et al. 2006).

This review will focus on a SBC style methodology used by our lab implemented as a series of preprocessing steps followed by classification using a previously trained multilayer neural network. This method uses prior information for the localization of RSNs across the brain, and requires careful denoising to exclude non-neural artifact from the data. An advantage of SBC in comparison to sICA is that using prior information provides a more robust mapping in individual patients with relatively high motion and relatively short scanning times that are more realistic in a population of patients with brain tumors (Lee et al. 2016).

19.2.3 General Preprocessing

The following preprocessing steps are performed on the raw fMRI data (Shulman et al. 2010):

1. Compensation for slice dependent time shifts: Although a typical TR is around 2 s (faster for the newer multi band sequences), each slice of the brain is acquired at a slightly different time and thus interpolation methods are used to create a full brain image that was acquired "simultaneously" at a single time point.
2. Elimination of systemic odd–even slice intensity differences due to interleaved acquisition.
3. Rigid body correction for head movement within and across runs using affine registration techniques (Fig. 19.4 demonstrates examples of head motion curves).
4. Intensity scaling (multiplicative factor applied to all voxels of all frames within each run) to obtain a mode value of 1000 (Ojemann et al. 1997). This facilitates assessment of voxel-wise variance for the purpose of quality assessment but does not affect computed correlation.
5. Head movement correction is achieved by atlas transformation using a composition of affine transforms connecting the fMRI volumes with the T1- and T2-weighted structural images. Figure 19.5 demonstrates examples of brain registration quality control. Head movement correction is included in a single resampling to generate a volumetric time series in 3 mm cubic atlas space.
6. Spatial smoothing using a 6 mm full width at half maximum Gaussian blur in each direction in order to increase the signal to noise with some loss of resolution.
7. Voxel-wise removal of linear trends over each run.
8. Temporal band pass filtering to retain frequencies between 0.01 and 0.1 Hz.
9. Reduction of spurious variance by regression of nuisance variables. These include waveforms derived from:
   (a) Signal of head motion correction.
   (b) Signal extracted from cerebrospinal fluid (CSF).
   (c) Signal extracted from white matter areas.

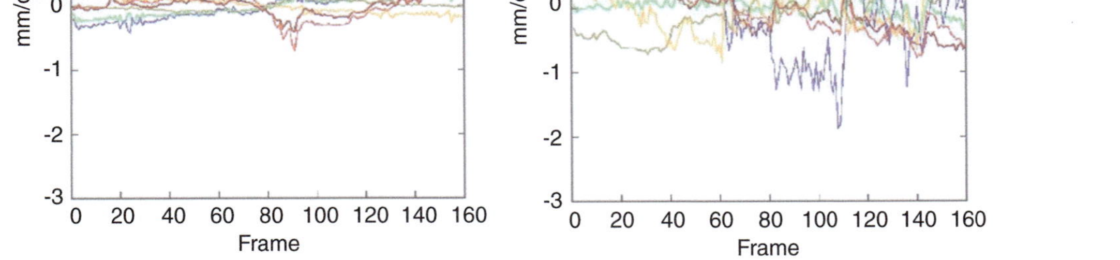

Fig. 19.4 Quality control head motion curves in a low motion (**a**), and high motion subject (**b**). The curves represent shifts in the *x*, *y*, and *z* position in millimeters, and rotations around the *x*, *y*, and *z* axis in degrees

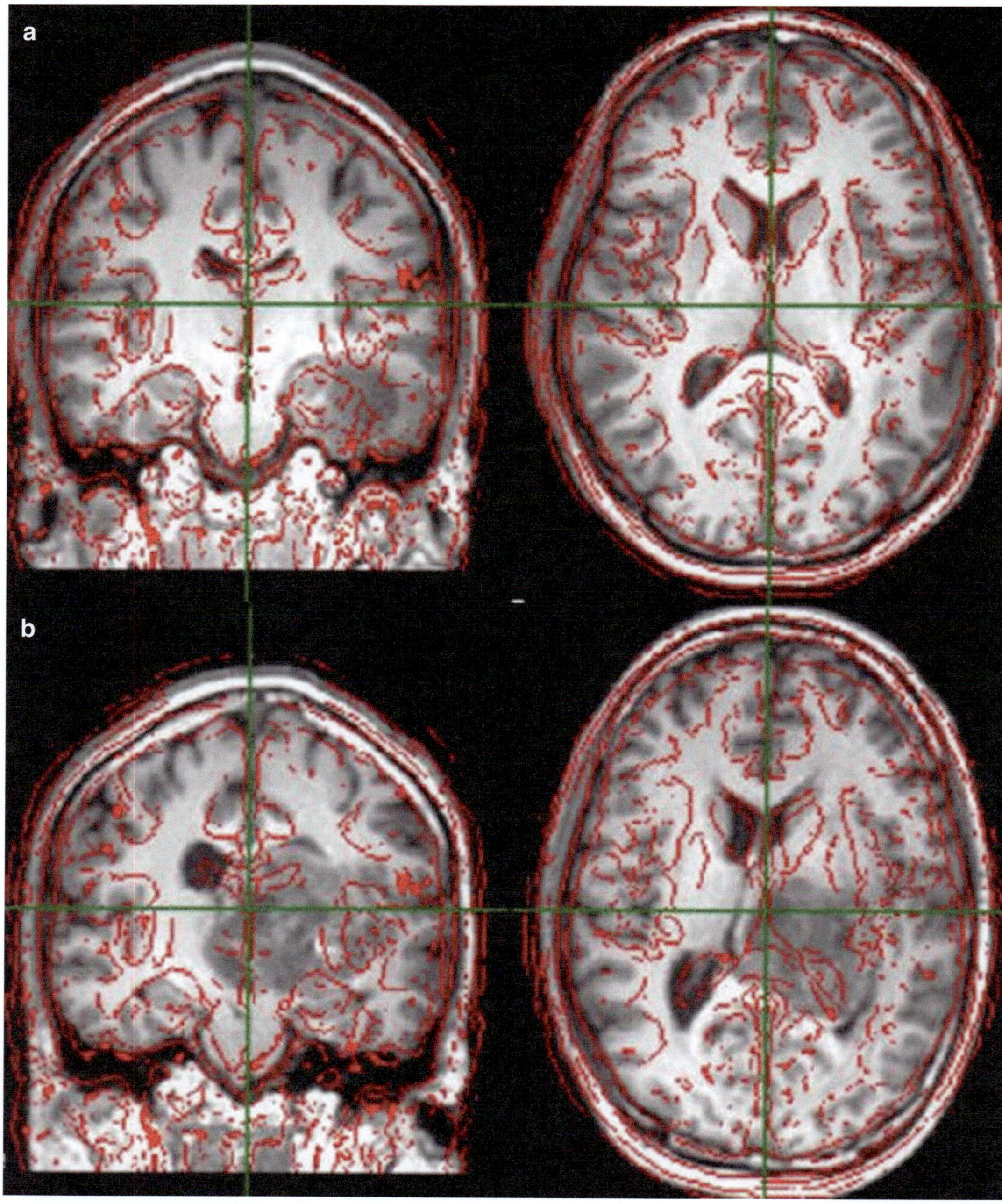

Fig. 19.5 Quality control images of image registration in atlas space in a patient with a small tumor with high quality registration (**a**), and in a patient with a large tumor with a low quality registration (**b**). The red outline represents key edge information in atlas space, such as the edge of the brain and ventricles and the gray–white matter boundary

(d) Global signal across the whole brain.

The last step of global signal regression (GSR) remains controversial and further detail is provided in the next section.

10. Removal/scrubbing of high motion time points to minimize the impact of head motion on the correlation results. Two common strategies to identify compromised frames include selection based on analysis of retrospective head motion correction time series (Power et al. 2014) or by voxel-wise evaluation over the whole brain of the differentiated fMRI time series (derivative of variance (DVARS) measure) (Power et al. 2011; Afyouni and Nichols 2018).

19.2.4 Global Signal Regression

Global signal regression (GSR) prior to correlation mapping is a highly effective means of reducing widely shared variance and thereby improving the spatial specificity of computed maps (Fox et al. 2009; Aguirre et al. 1998; Macey et al. 2004). Some part of the global signal is of neural origin (Scholvinck et al. 2010). However, much of the global signal represents non-neural artifact attributable to physical effects of head motion (Friston et al. 1996; Yan et al. 2013; Power et al. 2012; Satterthwaite et al. 2012) and variations in the partial pressure of arterial carbon dioxide (Wise et al. 2004). Absent GSR, all parts of the brain appear to be strongly positively correlated (Lowe et al. 1998; Vincent et al. 2006; Joel et al. 2011; Chai et al. 2012). GSR causes all subsequently computed correlation maps to be approximately zero-centered; in other words, positive and negative values are approximately balanced over the whole brain (Fox et al. 2009). Thus, GSR does negatively bias all computed correlations, although iso-correlation contours, that is, map topographies, remain unchanged. This negative bias has caused some to criticize GSR on the grounds that it induces artifactual anticorrelations (Anderson et al. 2011; Murphy et al. 2009). Although it has since been demonstrated that some parts of the brain appear to be truly anticorrelated in the resting state, as demonstrated using sICA (Liao et al. 2010; Zuo et al. 2010). More recent objections to GSR focus on the possibility that it can distort quantitative functional connectivity differences across diagnostic groups (Saad et al. 2012). However, this objection to GSR is irrelevant in the context of using rsfMRI for purposes of RSN mapping in individuals.

19.2.5 RSN Mapping Using a Trained Multilayer Perceptron (MLP)

Our early efforts at RSN mapping used simple seed-based correlation, similar to the first efforts of Biswal et al. (1995). Seed-based analyses require prior knowledge of the locations of regions of interest (ROI) and these can be obtained from previously determined atlas coordinates or from task-based fMRI data. As an example (Fig. 19.6), in a patient with a brain tumor adjacent to the motor region of the ipsilateral hemisphere a seed for the motor network could be placed in the contralateral, undistorted hemisphere based on the anatomic localization of the central sulcus and the resting state time courses from the rest of the brain compared with this region and a correlation map can be generated that is used to identify the location of the motor network in the distorted ipsilateral side containing the tumor (Zhang et al. 2009).

More recently we described a technique for mapping the topography of known RSNs in individuals using a multilayer perceptron (MLP) (Hacker et al. 2013). Perceptrons are machine-

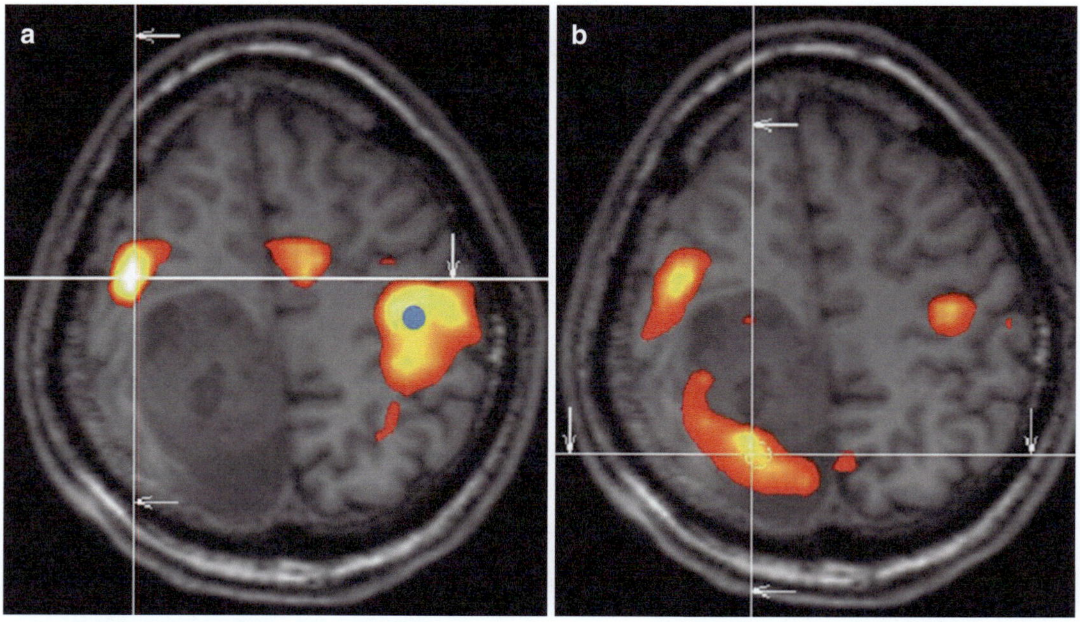

Fig. 19.6 (**a**) Structural MRI showing a mass in the right parietal cortex with resting state correlation mapping showing anterior displacement of the right motor cortex (intersection of white lines). The seed region is shown as a blue circle placed on the normal left motor cortex area. (**b**) Task-related mapping of the motor cortex in the same patient also demonstrates the anterior displacement of the motor cortex on the right; however, there is also a large area of activation, likely artifactual, posterior to the tumor (intersection of white lines)

learning algorithms that can be trained to associate specific input patterns with discrete output labels (Rumelhart et al. 1986). An MLP was trained to associate seed-based correlation maps with particular RSNs. Running the trained MLP on correlation maps corresponding to all voxels in the brain generates voxel-wise RSN membership estimates. Thus, RSN mapping using a trained MLP exemplifies supervised classification. It is critical to note that our MLP assigns RSN membership to rsfMRI correlation maps. Detailed quantitative evaluation of the MLP performance is presented in ref. (Hacker et al. 2013). MLP performance was also compared to alternative RSN estimation schemes, such as dual regression and linear discriminant analysis, and was found to provide improved area under the curve estimation, with better orthogonal estimates of RSN membership.

In summary, the MLP accurately generates RSN topography estimates in individuals consistent with previous studies, even in brain regions distorted by tumor and not represented in the training data. Most importantly, as it is a supervised classification procedure, the MLP provides a highly robust means of generating RSN maps in individuals.

19.3 Application to Presurgical Planning

19.3.1 Introduction

Multiple studies have demonstrated that maximal resection of a brain tumor while sparing nearby eloquent cortex leads to improved outcomes, with minimal morbidity (Lacroix et al. 2001; McGirt et al. 2009; Keles et al. 2001, 2006; Sanai et al. 2008). Historically, neurosurgeons have been concerned with localization of the motor and language system on the assumption that these parts of the brain ("eloquent" cortex) instantiate critical functionality. However, a broader understanding of brain function suggests that all parts of the brain contribute to important functionality

(Lee et al. 2012; Hacker et al. 2013; Golland et al. 2008; Yeo et al. 2011). Thus, improved functional mapping of multiple RSNs beyond motor and language could lead to further improvements in patient outcomes.

Multiple prior publications have explored the use of rsfMRI for presurgical planning. An early case report example of this technique used to localize the motor cortex in a patient with a brain tumor was presented in reference Shimony et al. (2009). Kokkonen et al. (2009) similarly compared motor task data to resting state data and showed that the motor functional network could be localized using resting state data in 8 tumor patients, as well as 10 healthy control subjects.

rsfMRI may also be used for presurgical planning in patients with epilepsy. The higher spatial resolution afforded by rsfMRI over electroencephalography could provide a distinct advantage in mapping epileptic foci or networks. Seed-based methods were used by Liu et al. (2009) to successfully locate sensorimotor areas by using rsfMRI in patients with tumors or epileptic foci close to sensorimotor areas. They found agreement between rsfMRI, task-based fMRI, and intraoperative cortical stimulation data. In another study from the same laboratory, Stufflebeam and colleagues (Stufflebeam et al. 2011) were able to localize areas of increased functional connectivity in 5 of 6 patients that overlapped with epileptogenic areas identified by invasive encephalography. Zhang et al. (2011) used graph methods and a pattern classifier applied to rsfMRI data to identify subjects as either having medial temporal lobe epilepsy or as normal controls. Using data from 16 patients with intractable medial temporal lobe epilepsy and 52 normal controls, they achieved an average sensitivity of 77.2% and a specificity of 83.86% in classification. Bettus et al. (2010) reported that increases in basal functional connectivity were a specific marker of the location of the epileptogenic zone in 22 patients with mesial temporal lobe epilepsy. Weaver et al. (2013) studied 4 nonlesion, focal epileptic patients along with 16 control subjects to determine whether the seizure focus could be found using the functional patterns near the epileptogenic zone. By averaging voxel homogeneity across regions of interest and comparing that with other regions, they were able to accurately identify the epileptic focus. Tie et al. (2014) used structural independent component analysis (sICA) on a training group of 14 healthy subjects to identify the language network from the rsfMRI data. The result of that analysis was then used to identify the language network in a second group of 18 healthy subjects at the individual level. They further proposed an automated system for determining the language network in individual patients using sICA.

19.3.2 Differences Between Mapping of Task and Resting State fMRI

Although both the methods of task fMRI and rsfMRI are based on fMRI, they each measure different aspects of brain function. Task fMRI imposes a behavior on the patient and provides the representation of a fixed sensory, motor, or cognitive process. Each paradigm yields a multifocal response mapped onto the brain's anatomy. This strategy cannot be used with rsfMRI since there is no imposed task and no response, only fluctuations of the fMRI signal. rsfMRI measures a network, that is topography of temporally synchronous spontaneous BOLD fluctuations.

19.3.2.1 Somatomotor

When evaluating the somatomotor systems task fMRI is limited to the area of activation, for example, the hand area when the task is a finger tapping, as compared to the motor network revealed by rsfMRI which is more extensive and includes Brodmann areas 1–4 as well as the supplemental motor cortex (Dierker et al. 2017). This distribution is illustrated in Fig. 19.7a.

19.3.2.2 Language

The language system is more complicated with many different components. Language tasks can emphasize expressive language (Broca's area, Brodmann 44–45) or receptive language (Wernicke's area, Brodmann 22), but also can involve parietal regions (Price 2012), and also the visual (reading), auditory (listening to language),

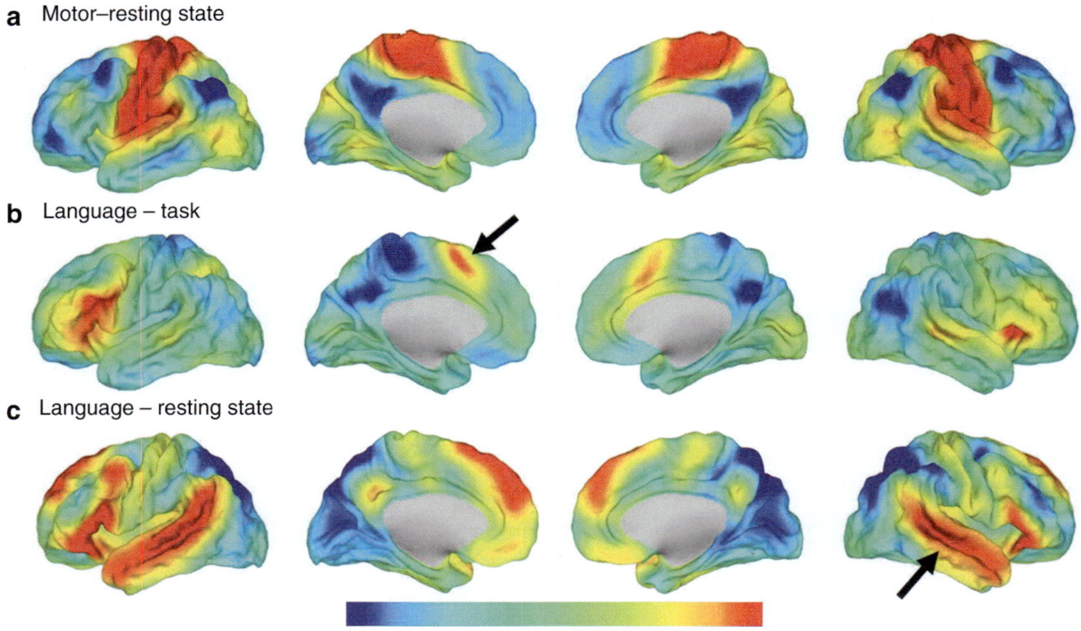

Fig. 19.7 (**a**) Average somatomotor RSN. The motor topography seen with the RSN is more extensive than a more focal task response, such as the hand area activated with finger tapping. (**b**) Average language response to word generation task. Broca's area is strongly activated. The arrow points to the dorsal cingulate area that is also activated with many tasks and is not considered a traditional language area. (**c**) Average language RSN. Note the more robust response on the right side (arrow)

and even the motor system (speaking). Due to the specificity of any language task many centers will do several language tasks in order to provide the surgeon with more comprehensive coverage of the language areas. This comes at the cost of longer time in the scanner. It is uncertain whether all regions activated by language tasks are language specific or simply parts of the brain ubiquitously recruited by intentional performance of any task. These effects are illustrated in Fig. 19.7b and c with activation of the dorsal cingulate, an area known to belong to the cingulo-opercular and/or salience networks (Seeley et al. 2007; Dosenbach et al. 2007). Resting state language maps are more specific to language functionality. However, resting state networks generally, including the "language network," are less lateralized than responses induced by language tasks. Hence, task-activation protocols may be preferable if determination of hemispheric dominance is the primary objective.

Finally, for a given surgical situation, not all of these regions will be equally relevant and the judgment of the surgeon is critical during the presurgical planning phase. Familiarity with these effects is important and can help the surgeon identify false positive or negative areas delineated on the localization maps.

19.4 Conclusion

This chapter presents an introduction to rsfMRI and RSNs and their application in presurgical planning. We briefly covered RSN imaging methods and then presented some examples of MLP-based RSN mapping, as this is our current method of choice for simultaneously mapping multiple RSNs to provide the surgeon with an accurate map of the resting state architecture of the brain prior to surgery. This experience suggests how MLP-based RSN mapping should be applied to minimize surgical morbidity.

As these results demonstrate, rsfMRI is a promising technique for presurgical planning with the objective of decreasing morbidity while maximizing complete resection of pathological tissue. However, the methodology is still in early stages of development. Further research is necessary to make these tools more accurate and more widely available in the operating room. Additional research is needed to explore the differences between rsfMRI, task-based MRI, and elastic common schema mapping, and to better understanding the consequences of disrupted RSNs other than the motor and language systems. Related engineering development should incorporate the presurgical MRI results into intraoperative neuronavigation systems, including the rsfMRI results in conjunction with white matter fiber bundle anatomy derived from diffusion tensor imaging. An additional possibility is real-time intraoperative rsfMRI during surgery using intraoperative MRI systems that currently are becoming more common. Our current efforts in the lab are devoted to several of these projects.

Acknowledgments We wish to thank the National Institutes of Health for its generous support of this project via NIH R01 CA203861. Dr. Shimony is additionally supported by the Eunice Kennedy Shriver National Institute of Child Health & Human Development of the National Institutes of Health under Award Number U54 HD087011 to the Intellectual and Developmental Disabilities Research Center at Washington University. Dr. Snyder is supported by P30 NS098577-01. Dr. Leuthardt is additionally supported by the Christopher Davidson Foundation.

References

Ackman JB, Crair MC (2014) Role of emergent neural activity in visual map development. Curr Opin Neurobiol 24(1):166–175

Afyouni S, Nichols TE (2018) Insight and inference for DVARS. NeuroImage 172:291–312

Aguirre GK, Zarahn E, D'Esposito M (1998) The inferential impact of global signal covariates in functional neuroimaging analyses. NeuroImage 8(3):302–306

Anderson JS (2008) Origin of synchronized low-frequency blood oxygen level-dependent fluctuations in the primary visual cortex. AJNR Am J Neuroradiol 29(9):1722–1729

Anderson JS et al (2011) Network anticorrelations, global regression, and phase-shifted soft tissue correction. Hum Brain Mapp 32(6):919–934

Bettus G et al (2010) Role of resting state functional connectivity MRI in presurgical investigation of mesial temporal lobe epilepsy. J Neurol Neurosurg Psychiatry 81(10):1147–1154

Bianciardi M et al (2009) Modulation of spontaneous fMRI activity in human visual cortex by behavioral state. NeuroImage 45(1):160–168

Biswal B et al (1995) Functional connectivity in the motor cortex of resting human brain using echo-planar MRI. Magn Reson Med 34(4):537–541

Chai XJ et al (2012) Anticorrelations in resting state networks without global signal regression. NeuroImage 59(2):1420–1428

Cohen AL et al (2008) Defining functional areas in individual human brains using resting functional connectivity MRI. NeuroImage 41(1):45–57

Cordes D, Nandy RR (2006) Estimation of the intrinsic dimensionality of fMRI data. NeuroImage 29(1):145–154

Cox RW (2012) AFNI: what a long strange trip it's been. NeuroImage 62(2):743–747

Damoiseaux JS et al (2006) Consistent resting-state networks across healthy subjects. Proc Natl Acad Sci U S A 103(37):13848–13853

Dandy WE (1921) The treatment of brain tumors. JAMA 77:1853–1859

Dierker D et al (2017) Resting-state functional magnetic resonance imaging in presurgical functional mapping: sensorimotor localization. Neuroimaging Clin N Am 27(4):621–633

Dosenbach NU et al (2007) Distinct brain networks for adaptive and stable task control in humans. Proc Natl Acad Sci U S A 104(26):11073–11078

Doucet G et al (2011) Brain activity at rest: a multiscale hierarchical functional organization. J Neurophysiol 105(6):2753–2763

Fox MD et al (2005) The human brain is intrinsically organized into dynamic, anticorrelated functional networks. Proc Natl Acad Sci U S A 102(27):9673–9678

Fox MD et al (2006) Spontaneous neuronal activity distinguishes human dorsal and ventral attention systems. Proc Natl Acad Sci U S A 103(26):10046–10051

Fox MD et al (2009) The global signal and observed anticorrelated resting state brain networks. J Neurophysiol 101(6):3270–3283

Fransson P (2006) How default is the default mode of brain function? Further evidence from intrinsic BOLD signal fluctuations. Neuropsychologia 44(14):2836–2845

Friston KJ et al (1996) Movement-related effects in fMRI time-series. Magn Reson Med 35(3):346–355

Golland Y et al (2008) Data-driven clustering reveals a fundamental subdivision of the human cortex into two global systems. Neuropsychologia 46(2):540–553

Gulati S et al (2011) The risk of getting worse: surgically acquired deficits, perioperative complications, and functional outcomes after primary resection of glioblastoma. World Neurosurg 76(6):572–579

Hacker CD et al (2013) Resting state network estimation in individual subjects. NeuroImage 82:616–633

He BJ (2011) Scale-free properties of the functional magnetic resonance imaging signal during rest and task. J Neurosci 31(39):13786–13795

He BJ (2013) Spontaneous and task-evoked brain activity negatively interact. J Neurosci 33(11):4672–4682
Hubel DH, Wiesel TN, LeVay S (1977) Plasticity of ocular dominance columns in monkey striate cortex. Philos Trans R Soc Lond Ser B Biol Sci 278(961):377–409
Hutchison RM et al (2012) Functional connectivity of the frontal eye fields in humans and macaque monkeys investigated with resting-state fMRI. J Neurophysiol 107(9):2463–2474
Jenkinson M et al (2012) Fsl. NeuroImage 62(2):782–790
Joel SE et al (2011) On the relationship between seed-based and ICA-based measures of functional connectivity. Magn Reson Med 66(3):644–657
Keles GE, Lamborn KR, Berger MS (2001) Low-grade hemispheric gliomas in adults: a critical review of extent of resection as a factor influencing outcome. J Neurosurg 95(5):735–745
Keles GE et al (2006) Volumetric extent of resection and residual contrast enhancement on initial surgery as predictors of outcome in adult patients with hemispheric anaplastic astrocytoma. J Neurosurg 105(1):34–40
Kokkonen SM et al (2009) Preoperative localization of the sensorimotor area using independent component analysis of resting-state fMRI. Magn Reson Imaging 27(6):733–740
Lacroix M et al (2001) A multivariate analysis of 416 patients with glioblastoma multiforme: prognosis, extent of resection, and survival. J Neurosurg 95(2):190–198
Larson-Prior LJ et al (2009) Cortical network functional connectivity in the descent to sleep. Proc Natl Acad Sci U S A 106(11):4489–4494
Laumann TO et al (2017) On the Stability of BOLD fMRI Correlations. Cereb Cortex 27(10):4719–4732
Lee MH et al (2012) Clustering of resting state networks. PLoS One 7(7):e40370
Lee MH et al (2016) Clinical resting-state fMRI in the preoperative setting: are we ready for prime time? Top Magn Reson Imaging 25(1):11–18
Liao W et al (2010) Evaluating the effective connectivity of resting state networks using conditional Granger causality. Biol Cybern 102(1):57–69
Liu H et al (2009) Task-free presurgical mapping using functional magnetic resonance imaging intrinsic activity. J Neurosurg 111(4):746–754
Lowe MJ, Mock BJ, Sorenson JA (1998) Functional connectivity in single and multislice echoplanar imaging using resting-state fluctuations. NeuroImage 7(2):119–132
Macey PM et al (2004) A method for removal of global effects from fMRI time series. NeuroImage 22(1):360–366
Maffei A, Fontanini A (2009) Network homeostasis: a matter of coordination. Curr Opin Neurobiol 19(2):168–173
Marcus DS et al (2007) The extensible neuroimaging archive Toolkit: an informatics platform for managing, exploring, and sharing neuroimaging data. Neuroinformatics 5(1):11–34
Marrelec G et al (2006) Partial correlation for functional brain interactivity investigation in functional MRI. NeuroImage 32(1):228–237
McAvoy M et al (2008) Resting states affect spontaneous BOLD oscillations in sensory and paralimbic cortex. J Neurophysiol 100(2):922–931
McGirt MJ et al (2009) Independent association of extent of resection with survival in patients with malignant brain astrocytoma. J Neurosurg 110(1):156–162
McKeown MJ, Hansen LK, Sejnowsk TJ (2003) Independent component analysis of functional MRI: what is signal and what is noise? Curr Opin Neurobiol 13(5):620–629
Mhuircheartaigh RN et al (2010) Cortical and subcortical connectivity changes during decreasing levels of consciousness in humans: a functional magnetic resonance imaging study using propofol. J Neurosci 30(27):9095–9102
Murphy K et al (2009) The impact of global signal regression on resting state correlations: are anti-correlated networks introduced? NeuroImage 44(3):893–905
Nasrallah FA, Tay HC, Chuang KH (2013) Detection of functional connectivity in the resting mouse brain. NeuroImage 163:419–436
Ojemann GA (1993) Functional mapping of cortical language areas in adults. Intraoperative approaches. Adv Neurol 63:155–163
Ojemann JG et al (1997) Imaging studies of memory and attention. Neurosurg Clin N Am 8(3):307–319
Petrella JR et al (2006) Preoperative functional MR imaging localization of language and motor areas: effect on therapeutic decision making in patients with potentially resectable brain tumors. Radiology 240(3):793–802
Pizoli CE et al (2011) Resting-state activity in development and maintenance of normal brain function. Proc Natl Acad Sci U S A 108(28):11638–11643
Power JD et al (2011) Functional network organization of the human brain. Neuron 72(4):665–678
Power JD et al (2012) Spurious but systematic correlations in functional connectivity MRI networks arise from subject motion. NeuroImage 59(3):2142–2154
Power JD et al (2014) Methods to detect, characterize, and remove motion artifact in resting state fMRI. NeuroImage 84:320–341
Price CJ (2012) A review and synthesis of the first 20 years of PET and fMRI studies of heard speech, spoken language and reading. NeuroImage 62(2):816–847
Raichle ME (2009) A paradigm shift in functional brain imaging. J Neurosci 29(41):12729–12734
Raichle ME (2010) Two views of brain function. Trends Cogn Sci 14(4):180–190
Rumelhart DE, Hinton GE, Williams RJ (1986) Learning representations by back-propagating errors. Nature 323:533–536
Saad ZS et al (2012) Trouble at rest: how correlation patterns and group differences become distorted after global signal regression. Brain Connect 2(1):25–32

Salvador R et al (2005) Neurophysiological architecture of functional magnetic resonance images of human brain. Cereb Cortex 15(9):1332–1342
Samann PG et al (2010) Increased sleep pressure reduces resting state functional connectivity. MAGMA 23(5–6):375–389
Sanai N, Mirzadeh Z, Berger MS (2008) Functional outcome after language mapping for glioma resection. N Engl J Med 358:18–27
Satterthwaite TD et al (2012) Impact of in-scanner head motion on multiple measures of functional connectivity: relevance for studies of neurodevelopment in youth. NeuroImage 60(1):623–632
Scholvinck ML et al (2010) Neural basis of global resting-state fMRI activity. Proc Natl Acad Sci U S A 107(22):10238–10243
Schwarz AJ et al (2013) Anti-correlated cortical networks of intrinsic connectivity in the rat brain. Brain Connect 3(5):503–511
Seeley WW et al (2007) Dissociable intrinsic connectivity networks for salience processing and executive control. J Neurosci 27(9):2349–2356
Shatz CJ (1990) Competitive interactions between retinal ganglion cells during prenatal development. J Neurobiol 21(1):197–211
Shimony JS et al (2009) Resting-state spontaneous fluctuations in brain activity: a new paradigm for presurgical planning using fMRI. Acad Radiol 16(5):578–583
Shulman GL et al (2010) Right hemisphere dominance during spatial selective attention and target detection occurs outside the dorsal frontoparietal network. J Neurosci 30(10):3640–3651
Smith SM et al (2009) Correspondence of the brain's functional architecture during activation and rest. Proc Natl Acad Sci U S A 106(31):13040–13045
Smyser CD et al (2010) Longitudinal analysis of neural network development in preterm infants. Cereb Cortex 20(12):2852–2862
Spitzer M et al (1995) Category-specific brain activation in fMRI during picture naming. Neuroreport 6(16):2109–2112
Stufflebeam SM et al (2011) Localization of focal epileptic discharges using functional connectivity magnetic resonance imaging. J Neurosurg 114(6):1693–1697
Tie Y et al (2014) Defining language networks from resting-state fMRI for surgical planning-a feasibility study. Hum Brain Mapp 35(3):1018–1030
Tononi G, Cirelli C (2014) Sleep and the price of plasticity: from synaptic and cellular homeostasis to memory consolidation and integration. Neuron 81(1):12–34
Turrigiano G (2011) Too many cooks? Intrinsic and synaptic homeostatic mechanisms in cortical circuit refinement. Annu Rev Neurosci 34:89–103
Vincent JL et al (2006) Coherent spontaneous activity identifies a hippocampal-parietal memory network. J Neurophysiol 96(6):3517–3531
Vitureira N, Letellier M, Goda Y (2012) Homeostatic synaptic plasticity: from single synapses to neural circuits. Curr Opin Neurobiol 22(3):516–521
Weaver KE et al (2013) Local functional connectivity as a pre-surgical tool for seizure focus identification in non-lesion, focal epilepsy. Front Neurol 4:43
Wig GS, Laumann TO, Petersen SE (2014) An approach for parcellating human cortical areas using resting-state correlations. NeuroImage 93(Pt 2):276–291
Wise RG et al (2004) Resting fluctuations in arterial carbon dioxide induce significant low frequency variations in BOLD signal. NeuroImage 21(4):1652–1664
Yan CG et al (2013) A comprehensive assessment of regional variation in the impact of head micromovements on functional connectomics. NeuroImage 76:183–201
Yeo BT et al (2011) The organization of the human cerebral cortex estimated by intrinsic functional connectivity. J Neurophysiol 106(3):1125–1165
Zhang D et al (2009) Preoperative sensorimotor mapping in brain tumor patients using spontaneous fluctuations in neuronal activity imaged with functional magnetic resonance imaging: initial experience. Neurosurgery 65(Suppl 6):226–236
Zhang X et al (2011) Social network theory applied to resting-state fMRI connectivity data in the identification of epilepsy networks with iterative feature selection. J Neurosci Methods 199(1):129–139
Zuo XN et al (2010) Reliable intrinsic connectivity networks: test-retest evaluation using ICA and dual regression approach. NeuroImage 49(3):2163–2177

20 Functional Magnetic Resonance-Guided Resection of Intra-Axial Brain Tumors

Alexa Bodman and Walter Hall

20.1 Introduction

In the surgical treatment of brain tumors, the goal is maximal surgical resection without the development of a new permanent neurological deficit after surgery. For the most common primary brain tumor, glioblastoma, the extent of the surgical resection, correlates with the overall survival. In one of the landmark studies addressing this issue, a greater than 98% surgical resection of a glioblastoma was associated with increased survival time (Lacroix et al. 2001). Additional studies showed that this survival benefit can be seen in just a 78% extent of tumor resection, but this result improves with an increased extent of resection with gross total resection having the greatest survival benefit (Sanai et al. 2011). In low grade gliomas, a maximal safe surgical resection is also the goal of surgery because an increased extent of resection is beneficial (Aghi et al. 2015). For both primary brain tumors and metastatic brain lesions, maximal safe resection is the goal. For solitary metastatic lesions to the brain, surgical resection followed by radiation therapy remains the main focus of treatment in order to improve survival (Kalkanis et al. 2009; Patchell et al. 1990).

Though aggressive surgical resection of glioblastoma is recommended, location within or adjacent to eloquent cortex can be a limiting factor for obtaining a gross total resection. Resection of eloquent cortex can leave patients with significant neurologic deficits, such as aphasia and hemiplegia, which lower a patient's quality of life. Neurologic deficits can delay a patient's postoperative chemotherapy and radiation therapy treatments (Gulati et al. 2011). Surgically acquired neurologic deficits have also been associated with a decreased overall survival (Gulati et al. 2011; McGirt et al. 2009).

Functional magnetic resonance imaging (fMRI) is a noninvasive method in determining the dominant hemisphere in surgical planning and it is better tolerated by patients than the traditional Wada test (Wada and Rasmussen 1960; Silva et al. 2017). Functional MRI for resection of brain tumors is obtained through blood oxygenation level-dependent (BOLD) contrast (Ogawa et al. 1993). It allows for mapping of a patient's eloquent cortex. The study can be used to determine the safety and feasibility of tumor resection. This imaging technique can also be used in conjunction with frameless neuronavigation for surgical resection of brain tumors. Frameless neuronavigation is a revolutionary tool in the neurological surgeon's armamentarium that has become a standard tool in neurosurgical oncology cases (Kim et al. 2010).

A. Bodman
Austin Brain and Spine, St. David's Health Care, Austin, TX, USA

W. Hall (✉)
Department of Neurosurgery, SUNY Upstate Medical University, Syracuse, NY, USA
e-mail: hallw@upstate.edu

S. Ulmer, O. Jansen (eds.), *fMRI*, https://doi.org/10.1007/978-3-030-41874-8_20

For preoperative planning, the primary motor cortex is typically mapped using the tasks of finger tapping, lip pouting, and flexion and extension of the toes during the MRI. The supplementary motor area and the premotor area can also be mapped (Castellano et al. 2017). In a comparison of healthy volunteers to patients with brain tumors, fMRI has been shown to reliably map the sensorimotor cortex in the presence of a distorting lesion (Krings et al. 1998). Additionally, fMRI has been shown to have a high degree of reproducibility in patients with brain tumors (Agarwal et al. 2018). During presurgical planning, fMRI is also useful in showing areas of cortical reorganization due to the tumor (Belyaev et al. 2013; Gunal et al. 2018). There are several other benefits to fMRI-guided brain tumor resection. Using this technique, one can avoid performing an awake craniotomy thereby avoiding cortical stimulation which can cause seizures (Kim et al. 2010; Qiu et al. 2017). General anesthesia also increases patient comfort and does not require specialized anesthesiologists. Although awake craniotomies have drawbacks, this method allows for direct assessment of the functionality of the brain tissue to be resected and is necessary in some cases. Functional MRI can aid in determining the need for an awake craniotomy or the ability to avoid it all together (Kim et al. 2010). Due to the importance of mapping eloquent cortex in planning and performing surgical resection of brain tumors located in these regions, fMRI has become an invaluable tool for the neurosurgeon.

20.2 Functional MRI Use with Neuronavigation in Resection

Frameless neuronavigation systems are a standard tool used in resection of brain tumors. Functional MRI obtained prior to surgery can be merged with the navigation imaging to allow for direct fMRI guidance during immediate presurgical planning of the approach and intraoperative use. Intraoperative navigation fused with fMRI data has been shown to aid in guiding the surgical resection, though partial resection with this method to avoid a neurologic deficit is common (Gumprecht et al. 2002). Intraoperative cortical stimulation can also be combined with neuronavigation fused with fMRI in surgical resection of tumors located in or near eloquent cortex (Roessler 2005). In one series of 16 patients with low grade glial tumors located in eloquent cortex, fMRI-guided surgical resection allowed for gross total resection in 10 patients and partial resection, as intended because the tumor was deemed to involve eloquent areas, in the remaining patients (Kim et al. 2010). None of the patients experienced permanent neurologic deficits postoperatively (Kim et al. 2010).

The distance from the tumor to eloquent cortex on fMRI impacts the risk of a new neurological deficit postoperatively. In one early study of fMRI-guided resection of 25 patients with brain tumors near eloquent cortex, a lesion located a distance of 10 mm or more from an eloquent area was associated with a significantly lower risk of postoperative neurologic deficit. This study was performed on an MRI with a 1.5 T magnet (Håberg et al. 2004). In another study of 33 glioma patients undergoing fMRI and diffusion tensor imaging (DTI)-guided resection of tumors located in or near eloquent cortex, 11% had residual tumor, 42% of patients had gross total resection, and 12% had greater than 40% residual tumor due to the proximity to eloquent cortex or white matter tracts. This study was performed using MRI scanners with a 3.0 T magnet. In this series 88% of patients remained neurologically stable and 12% suffered neurologic deterioration. At 3-month follow-up, 61% had improvement of their neurologic function, 30% were stable, and 9% deteriorated. The rate of clinical worsening postoperatively was higher in patients with less than 5 mm of distance from the lesion to the eloquent area. As expected, the rate of gross total resection was also decreased in this group in order to preserve neurologic function (Berntsen et al. 2010). Other studies have also shown lesions within 5 mm of eloquent cortex have higher rates of new deficits after resection (Krishnan et al. 2004). High magnetic field MRI (3 T) has also been shown to have an improved correlation with direct cortical stimulation (Roessler 2005).

In one study of neurologic and cognitive functional outcomes after fMRI-guided surgical resection of low-grade gliomas within eloquent cortex, patients showed a transient worsening in neurologic function in the early postoperative period but 44.4% improved at follow-up, while 36.1% remained stable, and 27.8% worsened. Patients with a greater extent of resection had a better functional outcome. Of the patients who worked before surgery, 82.4% returned to work within 6 months of surgery (Muto et al. 2018).

20.3 Resection in Sensorimotor Cortex Using fMRI Guidance

For patients with lesions in or near the sensorimotor cortex, fMRI is a useful tool in preoperative planning to help determine the feasibility of resection as well as the surgical approach (Fig. 20.1) (Lee et al. 1999). In a series of 54 patients with tumors located near the motor strip, fMRI in conjunction with neuronavigation resulted in gross total resection for 45 tumors though neurologic deterioration was observed in 9 patients (Krishnan et al. 2004). In another study by Tymowski et al., 28 patients who underwent surgical resection of a brain tumor guided by fMRI navigation within the sensorimotor cortex were compared to 30 historical control patients who were resected without undergoing a preoperative fMRI. At discharge only 13 of the 28 patients with fMRI-guided resection experienced neurologic decline. In the control group, 22 patients showed neurologic decline at discharge. In comparing motor deficits using a special scale, fMRI-guided resection leads to an 18% reduction in severity of motor deficits postoperatively (Tymowski et al. 2013).

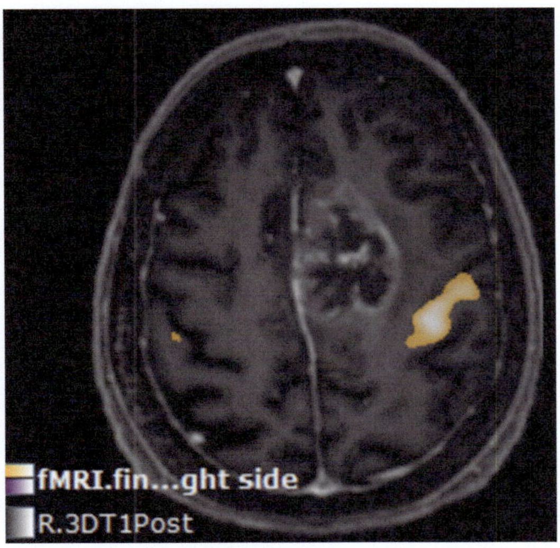

Fig. 20.1 Axial brain activation study performed at 3 T demonstrating the location of the functional area of the cortex for finger tapping of the right hand. The area of activation is just posterior and lateral to the contrast-enhancing tumor on this T1-weighted axial magnetic resonance imaging scan that was found to be a glioblastoma multiforme at surgery

20.4 Brain Tumor Resection within Language Areas Using fMRI

Patient variability in the location of language areas is well established, preventing surgical resection of brain tumors based on anatomical landmarks alone without a substantial risk of postoperative language deficits (Ojemann 1979).

In brain tumors involving the language areas, fMRI-guided surgery is useful in decreasing postoperative aphasia. One prospective study of 217 right-handed patients with gliomas located within 2 cm of language areas compared a study group of fMRI-guided tumor resection combined with intraoperative MRI to conventional navigation-guided tumor resection. The investigators found that in the study group, only 2.3% of patients developed postoperative aphasia whereas 34.8% of the conventional group developed this deficit. Additionally, the extent of resection was significantly higher in the study group, 95.5% compared to 89.9%, with an associated higher rate of gross total resection and increased overall survival, 19.6 months compared to 13 months (Zhang et al. 2014). These results may not be applicable to all institutions because there is significant heterogeneity in the task paradigms executed to map language on task-based fMRI between institutions, which may affect fMRI results used for presurgical planning (Binder et al. 2008).

20.5 Diffusion Tensor Imaging and fMRI-Guided Tumor Resection

Data from task-based fMRI alone is limited when the tumor extends into the deep white matter. In these cases, fMRI can be combined with diffusion tensor imaging (DTI) to aid in surgical resection (Kamada et al. 2007). DTI with MR tractography can also aid in determining if gross total resection is feasible without causing neurological deficits. In patients with intact tractography, there is a higher probability of gross total resection. If there is infiltration of the white matter tracts by tumor, this lowers the probability of a gross total resection (Castellano et al. 2017). Intraoperative DTI can compensate for brain shift during craniotomy and help to minimize deficits in brain tumor resection (D'Andrea et al. 2017). MRI tractography with fMRI is useful in the presurgical planning in pediatric patients with brain tumors (Lorenzen et al. 2018).

MR tractography in the context of language mapping is particularly useful during resection of lesions within language areas as it can delineate the arcuate fasciculus (Kamada et al. 2007). Approaching deeper lesions is also aided by the use of fMRI and DTI because the combination can reveal the safest corridor to safely reach the tumor (Frati et al. 2018).

20.6 Resting-State fMRI in Brain Tumor Resection

Patients with brain tumors may have symptoms that limit the usefulness of task-based fMRI, such as confusion, agitation, decreased attention span, hemiparesis, aphasia, and coma. Additionally, pediatric patients may also have limited cooperation with task-based fMRI (Roland et al. 2017). In these situations, resting-state fMRI can be useful since it does not require patient participation (Leuthardt et al. 2016). Resting-state fMRI obtains the topography of functionally connected areas of which the major ones are the default mode network, somatomotor network, visual network, auditory network, language network, dorsal attention network, and ventral attention network (Leuthardt et al. 2016). Resting-state fMRI can obtain multiple networks in a single image, resulting in it having a shorter acquisition time that task-based fMRI as well as it being simpler for the patients to undergo (Agarwal et al. 2017). Resting-state fMRI can also be reliably performed in sedated or unconscious patients (Leuthardt et al. 2016). Resting-state fMRI may be particularly useful in patients with tumors within the language area who present with deficits in their speech since they are hindered in their ability to participate in task-based fMRI. One study compared task-based fMRI of language areas with resting-state fMRI in patients with brain tumors and found that resting-state fMRI produced similar results to task-based fMRI (Branco et al. 2016). In another study of 38 patients, resting-state fMRI was obtained alongside task-based fMRI and resting-state fMRI was found to reliably map the sensorimotor cortex, although the maps are not comparable as expected (Dierker et al. 2017).

Resting-state fMRI can also be obtained during intraoperative MRI to guide further surgical resection. One study of 30 patients using this method showed its feasibility and correlation with direct cortical stimulation (Qiu et al. 2017). This method would also be ideal for patients who are unable to undergo an awake craniotomy. Resting-state fMRI, like task-based fMRI, has limitations and can be affected by the neovasculature associated with high grade gliomas resulting in a muted BOLD signal as well as having the standard limitations of MRI, such as head motion (Agarwal et al. 2017).

20.7 Limitations to Tumor Resection Guided by fMRI

Functional MRI has shown good but not perfect concordance rates with direct cortical stimulation (DCS) during surgery (Bizzi et al. 2008; Roux et al. 2003; Kuchcinski et al. 2015; Weng et al. 2018). The correlation with DCS and fMRI is higher for lower grade gliomas than for high grade gliomas (Bizzi et al. 2008). Due to this, for certain tumors within eloquent cortex, the surgeon may elect to perform an awake craniotomy (Roux et al. 2003). Brain tumors may alter the fMRI imaging accuracy as glioma development leads to an increase in neovasculature that alters the cerebral blood volume in an area which may mute the BOLD signal (Giussani et al. 2010). This can lead to a smaller area of activation volume that would have been found in normal tissue (Belyaev et al. 2013). Another factor in the discrepancies between direct cortical stimulation and fMRI is that stimulation is an inhibitory technique whereas fMRI is obtained through activation of areas (Silva et al. 2017). Certain medications can also interfere with the BOLD signal such as acetazolamide and specific habits of patients that include alcohol, caffeine, and tobacco use (Silva et al. 2017). Sleep deprivation may also disturb task-based fMRI (Silva et al. 2017).

20.8 Conclusion

Brain tumor surgery near eloquent brain tissue has become a safer practice since the advent of fMRI. Although several limitations exist, when combined with frameless neuronavigation, a safe approach and increased extent of tumor resection can be performed while minimizing the risks of a postoperative decline in neurologic function. Intraoperative MRI can further improve the extent of resection in these patients, improving their overall prognosis. The addition of MR tractography has allowed for safer resections into the white matter adjacent to eloquent cortex. New techniques such as resting-state fMRI may lead to further improvements in fMRI-guided brain tumor surgery.

References

Agarwal S, Hua J, Sair HI, Gujar S, Bettegowda C, Lu H et al (2018) Repeatability of language fMRI lateralization and localization metrics in brain tumor patients. Hum Brain Mapp 18(10):423–410

Agarwal S, Sair HI, Pillai JJ (2017) Limitations of resting-state functional MR imaging in the setting of focal brain lesions. Neuroimaging Clin N Am 27(4):645–661

Aghi MK, Nahed BV, Sloan AE, Ryken TC, Kalkanis SN, Olson JJ (2015) The role of surgery in the management of patients with diffuse low grade glioma. J Neurooncol 125(3):503–530

Belyaev AS, Peck KK, Petrovich Brennan NM, Holodny AI (2013) Clinical applications of functional MR imaging. Magn Reson Imaging Clin 21(2):269–278

Berntsen EM, Gulati S, Solheim O, Kvistad KA, Torp SH, Selbekk T et al (2010) Functional magnetic resonance imaging and diffusion tensor tractography incorporated into an intraoperative 3-dimensional ultrasound-based neuronavigation system. Neurosurgery 67(2):251–264

Binder JR, Swanson SJ, Hammeke TA, Sabsevitz DS (2008) A comparison of five fMRI protocols for mapping speech comprehension systems. Epilepsia 49(12):1980–1997

Bizzi A, Blasi V, Falini A, Ferroli P, Cadioli M, Danesi U et al (2008) Presurgical functional MR imaging of language and motor functions: validation with intraoperative electrocortical mapping. Radiology 248(2):579–589

Branco P, Seixas D, Deprez S, Kovacs S, Peeters R, Castro SL et al (2016) Resting-state functional magnetic resonance imaging for language preoperative planning. Front Hum Neurosci 10(19):137–114

Castellano A, Cirillo S, Bello L, Riva M, Falini A (2017) Functional MRI for surgery of gliomas. Curr Treat Options Neurol 19(10):34

D'Andrea G, Trillo G, Picotti V, Raco A (2017) Functional magnetic resonance imaging (fMRI), pre-intraoperative tractography in neurosurgery: the experience of Sant' Andrea Rome University Hospital. In: Trends in reconstructive neurosurgery. Springer International Publishing, Cham, pp 241–250. (Acta Neurochirurgica Supplement; vol. 124)

Dierker D, Roland JL, Kamran M, Rutlin J, Hacker CD, Marcus DS et al (2017) Resting-state functional magnetic resonance imaging in presurgical functional mapping. Neuroimaging Clin North Am 27(4):621–633

Frati A, Pesce A, D'Andrea G, Fraschetti F, Salvati M, Cimatti M et al (2018) A purely functional imaging based approach for transcortical resection of lesion involving the dominant atrium: towards safer, imaging-guided, tailored cortico-leucotomies. J Clin Neurosci 50:252–261

Giussani C, Roux F-E, Ojemann J, Sganzerla EP, Pirillo D, Papagno C (2010) Is preoperative functional magnetic resonance imaging reliable for language areas mapping in brain tumor surgery? Review of language functional magnetic resonance imaging and direct cortical stimulation correlation studies. Neurosurgery 66(1):113–120

Gulati S, Jakola AS, Nerland US, Weber C, Solheim O (2011) The risk of getting worse: surgically acquired deficits, perioperative complications, and functional outcomes after primary resection of glioblastoma. World Neurosurg 76(6):572–579

Gumprecht H, Ebel GK, Auer DP, Lumenta CB (2002) Neuronavigation and functional MRI for surgery in patients with lesion in eloquent brain areas. Minim Invasive Neurosurg 45(3):151–153

Gunal V, Savardekar A, Devi B, Bharath R (2018) Preoperative functional magnetic resonance imaging in patients undergoing surgery for tumors around left (dominant) inferior frontal gyrus region. Surg Neurol Int 9(1):126–116

Håberg A, Kvistad KA, Unsgård G, Haraldseth O (2004) Preoperative blood oxygen level-dependent functional magnetic resonance imaging in patients with primary brain tumors: clinical application and outcome. Neurosurgery 54(4):902–915

Kalkanis SN, Kondziolka D, Gaspar LE, Burri SH, Asher AL, Cobbs CS et al (2009) The role of surgical resection in the management of newly diagnosed brain metastases: a systematic review and evidence-based clinical practice guideline. J Neurooncol 96(1):33–43

Kamada K, Todo T, Masutani Y, Aoki S, Ino K, Morita A et al (2007) Visualization of the frontotemporal language fibers by tractography combined with functional magnetic resonance imaging and magnetoencephalography. J Neurosurg 106(1):90–98

Kim PD, Truwit CL, Hall WA (2010) Functional magnetic resonance-guided brain tumor resection. In: fMRI. Springer, Berlin, Heidelberg, Berlin, Heidelberg, pp 107–120

Krings T, Reul J, Spetzger U, Klusmann A, Roessler F, Gilsbach JM et al (1998) Functional magnetic resonance mapping of sensory motor cortex for image-guided neurosurgical intervention. Acta Neurochir 140(3):215–222

Krishnan R, Raabe A, Hattingen E, Szelényi A, Yahya H, Hermann E et al (2004) Functional magnetic resonance imaging-integrated neuronavigation: correlation between lesion-to-motor cortex distance and outcome. Neurosurgery 55(4):904–915

Kuchcinski G, Mellerio C, Pallud J, Dezamis E, Turc G, Rigaux-Viode O et al (2015) Three-tesla functional MR language mapping: comparison with direct cortical stimulation in gliomas. Neurology 84(6):560–568

Lacroix M, Abi-Said D, Fourney DR, Gokaslan ZL, Shi W, DeMonte F et al (2001) A multivariate analysis of 416 patients with glioblastoma multiforme: prognosis, extent of resection, and survival. J Neurosurg 95(2):190–198

Lee CC, Ward HA, Sharbrough FW, Meyer FB, Marsh WR, Raffel C et al (1999) Assessment of functional MR imaging in neurosurgical planning. AJNR Am J Neuroradiol 20(8):1511–1519

Leuthardt EC, Allen M, Kamran M, Hawasli AH, Snyder AZ, Hacker CD et al (2016) Resting-state blood oxygen level-dependent functional MRI: a paradigm shift in preoperative brain mapping. Stereotact Funct Neurosurg 93(6):427–439

Lorenzen A, Groeschel S, Ernemann U, Wilke M, Schuhmann MU (2018) Role of presurgical functional MRI and diffusion MR tractography in pediatric low-grade brain tumor surgery: a single-center study. Childs Nerv Syst 34(11):2241–2248

McGirt MJ, Mukherjee D, Chaichana KL, Than KD, Weingart JD, Quinones-Hinojosa A (2009) Association of surgically acquired motor and language deficits on overall survival after resection of glioblastoma multiforme. Neurosurgery 65(3):463–469; discussion 469–70

Muto J, Dezamis E, Rigaux-Viode O, Peeters S, Roux A, Zanello M et al (2018) Functional-based resection does not worsen quality of life in patients with a diffuse low-grade glioma involving eloquent brain regions: a prospective cohort study. World Neurosurg 113:e200–e212

Ogawa S, Menon RS, Tank DW, Kim SG, Merkle H, Ellermann JM et al (1993) Functional brain mapping by blood oxygenation level-dependent contrast magnetic resonance imaging. A comparison of signal characteristics with a biophysical model. Biophys J 64(3):803–812

Ojemann GA (1979) Individual variability in cortical localization of language. J Neurosurg 50(2): 164–169

Patchell RA, Tibbs PA, Walsh JW, Dempsey RJ, Maruyama Y, Kryscio RJ et al (1990) A randomized trial of surgery in the treatment of single metastases to the brain. N Engl J Med 322(8):494–500

Qiu T-M, Gong F-Y, Gong X, Wu J-S, Lin C-P, Biswal BB et al (2017) Real-time motor cortex mapping for the safe resection of glioma: an intraoperative resting-state fMRI study. AJNR Am J Neuroradiol 38(11):2146–2152

Roessler K (2005) Evaluation of preoperative high magnetic field motor functional MRI (3 Tesla) in glioma patients by navigated electrocortical stimulation and postoperative outcome. J Neurol Neurosurg Psychiatry 76(8):1152–1157

Roland JL, Griffin N, Hacker CD, Vellimana AK, Akbari SH, Shimony JS et al (2017) Resting-state functional magnetic resonance imaging for surgical planning in pediatric patients: a preliminary experience. J Neurosurg Pediatr 20(6):583–590

Roux F-E, Boulanouar K, Lotterie J-A, Mejdoubi M, LeSage JP, Berry I (2003) Language functional magnetic resonance imaging in preoperative assessment of language areas: correlation with direct cortical stimulation. Neurosurgery 52(6):1335–1347

Sanai N, Polley M-Y, McDermott MW, Parsa AT, Berger MS (2011) An extent of resection threshold for newly diagnosed glioblastomas. J Neurosurg 115(1):3–8

Silva MA, See AP, Essayed WI, Golby AJ, Tie Y (2017) Challenges and techniques for presurgical brain mapping with functional MRI. Neuroimage 17:794–803

Tymowski M, Majchrzak K, Bobek-Billewicz B, Ladziński PÅ, Majchrzak H (2013) The use of functional magnetic resonance imaging in reducing a risk of postoperative neurological deficits in the patients with brain tumour. Neurol Neurochir Pol 47(6):547–554

Wada J, Rasmussen T (1960) Intracarotid injection of sodium amytal for the lateralization of cerebral speech dominance. J Neurosurg 17(2):266–282

Weng H-H, Noll KR, Johnson JM, Prabhu SS, Tsai Y-H, Chang S-W et al (2018) Accuracy of presurgical functional MR imaging for language mapping of brain tumors: a systematic review and meta-analysis. Radiology 286(2):512–523

Zhang J, Chen X, Zhao Y, Wang F, Li F, Xu B (2014) Impact of intraoperative magnetic resonance imaging and functional neuronavigation on surgical outcome in patients with gliomas involving language areas. Neurosurg Rev 38(2):319–330

Direct Cortical Stimulation and fMRI

21

H. Maximilian Mehdorn, Simone Goebel, and Arya Nabavi

21.1 Introduction

Intracranial space-occupying lesions, particularly glial tumors in or close to eloquent areas, may challenge the neurosurgeon who aims at preserving cerebral functions as much as possible while removing as much of the lesion as possible. It has been repeatedly questioned whether radical resection of gliomas is the method of choice because of their invasive nature, particularly more recently with the advent of additional classification of tumors based on their molecular parameters as formalized in the 2016 WHO classification (Louis et al. 2016), but it has also been shown recently that patients do benefit from radical resection both in primary (Stummer et al. 2006) and recurrent gliomas and in low-grade gliomas (Claus and Black 2006; Sanai and Berger 2008), as far as length of survival is concerned. Radical resection of glial tumors, however, is hampered by the risk of damaging neuronal functions, particularly of speech and motor functions. Therefore, early on in the development of modern neurosurgery, brain tumor surgery under local anesthesia (LA) was suggested in order to reduce the risk of immediate severe and nonreversible postoperative neurological deficit (Berger and Ojemann 1992; Black and Ronner 1987; Ojemann et al. 1989; Ojemann 1988). Most of the patients are initially frightened by the suggestion of undergoing brain tumor surgery under local anesthesia. However, they accept this method when the details are fully explained to them (Danks et al. 1998). Nevertheless, there are limitations, such as patients' inability to cooperate—in the case of very young and very old patients or a tumor located and extending in such a fashion that there is no good way to position the patient with sufficient comfort; patients with reduced cardiopulmonary functions or seizures related to the tumor should be particularly well taken care of. Taking these precautions into account, it has been shown by many centers that it is possible to reduce the risk of a focal neurological deficit while increasing the chance to completely remove a tumor located in eloquent areas (Danks et al. 2000; Duffau 2005a, b; Duffau et al. 2003; Ebeling et al. 1995; Pinsker et al. 2007).

H. M. Mehdorn (✉)
Klinik für Neurochirurgie, Kiel, Germany

Mehdorn Consilium, Kiel, Germany
e-mail: mehdorn@nch.uni-kiel.de; prof@mehdorn-consil.de

S. Goebel
Klinik für Neurochirurgie, Kiel, Germany

Mehdorn Consilium, Kiel, Germany

Department of Psychology, University of Kiel, Kiel, Germany

A. Nabavi
Klinik für Neurochirurgie, Kiel, Germany

Mehdorn Consilium, Kiel, Germany

International Neuroscience Institute, Nordstadtkrankenhaus, Hannover, Germany

S. Ulmer, O. Jansen (eds.), *fMRI*, https://doi.org/10.1007/978-3-030-41874-8_21

With the advent of magnetic resonance imaging (MRI) and particularly functional MRI (fMRI), this technique is now widely accepted as being able to precisely localize brain functions (Brannen et al. 2001; Naidich et al. 2001), with a high degree of sophistication and reliability (with a 53% regional specificity (FitzGerald et al. 1997)): even different brain functions requiring complex interactions between various active brain areas can be evaluated. While the latter may be further explored in research projects, some indications for its use in a clinical setting have emerged over the recent years and led to its implementation into routine MRI scanner software. In routine clinical neurosurgical practice, these techniques mainly concern the definition of the dominant hemisphere, the various speech areas, and motor cortex. Furthermore, relation between the most important areas can be demonstrated by fiber tracking, thus enabling the surgeon to prevent damage to the white matter tracts (Duffau 2005a, b, 2007; Nimsky et al. 2006a, b, c). However, there are certain limitations which may lead one to question the value of these fMRI results in relation to preoperative planning and intraoperative application. This chapter should elucidate some of the benefits and pitfalls of both techniques—fMRI and awake craniotomy—as experienced by the authors in clinical practice and review the pertinent modern literature.

21.2 Indications for Direct Cortical Stimulation and/or Functional Magnetic Resonance Imaging (fMRI): Patient Selection

Two factors determine the indication for either direct cortical stimulation (DCS) during surgery under awake conditions or fMRI:

1. The clinical condition of the patient, particularly his presenting symptoms and his neurological status

   If the patient's history and presenting symptoms, like temporary speech deficits or focal seizures, suggest a lesion affecting motor or speech areas and the diagnosis of an intrinsic brain tumor in these areas is ascertained, the patient is considered for awake craniotomy using DCS. Special attention should be given to the patient's problems of understanding and his/her capability and willingness to cooperate with the surgeon and the OR team; these factors need to be analyzed preoperatively by the neurosurgical staff members and dedicated neuropsychologists.

   These criteria obviously exclude the following patient groups from awake craniotomy: emergency tumor decompressions in comatose patients, small children, and geriatric patients who would be unable to cooperate fully.

   In all other patients with tumors in the abovementioned locations, the method of DCS was the method of choice, before fMRI was available in our institution as well as in others, to determine intraoperatively how much tumor could be removed safely without provoking too big a neurological deficit. In our experience as well in the experience of others, DCS has shown to improve surgical outcome when operating in functionally relevant areas, enhancing both the amount of tumor resection and the preserving function.

   Now, since the advancement of MRI technology and introduction of fMRI in the armamentarium of preoperative evaluation, this method needs to be taken into consideration and weighted against the DCS method.
2. Tumor localization and function of brain region

   Following the first diagnostic imaging of the tumor which is usually made in a 1,5 T MRI machine in order to grade it in a assumptive manner, its localization is analyzed further in a 3 T MRI scanner to determine whether functionally relevant ("eloquent") brain structures including fiber tracts are in vicinity to the tumor and could possibly be harmed during tumor removal. This grading should help to define the extent of surgical resection. Resection of a WHO grade III or IV glioma should be attempted with the intent to completely preserve function at the preoperative level for the rather limited survival time, but in grade I or II gliomas, complete resection should be attempted in order to optimize survival times without adjunctive therapy, taking into account the plasticity of the brain under certain conditions (Southwell et al. 2016). In these patients, particular workup is required in order to define the spatial relation between the tumor borders and the functionally relevant structures, i.e., speech and motor cortical areas, optical regions, and the fiber tracts, particularly the pyramidal tract and the fiber bundles between the motor and sensory speech areas as well as the optical fiber tracts, e.g., the Gratiolet tract.

While fMRI data acquisition can be applied to all patients who tolerate the narrow canal of MRI machines and who understand the need to cooperate while performing the neuropsychological paradigms, the DWI measurements required for representation of fiber bundles demand that a patient lie for some additional time without moving his/her head until the data are acquired.

The fMRI data need to be processed and transferred to the neuronavigation consoles in order to be used for surgical planning.

Additional information is often acquired using transcranial magnetic stimulation TMS), preferably as regional TMS (rTMS) (Ille et al. 2016; Qiu et al. 2014).

On the basis of the abovementioned criteria, the patient is advised to undergo surgery as awake or asleep craniotomy. Our experience in reviewing patient perception of awake craniotomy and intraoperative MRI scanning (Goebel et al. 2010) as well as the experience of others has alleviated much of the preoperative patients' fear and facilitated their management, even if they might claim claustrophobia.

21.3 Methods

21.3.1 Surgery Under Local Anesthesia: Awake Craniotomy

Details of this technique have been described by many groups (Danks et al. 2000; Duffau et al. 1999, 2003; Duffau 2005a, b; Pinsker et al. 2007; Tonn 2007). We have implemented awake craniotomy since 1993 in our department in order to remove as much tumor as possible in or close to eloquent areas while preserving function. Prerequisite for this technique is, in our opinion, a good (neuro-)psychological preparation of the patient. The majority of our brain tumor patients undergo formal preoperative neuropsychological testing by our dedicated neuropsychologists who not only evaluate the aspects of the dominant hemisphere and, in a very sophisticated manner, the neuropsychological deficits but also talk to the patients and relatives concerning their individual fears related to the tumor diagnosis and the upcoming surgery (Goebel et al. 2011, b, 2013, 2018; Goebel and Mehdorn 2018). These aspects should not be underestimated in the modern neurosurgical setting as they may affect efficacy of treatment! In the initial phase, we also brought the patients into the operating room and positioned them onto the OR table to make them familiar with the setting; due to time restraints, this is no longer possible, but the patients are well familiarized with this particular type of surgery. Anesthesiologists also play a special role in this setting; they have to take care of the patient during surgery and are essential in keeping a balance between sedation of the patient during some parts of surgery, e.g., craniotomy itself and having him/her awake for testing during tumor removal. Medications used in this regard are propofol and analgesics. Central lining is given to all our patients although this may not be the routine in other centers (Fig. 21.1).

LA is applied to the patient by the neurosurgeon using ropivacaine HCl (Naropin®) 0.75% for the blocks around the 3-pin headholder. Neuronavigation is used to define the optimal craniotomy site and delineation of the skin incision. Subsequently, the line of the skin incision is anesthetized additionally; when a curved incision is required, particular care is paid to apply sufficient anesthesia to the underlying muscles, usually the temporal muscle. After careful aseptic preparation, the surgical drapes are placed after having applied a semicircular or rectangular cage-like metal to hold the drapes with suffi-

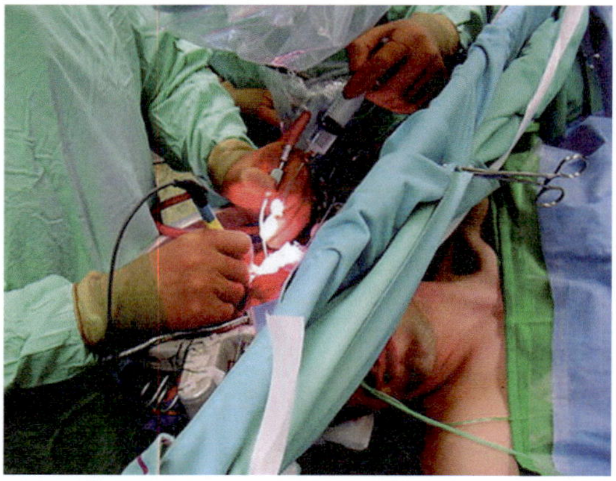

Fig. 21.1 Brain surgery in the awake patient. The patient is operated with standard microneurosurgical equipment while undergoing specific neurophysiologic and neuropsychological testing

cient comfort for the patient to whom every single step of draping him/her is explained carefully (Fig. 21.2).

Then, surgery is performed as usual while always talking to the patient and explaining all the steps and adding LA as required; particular care is taken while the craniotomy is performed. Until this step and a little bit longer, the patient is also allowed to sleep under anesthesiological supervision and with the help of sedation and/or analgesic short-lasting medication (propofol).

The dura is subsequently opened under the operating microscope and the brain inspected, and again with the help of the neuronavigation, the brain tumor is localized.

Fig. 21.2 Positioning the awake patient in the 3-pin headholder using local anesthesia. (**a**) Close-up view of the patient. (**b**) During surgery with the neuropsychologist calming and testing the patient

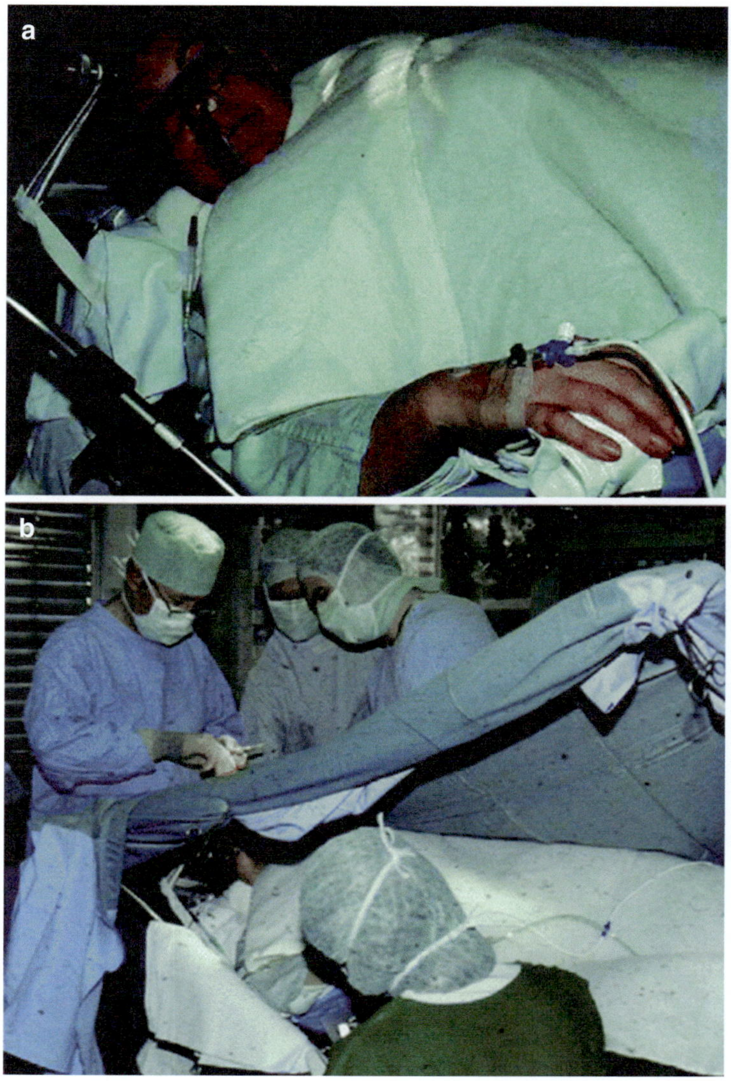

21.3.2 Stimulation

Once the tumor has been outlined with inspection and neuronavigation, the functional mapping is required to define cortical brain areas which are functionally relevant. These areas can be outlined in the fashion as described by Ojemann et al. (Ojemann et al. 1989; Ojemann 1988) and marked by cotton pledgets with numbers on it, or they can be virtually marked with neuronavigation. Results of preoperative fMRI studies defining functionally relevant areas can be implemented during surgery, using particular computer programs, as provided commercially by BrainLAB and other companies, which help to blend them into a particular computer screen adjacent to a surgical microscope or to implement them into light course of the microscope, thus overlaying them virtually onto the surgical field. Both methods are available, presenting the tumor either as outline onto the brain surface or the level of visual acuity or by defining the tumor as 3D volume (Fig. 21.3).

Stimulation itself is performed using the Ojemann stimulator with various settings and eliciting the patient's response to various levels of bipolar stimulation. The motor respective speech disturbances are carefully monitored by the neuropsychologist attending on the patient during the important phases of surgery, and this way, a mapping of cortical areas which are safe to remove and those whose removal may cause neu-

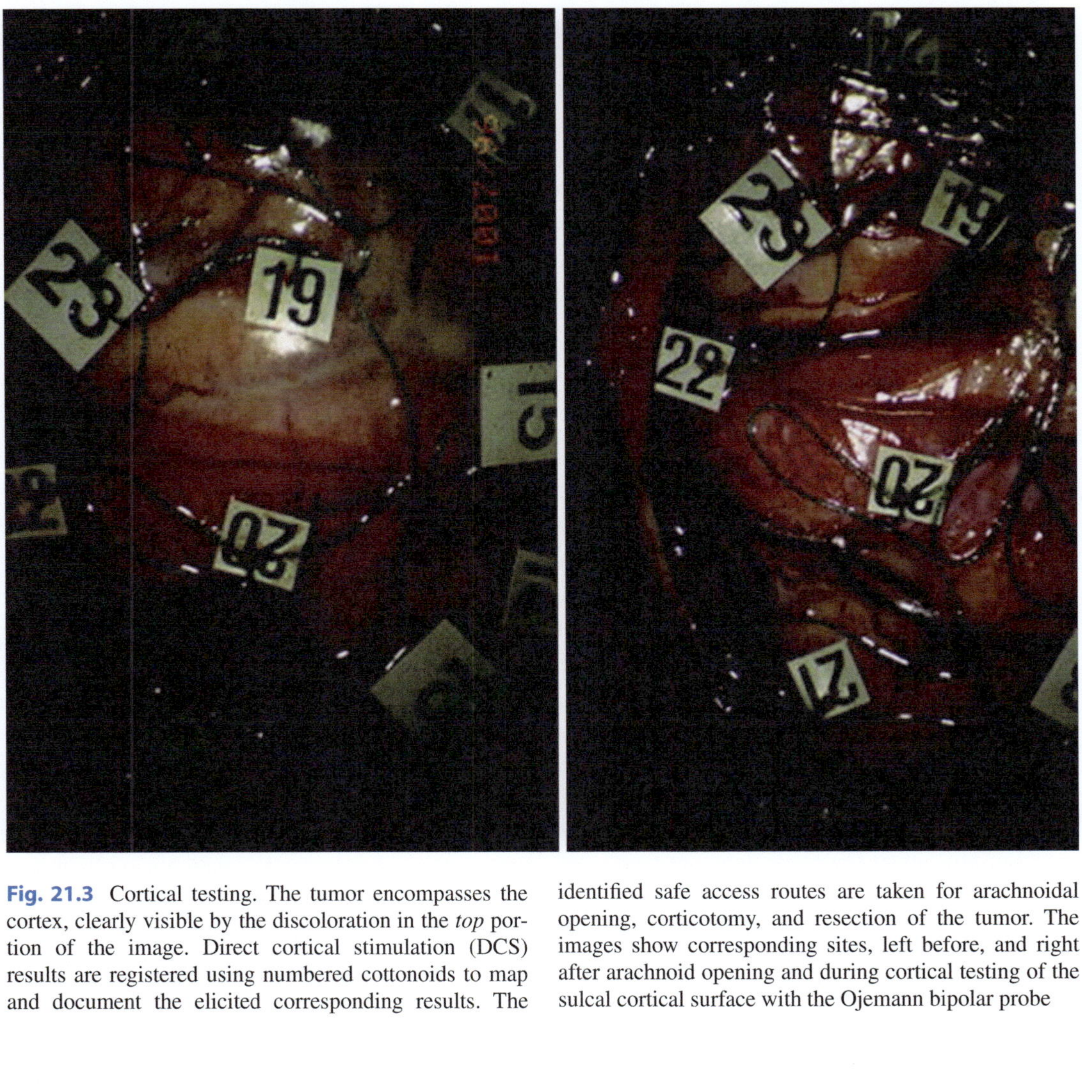

Fig. 21.3 Cortical testing. The tumor encompasses the cortex, clearly visible by the discoloration in the *top* portion of the image. Direct cortical stimulation (DCS) results are registered using numbered cottonoids to map and document the elicited corresponding results. The identified safe access routes are taken for arachnoidal opening, corticotomy, and resection of the tumor. The images show corresponding sites, left before, and right after arachnoid opening and during cortical testing of the sulcal cortical surface with the Ojemann bipolar probe

rological deficits, is ascertained. Particular attention needs to be paid to the vasculature of the cortical surface as it relates to the stimulated areas since one should always remind oneself that the cortical vessels, particularly the arteries, are nearly more important to be preserved than the cortical surface itself which they irrigate.

Once the area which can safely be removed has been defined, the interaction between the surgeon and the patient should not end. Care has to be taken depending on the correlation between the tumor borders and the white matter tracts, e.g., the pyramidal tract (Nimsky et al. 2006a, b, c) and further to language function connectivity (Henry et al. 2004; Moritz-Gasser et al. 2013). Stimulation should, therefore, be continued while the surgeon is entering the white matter, and combined with neuronavigation, in order to show the spatial correlation between these important structures (Bello et al. 2008; Duffau 2007; Duffau et al. 2002). In our experience, the voltage required to elicit some motor problems in the patient relates well with the distance to the pyramidal tract: the higher the voltage, the longer the distance to the tract. This means that one has to monitor this distance continuously as the tracts may be displaced during surgical removal of the tumor, when compared to their preoperative position.

21.3.3 Intraoperative MRI

The implementation of a high-field (1,5 T) MRI machine into a neurosurgical operating room (OR) has facilitated tumor removal further by allowing real-time imaging on a high level of imaging quality. This enables the surgeon to reestablish the true anatomical situation which changes permanently after opening of the dura due to CSF drainage and manipulation of the brain and during tumor removal (Nabavi et al. 2001; Nimsky et al. 2000). This phenomenon of brain shift is also of high importance concerning the accuracy of fMRI data acquired preoperatively. Once the surgeons think the tumor has been removed as radially as possible, the patient is taken back to the MRI scanner, and additional imaging is performed under light sedation as described previously in detail (Nabavi et al. 2009). Some centers (Pamir 2011; Lang et al. 2011; Qiu et al. 2012) have pioneered the use of 3 T MRI machine in the OR suite thus facilitating intraoperative spectroscopy and readily functional imaging including tractography.

21.4 Practical Considerations

In order to optimize the situation for the patient, we have developed a protocol for patients with tumors in or near to eloquent brain areas. Formal neuropsychological testing as an initial step and detailed neuroimaging using MRI (T1 and T2, DWI and DTI, and MPRage for 3D reconstruction and preparation for neuronavigation), fMRI data, and DWI images are performed in order to determine the spatial relationship between tumor and functionally relevant structures, and then the situation is discussed with the patient to see whether awake craniotomy should be suggested. If the patient agrees, he undergoes surgery under LA as usual and under intraoperative high-field MRI control. This allows for reregistration of functionally relevant data and update into the neuronavigation (Nabavi et al. 2003; Nimsky et al. 2006a, b, c). In the recent years, most patients with low- and high-grade gliomas underwent surgery under local anesthesia with intermittent control in the high-field MRI (Mehdorn et al. 2011).

21.5 Results

In a previous paper (Pinsker et al. 2007), we have compared the results of surgery performed between 1998 and 2002 in 80 patients with gliomas located in eloquent areas, using awake craniotomy in 37 primary operations and 18 operations for recurrent gliomas, while using—on the patients' request—general anesthesia in 27 patients. Comparing only patients with tumors located in the motor areas, patients operated using awake craniotomy had a higher rate of complete resection as evaluated by MRI scans within the 48 h postsurgery: 20 out of 26 (77%)

as compared to 4 out of 12 (33%). Worsening of motor functions occurred and lasted more than 3 months in three patients (12%) following awake craniotomy, while it happened in four patients (33%) operated under general anesthesia. Since the routine use of preoperative fMRI and fiber tracking and intraoperative high-field MRI, we have the "clinical feeling" that we may be less intense to persuade patients into awake craniotomy, but this feeling would need to be substantiated in a prospective fashion, and the results of this policy are presently evaluated with regard to long-term outcome. Having the possibilities, however, to use elaborate neuropsychological evaluation, intraoperative monitoring, intraoperative MRI scanning, and intraoperative application of local chemotherapy agents, the number of patients coming to us in a predetermined fashion has certainly risen, and such a study may be difficult to initiate.

Intraoperative guidance by preoperatively acquired data with regard to position of eloquent areas may certainly be helpful (Nimsky et al. 2004; Pinsker et al. 2007), but still the surgeon has to be aware of intraoperative brain deformation, i.e., "brain shift" (Nabavi et al. 2001; Nimsky et al. 2000), and must, therefore, still use his best surgical judgment while removing tumor tissue in or around eloquent areas. In this regard, intraoperative clinical control plays a substantial role in defining the extent of surgical resection around eloquent areas. A careful comparison of the location of eloquent areas as defined on fMRI studies (possibly with various modalities: Qiu et al. 2014) and the intraoperative definition of these areas using DCS should be helpful in determining the clinical value of each of the methods described in order to maximize extent of resection (Ottenhausen et al. 2015): Some authors have concluded that preoperative fMRI of language function was not helpful in preventing an intraoperative deficit (Trinh et al. 2014); others have described many pitfalls using 3 T fMRI mapping compared to DCS (Kuchcinski et al. 2016). Also, after a review of the pertinent literature, Morrison et al. (2016) have analyzed, although only in a small group of patients (n = 14), some of the most relevant pitfalls like statistical thresholds for fMRI and grid placement in DCS and awake craniotomy and compared fMRI and DCS data. They found that data for motor mapping correlate better than language mapping data and that clinically relevant discordances arise primarily from false-positive fMRI results. They submit that best results could be achieved using batteries of tasks that are standardized across both mapping methods. Duffau's group (Cochereau et al. 2016) has compared resting-state fMRI and responsive cortical stimulation in nearly 100 patients with diffuse low-grade gliomas and proposed that independent component analysis partly succeeded to distinguish between truly eloquent and surgically removable areas.

Further advanced technologies such as rTMS combined with navigation to make it navigated TMS (Coburger et al. 2012; Krieg et al. 2013; Sollmann et al. 2013) and further experience using direct brain electrostimulation in a variety of tumor locations (Moritz-Gasser et al. 2013; Li et al. 2015) may also push surgical limits further.

Direct electrical stimulation (DES) of subcortical fiber tracts (Gras-Combe et al. 2012; Duffau 2015) has also been suggested to further improve outcome. Moiyadi et al. (2018) have modified DCS techniques by adding continuous MEP monitoring, but they were able to perform it only in 75%. Still, they reported a radical resection rate of 68% with 10 out of 40 patients experiencing neurologic worsening, only 3 presenting with prolonged and 1 permanent deficit.

On the other hand, Qiu et al. (2017) have used, in their 3 T MRI, intraoperative resting-state fMRI and found it beneficial to avoid the risk of intraoperative seizures due to direct cortical stimulation.

Most certainly randomized studies will not be possible comparing the different modalities suggested in modern literature and briefly reviewed here such as to solve the issue of awake vs. asleep craniotomy resp. fMRI vs. direct electrical stimulation in its variations. At present, it may be summarized that many modalities have been suggested to optimize treatment results. They should be provided without financial interests of the involved medical personnel and be evaluated as scientifically as possible. The dilemma of unsolved superiority may indicate, on the other hand, that neurosurgery of these difficult-to-treat tumors will remain an art performed by individual surgeons as part of an interdisciplinary team.

21.6 Further Developments

The implementation of further advanced technologies has certainly refined our knowledge of functional anatomy of cortical structures and deep white matter and thereby extended the surgical indications for brain tumors of locations previously considered inoperable. Initial surgery is essential to remove as much tumor as possible and thereby determine long-term results, while second or third surgery often must take compromises to preserve remaining function.

Long-term follow-up of these patients in dedicated registries including neuropsychological evaluation and adequate support and measuring performance in daily life should further clarify the benefit of the various adjuncts to surgical excellence. With the advent of molecular imaging and preoperative classification of these tumors, other treatment ways may further prolong "useful survival." Yet, it remains obvious that this kind of sophisticated surgery and additional treatments should be concentrated in dedicated high-volume centers offering the full spectra of modern neuro-oncological options in order to both gain more experience and economize on dedicated manpower and machines. This progress should be guided resp. monitored more closely by appropriate organizations like scientific societies and not by insurance companies or else.

References

Bello L, Gambini A et al (2008) Motor and language DTI fiber tracking combined with intraoperative subcortical mapping for surgical removal of gliomas. Neuroimage 39(1):369–382

Berger MS, Ojemann GA (1992) Intraoperative brain mapping techniques in neurooncology. Stereotact Funct Neurosurg 58(1–4):153–161

Black PM, Ronner SF (1987) Cortical mapping for defining the limits of tumor resection. Neurosurgery 20(6):914–919

Brannen JH, Badie B et al (2001) Reliability of functional MR imaging with word-generation tasks for mapping Broca's area. AJNR Am J Neuroradiol 22(9):1711–1718

Claus EB, Black PM (2006) Survival rates and patterns of care for patients diagnosed with supratentorial low-grade gliomas: data from the SEER program, 1973–2001. Cancer 106(6):1358–1363

Coburger J, Karhu J, Bittl M, Hopf NJ (2012) First preoperative functional mapping via navigated transcranial magnetic stimulation in a 3-year-old boy. J Neurosurg Pediatr 9(6):660–664. https://doi.org/10.3171/2012.2.PEDS11426

Cochereau J, Deverdun J, Herbet G, Charroud C, Boyer A, Moritz-Gasser S, Le Bars E, Molino F, Bonafé A, Menjot de Champfleur N, Duffau H (2016) Comparison between resting state fMRI networks and responsive cortical stimulations in glioma patients. Hum Brain Mapp 37(11):3721–3732. https://doi.org/10.1002/hbm.23270

Danks RA, Aglio LS et al (2000) Craniotomy under local anesthesia and monitored conscious sedation for the resection of tumors involving eloquent cortex. J Neurooncol 49(2):131–139

Danks RA, Rogers M et al (1998) Patient tolerance of craniotomy performed with the patient under local anesthesia and monitored conscious sedation. Neurosurgery 42(1):28–34; discussion 34–36

Duffau H (2005a) Intraoperative cortico-subcortical stimulations in surgery of low-grade gliomas. Expert Rev Neurother 5(4):473–485

Duffau H (2005b) Lessons from brain mapping in surgery for low-grade glioma: insights into associations between tumour and brain plasticity. Lancet Neurol 4(8):476–486

Duffau H (2007) Contribution of cortical and subcortical electro-stimulation in brain glioma surgery: methodological and functional considerations. Neurophysiol Clin 37(6):373–382

Duffau H (2015) Stimulation mapping of white matter tracts to study brain functional connectivity. Nat Rev Neurol 11(5):255–265. https://doi.org/10.1038/nrneurol.2015.51. Epub 2015 Apr 7

Duffau H, Capelle L et al (1999) Intra-operative direct electrical stimulations of the central nervous system: the salpetriere experience with 60 patients. Acta Neurochir 141(11):1157–1167

Duffau H, Capelle L et al (2002) Intraoperative mapping of the subcortical language pathways using direct stimulations. An anatomo-functional study. Brain 125(Pt 1):199–214

Duffau H, Capelle L et al (2003) Usefulness of intraoperative electrical subcortical mapping during surgery for low-grade gliomas located within eloquent brain regions: functional results in a consecutive series of 103 patients. J Neurosurg 98(4):764–778

Ebeling U, Fischer M et al (1995) Surgery of astrocytomas in the motor and premotor cortex under local anesthesia: report of 11 cases. Minim Invasive Neurosurg 38(2):51–59

FitzGerald DB, Cosgrove GR et al (1997) Location of language in the cortex: a comparison between functional MR imaging and electrocortical stimulation. AJNR Am J Neuroradiol 18(8):1529–1539

Goebel S, Kaup L, Mehdorn HM (2011) Measuring preoperative anxiety in patients with intracranial tumors: the Amsterdam preoperative anxiety and information scale. J Neurosurg Anesthesiol 23(4):297–303. https://doi.org/10.1097/ANA.0b013e318222b787

Goebel S, Kaup L, Wiesner CD, Mehdorn HM (2013) Affective state and cognitive functioning in patients with intracranial tumors: validity of the neuropsychological baseline assessment. Psychooncology 22(6):1319–1327. https://doi.org/10.1002/pon.3142. Epub 2012 Jul 30

Goebel S, Mederer D, Mehdorn HM (2018) Surgery-related coping in surgery patients with intracranial tumors. World Neurosurg 116:e775–e782. https://doi.org/10.1016/j.wneu.2018.05.091. Epub 2018 May 23

Goebel S, Mehdorn HM (2018) Assessment of preoperative anxiety in neurosurgical patients: Comparison of widely used measures and recommendations for clinic and research. Clin Neurol Neurosurg 172:62–68. https://doi.org/10.1016/j.clineuro.2018.06.036. Epub 2018 July 2

Goebel S, Nabavi A, Schubert S, Mehdorn HM (2010) Patient perception of combined awake brain tumor surgery and intraoperative 1.5-T magnetic resonance imaging: the Kiel experience. Neurosurgery 67:594–600

Goebel S, Stark AM, Kaup L, von Harscher M, Mehdorn HM (2011) Distress in patients with newly diagnosed brain tumours. Psychooncology 20(6):623–630. https://doi.org/10.1002/pon.1958. Epub 2011 Mar 30

Gras-Combe G, Moritz-Gasser S, Herbet G, Duffau H (2012) Intraoperative subcortical electrical mapping of optic radiations in awake surgery for glioma involving visual pathways. J Neurosurg 117(3):466–473. https://doi.org/10.3171/2012.6.JNS111981. Epub 2012 July 13

Henry RG, Berman JI, Nagarajan SS, Mukherjee P, Berger MS (2004) Subcortical pathways serving cortical language sites: initial experience with diffusion tensor imaging fiber tracking combined with intraoperative language mapping. Neuroimage 21(2):616–622

Ille S, Sollmann N, Butenschoen VM, Meyer B, Ringel F, Krieg SM (2016) Resection of highly language-eloquent brain lesions based purely on rTMS language mapping without awake surgery. Acta Neurochir 158(12):2265–2275. Epub 2016 Sept 29

Krieg SM, Shiban E, Buchmann N, Meyer B, Ringel F (2013) Presurgical navigated transcranial magnetic brain stimulation for recurrent gliomas in motor eloquent areas. Clin Neurophysiol.124(3):522–7. https://doi.org/10.1016/j.clinph.2012.08.011. Epub 2012 Sep 15.

Kuchcinski G, Mellerio C, Pallud J, Dezamis E, Turc G, Rigaux-Viodé O, Malherbe C, Roca P, Leclerc X, Varlet P, Chrétien F, Devaux B, Meder JF, Oppenheim C (2016) Three-tesla functional MR language mapping: comparison with direct cortical stimulation in gliomas. Neurology 84(6):560–568

Lang MJ, Greer AD, Sutherland GR (2011) Intraoperative MRI at 3.0 Tesla: a moveable magnet. Acta Neurochir Suppl 109:151–156

Li T, Bai H, Wang G, Wang W, Lin J, Gao H, Wang L, Xia L, Xie X (2015) Glioma localization and excision using direct electrical stimulation for language mapping during awake surgery. Exp Ther Med 9(5):1962–1966. Epub 2015 Mar 16

Louis DN, Perry A, Reifenberger G, von Deimling A, Figarella-Branger D, Cavenee WK, Ohgaki H, Wiestler OD, Kleihues P, Ellison DW (2016) The 2016 World Health Organization classification of tumors of the central nervous system: a summary. Acta Neuropathol 131(6):803–820. https://doi.org/10.1007/s00401-016-1545-1. Epub 2016 May 9

Mehdorn HM, Schwartz F et al (2011) High-field MRI in glioblastoma surgery: improvement of resection radicality and survival for the patient? Acta Neurochir Suppl 109:103–106

Moiyadi A, Velayutham P, Shetty P, Seidel K, Janu A, Madhugiri V, Singh VK, Patil A, John R (2018) Combined motor evoked potential monitoring and subcortical dynamic mapping in motor eloquent tumors allows safer and extended resections. World Neurosurg 120:e259–e268. https://doi.org/10.1016/j.wneu.2018.08.046. Epub 2018 Aug 21

Moritz-Gasser S, Herbet G, Duffau H (2013) Mapping the connectivity underlying multimodal (verbal and non-verbal) semantic processing: a brain electrostimulation study. Neuropsychologia 51(10):1814–22. https://doi.org/10.1016/j.neuropsychologia.2013.06.007. Epub 2013 June 15

Morrison MA, Tam F, Garavaglia MM, Hare GM, Cusimano MD, Schweizer TA, Das S, Graham SJ (2016) Sources of variation influencing concordance between functional MRI and direct cortical stimulation in brain tumor surgery. Front Neurosci 10:461. eCollection

Nabavi A, Black PM et al (2001) Serial intraoperative magnetic resonance imaging of brain shift. Neurosurgery 48(4):787–797; discussion 797–798

Nabavi A, Gering DT et al (2003) Surgical navigation in the open MRI. Acta Neurochir Suppl 85:121–125

Nabavi A, Goebel S, Doerner L, Warneke N, Ulmer S, Mehdorn M (2009) Awake craniotomy and intraoperative magnetic resonance imaging: patient selection, preparation, and technique. Top Magn Reson Imaging 19(4):191–196. https://doi.org/10.1097/RMR.0b013e3181963b46

Naidich TP, Hof PR et al (2001) The motor cortex: anatomic substrates of function. Neuroimaging Clin N Am 11(2):171–193, vii–viii

Nimsky C, Ganslandt O et al (2000) Quantification of, visualization of, and compensation for brain shift using intraoperative magnetic resonance imaging. Neurosurgery 47(5):1070–1079; discussion 1079–1080

Nimsky C, Ganslandt O et al (2004) Functional neuronavigation and intraoperative MRI. Adv Tech Stand Neurosurg 29:229–263

Nimsky C, Ganslandt O et al (2006a) Intraoperative visualization for resection of gliomas: the role of functional neuronavigation and intraoperative 1.5 T MRI. Neurol Res 28(5):482–487

Nimsky C, Ganslandt O et al (2006b) Implementation of fiber tract navigation. Neurosurgery 58(4 Suppl 2):ONS-292–ONS-303; discussion ONS-303–304

Nimsky C, Ganslandt O et al (2006c) Intraoperative visualization of the pyramidal tract by diffusion–tensor-imaging-based fiber tracking. Neuroimage 30(4):1219–1229

Ojemann GA (1988) Effect of cortical and subcortical stimulation on human language and verbal memory. Res Publ Assoc Res Nerv Ment Dis 66:101–115

Ojemann G, Ojemann J et al (1989) Cortical language localization in left, dominant hemisphere. An electrical stimulation mapping investigation in 117 patients. J Neurosurg 71(3):316–326

Ottenhausen M, Krieg SM, Meyer B, Ringel F (2015) Functional preoperative and intraoperative mapping and monitoring: increasing safety and efficacy in glioma surgery. Neurosurg Focus 38(1):E3. https://doi.org/10.3171/2014.10.FOCUS14611

Pamir NM (2011) 3 T ioMRI: the Istanbul experience. Acta Neurochir Suppl 109:131–137

Pinsker MO, Nabavi A et al (2007) Neuronavigation and resection of lesions located in eloquent brain areas under local anesthesia and neuropsychological-neurophysiological monitoring. Minim Invasive Neurosurg 50(5):281–284

Qiu TM, Gong FY, Gong X, Wu JS, Lin CP, Biswal BB, Zhuang DX, Yao CJ, Zhang XL, Lu JF, Zhu FP, Mao Y, Zhou LF (2017) Real-time motor cortex mapping for the safe resection of glioma: an intraoperative resting-state fMRI study. AJNR Am J Neuroradiol 38(11):2146–2152. https://doi.org/10.3174/ajnr.A5369. Epub 2017 Sept 7

Qiu TM, Yan CG, Tang WJ, Wu JS, Zhuang DX, Yao CJ, Lu JF, Zhu FP, Mao Y, Zhou LF (2014) Localizing hand motor area using resting-state fMRI: validated with direct cortical stimulation. Acta Neurochir 156(12):2295–2302. https://doi.org/10.1007/s00701-014-2236-0. Epub 2014 Sept 24

Qiu TM, Yao CJ, Wu JS, Pan ZG, Zhuang DX, Xu G, Zhu FP, Lu JF, Gong X, Zhang J, Yang Z, Shi JB, Huang FP, Mao Y, Zhou LF (2012) Clinical experience of 3T intraoperative magnetic resonance imaging integrated neurosurgical suite in Shanghai Huashan Hospital. Chin Med J 125(24):4328–4333

Sanai N, Berger MS (2008) Glioma extent of resection and its impact on patient outcome. Neurosurgery 62(4):753–764; discussion 264–266

Sollmann N, Picht T, Mäkelä JP, Meyer B, Ringel F, Krieg SM (2013) Navigated transcranial magnetic stimulation for preoperative language mapping in a patient with a left frontoopercular glioblastoma. J Neurosurg 118(1):175–179. https://doi.org/10.3171/2012.9.JNS121053. Epub 2012 Oct 26

Southwell DG, Hervey-Jumper SL, Perry DW, Berger MS (2016) Intraoperative mapping during repeat awake craniotomy reveals the functional plasticity of adult cortex. J Neurosurg 124(5):1460–1469. https://doi.org/10.3171/2015.5.JNS142833. Epub 2015 Nov 6

Stummer W, Pichlmeier U et al (2006) Fluorescence-guided surgery with 5-aminolevulinic acid for resection of malignant glioma: a randomised controlled multicentre phase III trial. Lancet Oncol 7(5):392–401

Tonn JC (2007) Awake craniotomy for monitoring of language function: benefits and limits. Acta Neurochir 149(12):1197–1198

Trinh VT, Fahim DK, Maldaun MV, Shah K, McCutcheon IE, Rao G, Lang F, Weinberg J, Sawaya R, Suki D, Prabhu SS (2014) Impact of preoperative functional magnetic resonance imaging during awake craniotomy procedures for intraoperative guidance and complication avoidance. Stereotact Funct Neurosurg 92(5):315–322. https://doi.org/10.1159/000365224. Epub 2014 Sept 18

Modeling Connectivity in Health and Disease: Examples from the Motor System

22

Simon B. Eickhoff and Christian Grefkes

22.1 Principles of Brain Organization

Elucidating the neural correlates underlying dysfunction in neurological or psychiatric disease is one of the major long-term goals in systems neuroscience research. Knowing pathophysiological mechanisms giving rise to complex disorders like schizophrenia or Parkinson's disease will, however, remain futile without understanding physiological brain organization. The human brain, like that of other mammals, is organized according to two fundamental principles: *functional segregation* and *functional integration* (Friston 2002). The former emphasizes that the human brain—and in particular the cerebral cortex—is not a homogenous entity but can be subdivided into regionally distinct *modules* such as cortical areas or subcortical nuclei based on functional or microstructural properties. The idea of *functional integration*, conversely, is based on the observation that no brain region is by itself sufficient to perform any cognitive, sensory, or motor process. Rather, all of these mental capacities or *tasks* have to rely on a dynamic interplay and exchange of information between different regions sustaining different computational processes. Importantly, however, functional integration and functional segregation are not mutually exclusive, but rather complementary concepts of brain organization as any interaction will need to take place between specialized regions, each performing a distinct computational subprocess (Friston 2002; Eickhoff et al. 2009).

S. B. Eickhoff (✉)
Institute of Clinical Neuroscience and Medical Psychology, Heinrich-Heine-University Düsseldorf, Düsseldorf, Germany

JARA—Translational Brain Medicine, Aachen, Germany

Institute of Neurosciences and Medicine (INM-2), Research Centre Jülich, Jülich, Germany
e-mail: s.eickhoff@fz-juelich.de

C. Grefkes
Neuromodulation & Neurorehabilitation Group, Max Planck Institute for Neurological Research, Cologne, Germany

Department of Neurology, University of Cologne, Cologne, Germany

22.1.1 Specialized Modules in the Brain: The Nodes of Connectivity Models

In particular, invasive research in nonhuman primates with electrodes penetrating the cerebral cortex has demonstrated that the regional specialization of the brain, that is, the cognitive or sensory processes that are served by particular location of the cortex, is determined by both the intrinsic (structure) and extrinsic (connectivity) properties of a cortical area (Broca 1863; Brodmann 1909; Eickhoff et al. 2005; Schleicher et al. 2005; Grodzinsky and Santi 2008). In comparison to the

S. Ulmer, O. Jansen (eds.), *fMRI*, https://doi.org/10.1007/978-3-030-41874-8_22

fundamental distinction between functional segregation and functional integration outlined above, this evidence provides a slightly different focus as it suggests that specialization for a particular function or process is not necessarily an intrinsic property of a region independent of its connectivity. Rather, functional specialization of a cortical area is seen as a (potentially necessary) result of both its local anatomical and neurochemical features as well as its distinct pattern of inputs and outputs, that is, connectivity. A module of functional specialization may hence not be completely defined without its (potential) connectivity but is rather provided by the intersection of regionally specific architecture and connectivity patterns. Each cognitive, sensory, or motor task or mental capacity then relies on the coordinated activity and interaction of such modules.

Brain organization and disturbances thereof in neurological and psychiatric disorders might thus only be targeted by considering (1) the anatomical differentiation of the cerebral cortex into microstructurally distinct areas; (2) the specific response properties or, more general, the pattern of recruitment of brain regions during the performance of various mental operations; and, finally, (3) interaction with other brain regions. Research in nonhuman primates has a long tradition for such integrated analysis of regional brain organization (Kobbert et al. 2000; Le et al. 1986; Behrens et al. 2003; Friston 1994). Here, functional properties of a microstructurally distinct area (e.g., as determined by cytoarchitectonic, myeloarchitectonic, or receptorarchitectonic criteria) may be probed by recording single cells or local field potentials (LFPs). Axonal connectivity of the very same location may be revealed by injecting a tracing dye that is transported to interconnected brain regions. All of these techniques, however, ultimately entail sacrificing the examined animal and hence are not feasible in *human*s. Recent advances in neuroimaging techniques, however, have enabled not only the integration of structural and functional data on the organization of the human cerebral cortex but, in particular, also the modeling of functional interactions, thereby allowing a mechanistic insight into the dynamic interplay between cortical regions.

22.2 Structure-Function Relationships in the Brain

22.2.1 Regional Functional Specialization

Functional neuroimaging approaches such as positron emission tomography (PET) and functional magnetic resonance imaging (fMRI) are well established for the in vivo investigation of functional specialization in the human brain (Biswal et al. 1995; Fox and Raichle 2007; Greicius et al. 2003; Sporns et al. 2004; Buckner 2010). Based on the measurement of local changes in cerebral blood flow, glucose, or oxygen metabolism, these techniques allow the localization of regionally specific neural activation underlying a certain motor, sensory, or cognitive task. Although spatial precision in group activation studies is influenced by factors such as interindividual variability, averaging effects, and imperfect spatial normalization (Eickhoff et al. 2009), group fMRI studies enable localizing specific response patterns and testing hypotheses about, for example, a functional differentiation between two regions or a dichotomy between the neural correlates of two processes in the range of a centimeter or less.

22.2.2 Regional Structural Specialization

The structural examination of the human brain, in particular, the histological mapping of the cerebral cortex, has a long tradition in neuroscience (Brodmann 1909). These analyses rely on the investigation of human postmortem tissue, where cell bodies, myelinated fibers, or the presence of specific molecules may be visualized using cell staining, radioactive labeling, or in situ hybridization. More recently, high-field imaging methods also opened the possibility of assessing the microstructural properties of the human brain in vivo (Stephan et al. 2007a). However, currently, no in vivo imaging approach seems capable of providing a microstructural account of the human brain as precise as histological postmortem data. Therefore, combining functional imaging and histological maps has been proposed for an integrated description of regional segregation (Eickhoff et al. 2005). The currently prevalent approach for analyzing the correspondence between structure and function in the human brain is thus to perform both analyses separately (evidently in two groups of subjects) and then to integrate the obtained data by means of probabilistic brain atlases (Friston et al. 2003; Kiebel et al. 2006; Stephan et al. 2008). These atlases may be generated on the basis of automated analyses of histological sections in micrometer resolution (Schleicher et al. 2005), which are then warped to a common reference brain, for example, the MNI brain, to describe the location and variability of cortical areas on the group level in standard space. In contrast to classical anatomical brain atlases that present the observer-dependent parcellation of one or a few brains as drawings or schematic surface views, probabilistic atlases thus allow the direct and quantitative assessment of structure-function correlations (Fig. 22.1; Eickhoff et al. 2005).

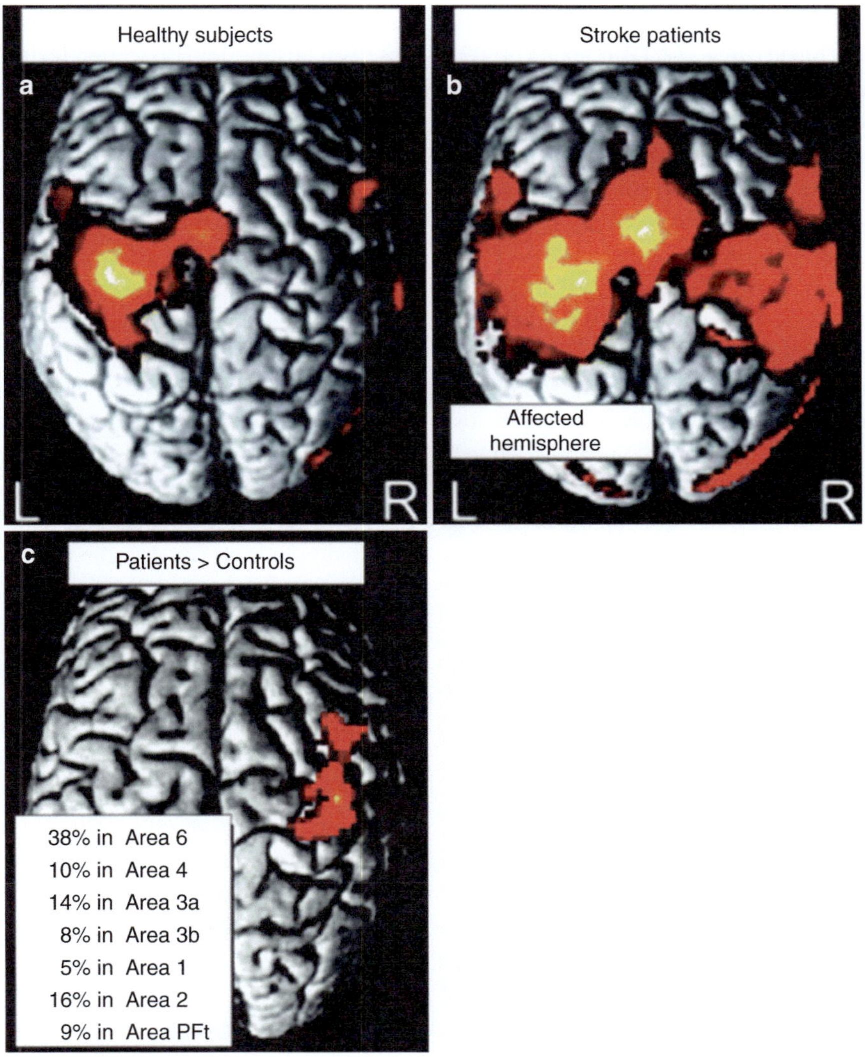

Fig. 22.1 Blood oxygenation level-dependent (BOLD) activity during a simple motor task. (**a**) In healthy subjects, rhythmic fist closures of the right hand activate a left-lateralized network of areas in frontal and parietal cortex. (**b**) BOLD activity in patients with motor deficits of the right hand is more widespread and also found in the unaffected (here right) hemisphere. (**c**) Using a probabilistic cytoarchitectonic atlas, enhanced activity can be localized in distinct cortical areas such as BA 6 (premotor cortex), BA 4 (primary motor cortex), primary somatosensory cortex (BA 3a and 3b), and higher-order somatosensory areas (BA1, BA2, and PFt). (Adopted from Grefkes et al. (2008b))

22.2.3 Regional Structure-Function Relationships

Advances in the mapping of regional specialization enable a description of the mental processes that recruit a specific, structurally defined area and have provided plenty of evidence that anatomical borders indeed constrain functional specialization (Friston et al. 2003). However, such a *localization approach* is not sufficient to describe brain function, as a single region may be *specialized* for a broad range of mental operations. For example, the inferior frontal gyrus hosts a distinct cytoarchitectonic area which Korbinian Brodmann coined *area 44* (Brodmann 1909). Pierre-Paul Broca already noticed that this part of the brain is strongly engaged in language production (Broca 1863). A number of neuroimaging studies, however, clearly showed that this region is not language specific but recruited by a broad range of tasks ranging from speech to working memory and motor production (Grodzinsky and Santi 2008). Does this contradict the fundamental idea of functional specialization? Not necessarily, when assuming that BA 44 is specialized toward a particular computational process rather to sustain any particular (psychologically defined) mental operations. These basic computations, however, which may be sequencing or temporospatial updating like, would then be integral parts of many different task-specific recruited networks. Hence, a network perspective seems to be much closer to the neurobiology underlying human brain function under both physiological and pathological conditions.

22.3 The Elusive Concept of Brain Connectivity

In spite of the pivotal role of connectivity analyses for the understanding of human brain organization, the concept of brain connectivity in itself has remained somewhat enigmatic. First, there is no such thing as *the* connectivity of a particular brain region. Rather, several conceptually different aspects of brain connectivity may be distinguished. In the following, we will provide a short outline of the major concepts and approaches and their strength and drawback and then focus on explicit network modeling as an approach to a mechanical understanding of the context-dependent interactions in health and disease.

22.4 Anatomical Connectivity

Anatomical connectivity in the strict sense denotes the presence of axonal connections between neurons in different brain regions. Several years ago, knowledge on the anatomical connectivity of the human brain was mostly based on postmortem dissection techniques or on extrapolations from invasive tract-tracing studies in nonhuman primates (Kobbert et al. 2000). The advent of diffusion-weighted imaging (DWI) and tractography approaches has more recently also enabled the in vivo explorations of anatomical connectivity in the human brain. DWI is based on the fact that in a structured tissue such as a fiber bundle, water does not diffuse isotropic but rather primarily along the direction of the fiber. By employing MR sequences sensitive to random motion of water molecules along a diffusion-encoding direction in a pulsed field gradient (Le et al. 1986), it becomes possible to characterize the diffusion characteristics and hence the fiber orientation in each voxel. From the fiber orientation directions in each voxel in combination with measures about diffusion uncertainty, it is possible to infer the course of a particular fiber tract in the brain. Such *tractography* (Fig. 22.2) may be deterministic (following the principal diffusion direction at each voxel) or probabilistic (by repeated sampling of the possible diffusion directions in each voxel as reflected by the uncertainty on orientation distributions; Behrens et al. 2003). Although it should be noted that such approaches only delineate fiber tracts running from one region to another (rather than axonal connections between neurons in these regions), anatomical connectivity as revealed by diffusion imaging represents the structural scaffold, on which any functional interaction may be realized. It also represents a truly independent aspect of interregional integration and brain networks that is

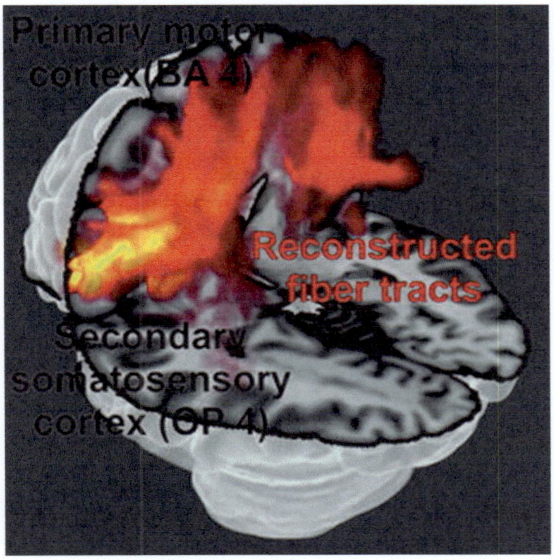

Fig. 22.2 Illustration of the fiber tracts running from area OP 4 of the secondary somatosensory cortex to the primary motor cortex, as delineated by probabilistic tractography based on diffusion-weighted imaging of 17 healthy subjects. Note that due to interindividual variability but also uncertainty about the fiber orientation in each voxel, there is a considerable variance in the data as demonstrated by the fact that only few voxels have high probabilities of belonging to this particular tract (coded in *bright yellow*)

not confounded by using the same source of data as investigations into functional specialization. Anatomical connectivity studies, however, do not allow any inference on information transfer and dynamics within the hereby defined networks.

22.5 Functional Connectivity

Functional connectivity is rather broadly defined as the temporal coincidence of spatially distant neurophysiological events (Friston 1994). That is, areas are presumed to be functionally coupled and hence components of the same network if their properties are consistently correlated. This definition already stresses a key aspect that must be considered when dealing with functional connectivity, that is, its correlative nature. Importantly, functional connectivity thus does not imply any causal relationship or a direct connection between functionally coupled areas. Rather, correlated activity in two regions may be mediated via additional structures relaying information from the first area to the second, including cortical-subcortical loops involving, for example, the basal ganglia or the cerebellum, or a third area may induce correlated activation in two regions not having any direct interaction. An example for the latter situation would be the feed-forward of stimulus-driven activity in sensory areas that is forwarded to parietal sensory areas for perceptual analysis and, in parallel, to premotor cortex for response preparation.

22.5.1 Resting-State Functional Connectivity

To date, functional connectivity in neuroimaging is mainly analyzed by assessing coherent low-frequency fluctuations in resting-state fMRI time series (Biswal et al. 1995). Given the richness of fMRI data, which usually consists of several hundred time points of voxel-wise data across the brain, this approach has the perspective to yield information on functional connectivity at the level of the entire brain. Resting-state fMRI time series are obtained while the subjects are scanned lying in the scanner without any imposed task. Given that raw MRI signal time courses are noisy due to scanner or motion-induced effects, there is an important need to reduce spurious correlations by multiple processing steps such as spatial and temporal filtering as well as removal of signal contributions from motion, physiological noise, and global signal fluctuations. A large number of different studies have used data-driven approaches, in particular, independent component analysis (ICA; Fox and Raichle 2007), to delineate large-scale systems of coherent MRI signal changes providing evidence for the existence of several distinct components (i.e., functional networks) in fMRI datasets obtained during a task-free, *resting* state, in particular, at lower frequencies (<0.1 Hz; Greicius et al. 2003). Most of these *resting-state networks* (RSNs) closely resemble networks that are commonly engaged in task-based fMRI studies (Fox and Raichle 2007). The relationship of these components to task-related networks, however, warrants further examination as intuitive associations may be premature (Rehme et al. 2013). There is also an ongoing debate on the physiological basis of such correlations. They have been suggested to arise from intrinsic activity events constrained by anatomical connections between the respective areas (Sporns et al. 2004), that is, anatomical connectivity. Other RSNs, however, are poorly explained by anatomical connections, and it remains unresolved what drives fluctuations of sufficient magnitude to propagate along anatomical connections (Buckner 2010). This has motivated a modified view, which de-empathizes the *resting* aspect by assuming that the brain is never at *rest* (Fox and Raichle 2007). Rather, the *resting* state should reflect ongoing activity composed of a vast variety of mental functions such as bodily perception, memories, emotions, and explicit cognitive thoughts, including inner speech (Eickhoff and Grefkes 2011). That is, when lying in an MRI scanner without a specific task, subjects are not resting but rather performing all sorts of mental operations in succession or parallel. The correlation in the MR signal-time course between two regions should thus reflect the degree to which these jointly participate in the various mental networks (Laird et al. 2011b). *Resting-state* activity would hence consist of a, more or less random, sampling of all the different task-related networks that the brain is capable of. It has hence been proposed to refrain from the term *resting state* in favor of *endogenous, task-free functional connectivity* or *functional connectivity in the absence of a structured task set*.

22.5.2 Task-Based Functional Connectivity

The notion of functional connectivity in the absence of a structured task easily leads to the complementary aspect of *task-based* or *task-dependent* functional connectivity which may be inferred from correlation analysis between time series from different brain regions while performing a particular task (Rehme et al. 2013). In this case, however, inference is limited to the task at hand or, more precisely, the particular experiment rather than addressing the core question about "which other regions do a particular area work with?" In other words, if a particular area is activated, which other brain regions are also co-activated more likely than chance? An answer to this question has emerged from the advent of large-scale databases on functional neuroimaging results (Fig. 22.3), which enabled new approaches to task-based functional connectivity analysis (Eickhoff et al. 2010). Such resources, like the BrainMap database (http://brainmap.org/; Logothetis 2000; Friston et al. 2003), contain a summary of the results of several thousands of functional neuroimaging experiments. Given the high standardization when reporting neuroimaging data and the ubiquitous adherence to standard coordinate systems, the results reported in these studies can be readily integrated to assess co-activation probabilities. In practice, functional connectivity of a seed region is established by retrieving all experiments from a database that feature at least one focus of activation within this seed region of interest (Eickhoff et al. 2010; Laird et al. 2009a, b). Coordinate-based meta-analysis is then performed over all activation foci reported in these experiments to test for significant convergence, which (outside the seed itself) reflects above-chance co-activation. In doing so, *meta-analytic connectivity mapping* (MACM) closely follows the definition of functional connectivity by testing for coincidences of neurophysiological events (Laird et al. 2011a, b). In MACM, however, unit of observation is not a specific point in an acquired (e.g., resting-state fMRI) time series but a particular neuroimaging experiment. Thus, functional connectivity is not expressed as coherent fluctuation across time but rather as coherent activation across experiments (Eickhoff and Grefkes 2011; Fig. 22.4).

The fact that functional connectivity analyses are fundamentally correlative in nature represents both their major strength and mostly severe drawback. As noted above, a correlation between neuroimaging signals on any scale does not imply a direct interaction. Moreover, given the absence of a specific model on the nature of the interactions,

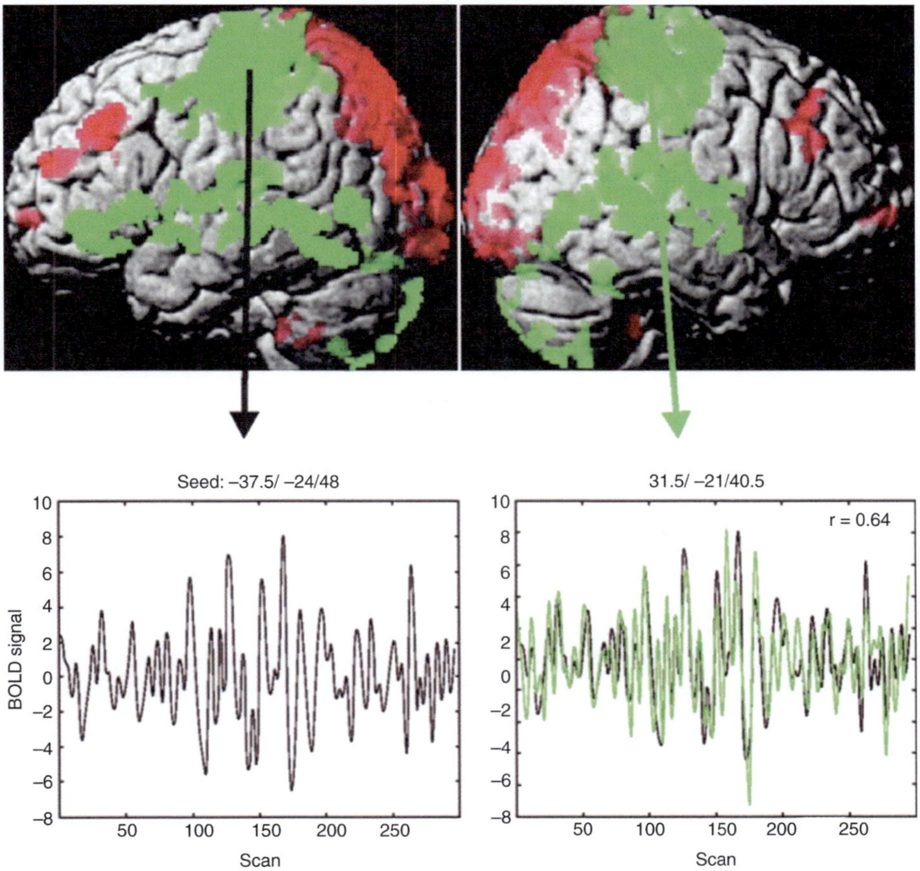

Fig. 22.3 Demonstration of resting-state functional connectivity analysis, seeding from the left primary motor cortex. Following spatial (realignment, spatial normalization, smoothing) and temporal (confound removal, band-pass filtering for the range of 0.001–0.008 Hz) preprocessing, the fMRI time series of the seed is extracted as displayed in the *lower left*. Subsequently, the similarly time series of all other voxels in the brain are correlated with the seed's time series. Significant correlations are shown in *green*, significant anti-correlations in *red*. The significantly correlated time series of the right motor cortex is displayed (*green*) on the seed time series (*black*) in the *lower right panel*

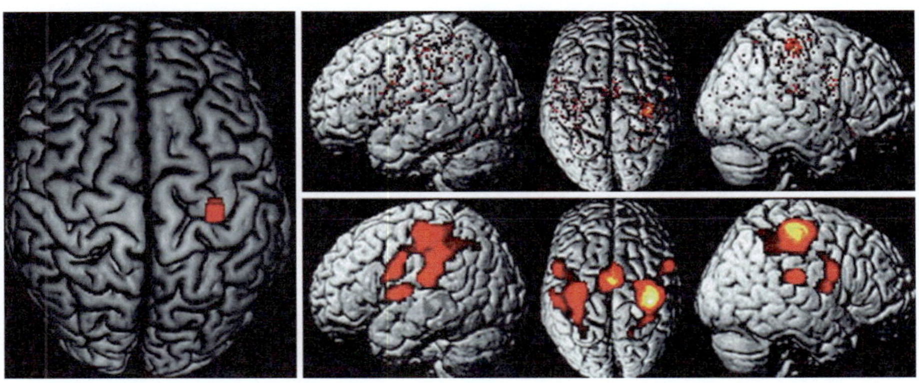

Fig. 22.4 Task-based functional connectivity of the right primary motor cortex. The *left panel* illustrates the location of the seed region on the MNI single subject template. Subsequently, the BrainMap database was filtered to identify all those experiments that featured at least one activation within this region of interest. The location of all foci of activation reported in the thus identified experiments is shown in the *upper-right panel*. By performing a quantitative meta-analysis over the identified experiments, locations where the reported foci significantly converge and which thus show significant above-chance co-activation likelihood with the seed may be identified

functional connectivity analyses tend to be rather susceptible to various physiological confounds or epiphenomena. On the other hand, the fact that only minimal assumptions need to be made for functional connectivity analyses also renders them a particularly unbiased and robust approach toward the mapping of interacting networks.

22.6 Effective Connectivity

Effective connectivity in the brain is defined as the causal influence one area exerts over another (Friston 1994), thus providing an approach toward to understanding how different brain regions affect another. Importantly, in contrast to the correlative nature of functional connectivity analyses, effective connectivity measurements are based on explicit models, how influences between brain regions are mediated. Model parameters are then fitted using the measured fMRI signal.

In spite of the considerable differences between methods and concepts for effective connectivity modeling, all approaches allow inference on directed influences. This has led to the common custom of representing effective connectivity analyses as directed graphs, where nodes represent the individual brain regions that were either included in the analysis or inferred from it (Bullmore and Sporns 2009). The directed edges of the graph then express the causal influences of one region on another, that is, effective connectivity. The dependency on an explicit model of interactions between areas is the major advantage of effective connectivity analyses. Since models reflect hypotheses about functional integration in the brain, the comparison of different models allows the comparison of competing hypotheses. Models of effective connectivity are thus hypothesis-driven investigations of how data are propagated and processed in and between different areas of the brain. However, the reliance on the explicit and implicit assumptions going into a particular model and its parameter estimation scheme has also been voiced as the most fundamental limitation of effective connectivity modeling. In particular, while model- and hypothesis-based analyses enable a mechanistic assessment of interaction processes, any inference drawn from these analyses crucially depends on the validity of the modeling assumptions. Moreover, estimating effective connectivity from fMRI time presents a major challenge, since fMRI measurements do not reflect any neuronal signal directly but rather after its convolution with a hemodynamic response function (HRF; Logothetis 2000). Inference hence has to be based on a constrained approximation or inference of neuronal responses based on the measured time series rather than on the hemodynamic observation (David et al. 2008).

Above these fundamental aspects that must be considered for all approaches for assessing effective connectivity, there are also major lines of conceptual and practical distinctions between them. Some methods such as psychophysiological interactions (PPI) or Granger causality mapping (GCM) enable spatial inference (Friston et al. 1997; Roebroeck et al. 2005). That is, given a particular seed region or a set of seed regions, areas showing functional connectivity with these, either by influencing the seed or being influenced by it, may be delineated. Other approaches, for example, dynamic causal modeling (DCM) or structural equation modeling (SEM), do not aim at localizing effects but rather model the interactions within a predefined network or regions (Friston et al. 2003; McIntosh and Gonzalez-Lima 1994; Stephan 2004). Models of effective connectivity also differ in whether external perturbations of a system are explicitly incorporated in a model, assumed to be stochastic, or in equilibrium. Examples for the former would be PPIs and DCM; the probably prime example for the latter is SEM. Finally, modeling schemes may also differ with respect to the level of hemodynamic modeling involved (David et al. 2008; Stephan et al. 2007b; Penny et al. 2004a, b).

22.6.1 Dynamic Causal Modeling

In contrast to other methods, which are rooted in non-brain imaging applications, dynamic causal modeling (DCM) represents an approach to effective connectivity modeling that has been specifically designed for the analysis of fMRI time series (Friston et al. 2003). Given this conceptual specificity and the fact that it represents by far the most common approach to fMRI-based effective connectivity analysis, we will hence here focus on the theory and application of DCM while referring the reader to specialized literature on other approaches (Stephan et al. 2007a; Kiebel et al. 2006).

The key concept behind DCM is to consider the brain as a nonlinear dynamic system in which external perturbations (inputs, which consist of the experimental manipulations) cause changes in neuronal activity or interregional coupling strength, that is, connectivity. The ensuing changes in neuronal activity states, which are explicitly modeled in DCM, in turn then cause changes in the blood oxygen level-dependent (BOLD) signal observable with fMRI. That is, DCM considers a hidden level of neuronal dynamics (neuronal states) which are driven by the experimental inputs (sensory stimulation or contextual influences such as task settings). These dynamics are explicitly modeled by a set of differential equations but, however, cannot be directly observed, that is, measured by fMRI. Rather, these neuronal dynamics give rise to externally assessable outputs such as BOLD signal changes through the hemodynamic response that they evoke. In DCM, the effective connectivity within the assessed dynamic neuronal system is, therefore, expressed in terms of coupling between unobservable brain states (e.g., the modeled neuronal activity in the different regions comprised in the model), rather than being inferred directly from the measured time series. It must be noted that the neuronal states, which are central to DCM as it is their dynamics and interactions that are at the heart of the model, do not directly correspond to a particular physiological quantity (Friston et al. 2003). Consequently, they do not represent multiunit activity, spike rates, or local field potentials. Rather, they represent the population dynamic of the represented area in an abstract form. The neuronal state of region k at a particular time t is given by $z_{k(t)}$. Aggregating the neuronal states of all modeled regions at a particular time then provides the neuronal state vector $z_{(t)}$, which describes the state of the entire system considered for a particular point in time. Key to the modeling is now to explain the change in the neuronal state variable of each region, which means the dynamic of activity as a function of (1) the influences other areas exert over it, (2) the modulations of these influences brought upon by the experimental manipulations, and (3) the direct driving input of the latter. This is implemented by a set of differential equations that reflect the change of the neuronal state vector z over time as a function of its current state (via the exerted effective connectivity) and the experimental perturbations that act on the neuronal system. For the purpose of the model, experimental factors are represented by a set of input functions u, with u_j corresponding to the time course (denoting presence or absence) of the jth condition or manipulation. In the standard form of DCM for fMRI, changes in neuronal states over time are represented in the following equation forming the generative model of the neuronal level (Stephan et al. 2008):

$$\frac{dx}{dt} = \left(A + \sum_{j=1}^{m} u_j B^{(j)} + xD \right) x + Cu$$

In this formulation of effective connectivity architecture, the endogenous connectivity matrix A (square matrix, whose size reflects the number of regions) represents the task- or process-independent component of interregional interactions, that is, the propagation of neuronal activity from one area to another expressed as the change of neuronal state as a function of the current state of the system. The task-dependent modulations in matrix B represent the changes in coupling strength brought upon by a particular stimulus or task. More specifically, $B^{(j)}$ (of the same size as A) reflects the additive effect that is present when the respective context u_j is present. If the respective context is not present, as reflected by a value of 0 in the input function, the term i_j $B^{(j)}$ becomes zero, and only the remaining components of the effective connectivity model become expressed. Nonlinear effects are modeled in D which represents the modulatory influence of a particular region on the coupling strength between two other regions (i.e., gating). That is, the change of neuronal states is modeled as a nonlinear (multiplicative) interaction between the activity in two other regions such that the current state of region *A* only influences the change in the neuronal state of region *B* (exerting effective connectivity) when activity is also present in region *C*. Finally, the driving inputs *C* reflect direct effects of experimental conditions, again separated according to the individual input functions $u_{(j)}$ on the different regions. These driving inputs are particularly relevant, as they inject activity into the system, which is then propagated between the different regions and returns back to baseline level due to negative self-coupling, that is, dampening of activity, within each region. In that context, it must be noted that while the driving inputs mostly reflect sensory stimuli, they are not limited to those. Rather, activity could also enter a particular *higher-order* brain region, like the SMA or the DLPFC, in a given endogenously driven context in the same manner that it could enter a sensory area in the case of an external, for example, visual stimulus.

The modeled neuronal dynamics are then linked to the observable changes in the BOLD response via a biophysically validated hemodynamic forward model translating neuronal states into predicted measurements (Friston et al. 2003). While this approach entails two separate layers of modeling, the neuronal and the hemodynamic, each of which has its own sets of parameters to be estimated, it has two major advantages. First, DCM allows building mechanistic models of neuronal dynamics, interactions, and causal effects at the neuronal level, which evidently is of primary interest. Second, by not de-convolving the observed MRI time series by a canonical hemodynamic response function but rather estimating the regionally specific HRF from the acquired data (under biological constraints), it may accommodate moderate deviations of the hemodynamic effects from their canonical form. The latter is, in particular, relevant in the application to clinical populations such as patient post-stroke, which may show generalized vascular changes that could impact the form of hemodynamic responses. In the conceptual framework of DCM, effective connectivity within a given brain network is inferred from the coupling parameters computed for the hidden neuronal states as detailed above. In this context, effects are deemed causal in the sense of control theory, describing how dynamics in one neuronal population cause dynamics in another and how such interactions are modulated by contextual manipulations. That is, rather than computing a measure of connectivity from the actual data, DCM fits a model of neuronal states; their interactions and evoked hemodynamics to the measured fMRI time series and effective connectivity in the modeled system are then given by the estimated parameters of the neuronal model.

22.6.1.1 Model Estimation

Estimation of the (in particular, neuronal) model parameters and hence inference on effective connectivity are based on perturbing the system through experimental manipulation, for example, by engaging subjects with different tasks while measuring the evoked effects on the BOLD time series of the regions included in the model. The parameters of the model that best translate the input functions based on the experimental design into the measured time series may be estimated by Bayesian inversion. For the hemodynamic parameters, the use of a Bayesian framework has the major advantage that it allows to incorporate prior knowledge about biophysically plausible ranges for the different parameters controlling the hemodynamic response such as vessel stiffness or transit time (Friston et al. 2003; Stephan et al. 2007a). For the neuronal parameters, in turn, shrinkage priors are employed, that is, the a priori expected effective connectivity for any connection in the model is zero. The precision of these shrinkage priors then determines how much the model is allowed to adapt the parameters to fit the observed data and plays a major role in ensuring model stability. In particular, the larger the model, that is, the more areas it contains, the higher the danger of activity *spiraling up* and the model becoming instable (Friston et al. 2003). Consequently, the precision of the shrinkage prior increases with model size, making the model more conservative as now the prior expectation of zero, that is, no connectivity, has a higher influence on the posterior parameter estimates.

22.6.1.2 Model Comparison

Bayesian model inversion does provide not only estimates (posterior densities) for the model parameters but also an approximation to the log evidence of the model for the observed data. This log evidence can be used to compare alternative DCMs of the same data, that is, to decide between alternative hypotheses on the architecture of the neuronal interactions underlying an observed pattern of activation (Penny et al. 2004a, b). This formal approach to comparing different hypothesis on the model structure has been conceptualized as one of the major advantages of DCM over other approaches to effective connectivity.

22.6.1.3 Deterministic and Stochastic Models

As noted above, perturbation is especially important in the classical formulation of DCM (Friston et al. 2003), as here the modeled neuronal network is considered completely deterministic and only driven by external inputs without which it would remain idle. Without such driving input, however, the system would stay and remain at rest. More recent developments, however, have added stochastic behavior and may thus alleviate the strong dependency of DCM analyses on the experimental manipulation and the assumption that neural population dynamics may be correctly captured from the modeled inputs (Daunizeau et al. 2009). In spite of these revisions, the mainstay of DCM analyses is still the modeling of task-specific contextual influences aiming at an interpretation of functional neuroimaging data in terms of the underlying connectivity patterns. As such, the model and its parameters obviously are strongly conditioned on the performed experimental task and its particular setup. DCM thus primarily represents as a tool providing an additional layer of insight into the causes of regionally specific activation patterns rather than revealing information about functional connectivity patterns that go beyond the particular experiment. In other words, DCM represents the most confirmative modeling approach currently available for effective connectivity modeling in healthy subjects and patients. However, it must be remembered that confirmatory models of connectivity like DCM strongly depend on a priori assumptions, for example, on the included regions, the assessed model space, and finally the assumptions underlying the modeling approach itself such as the form of the hemodynamic priors.

22.6.1.4 Application: Modeling Effective Connectivity in the Motor System

Models of effective connectivity like DCM can be used to explain activation patterns observed in conventional fMRI analyses. As shown in Fig. 22.1, simple unilateral hand movements elicit a typical lateralized activation pattern with highest BOLD activity in contralateral primary motor cortex (M1). Patients with motor deficits due to a brain lesion resulting from stroke show several changes in neural activity during movements of the affected hand, especially in the unaffected hemisphere. Applying DCM to the dataset of healthy subjects reveals that neural coupling among key motor areas is symmetrically organized (Fig. 22.5a). Estimating the constant part of connectivity, that is, coupling irrespective of moving the left or right hand (DCM A matrix), reveals that motor areas such as the supplementary motor area (SMA), lateral premotor cortex (PMC), and primary motor cortex (M1) show a strong positive coupling with each other, especially between SMA and M1 (Grefkes et al. 2008a). The interhemispheric coupling parameters between left and right M1 are negative, suggesting mutual inhibition in the absence of a particular hand movement (Fig. 22.5a). In contrast, moving the left or the right hand induces a side-specific modulation of interregional connectivity. Neural coupling is strongly enhanced in the hemisphere contralateral to the moving hand, while ipsilateral areas, especially ipsilateral M1, are inhibited (Fig. 22.5b). Patients suffering from stroke-induced motor deficits in the subacute phase (i.e., in the first few weeks and months poststroke) show several changes in this pattern of "normal" cortical connectivity within and across hemispheres (Grefkes

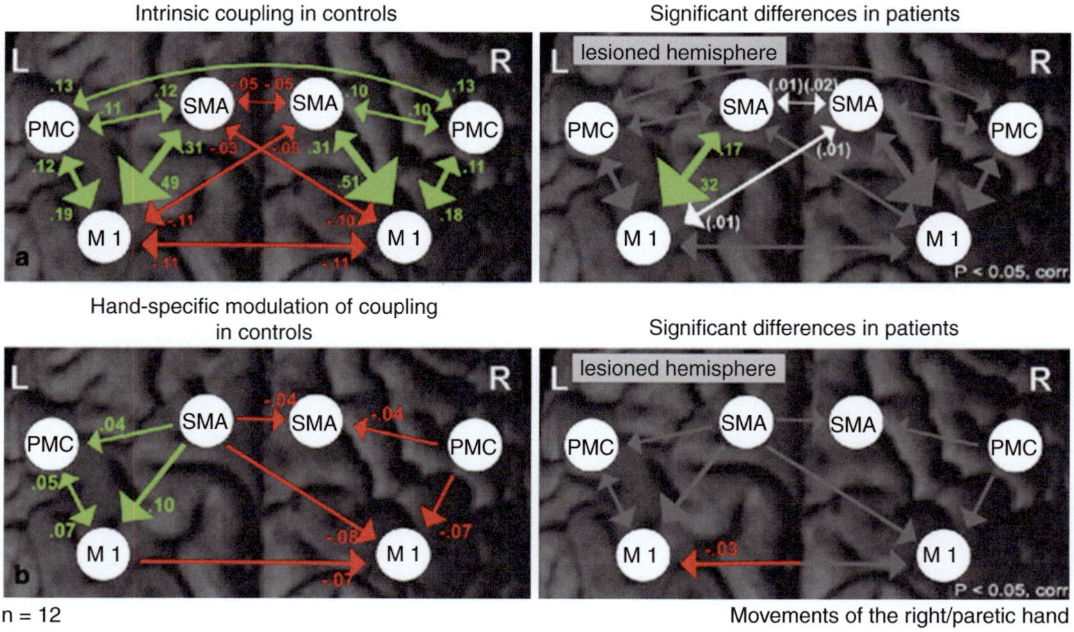

Fig. 22.5 Connectivity among motor regions in healthy subjects and patients with hemiparesis caused by subcortical stroke. Coupling parameters (rate constants in 1/s) indicate connection strength, which is also coded in the size and color of the *arrows* representing effective connectivity. Positive (*green*) values represent facilitatory, while negative (*red*) values inhibitory influences on neuronal activity. The greater the absolute value, the more predominant the effect one area has over another. (**a**) Neural coupling in healthy subjects: In healthy subjects, the intrinsic coupling of motor areas is well balanced within and across hemispheres, while movements of the right hand induce a hemispheric-specific modulation of interregional coupling. (**b**) Significant changes of coupling parameters in stroke patients. *Gray arrows* denote no significant difference to healthy control subjects, while *white arrows* indicate a loss of coupling in the patient group. Patients with subcortical stroke show a significant reduction in intrinsic SMA-M1 coupling in the lesioned hemisphere and a decoupling of ipsilesional areas from contralesional SMA (*white arrows*). Movements of the paretic hand are associated with a pathological inhibition of ipsilesional M1 exerted by contralesional M1, which does not occur in healthy subjects and correlate with the motor deficit of the paretic hand. (Adapted from Grefkes et al. (2008b) with permission)

et al. 2008b). Especially endogenous (i.e., movement-independent) coupling between ipsilesional SMA and ipsilesional M1 is significantly reduced compared to healthy control subjects (Fig. 22.5a, right panel). Importantly, the amount of *hypoconnectivity* between SMA and M1 correlates with the individual motor deficit, suggesting that reduced motor performance may—at least to some extent—be caused by ineffective processing between ipsilesional SMA and M1. Likewise, the negative coupling with contralesional SMA is significantly reduced in the group of stroke patients (Fig. 22.5a, right panel). As these disturbances in effective connectivity are independent from which hand was moved by the patients, they might explain the finding that the unaffected hand of stroke patients often shows subtle motor deficits when compared to healthy control subjects (Nowak et al. 2007). Apart from changes in movement-independent coupling, the DCM analysis also revealed significant changes in the modulation of interregional coupling evoked by moving the paretic or non-paretic hand. While in healthy subjects contralateral M1 exerts an inhibitory influence on M1 activity ipsilateral to the moving hand, stroke patients show an additional inhibitory influence on ipsilesional M1 originating from contralesional M1, which is not present in healthy subjects or when patients move their unaffected hand (Fig. 22.5b, right panel). Importantly, the strength of this pathological inhibition from contralesional M1 correlates with the motor impairment of the paretic hand (Grefkes et al. 2008b). This means that especially in patients with stronger motor deficits, ipsilesional M1 activity is negatively influenced by contralesional M1 which exerts a detrimental effect upon motor performance of the paretic hand. Reducing contralesional M1 excitability by means of repetitive transcranial magnetic stimulation (rTMS) is associated with a significant reduction of pathological coupling between contralesional and ipsilesional M1 compared to an rTMS control stimulation site (Grefkes et al. 2010). In addition, intrinsic neural coupling between ipsilesional SMA and ipsilesional M1 is significantly enhanced after rTMS applied over contralesional M1, and the increase in coupling correlates with the increase in motor performance of the paretic hand (Grefkes et al. 2010). Hence, a focal stimulation by means of TMS does alter connectivity not only of the region stimulated but also of areas distant to the stimulation site. This also implies that behavioral effects evolving after stimulation are based on a remodeling of the whole network rather than being caused by excitability changes of a single motor region. In particular, a more effective integration of ipsilesional M1 into the motor network architecture might constitute a key factor for improving motor performance of stroke patients by means of rTMS (Grefkes et al. 2010).

22.7 Conclusion

A connectivity-based approach of analyzing functional imaging data allows hypothesis-driven investigations of the interactions among brain regions under physiological and pathological conditions. In contrast to *classical* voxel-wise analyses of fMRI data aimed at localizing neural activity, models of connectivity make use of a network perspective in which the change of neural activity of a given brain region is explained by interactions with other brain regions. In this context, it is important to underline that there is no such thing as *the* connectivity in the brain, but rather several different characteristics may be assessed. Structural, task-based, and task-independent functional as well as effective connectivity all focus on different properties and aspects of network properties and may hence inform our knowledge on the physiological and pathological organization of the human brain.

References

Behrens TE, Woolrich MW et al (2003) Characterization and propagation of uncertainty in diffusion-weighted MR imaging. Magn Reson Med 50:1077–1088

Biswal B, Yetkin FZ et al (1995) Functional connectivity in the motor cortex of resting human brain using echo-planar MRI. Magn Reson Med 34:537–541

Broca P (1863) Localisations des fonctions cérébrales. Bull Soc Anthropol 4:200–208

Brodmann K (1909) Vergleichende Lokalisationslehre der Großhirnrinde. Barth, Leipzig

Buckner RL (2010) Human functional connectivity: new tools, unresolved questions. Proc Natl Acad Sci U S A 107:10769–10770

Bullmore E, Sporns O (2009) Complex brain networks: graph theoretical analysis of structural and functional systems. Nat Rev Neurosci 10:186–198

Daunizeau J, David O et al (2009) Dynamic causal modelling: a critical review of the biophysical and statistical foundations. Neuroimage 58(2):312–322

David O, Guillemain I et al (2008) Identifying neural drivers with functional MRI: an electrophysiological validation. PLoS Biol 6:2683–2697

Eickhoff SB, Grefkes C (2011) Approaches for the integrated analysis of structure, function and connectivity of the human brain. Clin EEG Neurosci 42:107–121

Eickhoff SB, Jbabdi S et al (2010) Anatomical and functional connectivity of cytoarchitectonic areas within the human parietal operculum. J Neurosci 30(18):6409–6421

Eickhoff SB, Laird AR et al (2009) Coordinate-based activation likelihood estimation meta-analysis of neuroimaging data: a random-effects approach based on empirical estimates of spatial uncertainty. Hum Brain Mapp 30:2907–2926

Eickhoff SB, Stephan KE et al (2005) A new SPM toolbox for combining probabilistic cytoarchitectonic maps and functional imaging data. Neuroimage 25:1325–1335

Fox MD, Raichle ME (2007) Spontaneous fluctuations in brain activity observed with functional magnetic resonance imaging. Nat Rev Neurosci 8:700–711

Friston KJ (1994) Functional and effective connectivity in neuroimaging: a synthesis. Hum Brain Mapp 2(1–2):56–78

Friston K (2002) Beyond phrenology: what can neuroimaging tell us about distributed circuitry? Annu Rev Neurosci 25:221–250

Friston KJ, Buechel C et al (1997) Psychophysiological and modulatory interactions in neuroimaging. Neuroimage 6:218–229

Friston KJ, Harrison L et al (2003) Dynamic causal modelling. Neuroimage 19:1273–1302

Grefkes C, Eickhoff SB et al (2008a) Dynamic intra- and interhemispheric interactions during unilateral and bilateral hand movements assessed with fMRI and DCM. Neuroimage 41:1382–1394

Grefkes C, Nowak DA et al (2008b) Cortical connectivity after subcortical stroke assessed with functional magnetic resonance imaging. Ann Neurol 63:236–246

Grefkes C, Nowak DA et al (2010) Modulating cortical connectivity in stroke patients by rTMS assessed with fMRI and dynamic causal modeling. Neuroimage 50:233–242

Greicius MD, Krasnow B et al (2003) Functional connectivity in the resting brain: a network analysis of the default mode hypothesis. Proc Natl Acad Sci U S A 100:253–258

Grodzinsky Y, Santi A (2008) The battle for Broca's region. Trends Cogn Sci 12:474–480

Kiebel SJ, David O et al (2006) Dynamic causal modelling of evoked responses in EEG/MEG with lead field parameterization. Neuroimage 30:1273–1284

Kobbert C, Apps R et al (2000) Current concepts in neuroanatomical tracing. Prog Neurobiol 62:327–351

Laird AR, Eickhoff SB et al (2009a) ALE meta-analysis workflows via the brainmap database: progress towards a probabilistic functional brain atlas. Front Neuroinform 3:23

Laird AR, Eickhoff SB et al (2009b) Investigating the functional heterogeneity of the default mode network using coordinate-based meta-analytic modeling. J Neurosci 29:14496–14505

Laird AR, Eickhoff S et al (2011a) The BrainMap strategy for standardization, sharing, and meta-analysis of neuroimaging data. BMC Res Notes 4:349

Laird AR, Fox PM et al (2011b) Behavioral interpretations of intrinsic connectivity networks. J Cogn Neurosci 23:4022–4037

Le BD, Breton E et al (1986) MR imaging of intravoxel incoherent motions: application to diffusion and perfusion in neurologic disorders. Radiology 161:401–407

Logothetis N (2000) Can current fMRI techniques reveal the micro-architecture of cortex? Nat Neurosci 3:413–414

McIntosh AR, Gonzalez-Lima F (1994) Structural equation modeling and its application to network analysis in functional brain imaging. Hum Brain Mapp 2:2–22

Nowak DA, Grefkes C et al (2007) Dexterity is impaired at both hands following unilateral subcortical middle cerebral artery stroke. Eur J Neurosci 25:3173–3184

Penny WD, Stephan KE et al (2004a) Comparing dynamic causal models. Neuroimage 22:1157–1172

Penny WD, Stephan KE et al (2004b) Modelling functional integration: a comparison of structural equation and dynamic causal models. Neuroimage 23(Suppl 1):S264–S274

Rehme AK, Eickhoff SB et al (2013) State-dependent differences between functional and effective connectivity of the human cortical motor system. Neuroimage 67:237–246

Roebroeck A, Formisano E et al (2005) Mapping directed influence over the brain using Granger causality and fMRI. Neuroimage 25:230–242

Schleicher A, Palomero-Gallagher N et al (2005) Quantitative architectural analysis: a new approach to cortical mapping. Anat Embryol (Berl) 210(5–6):373–386

Sporns O, Chialvo DR et al (2004) Organization, development and function of complex brain networks. Trends Cogn Sci 8:418–425

Stephan KE (2004) On the role of general system theory for functional neuroimaging. J Anat 205:443–470

Stephan KE, Harrison LM et al (2007a) Dynamic causal models of neural system dynamics:current state and future extensions. J Biosci 32:129–144

Stephan KE, Kasper L et al (2008) Nonlinear dynamic causal models for fMRI. Neuroimage 42(2):649–662

Stephan KE, Weiskopf N et al (2007b) Comparing hemodynamic models with DCM. Neuroimage 38:387–401

Resting-State fMRI in Multiple Sclerosis

23

Maria A. Rocca, Ermelinda De Meo, and Massimo Filippi

23.1 Introduction

23.1.1 General Considerations

Over the last decade, improvements of methods of acquisition and analysis of magnetic resonance imaging (MRI) techniques have extended the knowledge of the mechanisms underlying the clinical manifestations of several neurologic and psychiatric disorders. Structural MRI techniques have been widely used to study patients with multiple sclerosis (MS) with the aim of increasing the understanding of the mechanisms responsible for the accumulation of irreversible disability, including cognitive impairment (Filippi and Rocca 2004; Filippi et al. 2003). Despite this, measures derived from quantitative MR techniques, such as diffusion tensor (DT) and magnetization transfer imaging, to grade the presence and extent of microscopic disease-related structural damage in the central nervous system (CNS) have contributed only partially to explain MS clinical manifestations and variability of disease course (Filippi and Rocca 2004; Filippi et al. 2003).

Interindividual variability of response to CNS damage in terms of recovery from tissue damage (Franklin and Kotter 2008) and functional plasticity (Tomassini et al. 2012) can help explain that gap. Brain plasticity relies on molecular and cellular mechanisms (including increased axonal expression of sodium channels, synaptic changes, increased recruitment of parallel existing pathways or "latent" connections, and reorganization of distant sites) (Waxman 1998) with the potential to induce modifications in system-level functional responses. Functional MRI (fMRI) techniques based on changes in the blood-oxygenation-level-dependent (BOLD) signal provide an indirect measure of neural activity, thus representing a powerful tool to measure brain plasticity in vivo.

The application of fMRI has shown that functional reorganization does occur after CNS white matter (WM) injury of different etiology (including MS), that such functional changes are related to the extent of CNS damage, and that they can contribute to limit the clinical consequences of

M. A. Rocca (✉)
Division of Neuroscience, Neuroimaging Research Unit, Institute of Experimental Neurology, IRCCS San Raffaele Scientific Institute, Milan, Italy

Neurology Unit, IRCCS San Raffaele Scientific Institute, Milan, Italy
e-mail: rocca.mara@hsr.it

E. De Meo
Division of Neuroscience, Neuroimaging Research Unit, Institute of Experimental Neurology, IRCCS San Raffaele Scientific Institute, Milan, Italy

M. Filippi
Division of Neuroscience, Neuroimaging Research Unit, Institute of Experimental Neurology, IRCCS San Raffaele Scientific Institute, Milan, Italy

Neurology Unit, IRCCS San Raffaele Scientific Institute, Milan, Italy

Neurophysiology Unit, IRCCS San Raffaele Scientific Institute, Milan, Italy

Vita-Salute San Raffaele University, Milan, Italy

S. Ulmer, O. Jansen (eds.), *fMRI*, https://doi.org/10.1007/978-3-030-41874-8_23

widespread structural tissue damage (at least in some groups of patients) (Rocca and Filippi 2006, 2007). Conversely, the failure or the exhaustion of the adaptive properties of the cerebral cortex might be among the factors responsible for the accumulation of irreversible neurological deficits or the presence of specific symptoms (e.g., fatigue) in MS patients (Rocca and Filippi 2006, 2007).

While the majority of previous fMRI studies used active fMRI paradigms to investigate the patterns of recruitment within different functional systems (motor, visual, cognitive) in MS patients, the need for obtaining relevant pieces of information on functional reorganization also in patients with severe clinical (and cognitive) impairment has fuelled the use of resting-state (RS) fMRI paradigms. From its seminal description by Biswal et al. (1995), RS fMRI has been widely used in both healthy subjects and patients with various neurologic, neurosurgical, and psychiatric disorders (Fox et al. 2005). As previously mentioned, one of the features that makes RS fMRI particularly attractive is that it is a task-free approach, thus providing the unique opportunity to perform fMRI studies in MS patients who may have difficulty with task instructions and execution, as well as in pediatric MS patients who may have different compliance (not disease-related) when performing an active task.

23.1.2 Methodological Issues

The RS fMRI analysis examines correlations in slow (<0.1 Hz) spontaneous fluctuations in the BOLD signal (Cordes et al. 2001). There are multiple ways to analyze RS fMRI data, and each approach has different implications in terms of type of information that can be extracted from the data (Lv et al. 2018). Analysis approaches can be broadly grouped into two categories: functional segregation techniques, which rely on the analysis of RS fMRI focusing on local function of specific brain regions, and functional integration techniques, which rely on functional connectivity (FC) analysis looking at the brain as an integrated network (Liu et al. 1999; Tononi et al. 1994).

Methods commonly used for functional segregation analysis include amplitude of low-frequency fluctuations (ALFF), fractional ALFF, and regional homogeneity (ReHo). These methods reflect different aspects of regional neural activity. While ALFF is focused on measuring the strength of the activity, ReHo is more specific for coherence and centrality of regional activity (Lv et al. 2018). However, because the brain is more appropriately studied as an integrated network rather than isolated clusters, the excitement for stand-alone functional segregation methods has gradually receded in favor of functional integration methods, which measure the degree of synchrony of the BOLD time-series between different brain regions and can be the result of a direct anatomic connection, an indirect path (Lanting et al. 2014), or may have no anatomic connection. For assessing functional integration features, commonly used computational methods include FC density analysis, region of interest (ROI)-based FC analysis, independent component analysis (ICA), and graph analysis. FC density analysis attempts to identify the highly connected functional hubs, but it does not indicate which regions are connected (Tomasi and Volkow 2010). Seed-based FC, also called ROI-based FC, finds regions correlated with the activity in a seed region, requiring a priori determination of the seeds, which is often based on a hypothesis or prior results. ICA facilitates the effective extraction of distinct RS fMRI networks by employing mathematical algorithms to decompose the signal from whole-brain voxels to spatially and temporally independent components. ICA investigates multiple simultaneous voxel-to-voxel interactions of distinct networks in the brain, thus representing a powerful technique to perform group-level analysis as well as for the same group in different conditions (e.g., different psychological, physiological, and pharmacological conditions) (Smitha et al. 2017). Graph theory analysis of brain FC assesses different aspects of connectivity through different graph parameters (Bullmore and Sporns 2009), which provides measure of both functional integration and segregation.

Starting from this background, this chapter summarizes the major contribution of RS fMRI application to understand the pathophysiology of MS and its clinical manifestations, in terms of clinical disability and cognitive impairment as well as to monitor treatment, mostly in the field of rehabilitation.

23.2 Within-Network RS fMRI Abnormalities in MS

23.2.1 Sensorimotor Network

As previously discussed, many studies have applied active fMRI tasks to investigate the patterns of recruitment within the sensorimotor network in patients with MS, mainly focusing on the analysis of the performance of simple motor tasks with the dominant right upper limb (Lee et al. 2000; Reddy et al. 2000, 2002; Filippi et al. 2002b, 2004; Rocca et al. 2002a, b, 2003a, b, c, d, 2004a, b, 2005a, b, 2007a, b, 2008; Pantano et al. 2002a, b; Lowe et al. 2002; Mezzapesa et al. 2008). More recently, sensorimotor network reorganization has been explored using RS fMRI.

In line with the evidence of the one-to-one functional link of motor network regions of one hemisphere to their homolog in the contralateral hemisphere, with a somatotopic organization (van den Heuvel and Hulshoff Pol 2010), a decreased RS FC has been shown, using a ROI approach, between right- and left-hemisphere primary motor cortices in MS patients in comparison to healthy controls (HC) (Lowe et al. 2002). Using ICA, another study demonstrated that motor network functional reorganization occurs relatively early in the course of the disease, already in patients presenting with a clinically isolated syndrome (CIS), and tends to decrease with disease progression, in relapsing-remitting (RR) MS. Compared to HC, CIS patients showed areas of significantly higher RS FC in the sensorimotor network (right premotor and sensory cortices) of nondominant hemisphere as well as a subthreshold increased RS FC in the dominant premotor cortex and in supplementary motor area (Fig. 23.1), whereas

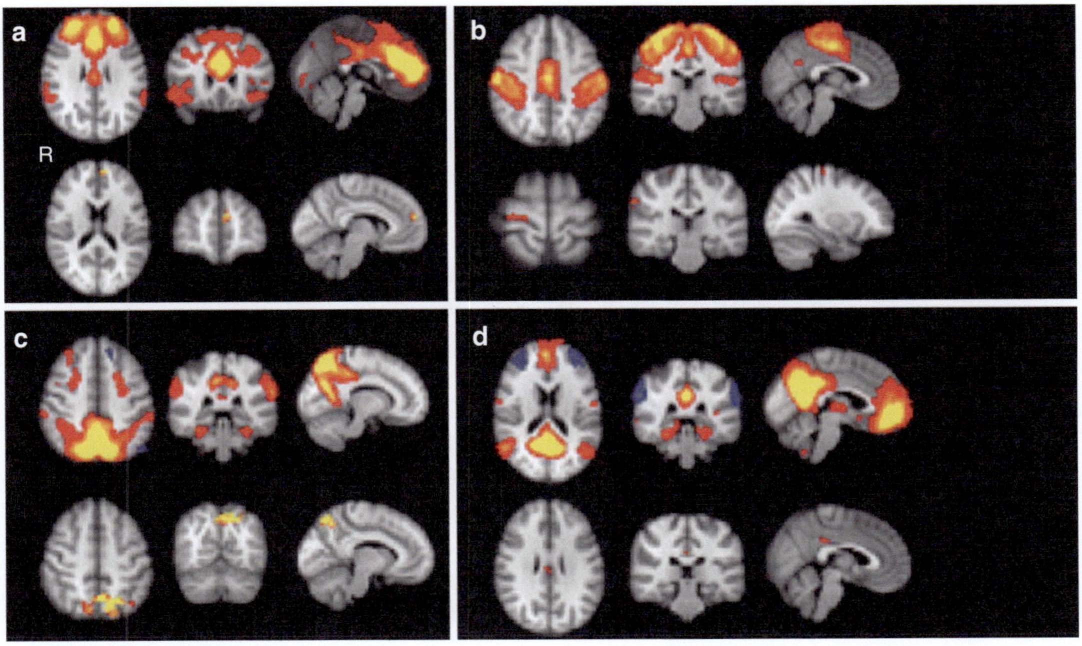

Fig. 23.1 Resting-state (RS) networks identified with independent component analysis in healthy controls (upper rows) and patients with clinically isolated syndromes (lower rows). (**a**) Executive functioning network; RS functional connectivity (FC) was increased compared to controls in the left mesial prefrontal cortex. (**b**) Sensorimotor network: increased RS FC compared to controls in the right premotor cortex and inferior parietal gyrus. (**c**) Ventral and dorsal attention system: increased RS FC compared to controls in the bilateral precuneus. RS FC was also increased compared to relapsing-remitting (RR) multiple sclerosis (MS) patients in the precuneus. (**d**) Default mode network: increased RS FC compared to RRMS patients in the posterior cingulate gyrus. (**e**) Right frontoparietal network: increased RS FC compared to RRMS patients in the left inferior temporal gyrus and right superior temporal gyrus. (**f**) Left frontoparietal network: increased RS FC compared to RRMS patients in the left superior parietal gyrus and the occipital lobe. (**g**) Visual processing and (**h**) auditory and language processing: no significant differences between groups. (Reproduced from Roosendaal et al. (2010) with permission)

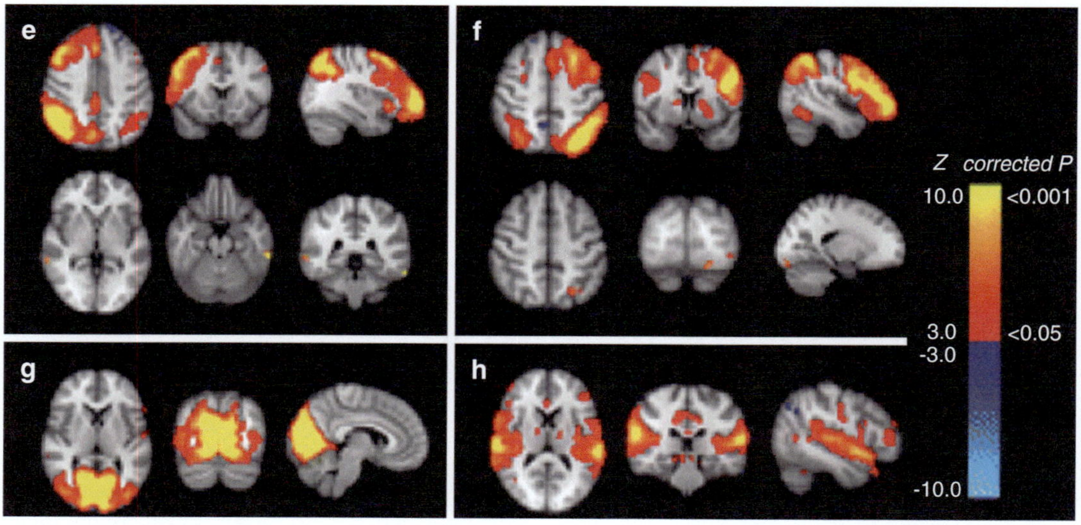

Fig. 23.1 (continued)

no RS FC modifications were detected in RRMS patients (Roosendaal et al. 2010). In the whole group of patients, increased RS FC of the right premotor cortex was significantly correlated with reduction of WM fractional anisotropy (FA) (a measure of microstructural integrity), which was prominent in RRMS and almost absent in CIS patients, suggesting that functional reorganization might be a finite phenomenon, modulated by the progressive accumulation of disease-related structural damage. Additional studies have confirmed the presence of increased sensorimotor network RS FC in RRMS patients at disease onset (Faivre et al. 2012), including pediatric patients (Rocca et al. 2014), as well as stronger functional coupling between the left dorsal premotor cortex and the motor RS network with increasing disability in RRMS (Dogonowski et al. 2013a).

In progressive MS patients (both primary progressive [PP] and secondary progressive [SP] phenotypes), reduced sensorimotor network RS FC has been shown by several studies, suggesting that functional reorganization might reach a plateau with the progressive accumulation of CNS structural damage and that this might be an additional phenomenon contributing to disability accumulation over time (Rocca et al. 2012, 2018; Basile et al. 2014).

RS fMRI has been also applied to study FC of deep gray matter (DGM) structures, such as the basal ganglia. Compared to HC, MS patients had more widespread motor connectivity in the basal ganglia and a preservation of cortical motor RS FC, which was attributed to a less efficient funneling of neural processing in the motor cortico-basal ganglia-thalamo-cortical loops (Dogonowski et al. 2013b). Subcortical expansion of RS FC did not differ between RRMS and SPMS, suggesting that this altered subcortical motor RS FC could represent a disease-state marker rather than a phenotypical marker (Dogonowski et al. 2013b).

23.2.2 Default-Mode Network

The default-mode network (DMN) is a medial cortical network including several brain regions (medial prefrontal cortex [mPFC], rostral anterior cingulate cortex [ACC], posterior cingulate cortex [PCC], precuneus, and lateral parietal cortex), which has been found to be active at rest (Raichle et al. 2001) and deactivated when subjects perform attention-demanding or goal-oriented tasks (Shulman et al. 1997). The first observations of DMN alterations in MS come from fMRI studies conducted during active tasks demonstrating that MS patients required greater deactivation of the DMN (and increased prefrontal recruitment) to perform the same cognitive tasks of HC (Sweet et al. 2006; Morgen et al. 2007). This led to the assumption that DMN recruitment could be considered as a marker of cerebral efficiency, which was investigated by subsequent RS fMRI studies.

In the study by Roosendaal et al. (2010), DMN RS FC had the same behavior of the sensorimotor network, with an increased RS FC of the cingulate cortex in CIS patients compared to HC, which was lost in RRMS patients (Fig. 23.1). Reduced DMN RS FC, particularly in the anterior node of the network, contributed to explain the presence of cognitive impairment, both in RRMS (Bonavita et al. 2011) and progressive MS patients (Rocca et al. 2010). In this latter study (Rocca et al. 2010), the extent of DMN RS FC reduction correlated with the severity of structural damage of the cingulum and corpus callosum, measured using DT tractography, pointing to WM structural damage as one of the substrates of the maladaptive functional reorganization occurring in the DMN in progressive MS patients. Differently from adults, pediatric MS patients with cognitive impairment showed decreased RS FC in the posterior regions of the DMN (Rocca et al. 2014), suggesting that onset of the disease in pediatric subjects might impair network maturational trajectories.

Another study compared RRMS to SPMS and found higher RS FC in SPMS patients in the right supramarginal gyrus, left PCC, ITG, and middle temporal gyrus (MTG) (Basile et al. 2013). The previous regions are involved in a number of cognitive processes, including language and visual perception (Cabeza and Nyberg 2000), and fall out the DMN, indicating that the re-allocation of neuronal resources is another mechanism contributing to counteract structural damage in these patients.

A combined DT MRI and RS fMRI study explored alterations of long WM tracts in paired DMN subregions and their RS FC in RRMS patients (Zhou et al. 2014). Structural and functional connectivity measures were significantly correlated in the connection between the PCC/precuneus and mPFC and between PCC/precuneus and bilateral medial temporal lobes. More interesting, three different patterns of structural and functional connectivity relationship were identified: (a) a slightly increased RS FC positively correlated with structural connection damage, (b) significantly increased RS FC negatively correlated with structural connection damage, and (c) a dissociation of structural and functional connectivity coupling. These results contribute to support the previous speculations, demonstrating how in minimally disabled MS patients, increased DMN RS FC may represent a finite compensatory mechanism in response to structural damage.

23.2.3 Visual Network

Optic neuritis (ON) is one of the most common clinical manifestations of MS. As a consequence, several studies have investigated the effect of ON on visual network reorganization. Studies using active fMRI paradigms have consistently shown relevant and dynamic functional changes taking place in the primary and secondary visual areas following acute ON (Toosy et al. 2005; Rombouts et al. 1998; Werring et al. 2000).

Using RS fMRI, several studies have demonstrated modification of FC within the visual network in CIS and RRMS patients with an acute (Wu et al. 2015; Backner et al. 2018) or chronic (Gallo et al. 2012) ON, mainly characterized by altered RS FC of primary visual processing areas and extra-striate motion processing regions. A collective interpretation of these findings suggests that even a single episode of ON is sufficient to induce RS FC changes within the visual network, resulting in reduced RS FC in the acute stage (Wu et al. 2015), and increased connectivity (probably as a compensatory mechanism) during the recovery stage (Backner et al. 2018). However, also for this system, the compensatory capabilities may tend to decrease over time, as supported by the correlation found in RRMS patients between the number of ON and reduced FC (Gallo et al. 2012).

A recent study (Backner et al. 2018) has investigated visual network anatomical and functional connectivity abnormalities in CIS patients with and without ON. Patients with ON had a higher RS FC within the visual network (calcarine cortex and visual motion processing areas) in the presence of an intact postgeniculate anatomical network, suggesting that functional network changes may be part of the recovery process, independently from structural damage.

23.2.4 Cognitive Networks

A few studies in MS patients have analyzed modifications of RS FC of networks involved in specific cognitive processes.

The executive control network (ECN), constituted by the medial frontal gyrus (MFG), superior frontal gyrus (SFG), and ACC, is involved in executive functions, such as control processes and working memory. The seminal study by Roosendaal et al. (Roosendaal et al. 2010) found ECN RS FC abnormalities in CIS patients compared to HC, but not in RRMS patients. However, these results have not been confirmed by more recent studies, which detected ECNS alterations also in patients with RRMS (Rocca et al. 2012; Sbardella et al. 2015).

Studies aimed at exploring other networks involved in cognitive functioning, such as the salience network (SN), working memory network (WMN), dorsal attention network (DAN), and frontoparietal network (FPN), are still scanty and provided inconclusive and sometime discordant results (Roosendaal et al. 2010; Faivre et al. 2012; Rocca et al. 2012; Smith et al. 2009).

23.2.5 Deep Gray Matter RS FC

Structural involvement of DGM structures, in terms of focal lesions, microscopic abnormalities, and atrophy, is frequent and occurs early during the course of MS. Only recently these structures have become topic of functional investigations.

In a large cohort of 295 MS patients (121 early RRMS patients, 122 late RRMS, and 52 SPMS), Meijer et al. (2018) explored whether RS FC abnormalities follow the atrophy pattern observed with disease progression, that is, moving from the DGM toward the cortex. SPMS patients had higher within-DGM connectivity compared with patients with late and early RRMS, higher DGM-cortex connectivity compared with patients with early RRMS and HCs, and lower within-cortex connectivity compared with patients with early RRMS. Late RRMS showed higher within-DGM and DGM-cortex connectivity than early RRMS (Fig. 23.2). These results suggested that RS FC changes might start with disturbances in the interaction between DGM structures that, on turn, could lead to an improper filtering of irrelevant information, resulting in strong and maladaptive connections between the DGM and cortex. After a long period of increasing structural damage and inefficient network connections, RS FC between cortical regions is likely to decrease in SPMS, a sign of incipient cortical network collapse that may be specific to this disease stage.

Another study (Cui et al. 2017) used a seed-based technique to explore RS FC of six striatal subregions for each hemisphere with the remaining brain regions. Compared to HC, MS patients had a significant increase of RS FC of dorsal caudal putamen with premotor area, dorsal PFC, insula, precuneus, and superior parietal lobule as well as increased RS FC of superior ventral striatum and PCC, indicating the importance of this region in the pathophysiology of MS.

Among DGM structures, the thalamus represents the most frequently studied region, due to its early and clinically relevant involvement in the disease, according to the literature derived from the use of structural MRI techniques. On the other hand, the application of RS fMRI has provided heterogeneous and conflicting results. While some studies described a decreased RS FC between the thalami and several brain regions (Liu et al. 2015; De Giglio et al. 2016), others reported both increased and decreased RS FC between the thalamus and different cortical regions in MS patients (Prosperini et al. 2014). In one study (De Giglio et al. 2016), increased thalamo-cortical RS FC correlated with poor cognitive performance, suggesting that this might reflect a maladaptive mechanism contributing to cognitive deficits.

The heterogeneity of these results might be explained by a recent study that, by using a connectivity-based parcellation of the thalamus, showed that the main thalamic subregions have

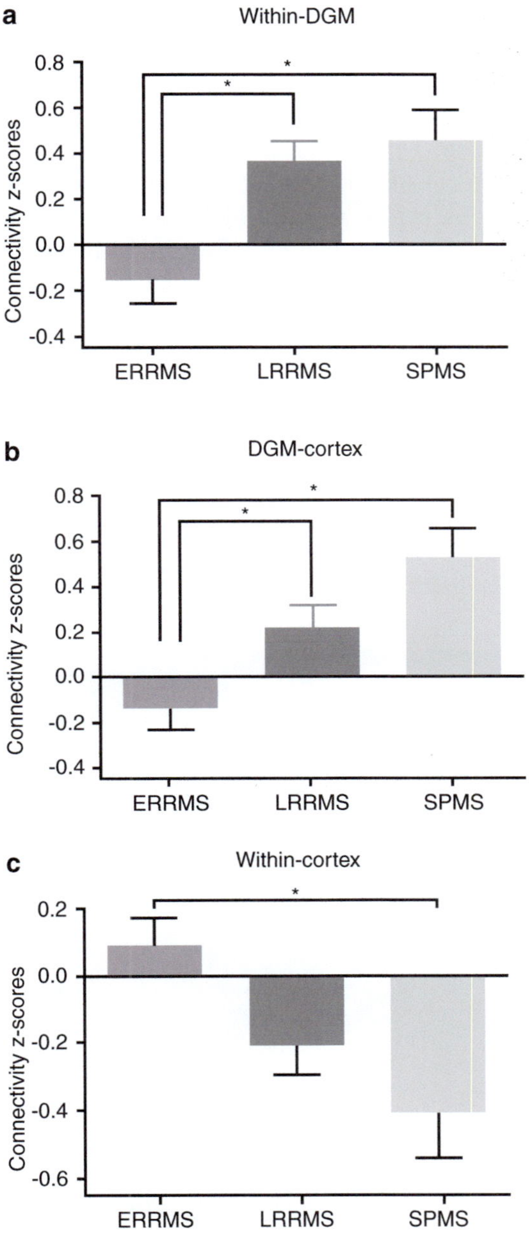

Fig. 23.2 Resting-state (RS) functional connectivity (FC) within deep gray matter (DGM) structures, between DGM and the cortex, and within cortex in the different stages of relapse-onset multiple sclerosis (MS). (**a**) Connectivity within DGM. (**b**) Connectivity between DGM and cortex. (**c**) Connectivity within the cortex. Positive connectivity *z*-scores reflect increases in the level of connectivity, whereas negative connectivity *z*-scores reflect decreases in the level of connectivity. Asterisk (∗) indicates significant differences and error bars reflect standard error of the mean. *ERRMS* early relapsing-remitting MS, *LRRMS* late relapsing-remitting MS, *SPMS* secondary progressive MS. (Reproduced from Meijer et al. (2018) with permission)

different RS FC abnormalities in MS patient (d'Ambrosio et al. 2017). In details, compared to HC, MS patients had increased intra- and inter-thalamic RS FC for almost all thalamic subregions and increased RS FC between all thalamic subregions and the left insula. Reduced RS FC was also found between frontal and motor thalamic subregions and the caudate nucleus as well as between the temporal thalamic subregions and the ipsilateral thalamus, anterior and middle cingulate cortex, and cerebellum. RS FC abnormalities contributed to explain the different clinical features, since lower thalamic RS FC correlated with worse motor performance, whereas higher thalamic RS FC correlated with better motor performance.

23.2.6 Cerebellar RS FC

The cerebellum plays a crucial role in motor and cognitive functions. Using a ReHo analysis, compared to HC, MS patients had reduced ReHo in the left cerebellar hemisphere, including left superior cerebellar lobe, which was correlated with higher T2 lesion load (Dogonowski et al. 2014). Another study (Sbardella et al. 2017) detected higher RS FC between the dentate nucleus and several frontal and parietal areas in MS patients in comparison to HC. Within the previous areas, higher RS FC correlated with less severe disability, suggesting an adaptive mechanism contributing to preserved clinical function.

Cerebellar dentate nuclei RS FC has been also investigated in pediatric patients with MS (Cirillo et al. 2016), who experienced patterns of both increased and decreased RS FC. Decreased RS FC was correlated with longer disease duration, higher T2 lesion volumes, and cognitive impairment, suggesting a maladaptive mechanism. On the other hand, increased RS FC correlated with shorter disease duration, lower T2 lesion volume, and a better motor performance.

23.2.7 Spinal Cord RS FC

Using ultra-high field MRI, recent studies have provided evidence of RS FC in the human spinal cord (Barry et al. 2014, 2016). RS FC in spinal cord was highly reproducible within and across human HC and was mainly constituted by two networks: a ventral motor and a dorsal sensory network, whose organization and spatial distribution appeared consistent with those detected with task-based fMRI studies (Maieron et al. 2007; Cadotte et al. 2012; Eippert et al. 2017; Stroman et al. 2012). To date, only one study has assessed RS fMRI abnormalities at the level of the spinal cord in MS patients using a 7 T scanner (Conrad et al. 2018). In HC, a pattern of connectivity among ventral GM regions and a distinct network among dorsal regions were detected, with higher ventral network connectivity in female. No differences were detected between MS patients and controls. However, a significant effect of focal lesions on local alterations in connectivity was found in patients, with differential effects depending on columnar location.

23.3 Between-Network RS fMRI Abnormalities

Brain functioning requires high level of integration between functionally relevant networks to subserve higher functional processes. In this perspective, in addition to the previous approaches that provide a FC measure for each single network, functional interactions among the RS networks were also explored. In RRMS patients, compared to HC, the ECN had an increased connectivity with the SN and a decreased connectivity with the DMN. An abnormal connectivity between the WMNs and sensory networks was also found (Fig. 23.3) (Rocca et al. 2012). These findings supported the hypothesis that MS alters CNS functioning in a distributed manner.

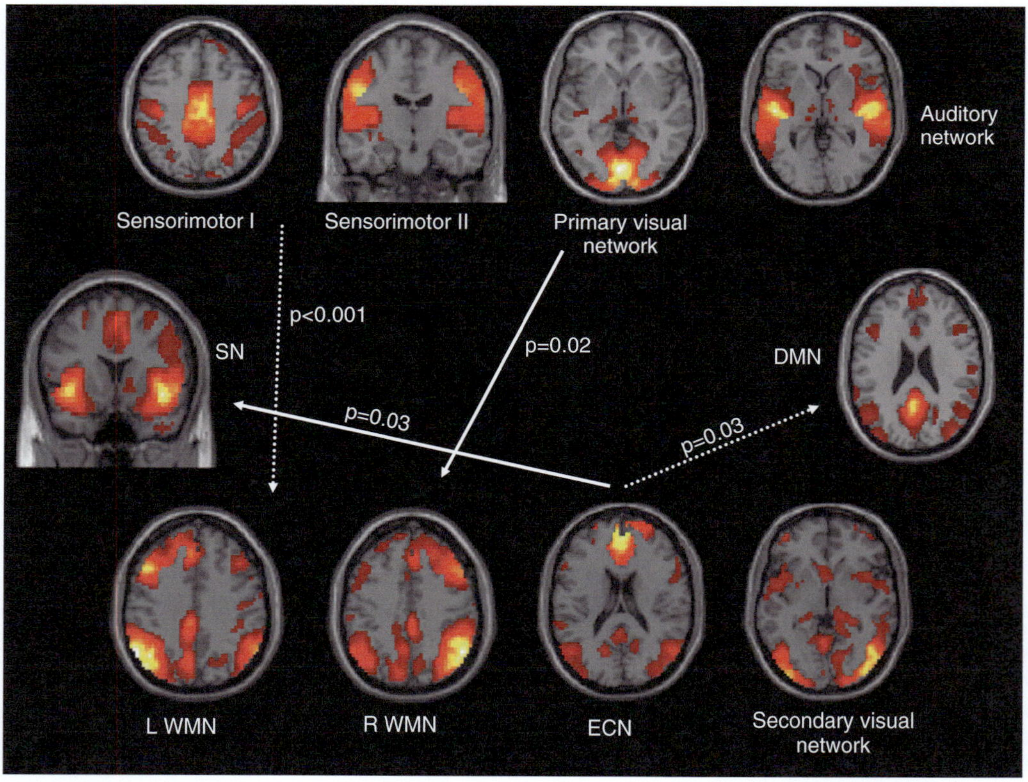

Fig. 23.3 Internetwork connectivity of resting-state networks in patients with relapsing-remitting multiple sclerosis. Diagram showing resting-state networks with a significantly different pairwise connectivity between healthy controls and patients with relapsing-remitting multiple sclerosis (RRMS), as assessed using a functional network connectivity analysis. Solid arrows indicate increased network connectivity in patients with RRMS vs controls; dotted arrows indicate decreased network connectivity in patients with RRMS vs controls. *DMN* default mode network, *ECN* executive control network, *SN* salience network, *WMN* working memory network. (Reproduced from Rocca et al. (2012) with permission)

Starting from the observation that the anticorrelation existing between the DMN and the DAN represents an intrinsic aspect of brain functional organization, whose strength varies across individuals and appears determinant for behavioral performance (Kelly et al. 2008), a recent study (Huang et al. 2018) explored the relationship between these two networks in RRMS patients. A stable relationship between DMN and DAN was detected in RRMS patients, with a significantly increased driving connectivity from DAN to DMN, which may represent an adaptive mechanism contributing to the maintenance of a stable interaction by increasing the information transmission capacity.

A distributed pattern of FC abnormalities within large-scale neuronal networks has also been detected in pediatric MS patients and has been shown to be influenced by focal WM lesions and to contribute to their cognitive status (Rocca et al. 2014). To explore whether functional reorganization mechanisms have a protective role over time in pediatric MS patients, another study assessed brain alterations in pediatric-onset MS patients in their early adulthood in comparison with age- and disability-matched adult-onset MS patients. Compared to adult-onset patients and HC, pediatric-onset MS patients had reduced long-range RS FC between DMN and secondary visual network, whose interaction subserves important cognitive functions. They also had more severe structural damage, measured with DT MRI, in clinically eloquent regions for physical disability (Giorgio et al. 2017). These data suggest that occurrence of functional and structural abnormalities early in the disease course may confer higher vulnerability to unfavorable clinical outcome in the long term.

23.4 Large-Scale Network Connectivity by Means of Graph Analysis

A large body of literature in neuroscience has analyzed brain networks from the perspective of graph theory, where network graphs can be quantified with a wide range of simple yet "neuro-biologically" meaningful measures (Rubinov and Sporns 2010). Considering MS as a disconnection syndrome, graph theoretical analysis is a promising approach to detect functional changes occurring at different stages of the disease, characterized by both global and local network measure alterations.

Graph analysis studies in patients at the earliest stages of MS have so far provided conflicting results. While some authors found no abnormalities of network measures in CIS patients in comparison to HC (Shu et al. 2016), others (Liu et al. 2017; Abidin et al. 2017) found that CIS patients had decreased whole-brain network efficiency, which was, however, less pronounced than what observed in RRMS patients. Conversely, at regional analysis, alterations in nodal efficiency and RS FC detected in CIS patients were similar to those found in MS patients, supporting the hypothesis that regional network degeneration is already present in CIS.

By applying a graph theoretical approach, Rocca et al. (2016) investigated the topological organization of the functional brain connectome in a large cohort of MS patients including RRMS, benign MS (BMS), and SPMS. A disruption of global functional organization was observed in the whole group of MS patients and contributed to distinguish cognitively impaired MS patients from HC, but not the main MS clinical phenotypes. Compared to HC, MS patients also had modifications of regional network properties, which contributed to cognitive impairment and phenotypic variability of MS.

In a large group of MS patients at 6 years from the diagnosis, Schoonheim et al. (2014) reported an increase in centrality in the PCC and decreased centrality in the sensorimotor and ventral stream areas. Since the thalamus, an area exhibiting increased centrality, showed a higher connectivity to areas with decreased centrality, the authors hypothesized a rerouting of thalamic connections as a response to continuous inflammatory activity.

23.5 Clinical Relevance of Functional Network Abnormalities

23.5.1 Diagnosis and Differential Diagnosis

The potential of RS fMRI analysis as a tool for diagnosis and differential diagnosis has been only marginally explored. One study has investigated the utility of graph theoretical network measures to differentiate CIS and MS patients from HC (Liu et al. 2017). Among the metrics analyzed, the mean connectivity strength exhibited the highest power in distinguishing MS (AUC = 0.825, $P < 0.001$) and CIS (AUC = 0.789, $P < 0.001$) patients from HC, with sensitivity of 88.2% (30 of 34 patients) and 61.8% (21 of 34 patients) and specificity of 66.7% (24 of 36 control subjects) and 91.7% (33 of 36 control subjects), respectively. This yielded an accuracy of 77.1% for the classification of MS patients vs HC and of 77.1% for the classification of CIS patients vs HC.

Another study (Eshaghi et al. 2015) combined RS fMRI, structural MRI, and clinical measures to automatically differentiate MS from neuromyelitis optica (NMO) patients. RS fMRI resulted the second modality (after WM lesions) able to distinguish HC, MS, and NMO patients.

Using a whole brain connectivity analysis, Richiardi et al. (2012) demonstrated that a multivariate approach, based on predictive modeling of brain RS FC, allows a reliable differentiation of minimally disabled MS patients and HCs. In this model, only 4% of the analyzed connections (90 × 90) resulted discriminative. Classification performance yielded a sensitivity of 82% and specificity of 86% to distinguish between MS patients and HC. The most discriminative connectivity changes were found in subcortical and temporal regions, and contralateral connections were more discriminative than ipsilateral ones.

23.5.2 Phenotype-Specific RS fMRI Patterns and Clinical Disability, Ambulation, and Balance

Many of the studies previously discussed have assesses the correlations between RS FC abnormalities and clinical disability. In the majority of studies, a negative correlation between RS FC strength and clinical impairment, measured with the Expanded Disability Status Scale (EDSS), has been reported (Roosendaal et al. 2010; Faivre et al. 2012; Rocca et al. 2012; Richiardi et al. 2012), whereas a few studies found a positive correlation between increased RS FC strength and more severe clinical impairment (Dogonowski et al. 2013a; Rocca et al. 2010). These discrepancies may be due not only to differences in patient populations and methods of analysis but also to the clinical function considered and the network investigated.

Several studies tried to define whether RS FC modifications might have different expression and might correlated differently with clinical disability according to the clinical phenotype of the disease. Studies in patients with RRMS have consistently shown a correlation between reduced RS FC within selected brain networks and higher EDSS (reflecting more severe disability) (Rocca et al. 2012; Schoonheim et al. 2014; Janssen et al. 2013). A recent study (Rocca et al. 2018) included 215 MS patients with the main disease clinical phenotypes (from CIS to progressive MS) and demonstrated a progressive reduction of RS FC from the earliest to the progressive phenotypes in parietal, frontal, and cerebellar regions of cognitive, sensory, and motor networks, which may reflect an exhaustion of functional plasticity with progressive accumulation of disease-related structural damage.

Other studies focused their analysis to specific clinical deficits, such as ambulation and balance. A study (Bollaert et al. 2018) examined the correlation between RS FC in cortical motor and non-motor networks and walking performance, assessed by timed 25-foot walk (T25FW) in MS patients. T25FW performance correlated with RS FC of brain regions that are part of the sensorimotor network as well as with FC of regions that have a major role in visual perception, spatial orientation, and navigation, indicating that MS clinical manifestations are influenced by functional abnormalities of critical regions part of interconnected networks.

Balance deficits affect almost 75% of MS patients during the course of the disease (Cameron and Lord 2010). Using a seed-based analysis, reduced RS FC between the dentate nucleus and the left caudate nucleus within the cerebellar network was found to correlate with worse balance measures in RRMS patients, suggesting that a functional disconnection between these two regions may impair high-level control of balance (Tona et al. 2018).

23.5.3 Cognitive Impairment, Depression, and Fatigue

Cognitive impairment affects a large proportion of MS patients, with prevalence ranging from 40% to 70%, depending on the population studied, the tests used, and the cut-off values applied (Chiaravalloti and DeLuca 2008). A prominent involvement of information processing speed and episodic memory domain has been observed, while less frequently impairment in executive functions, including verbal fluency, and word list generation have been described (Benedict et al. 2002; Benedict and Zivadinov 2006).

RS FC of the DMN and its relation with cognitive impairment have been previously discussed (see Sect. 23.2.2). Using a whole-brain connectivity approach, a recent graph analysis study (Eijlers et al. 2017) measured the overall importance for cognition of individual brain regions in 332 MS patients. Both degree and eigenvector centrality were assessed in order to respectively measure the quantity and quality of functional connections. Cognitively impaired (CI) MS patients had widespread centrality increases compared to both HC and cognitively preserved (CP) MS patients mainly in regions making up the DMN, while all patient groups showed decreased centrality in occipital and sensorimotor areas. This study provides evidence that under pressure of disease, the hierarchy of the entire brain network shifts, and the DMN becomes of central importance in CI MS patients.

Despite less frequently object of investigation, depression is another frequent symptom of MS (Feinstein et al. 2014). The clinical manifestations of depression in MS patients are very similar to those of patients with major depressive disorder, but its etiology, potentially related to specific MS pathology, is still poorly understood. Starting from the observation of abnormal RS FC between limbic and frontal regions in patients with major depressive disorder (Northoff et al. 2011), a recent study explored frontolimbic system RS FC in MS patients with and without depression (van Geest et al. 2019). Compared to non-depressed MS patients, MS patients with depression had decreased RS FC between the amygdala and frontal regions, which correlated with higher depression rank scores. These results are in line with those from a previous study, which detected a correlation between higher depression scores and reduced RS FC between the hippocampus and the orbitofrontal cortex (Rocca et al. 2015).

Another study (Colasanti et al. 2016) explored the hippocampus in terms of neuroinflammation and RS FC as possible substrates of depressive symptoms in MS. Hippocampal RS FC to the subgenual cingulate and prefrontal and parietal regions correlated with depression severity and metabolic changes as assessed by positron emission tomography (PET). These results not only confirmed the central role of this set of regions in determining affective disorders in MS patients but also identified chronic neuroinflammation as potential pathogenic substrate of RS FC abnormalities.

Fatigue is one of the most disabling MS symptoms, significantly impacting patients' daily activities and quality of life and affecting up to 80% of patients. Several studies investigated the anatomical substrates of fatigue, identifying dysfunction in the sensorimotor network and basal ganglia as pathobiological basis of this symptom. Using regions of GM atrophy in fatigued (F) MS patients as seeds, F MS patients had decreased RS FC between the primary motor and somatosensory cortices, which correlated with the severity of fatigue. Non-fatigued (NF) MS patients presented higher RS FC in the premotor cortex compared to F MS and in the primary motor cortex compared to HC (Cruz Gomez et al. 2013). Based on these results, the authors suggested that the increased RS FC observed in NF MS patients could reflect a compensatory mechanism associated with subclinical fatigue. Another study (Bisecco et al. 2018) found that abnormalities of RS FC within both the sensorimotor network and DMN contributed to the presence and severity of fatigue in MS patients.

The investigation of basal ganglia RS FC has been substantiated by neuroimaging studies showing structural and functional changes of this level in F MS patients, including atrophy, reduced perfusion, reduced glucose metabolism, and reduced activation during the performance of motor tasks (DeLuca et al. 2008; Roelcke et al. 1997; Inglese et al. 2007; Filippi et al. 2002a). In RRMS patients, higher fatigue scores were correlated with reduced RS FC of caudate nucleus, putamen, and pallidum with frontal and parietal areas, but also positively correlated with RS FC between caudate nucleus and the motor cortex bilaterally (Finke et al. 2015). This latter finding was interpreted as a compensatory mechanism contributing to maintain a normal function.

By performing a RS FC analysis of the different thalamic subregions, a recent investigation (Hidalgo de la Cruz et al. 2018) demonstrated that regional thalamic RS FC abnormalities may contribute to explain the different components of fatigue in MS patients. In particular, abnormal thalamic connectivity with the precuneus and posterior lobe of the cerebellum explained cognitive fatigue, whereas altered connectivity with the sensorimotor network had a role in explaining physical and psychosocial fatigue.

23.6 Structural Substrates of RS fMRI Abnormalities

The majority of available RS fMRI studies has included different measures derived from structural MRI (e.g., T2 lesion volume, measures of WM integrity, measures of volume loss of the whole brain or of selected CNS regions) to investigate the correlation between structural and functional MRI abnormalities in patients with MS. Independently from the measure analyzed, all of them have consistently demonstrated that there is a relationship between structural damage and functional reorganization. Studies of patients at different stages of the disease have suggested that such a relationship might have an inverted U-shape, with increased functional reorganization with accumulation of brain structural damage until a certain level of the disease (adaptive functional reorganization), followed by collapse of functional reorganization when a plateauing level is reached. At this stage, functional reorganization becomes maladaptive and contributes, together with progression of structural damage, to clinical (and cognitive) worsening (Roosendaal et al. 2010; Rocca et al. 2010; Hawellek et al. 2011).

A combined analysis of structural and functional network alterations in CIS and RRMS patients has suggested that structural network modifications may precede (and maybe influence) those of network function, as CIS patients only showed structural network abnormalities, whereas RRMS had concomitant structural and functional abnormalities (Fig. 23.4) (Shu et al. 2016).

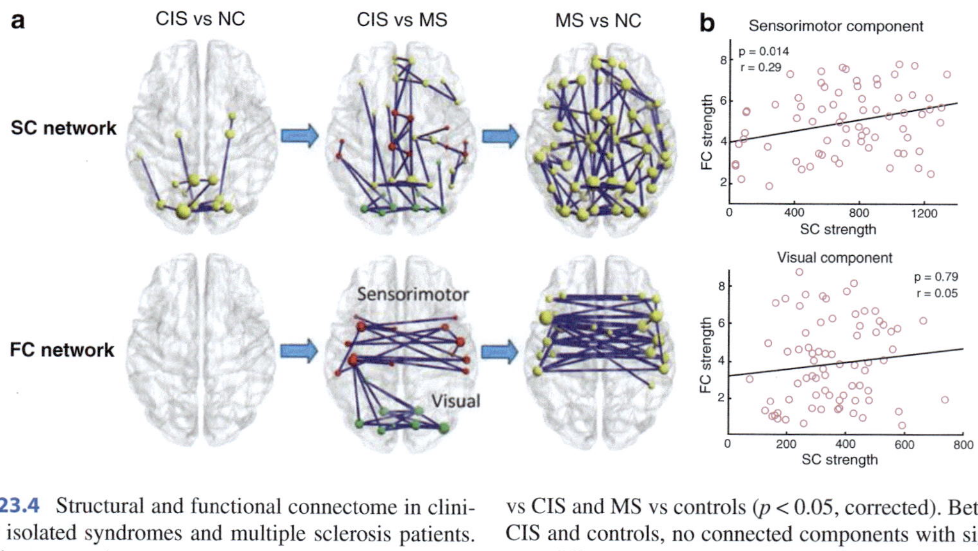

Fig. 23.4 Structural and functional connectome in clinically isolated syndromes and multiple sclerosis patients. (**a**) The top panel represents connected networks showing decreased structural connections in CIS vs controls, MS vs CIS, and MS vs controls. The regional pairs showed decreased connections in the patient groups ($p < 0.05$, corrected). The bottom panel represents the connected networks, showing decreased functional connections in MS vs CIS and MS vs controls ($p < 0.05$, corrected). Between CIS and controls, no connected components with significant differences were found. (**b**) Correlation between the structural and functional connection strength within sensorimotor and visual components across all patients while removing the effects of age and gender. (Reproduced from Shu et al. (2016) under a Creative Commons Attribution 4.0 International License)

23.7 RS fMRI and Treatment

23.7.1 Pharmaceutical Treatment

Only a few fMRI studies have been performed to monitor the effects of symptomatic treatments in MS patients (Parry et al. 2003; Mainero et al. 2004; Cader et al. 2009), mainly adopting active fMRI paradigms. Recently, the effects of smoke cannabis on cognition, as well as their possible functional and structural MRI correlates, have been investigated (Pavisian et al. 2014). MS patients who smoked cannabis on a regular basis showed more cognitive deficits than MS patients who were drug-free. Cannabis-related cognitive problems were associated with a different pattern of cerebral activation during the N-back on fMRI, whereas no relation was found with structural measures or with RS fMRI measures.

23.7.2 Motor Rehabilitation

Promoting restoration of function and competence of dysfunctional brain networks is one of the main goals of motor and cognitive rehabilitation. Even though the mechanisms underlying clinical improvement after rehabilitation are not yet fully understood, by applying different rehabilitation procedures, several studies in MS patients have consistently demonstrated that motor and cognitive rehabilitation results in an improvement of the rehabilitated function (i.e., motor functions, attention, memory, and executive function) and that this improvement is somehow mediated by modification of recruitment and/or functional connectivity occurring in function-related networks.

Improved gait performance following 4 weeks of motor rehabilitation was associated with RS FC modifications in the sensorimotor network in MS patients with mild-to-moderate disability (Tavazzi et al. 2018). All these changes disappeared 3 months after the termination of motor rehabilitation, suggesting the need of continuous training (or bouts of training) in order to maintain the benefits of motor rehabilitation.

Recent evidence has suggested that repetitive transcranial magnetic stimulation (rTMS) of the motor cortex may be effective to reduce spasticity and promoting motor function recovery in MS patients (Centonze et al. 2007; Mori et al. 2011). A recent study (Boutière et al. 2017) tested the effect on RS FC of 5-week intermittent theta burst stimulation (iTBS) applied over the primary motor cortex combined with physical rehabilitation. No effects of iTBS on global topology of brain network was observed, while changes of interhemispheric balance were observed in bilateral homologous primary cortices (connectivity degree decreased in the stimulated region of 38% and increased in the contralateral regions of 52%). Based on these findings, the authors concluded that the relative decrease in connectivity of the stimulated primary motor cortex with other brain areas could in turn promote corticospinal descending activity, resulting in improvement of spasticity.

23.7.3 Cognitive Rehabilitation

In patients with RRMS with selective deficits of attention, information processing, and executive functions, 3 months of computer-assisted cognitive rehabilitation of these functions resulted in cognitive improvement through enhanced recruitment of brain networks subserving the trained functions (Filippi et al. 2012). To investigate the persistence of treatment efficacy after treatment termination and its possible pathobiological substrates, the same cohort of patients was reevaluated 6 months after the termination of rehabilitation (Parisi et al. 2014). The positive effects of cognitive rehabilitation on cognitive tests were still present. There were some additional improvements at depression and quality of life scales, which were not detected immediately after the termination of cognitive rehabilitation. Interestingly enough, measures derived from RS fMRI during the rehabilitation phase of the study were the only predictors of these effects at 6 months, suggesting that cognitive rehabilitation may act by optimizing cognitive network recruitment, resulting in a generalized functional improvement.

Interestingly, since the results of fMRI analysis of the previous study (Filippi et al. 2012) pointed toward a role for the left dorsolateral PFC in improving cognitive functions, this region was selected, in a subsequent study, as a target for an anodal transcranial direct current stimulation, in combination with attention training in MS patients impaired in attention/speed of information processing (Mattioli et al. 2016). In the study of MS patients, the combination of cognitive training with an anodal transcranial direct current stimulation over the left dorsolateral PFC during ten daily sessions fostered improvements in attention and executive function, which persisted up to 6 months after the intervention (Mattioli et al. 2016).

The beneficial effect of cognitive rehabilitation and its modulation of RS FC have been confirmed by several subsequent studies, not only on information processing speed and executive functions (Pareto et al. 2018; Bonavita et al. 2015; Cerasa et al. 2013) but also on memory (Leavitt et al. 2014; Dobryakova et al. 2014). The effects of video-game-based cognitive rehabilitation on RS FC of the thalamus have also been shown (De Giglio et al. 2016).

Starting from the consideration that exercise training has been proposed as an approach for managing the cognitive consequences of MS, RS FC changes after a pilot treadmill walking exercise training intervention for improving cognitive processing speed in MS have been explored (Sandroff et al. 2018). After 12 weeks of treadmill walking exercise training, increase in thalamocortical RS FC, which correlated with cognitive processing speed improvement, was observed.

23.8 Future Perspectives

All fMRI studies discussed in this chapter have been based on the assumption that brain RS FC is static across the whole duration of image acquisition (usually taking about 10 min), and thus the strength of the interaction between different brain regions is considered to be constant over time. However, RS FC between two or more regions changes dynamically over time (Calhoun et al. 2014; Allen et al. 2014). This has led to a shift from measuring static to measuring time-varying (dynamic) FC between different brain regions (Calhoun et al. 2014). Analysis of dynamic FC allows capturing reoccurring patterns of interaction among intrinsic networks at rest (Calhoun et al. 2014; Allen et al. 2014). Studies that have used dynamic RS FC analysis have shown the utility of this method in shedding light not only on the physiological processes in HC (Allen et al. 2012) but also in diseased subjects, for diagnostic purposes (Jones et al. 2012) or to improve the understanding of their clinical manifestations (Rashid et al. 2014).

A preliminary study (Leonardi et al. 2013) has assessed dynamic RS FC abnormalities in 15 minimally disabled RRMS patients and found altered dynamic FC in a network of connections centered on the DMN. The clinical relevance of these abnormalities, particularly for cognition, deserves further investigations.

23.9 Conclusions

RS fMRI studies conducted in MS patients have demonstrated that this technique contributes to provide important insights into the role of functional reorganization following CNS structural injury. Being a task-free approach, this tool complements and sometime replaces active fMRI acquisitions, allowing the generalization of the results to the whole spectrum of MS clinical phenotypes or clinical manifestations.

It is now established that clinical and cognitive features of MS patients are likely to represent the output of the complex interplay existing between structural damage and RS FC changes, indicating that the rate of accumulation of disability in MS is a function not only of tissue loss but also of the progressive failure of the adaptive capacity of the brain with increasing tissue damage. All of this is pivotal for the development of intervention strategies for the preservation or restoration of function.

References

Abidin AZ, Chockanathan U, DSouza AM, Inglese M, Wismüller A (2017) Using large-scale granger causality to study changes in brain network properties in the clinically isolated syndrome (CIS) stage of multiple sclerosis. Proc SPIE Int Soc Opt Eng 10137. https://doi.org/10.1117/12.2254395

Allen EA, Damaraju E, Plis SM, Erhardt EB, Eichele T, Calhoun VD (2014) Tracking whole-brain connectivity dynamics in the resting state. Cereb Cortex 24(3):663–676

Allen EA, Erhardt EB, Wei Y, Eichele T, Calhoun VD (2012) Capturing inter-subject variability with group independent component analysis of fMRI data: a simulation study. Neuroimage 59(4):4141–4159

Backner Y, Kuchling J, Massarwa S, Oberwahrenbrock T, Finke C, Bellmann-Strobl J et al (2018) Anatomical wiring and functional networking changes in the visual system following optic neuritis. JAMA Neurol 75(3):287–295

Barry RL, Rogers BP, Conrad BN, Smith SA, Gore JC (2016) Reproducibility of resting state spinal cord networks in healthy volunteers at 7 Tesla. Neuroimage 133:31–40

Barry RL, Smith SA, Dula AN, Gore JC (2014) Resting state functional connectivity in the human spinal cord. Elife 3:e02812

Basile B, Castelli M, Monteleone F, Nocentini U, Caltagirone C, Centonze D et al (2013) Functional connectivity changes within specific networks parallel the clinical evolution of multiple sclerosis. Mult Scler J 20(8):1050–1057

Basile B, Castelli M, Monteleone F, Nocentini U, Caltagirone C, Centonze D et al (2014) Functional connectivity changes within specific networks parallel the clinical evolution of multiple sclerosis. Mult Scler 20(8):1050–1057

Benedict RH, Fischer JS, Archibald CJ, Arnett PA, Beatty WW, Bobholz J et al (2002) Minimal neuropsychological assessment of MS patients: a consensus approach. Clin Neuropsychol 16(3):381–397

Benedict RH, Zivadinov R (2006) Predicting neuropsychological abnormalities in multiple sclerosis. J Neurol Sci 245(1–2):67–72

Bisecco A, Nardo FD, Docimo R, Caiazzo G, d'Ambrosio A, Bonavita S et al (2018) Fatigue in multiple sclerosis: the contribution of resting-state functional connectivity reorganization. Mult Scler 24(13):1696–1705. https://doi.org/10.1177/1352458517730932

Biswal B, Yetkin FZ, Haughton VM, Hyde JS (1995) Functional connectivity in the motor cortex of resting human brain using echo-planar MRI. Magn Reson Med 34(4):537–541

Bollaert RE, Poe K, Hubbard EA, Motl RW, Pilutti LA, Johnson CL et al (2018) Associations of functional connectivity and walking performance in multiple sclerosis. Neuropsychologia 117:8–12

Bonavita S, Gallo A, Sacco R, Corte MD, Bisecco A, Docimo R et al (2011) Distributed changes in default-mode resting-state connectivity in multiple sclerosis. Mult Scler J 17(4):411–422

Bonavita S, Sacco R, Della Corte M, Esposito S, Sparaco M, d'Ambrosio A et al (2015) Computer-aided cognitive rehabilitation improves cognitive performances and induces brain functional connectivity changes in relapsing remitting multiple sclerosis patients: an exploratory study. J Neurol 262(1):91–100

Boutière C, Rey C, Zaaraoui W, Le Troter A, Rico A, Crespy L et al (2017) Improvement of spasticity following intermittent theta burst stimulation in multiple sclerosis is associated with modulation of resting-state functional connectivity of the primary motor cortices. Mult Scler J 23(6):855–863

Bullmore ET, Sporns O (2009) Complex brain networks: graph theoretical analysis of structural and functional systems. Nat Rev Neurosci 10(3):186–198

Cabeza R, Nyberg L (2000) Imaging cognition II: an empirical review of 275 PET and fMRI studies. J Cogn Neurosci 12(1):1–47

Cader S, Palace J, Matthews PM (2009) Cholinergic agonism alters cognitive processing and enhances brain functional connectivity in patients with multiple sclerosis. J Psychopharmacol 23(6):686–696

Cadotte DW, Stroman PW, Mikulis D, Fehlings MG (2012) A systematic review of spinal fMRI research: outlining the elements of experimental design. J Neurosurg Spine 17(Suppl 1):102–118

Calhoun VD, Miller R, Pearlson G, Adali T (2014) The chronnectome: time-varying connectivity networks as the next frontier in fMRI data discovery. Neuron 84(2):262–274

Cameron MH, Lord S (2010) Postural control in multiple sclerosis: implications for fall prevention. Curr Neurol Neurosci Rep 10(5):407–412

Centonze D, Koch G, Versace V, Mori F, Rossi S, Brusa L et al (2007) Repetitive transcranial magnetic stimulation of the motor cortex ameliorates spasticity in multiple sclerosis. Neurology 68(13):1045–1050

Cerasa A, Gioia MC, Valentino P, Nistico R, Chiriaco C, Pirritano D et al (2013) Computer-assisted cognitive rehabilitation of attention deficits for multiple sclerosis: a randomized trial with fMRI correlates. Neurorehabil Neural Repair 27(4):284–295

Chiaravalloti ND, DeLuca J (2008) Cognitive impairment in multiple sclerosis. Lancet Neurol 7(12):1139–1151

Cirillo S, Rocca MA, Ghezzi A, Valsasina P, Moiola L, Veggiotti P et al (2016) Abnormal cerebellar functional MRI connectivity in patients with paediatric multiple sclerosis. Mult Scler 22(3):292–301

Colasanti A, Guo Q, Giannetti P, Wall MB, Newbould RD, Bishop C et al (2016) Hippocampal neuroinflammation, functional connectivity, and depressive symptoms in multiple sclerosis. Biol Psychiatry 80(1):62–72

Conrad BN, Barry RL, Rogers BP, Maki S, Mishra A, Thukral S et al (2018) Multiple sclerosis lesions affect intrinsic functional connectivity of the spinal cord. Brain 141(6):1650–1664

Cordes D, Haughton VM, Arfanakis K, Carew JD, Turski PA, Moritz CH et al (2001) Frequencies contributing to functional connectivity in the cerebral cortex in "resting-state" data. AJNR Am J Neuroradiol 22(7):1326–1333

Cruz Gomez AJ, Ventura Campos N, Belenguer A, Avila C, Forn C (2013) Regional brain atrophy and functional connectivity changes related to fatigue in multiple sclerosis. PLoS One 8(10):e77914

Cui F, Zhou L, Wang Z, Lang C, Park J, Tan Z et al (2017) Altered functional connectivity of striatal subregions in patients with multiple sclerosis. Front Neurol 8:129

d'Ambrosio A, Hidalgo de la Cruz M, Valsasina P, Pagani E, Colombo B, Rodegher M et al (2017) Structural connectivity-defined thalamic subregions have different functional connectivity abnormalities in multiple sclerosis patients: implications for clinical correlations. Hum Brain Mapp 38(12):6005–6018

De Giglio L, Tona F, De Luca F, Petsas N, Prosperini L, Bianchi V et al (2016) Multiple sclerosis: changes in thalamic resting-state functional connectivity induced by a home-based cognitive rehabilitation program. Radiology 280(1):202–211

DeLuca J, Genova HM, Hillary FG, Wylie G (2008) Neural correlates of cognitive fatigue in multiple sclerosis using functional MRI. J Neurol Sci 270(1–2):28–39

Dobryakova E, Wylie GR, DeLuca J, Chiaravalloti ND (2014) A pilot study examining functional brain activity 6 months after memory retraining in MS: the MEMREHAB trial. Brain Imaging Behav 8(3):403–406

Dogonowski AM, Andersen KW, Madsen KH, Sorensen PS, Paulson OB, Blinkenberg M et al (2014) Multiple sclerosis impairs regional functional connectivity in the cerebellum. Neuroimage Clin 4:130–138

Dogonowski AM, Siebner HR, Soelberg Sorensen P, Paulson OB, Dyrby TB, Blinkenberg M et al (2013a) Resting-state connectivity of pre-motor cortex reflects disability in multiple sclerosis. Acta Neurol Scand 128(5):328–335

Dogonowski AM, Siebner HR, Sorensen PS, Wu X, Biswal B, Paulson OB et al (2013b) Expanded functional coupling of subcortical nuclei with the motor resting-state network in multiple sclerosis. Mult Scler 19(5):559–566

Eijlers AJ, Meijer KA, Wassenaar TM, Steenwijk MD, Uitdehaag BM, Barkhof F et al (2017) Increased default-mode network centrality in cognitively impaired multiple sclerosis patients. Neurology 88(10):952–960

Eippert F, Kong Y, Winkler AM, Andersson JL, Finsterbusch J, Büchel C et al (2017) Investigating resting-state functional connectivity in the cervical spinal cord at 3T. Neuroimage 147:589–601

Eshaghi A, Riyahi-Alam S, Saeedi R, Roostaei T, Nazeri A, Aghsaei A et al (2015) Classification algorithms with multi-modal data fusion could accurately distinguish neuromyelitis optica from multiple sclerosis. Neuroimage Clin 7:306–314

Faivre A, Rico A, Zaaraoui W, Crespy L, Reuter F, Wybrecht D et al (2012) Assessing brain connectivity at rest is clinically relevant in early multiple sclerosis. Mult Scler 18(9):1251–1258

Feinstein A, Magalhaes S, Richard JF, Audet B, Moore C (2014) The link between multiple sclerosis and depression. Nat Rev Neurol 10(9):507–517

Filippi M, Riccitelli G, Mattioli F, Capra R, Stampatori C, Pagani E et al (2012) Multiple sclerosis: effects of cognitive rehabilitation on structural and functional MR imaging measures—an explorative study. Radiology 262(3):932–940

Filippi M, Rocca MA (2004) Magnetization transfer magnetic resonance imaging in the assessment of neurological diseases. J Neuroimaging 14(4):303–313

Filippi M, Rocca MA, Colombo B, Falini A, Codella M, Scotti G et al (2002a) Functional magnetic resonance imaging correlates of fatigue in multiple sclerosis. Neuroimage 15(3):559–567

Filippi M, Rocca MA, Comi G (2003) The use of quantitative magnetic-resonance-based techniques to monitor the evolution of multiple sclerosis. Lancet Neurol 2(6):337–346

Filippi M, Rocca MA, Falini A, Caputo D, Ghezzi A, Colombo B et al (2002b) Correlations between structural CNS damage and functional MRI changes in primary progressive MS. Neuroimage 15(3):537–546

Filippi M, Rocca MA, Mezzapesa DM, Ghezzi A, Falini A, Martinelli V et al (2004) Simple and complex movement-associated functional MRI changes in patients at presentation with clinically isolated syndromes suggestive of multiple sclerosis. Hum Brain Mapp 21(2):108–117

Finke C, Schlichting J, Papazoglou S, Scheel M, Freing A, Soemmer C et al (2015) Altered basal ganglia functional connectivity in multiple sclerosis patients with fatigue. Mult Scler J 21(7):925–934

Fox MD, Snyder AZ, Vincent JL, Corbetta M, Van Essen DC, Raichle ME (2005) The human brain is intrinsically organized into dynamic, anticorrelated functional networks. Proc Natl Acad Sci U S A 102(27):9673–9678

Franklin RJ, Kotter MR (2008) The biology of CNS remyelination: the key to therapeutic advances. J Neurol 255(Suppl 1):19–25

Gallo A, Esposito F, Sacco R, Docimo R, Bisecco A, Della Corte M et al (2012) Visual resting-state network in relapsing-remitting MS with and without previous optic neuritis. Neurology 79(14):1458–1465

Giorgio A, Zhang J, Stromillo ML, Rossi F, Battaglini M, Nichelli L et al (2017) Pronounced structural and functional damage in early adult pediatric-onset multiple sclerosis with no or minimal clinical disability. Front Neurol 8:608

Hawellek DJ, Hipp JF, Lewis CM, Corbetta M, Engel AK (2011) Increased functional connectivity indicates the severity of cognitive impairment in multiple sclerosis. Proc Natl Acad Sci U S A 108(47):19066–19071

Hidalgo de la Cruz M, d'Ambrosio A, Valsasina P, Pagani E, Colombo B, Rodegher M et al (2018) Abnormal functional connectivity of thalamic sub-regions contributes to fatigue in multiple sclerosis. Mult Scler 24(9):1183–1195. https://doi.org/10.1177/1352458517717807

Huang MH, Zhou FQ, Wu L, Wang B, Wan H, Li FJ et al (2018) Synchronization within, and interactions between, the default mode and dorsal attention networks in relapsing-remitting multiple sclerosis. Neuropsychiatr Dis Treat 14:1241–1252

Inglese M, Park SJ, Johnson G, Babb JS, Miles L, Jaggi H et al (2007) Deep gray matter perfusion in multiple sclerosis: dynamic susceptibility contrast perfusion magnetic resonance imaging at 3 T. Arch Neurol 64(2):196–202

Janssen AL, Boster A, Patterson BA, Abduljalil A, Prakash RS (2013) Resting-state functional connectivity in multiple sclerosis: an examination of group differences and individual differences. Neuropsychologia 51(13):2918–2929

Jones DT, Vemuri P, Murphy MC, Gunter JL, Senjem ML, Machulda MM et al (2012) Non-stationarity in the "resting brain's" modular architecture. PLoS One 7(6):e39731

Kelly AM, Uddin LQ, Biswal BB, Castellanos FX, Milham MP (2008) Competition between functional brain networks mediates behavioral variability. Neuroimage 39(1):527–537

Lanting CP, de Kleine E, Langers DRM, van Dijk P (2014) Unilateral tinnitus: changes in connectivity and response lateralization measured with fMRI. PLoS One 9(10):e110704

Leavitt VM, Wylie GR, Girgis PA, DeLuca J, Chiaravalloti ND (2014) Increased functional connectivity within memory networks following memory rehabilitation in multiple sclerosis. Brain Imaging Behav 8(3):394–402

Lee M, Reddy H, Johansen-Berg H, Pendlebury S, Jenkinson M, Smith S et al (2000) The motor cortex shows adaptive functional changes to brain injury from multiple sclerosis. Ann Neurol 47(5):606–613

Leonardi N, Richiardi J, Gschwind M, Simioni S, Annoni JM, Schluep M et al (2013) Principal components of functional connectivity: a new approach to study dynamic brain connectivity during rest. Neuroimage 83:937–950

Liu Y, Duan Y, Huang J, Ren Z, Ye J, Dong H et al (2015) Multimodal quantitative MR imaging of the thalamus in multiple sclerosis and neuromyelitis optica. Radiology 277(3):784–792

Liu Y, Gao JH, Liotti M, Pu Y, Fox PT (1999) Temporal dissociation of parallel processing in the human subcortical outputs. Nature 400(6742):364–367

Liu Y, Wang H, Duan Y, Huang J, Ren Z, Ye J et al (2017) Functional brain network alterations in clinically isolated syndrome and multiple sclerosis: a graph-based connectome study. Radiology 282(2):534–541

Lowe MJ, Phillips MD, Lurito JT, Mattson D, Dzemidzic M, Mathews VP (2002) Multiple sclerosis: low-frequency temporal blood oxygen level-dependent fluctuations indicate reduced functional connectivity initial results. Radiology 224(1):184–192

Lv H, Wang Z, Tong E, Williams LM, Zaharchuk G, Zeineh M et al (2018) Resting-state functional MRI: everything that nonexperts have always wanted to know. AJNR Am J Neuroradiol 39(8):1390–1399

Maieron M, Iannetti GD, Bodurka J, Tracey I, Bandettini PA, Porro CA (2007) Functional responses in the human spinal cord during willed motor actions: evidence for side- and rate-dependent activity. J Neurosci 27(15):4182–4190

Mainero C, Inghilleri M, Pantano P, Conte A, Lenzi D, Frasca V et al (2004) Enhanced brain motor activity in patients with MS after a single dose of 3,4-diaminopyridine. Neurology 62(11):2044–2050

Mattioli F, Bellomi F, Stampatori C, Capra R, Miniussi C (2016) Neuroenhancement through cognitive training and anodal tDCS in multiple sclerosis. Mult Scler 22(2):222–230

Meijer KA, Eijlers AJC, Geurts JJG, Schoonheim MM (2018) Staging of cortical and deep grey matter functional connectivity changes in multiple sclerosis. J Neurol Neurosurg Psychiatry 89(2):205–210

Mezzapesa DM, Rocca MA, Rodegher M, Comi G, Filippi M (2008) Functional cortical changes of the sensorimotor network are associated with clinical recovery in multiple sclerosis. Hum Brain Mapp 29(5):562–573

Morgen K, Sammer G, Courtney SM, Wolters T, Melchior H, Blecker CR et al (2007) Distinct mechanisms of altered brain activation in patients with multiple sclerosis. Neuroimage 37(3):937–946

Mori F, Ljoka C, Magni E, Codeca C, Kusayanagi H, Monteleone F et al (2011) Transcranial magnetic stimulation primes the effects of exercise therapy in multiple sclerosis. J Neurol 258(7):1281–1287

Northoff G, Wiebking C, Feinberg T, Panksepp J (2011) The 'resting-state hypothesis' of major depressive disorder-a translational subcortical-cortical framework for a system disorder. Neurosci Biobehav Rev 35(9):1929–1945

Pantano P, Iannetti GD, Caramia F, Mainero C, Di Legge S, Bozzao L et al (2002a) Cortical motor reorganization after a single clinical attack of multiple sclerosis. Brain 125(Pt 7):1607–1615

Pantano P, Mainero C, Iannetti GD, Caramia F, Di Legge S, Piattella MC et al (2002b) Contribution of corticospinal tract damage to cortical motor reorganization after a single clinical attack of multiple sclerosis. Neuroimage 17(4):1837–1843

Pareto D, Sastre-Garriga J, Alonso J, Galan I, Arevalo MJ, Renom M et al (2018) Classic block design "pseudo"-resting-state fMRI changes after a neurorehabilitation program in patients with multiple sclerosis. J Neuroimaging 28(3):313–319

Parisi L, Rocca MA, Mattioli F, Copetti M, Capra R, Valsasina P et al (2014) Changes of brain resting state functional connectivity predict the persistence of cognitive rehabilitation effects in patients with multiple sclerosis. Mult Scler 20(6):686–694

Parry AM, Scott RB, Palace J, Smith S, Matthews PM (2003) Potentially adaptive functional changes in cognitive processing for patients with multiple sclerosis and their acute modulation by rivastigmine. Brain 126(Pt 12):2750–2760

Pavisian B, MacIntosh BJ, Szilagyi G, Staines RW, O'Connor P, Feinstein A (2014) Effects of cannabis on cognition in patients with MS: a psychometric and MRI study. Neurology 82(21):1879–1887

Prosperini L, Fanelli F, Petsas N, Sbardella E, Tona F, Raz E et al (2014) Multiple sclerosis: changes in microar-

chitecture of white matter tracts after training with a video game balance board. Radiology 273(2):529–538
Raichle ME, MacLeod AM, Snyder AZ, Powers WJ, Gusnard DA, Shulman GL (2001) A default mode of brain function. Proc Natl Acad Sci U S A 98(2):676–682
Rashid B, Damaraju E, Pearlson GD, Calhoun VD (2014) Dynamic connectivity states estimated from resting fMRI Identify differences among Schizophrenia, bipolar disorder, and healthy control subjects. Front Hum Neurosci 8:897
Reddy H, Narayanan S, Matthews PM, Hoge RD, Pike GB, Duquette P et al (2000) Relating axonal injury to functional recovery in MS. Neurology 54(1):236–239
Reddy H, Narayanan S, Woolrich M, Mitsumori T, Lapierre Y, Arnold DL et al (2002) Functional brain reorganization for hand movement in patients with multiple sclerosis: defining distinct effects of injury and disability. Brain 125(Pt 12):2646–2657
Richiardi J, Gschwind M, Simioni S, Annoni JM, Greco B, Hagmann P et al (2012) Classifying minimally disabled multiple sclerosis patients from resting state functional connectivity. Neuroimage 62(3):2021–2033
Rocca MA, Absinta M, Amato MP, Moiola L, Ghezzi A, Veggiotti P et al (2014) Posterior brain damage and cognitive impairment in pediatric multiple sclerosis. Neurology 82(15):1314–1321
Rocca MA, Agosta F, Colombo B, Mezzapesa DM, Falini A, Comi G et al (2007a) fMRI changes in relapsing-remitting multiple sclerosis patients complaining of fatigue after IFNbeta-1a injection. Hum Brain Mapp 28(5):373–382
Rocca MA, Agosta F, Mezzapesa DM, Falini A, Martinelli V, Salvi F et al (2004a) A functional MRI study of movement-associated cortical changes in patients with Devic's neuromyelitis optica. Neuroimage 21(3):1061–1068
Rocca MA, Colombo B, Falini A, Ghezzi A, Martinelli V, Scotti G et al (2005b) Cortical adaptation in patients with MS: a cross-sectional functional MRI study of disease phenotypes. Lancet Neurol 4(10):618–626
Rocca MA, Falini A, Colombo B, Scotti G, Comi G, Filippi M (2002b) Adaptive functional changes in the cerebral cortex of patients with nondisabling multiple sclerosis correlate with the extent of brain structural damage. Ann Neurol 51(3):330–339
Rocca MA, Filippi M (2006) Functional MRI to study brain plasticity in clinical neurology. Neurol Sci 27(Suppl 1):S24–S26
Rocca MA, Filippi M (2007) Functional MRI in multiple sclerosis. J Neuroimaging 17(Suppl 1):36S–41S
Rocca MA, Gallo A, Colombo B, Falini A, Scotti G, Comi G et al (2004b) Pyramidal tract lesions and movement-associated cortical recruitment in patients with MS. Neuroimage 23(1):141–147
Rocca MA, Gavazzi C, Mezzapesa DM, Falini A, Colombo B, Mascalchi M et al (2003a) A functional magnetic resonance imaging study of patients with secondary progressive multiple sclerosis. Neuroimage 19(4):1770–1777
Rocca MA, Matthews PM, Caputo D, Ghezzi A, Falini A, Scotti G et al (2002a) Evidence for widespread movement-associated functional MRI changes in patients with PPMS. Neurology 58(6):866–872
Rocca MA, Mezzapesa DM, Falini A, Ghezzi A, Martinelli V, Scotti G et al (2003b) Evidence for axonal pathology and adaptive cortical reorganization in patients at presentation with clinically isolated syndromes suggestive of multiple sclerosis. Neuroimage 18(4):847–855
Rocca MA, Mezzapesa DM, Ghezzi A, Falini A, Agosta F, Martinelli V et al (2003c) Cord damage elicits brain functional reorganization after a single episode of myelitis. Neurology 61(8):1078–1085
Rocca MA, Mezzapesa DM, Ghezzi A, Falini A, Martinelli V, Scotti G et al (2005a) A widespread pattern of cortical activations in patients at presentation with clinically isolated symptoms is associated with evolution to definite multiple sclerosis. AJNR Am J Neuroradiol 26(5):1136–1139
Rocca MA, Pagani E, Absinta M, Valsasina P, Falini A, Scotti G et al (2007b) Altered functional and structural connectivities in patients with MS: a 3-T study. Neurology 69(23):2136–2145
Rocca MA, Pagani E, Ghezzi A, Falini A, Zaffaroni M, Colombo B et al (2003d) Functional cortical changes in patients with multiple sclerosis and nonspecific findings on conventional magnetic resonance imaging scans of the brain. Neuroimage 19(3):826–836
Rocca MA, Pravata E, Valsasina P, Radaelli M, Colombo B, Vacchi L et al (2015) Hippocampal-DMN disconnectivity in MS is related to WM lesions and depression. Hum Brain Mapp 36(12):5051–5063
Rocca MA, Tortorella P, Ceccarelli A, Falini A, Tango D, Scotti G et al (2008) The "mirror-neuron system" in MS: a 3 tesla fMRI study. Neurology 70(4):255–262
Rocca MA, Valsasina P, Absinta M, Riccitelli G, Rodegher ME, Misci P et al (2010) Default-mode network dysfunction and cognitive impairment in progressive MS. Neurology 74(16):1252–1259
Rocca MA, Valsasina P, Leavitt VM, Rodegher M, Radaelli M, Riccitelli GC et al (2018) Functional network connectivity abnormalities in multiple sclerosis: correlations with disability and cognitive impairment. Mult Scler 24(4):459–471
Rocca MA, Valsasina P, Martinelli V, Misci P, Falini A, Comi G et al (2012) Large-scale neuronal network dysfunction in relapsing-remitting multiple sclerosis. Neurology 79(14):1449–1457
Rocca MA, Valsasina P, Meani A, Falini A, Comi G, Filippi M (2016) Impaired functional integration in multiple sclerosis: a graph theory study. Brain Struct Funct 221(1):115–131
Roelcke U, Kappos L, Lechner-Scott J, Brunnschweiler H, Huber S, Ammann W et al (1997) Reduced glucose metabolism in the frontal cortex and basal ganglia of multiple sclerosis patients with fatigue: a 18F-fluorodeoxyglucose positron emission tomography study. Neurology 48(6):1566–1571

Rombouts SA, Lazeron RH, Scheltens P, Uitdehaag BM, Sprenger M, Valk J et al (1998) Visual activation patterns in patients with optic neuritis: an fMRI pilot study. Neurology 50(6):1896–1899

Roosendaal SD, Schoonheim MM, Hulst HE, Sanz-Arigita EJ, Smith SM, Geurts JJ et al (2010) Resting state networks change in clinically isolated syndrome. Brain 133(Pt 6):1612–1621

Rubinov M, Sporns O (2010) Complex network measures of brain connectivity: uses and interpretations. Neuroimage 52(3):1059–1069

Sandroff BM, Wylie GR, Sutton BP, Johnson CL, DeLuca J, Motl RW (2018) Treadmill walking exercise training and brain function in multiple sclerosis: preliminary evidence setting the stage for a network-based approach to rehabilitation. Mult Scler J Exp Transl Clin 4(1):2055217318760641

Sbardella E, Tona F, Petsas N, Upadhyay N, Piattella MC, Filippini N et al (2015) Functional connectivity changes and their relationship with clinical disability and white matter integrity in patients with relapsing–remitting multiple sclerosis. Mult Scler J 21(13):1681–1692

Sbardella E, Upadhyay N, Tona F, Prosperini L, De Giglio L, Petsas N et al (2017) Dentate nucleus connectivity in adult patients with multiple sclerosis: functional changes at rest and correlation with clinical features. Mult Scler 23(4):546–555

Schoonheim MM, Geurts J, Wiebenga OT, De Munck JC, Polman CH, Stam CJ et al (2014) Changes in functional network centrality underlie cognitive dysfunction and physical disability in multiple sclerosis. Mult Scler 20(8):1058–1065

Shu N, Duan Y, Xia M, Schoonheim MM, Huang J, Ren Z et al (2016) Disrupted topological organization of structural and functional brain connectomes in clinically isolated syndrome and multiple sclerosis. Sci Rep 6:29383

Shulman GL, Corbetta M, Buckner RL, Raichle ME, Fiez JA, Miezin FM et al (1997) Top-down modulation of early sensory cortex. Cereb Cortex 7(3):193–206

Smith SM, Fox PT, Miller KL, Glahn DC, Fox PM, Mackay CE et al (2009) Correspondence of the brain's functional architecture during activation and rest. Proc Natl Acad Sci U S A 106(31):13040–13045

Smitha KA, Raja KA, Arun KM, Rajesh PG, Thomas B, Kapilamoorthy TR et al (2017) Resting state fMRI: a review on methods in resting state connectivity analysis and resting state networks. Neuroradiol J 30(4):305–317

Stroman PW, Bosma RL, Tsyben A (2012) Somatotopic arrangement of thermal sensory regions in the healthy human spinal cord determined by means of spinal cord functional MRI. Magn Reson Med 68(3):923–931

Sweet LH, Rao SM, Primeau M, Durgerian S, Cohen RA (2006) Functional magnetic resonance imaging response to increased verbal working memory demands among patients with multiple sclerosis. Hum Brain Mapp 27(1):28–36

Tavazzi E, Bergsland N, Cattaneo D, Gervasoni E, Lagana MM, Dipasquale O et al (2018) Effects of motor rehabilitation on mobility and brain plasticity in multiple sclerosis: a structural and functional MRI study. J Neurol 265(6):1393–1401

Tomasi D, Volkow ND (2010) Functional connectivity density mapping. Proc Natl Acad Sci U S A 107(21):9885–9890

Tomassini V, Matthews PM, Thompson AJ, Fuglo D, Geurts JJ, Johansen-Berg H et al (2012) Neuroplasticity and functional recovery in multiple sclerosis. Nat Rev Neurol 8(11):635–646

Tona F, De Giglio L, Petsas N, Sbardella E, Prosperini L, Upadhyay N et al (2018) Role of cerebellar dentate functional connectivity in balance deficits in patients with multiple sclerosis. Radiology 287(1):267–275

Tononi G, Sporns O, Edelman GM (1994) A measure for brain complexity: relating functional segregation and integration in the nervous system. Proc Natl Acad Sci U S A 91(11):5033–5037

Toosy AT, Hickman SJ, Miszkiel KA, Jones SJ, Plant GT, Altmann DR et al (2005) Adaptive cortical plasticity in higher visual areas after acute optic neuritis. Ann Neurol 57(5):622–633

van den Heuvel MP, Hulshoff Pol HE (2010) Specific somatotopic organization of functional connections of the primary motor network during resting state. Hum Brain Mapp 31(4):631–644

van Geest Q, Boeschoten RE, Keijzer MJ, Steenwijk MD, Pouwels PJ, Twisk JW et al (2019) Fronto-limbic disconnection in patients with multiple sclerosis and depression. Mult Scler 25(5):715–726. https://doi.org/10.1177/1352458518767051

Waxman SG (1998) Demyelinating diseases—new pathological insights, new therapeutic targets. N Engl J Med 338(5):323–325

Werring DJ, Bullmore ET, Toosy AT, Miller DH, Barker GJ, MacManus DG et al (2000) Recovery from optic neuritis is associated with a change in the distribution of cerebral response to visual stimulation: a functional magnetic resonance imaging study. J Neurol Neurosurg Psychiatry 68(4):441–449

Wu GF, Brier MR, Parks CA, Ances BM, Van Stavern GP (2015) An eye on brain integrity: acute optic neuritis affects resting state functional connectivity. Invest Ophthalmol Vis Sci 56(4):2541–2546

Zhou F, Zhuang Y, Gong H, Wang B, Wang X, Chen Q et al (2014) Altered inter-subregion connectivity of the default mode network in relapsing remitting multiple sclerosis: a functional and structural connectivity study. PLoS One 9(7):e101198

24 The Perirhinal, Entorhinal, and Parahippocampal Cortices and Hippocampus: An Overview of Functional Anatomy and Protocol for Their Segmentation in MR Images

Sasa L. Kivisaari, Alphonse Probst, and Kirsten I. Taylor

Abbreviations

A	Anterior
Ab	Angular bundle (PHg white matter)
aCf	Anterior calcarine fissure
AD	Alzheimer's disease
al	Alveus
Am	Amygdala
bG	Band of Giacomini
cf.	Crus of the fornix
Cs	Collateral sulcus
di	Hippocampal digitations
ERc	Entorhinal cortex
Fg	Fusiform gyrus
fi	Fimbria
gA	Gyrus ambiens
gS	Gyrus of Schwalbe
HB	Hippocampal body
Hf	Hippocampal fissure
HH	Hippocampal head
Hs	Hippocampal sulcus
HT	Hippocampal tail
I	Inferior
ILg	Intralimbic gyrus
Is	Isthmus
ITg	Inferotemporal gyrus
L	Lateral
Lg	Lingual gyrus
li-gm	Limen insulae gray matter
li-wm	Limen insulae white matter
M	Medial
Mb	Mammillary body
MTL	Medial temporal lobe
OTs	Occipitotemporal sulcus
P	Posterior
PHc	Parahippocampal cortex
PHg	Parahippocampal gyrus
PRc	Perirhinal cortex
Pu	Pulvinar
qgc	Quadrigeminal cistern
Rs	Rhinal sulcus
S	Superior
SAs	Semiannular sulcus

S. L. Kivisaari (✉)
Department of Neuroscience and Biomedical Engineering, Aalto University, Espoo, Finland
e-mail: sasa.kivisaari@aalto.fi

A. Probst
Department of Geriatrics, Memory Clinic, University Hospital Basel, Basel, Switzerland

Department of Neuropathology, University Hospital Basel, Basel, Switzerland
e-mail: aprobst@uhbs.ch

K. I. Taylor
Neuroscience, Ophthalmology, and Rare Diseases, Roche Pharma Research and Early Development, Roche Innovation Center Basel, F. Hoffmann-La Roche Ltd, Basel, Switzerland

Faculty of Psychology, University of Basel, Basel, Switzerland
e-mail: kirsten.taylor@roche.com

S. Ulmer, O. Jansen (eds.), *fMRI*, https://doi.org/10.1007/978-3-030-41874-8_24

SLg	Semilunar gyrus
Sp	Splenium
su	Subiculum
TLV	Temporal horn of lateral ventricle
TP	Temporal pole
TR	Transentorhinal cortex
U	Uncus
Ug	Uncinate gyrus
un	Uncal notch

24.1 Introduction

Medial temporal lobe (MTL)) damage severely disrupts our ability to form new memories (Scoville and Milner 1957). Indeed, memory dysfunction is the hallmark of Alzheimer's disease (AD; e.g., Salmon 2011), a progressive neurodegenerative disorder which begins in and most prominently affects the MTL region (Braak and Braak 1991). Accordingly, the classical model of memory claims that the MTL functions as a single system subserving memory formation and not other kinds of cognitive processes (Squire and Zola-Morgan 1988; Squire and Zola 1998; Squire and Wixted 2011).

Converging evidence from animal and human cognitive neuroscience research suggests a more differentiated picture, one of functional diversity in the MTL subregions (e.g., Lee et al. 2005; Davachi 2006). Thus, in addition to supporting the formation of memories, each MTL subregion may also perform other specific functions. A first section briefly describes the putative specialized functional roles of the MTL subregions, namely, the perirhinal cortex (PRc; Broadmann areas [BA] 35/36), the entorhinal cortex (ERc; BA 28/34), the posteriorly situated parahippocampal cortex (PHc; BA 36; also known as posterior parahippocampal cortex), and the hippocampus proper, highlighting recent findings from animal and human cognitive neuroscience research.

The functional neuroanatomy of the MTL, including but not limited to the domain of memory, has implications for the clinical interpretation of circumscribed MTL lesions as well as the interpretation of functional impairments in patients with neurodegenerative disorders, most notably AD. A second section, therefore, describes the neuropsychology of the early AD syndrome including amnestic mild cognitive impairment (aMCI; Winblad et al. 2004).

The prerequisite for advancements in this important area of research is the valid and reliable identification of these regions on structural brain imaging scans. Indeed, many of the controversies in current human neuropsychological research may stem from inadequate control of lesion extent and location, as noted by Squire and Wixted: "The importance of thorough neuroanatomical measurement in neuropsychological studies of memory cannot be overstated. Many current disagreements about the facts and ideas emerging from neuropsychological research on human memory can be traced to concerns about the locus and extent of lesions. […] There is no substitute for thorough, quantitative descriptions of damage based on magnetic resonance imaging, as well as (where possible) detailed neurohistological description of the postmortem brain" (Squire and Wixted 2011, p. 268). The identification of MTL subregions is challenging because of the uncertainty or obscurity of anatomical landmarks, a difficulty compounded by the fact that some MTL gyri and sulci are interindividually highly variable. A third section, therefore, describes the gross anatomy of the MTL and, building upon previous seminal work of especially Insausti and colleagues (Insausti et al. 1998), presents a method for delineating the PRc, ERc, PHc, and the hippocampus proper on structural MR images (see also Watson et al. 1992; Insausti et al. 1998; Pruessner et al. 2000; Van Hoesen et al. 2000; Vogt et al. 2006; Malykhin et al. 2007; Taylor and Probst 2008; Van Hoesen 1995).

24.2 Functional Neuroanatomy of the MTL

The MTL has been irrevocably linked with the formation of long-term memory traces since Scoville and Milner's (Scoville and Milner 1957) description of the patient H.M., who became severely amnesic following an experimental bilateral MTL resection to treat his intractable epilepsy. H.M.'s surgical lesion included the intraventricular portions of the bilateral hippocampi (see Fig. 24.7), the amygdalae, and the medial temporal poles and extended laterally to the ERc, with relative sparing of the PRc and PHc (Corkin et al. 1997). Following the procedure, H.M. suffered from a persistent and profound anterograde amnesia, that is, an inability to remember events occurring after the operation, and a temporally graded retrograde amnesia, that is, difficulty remembering events that occurred within the 11 years preceding the MTL resection. He also suffered from partial anosmia, a lack of initiative and emotional bluntness (Corkin 1984). Strikingly, H.M.'s intellectual functions were relatively preserved, as were other forms of memory such as perceptual and motor skill learning, priming, habit formation, working memory, and memories for facts, events, and verbal semantic memories remote from his surgery (Corkin 1984). These functions enabled him to perform normally in many tasks including his avid crossword puzzle hobby (Skotko et al. 2008).

Cases such as H.M. were remarkable on many fronts. Most importantly, they demonstrated that memory indeed had a circumscribed anatomic basis in the MTL (*cf.* Lashley 1929).[1] It became clear that the type of memory typically affected in the MTL amnesia syndrome was the acquisition of declarative memories, that is, explicit memories of events from an individual's autobiography (episodic memory) and for facts and world knowledge (semantic memory), all of which are available to conscious awareness. The case of H.M. also sparked intensive work on rodents and nonhuman primates. The strategy used in this research was to ablate cytoarchitectonically distinct regions of the MTL and measure ensuing memory performance, research which critically relied on the delayed (non) matching-to-sample recognition memory paradigm.[2] This work led to the development of an animal model of amnesia where bilateral lesions of the hippocampus, parahippocampal gyrus, and amygdala were associated with severe recognition memory impairments with otherwise apparently preserved cognitive functions (Mahut et al. 1982; Mishkin 1978). More specific ablation studies refined these early results by demonstrating that lesions restricted to the hippocampus (Mahut et al. 1982; Zola-Morgan et al. 1989a; but see also Murray and Mishkin 1998) or to the parahippocampal gyrus (Zola-Morgan et al. 1989c; Meunier et al. 1993), but not amygdala (Zola-Morgan et al. 1989b) or mammillary bodies (Aggleton and Mishkin 1985), were sufficient to produce a severe recognition memory disorder. Moreover, the effects of lesions to different subregions appeared to be additive, and the most severe recognition memory impairment was measured following PRc lesions (Meunier et al. 1993; Zola-Morgan et al. 1989b). Drawing on these seminal experiments, Squire and colleagues developed the classical, single-process model of human memory functioning, which posited that the MTL subregions represent a single memory system in which each area is critical for forming declarative memories but do not participate in other cognitive functions (Zola-Morgan et al. 1986; Squire and Zola-Morgan 1988; Squire and Zola 1998; Squire and Wixted 2011). This classical, single-process model of MTL function has remained highly influential.

The field of MTL research has since burgeoned and now uses multimodal imaging methods with increasingly more detailed cognitive paradigms to study multidimensional aspects of MTL functioning. This work has led many authors to reconceptualize the MTL as a group of functionally specialized subregions (Mishkin et al. 1997; Aggleton and Brown 1999; Lavenex and Amaral

[1] Later research demonstrated that profound memory impairments were also associated with damage to diencephalic regions such as mammillary bodies or mediodorsal nucleus of the thalamus (Squire and Zola-Morgan 1988; Victor et al. 1989), although the nature of the memory impairment differed from amnesia following MTL damage.

[2] In these experiments, an animal is presented with a sample stimulus during a learning phase. After a delay, the sample stimulus is presented again together with a novel stimulus. Intact recognition memory is demonstrated by the animal displacing either the sample object (delayed matching to sample) or the novel object (delayed non-matching to sample).

2000; Davachi 2006; Henke 2010; Montaldi and Mayes 2010; Ranganath 2010), with different models emphasizing different aspects of functional specialization. For example, the two-process model argues for specialized memory functions within the MTL, with the PRc supporting context-free item familiarity (i.e., a feeling of knowing that an item was previously encountered) and the hippocampus and PHc explicit, context-rich item recollection (Aggleton and Brown 1999, 2006; Brown and Aggleton 2001; Yonelinas 2002; Montaldi and Mayes 2010). Other authors highlight functional-neuroanatomical relationships specific to object and spatial information processing (e.g., Davachi 2006; Lee et al. 2008) or item and relational information processing (e.g., Eichenbaum et al. 1999; Davachi and Wagner 2002; Davachi 2006; Henke 2010). Common to these models is the idea that while the entire network of highly interconnected subregions is typically engaged during declarative memory formation, each subregion may be specialized for processing a unique aspect of the event or concept (for reviews, see, e.g., Aggleton and Brown 1999, 2006; Eichenbaum et al. 1999, 2007; Squire et al. 2004; Moscovitch et al. 2005; Henson 2005; Davachi 2006; Henke 2010; Montaldi and Mayes 2010, 2011; Kravitz et al. 2011).

Many researchers of MTL function rely on an anatomically driven connectivity approach based on nonhuman primate data (Mishkin et al. 1983; Lavenex and Amaral 2000) to generate novel hypotheses of human MTL function. Nonhuman primate MTL connectivity demonstrates that each subregion receives information from different sensory and polymodal cortices and integrates the information it receives in intrinsic associational connections and in a hierarchical system from the PRc and PHc to the ERc and from the ERc to the hippocampus (Mishkin et al. 1983, 1997; Lavenex and Amaral 2000). The first basic premise of this account is that each MTL subregion is specialized to process the information it receives and integrates in intrinsic associational connections (Lavenex and Amaral 2000; Lavenex et al. 2004). The second basic premise is that each processing level – from PRc/PHc to ERc and from ERc to the hippocampus – is characterized by an increasing amount of convergence of information and a higher level of associativity of the coded representation (a "hierarchy of associativity"; Lavenex and Amaral 2000). Further, we outline the functional neuroanatomy of the PRc, PHc, ERc, and hippocampus based on this approach.

The *perirhinal cortex* receives prominent afferents from the ventral visual object-processing stream (the "what" stream) and less dense inputs from other unimodal and polymodal sensory systems, the orbitofrontal, insula, and cingulate cortex (Suzuki and Amaral 1994a). Tracing studies have also demonstrated a rich network of intrinsic associational connections within the PRc, which presumably bind this multimodal information together (Lavenex et al. 2004). In line with this connectivity pattern, numerous animal lesions studies have demonstrated that the PRc plays an essential role in visual object recognition memory (Meunier et al. 1993; Zola-Morgan et al. 1989c) and multimodal object memory (e.g., by forming flavor-visual and tactile-visual associations; see Murray and Richmond 2001; Murray et al. 1998 for overviews). Bussey, Saksida, Murray, and colleagues suggested that the PRc represents the apex of the ventral occipital-temporal visual processing pathway, which computes increasingly more complex combinations of visual features from posterior to anterior sites. Thus, the PRc may be engaged during demanding visual perceptual task, e.g., discriminating between objects who share many features with one another (Bussey and Saksida 2002; Bussey et al. 2005).

Research on human PRc functioning has been hampered by the paucity of naturally occurring lesions restricted to this region, although PRc damage does occur in the context of more widespread lesions. Moreover, fMRI studies are confronted with signal dropout around the PRc due to nearby air-tissue interfaces which induce susceptibility artifacts in gradient-echo sequences (Cusack et al. 2005; Schmidt et al. 2005; Bellgowan et al. 2006; Schwarzbauer et al. 2010). Nonetheless, converging evidence from human functional imaging and patient studies broadly support the nonhuman primate findings described above. In fMRI studies, PRc activity in healthy controls has been associated with memorizing individual items (Davachi and Wagner 2002), changes in object identity (Pihlajamäki et al. 2004; Köhler et al. 2005; O'Neil et al. 2009), fine-grained analyses of visual objects (Tyler et al. 2004), the recognition of ambiguous visual objects (Moss et al. 2005), demanding visual discrimination tasks (Barense et al. 2005), and the integration of object features from different sensory modalities (Taylor et al. 2006). In the same vein, patients with brain damage in the parahippocampal gyrus including the PRc were impaired in discriminating highly similar, complex visual stimuli (Barense et al. 2007, 2010; Moss et al. 2005) and integrating crossmodal object features (Taylor et al. 2009, 2011a), even in the absence of memory demands. Finally, difficulties in visual object recognition memory were observed in patients with aMCI (Barbeau et al. 2004), commonly considered a possible AD prodrome with putative PRc pathology (Braak and Braak 1991).

The nature of information integrated in the PRc – multimodal and potentially non-sensory motivational features (Liu et al. 2000) associated with individual objects – has led some authors to suggest that the PRc codes for semantic object memories, that is, our knowledge about individual objects (Murray and Richmond 2001). For example, despite H.M.'s profound amnesia, he was able to acquire fragments of conceptual information, a feat attributed to his relatively intact PRc (*cf.* Corkin et al. 1997). When presented with the names of people who became famous after his MTL resection, H.M. was able to correctly distinguish these names from unfamiliar foil names, showing only a mild impairment relative to control participants (O'Kane et al. 2004). In an influential study, Vargha-Khadem et al. (1997) studied four patients with selective hippocampal damage acquired at an early age, who were nonetheless able to acquire normal levels of language comprehension and perform relatively well in school, that is, acquire semantic-like knowledge. Thus, although these individuals were significantly impaired at encoding the events in their lives, they were able to acquire world knowledge (semantic memories), an ability attributed to the intact parahippocampal gyrus (Mishkin et al. 1997; Vargha-Khadem et al. 1997).

MRI studies in humans provide additional support for the role of the PRc in processing the meaning of individual objects: fMRI studies showed that PRc activity was related to the meaning of object stimuli (Moss et al. 2005; Taylor et al. 2006; see also Wang et al. 2010), while voxel-based correlation studies (Hirni et al. 2011; Taylor et al. 2011b) and a cortical thickness study (Kivisaari et al. 2012) demonstrated significant relationships between gray matter integrity in the MTL, including the PRc and performance on semantic object tasks. Semantic object processing in the PRc may also manifest itself as the feeling of familiarity about having previously encountered an object in the absence of recall about specific contextual details (two-process models; see Eichenbaum et al. 2007; Montaldi and Mayes 2010 for reviews). Taken together, these findings suggest that the PRc integrates the visual and multimodal information it receives to support complex visual discriminations (Bussey et al. 2002, 2005) and to form visual and multimodal memories of meaningful objects, that is, semantic object memories.

The *parahippocampal cortex* lies posterior to the PRc and receives afferent projections primarily from the dorsal ("where") processing system in the posterior parietal cortex (Suzuki and Amaral 1994a). This "parieto-medial temporal pathway" has been implicated in visuospatial processing (Kravitz et al. 2011). It begins in the posterior inferior parietal lobule and sends direct connections to the PHc and hippocampus as well as indirect connections via the posterior cingulate and retrosplenial cortices to the PHc and same hippocampal fields. Thus, the PHc is attributed a central role in processing visuospatial and landmark information. Accordingly, in nonhuman primate studies, PHc damage has been linked with the impaired recognition of novel object locations and object-place associations (Alvarado and Bachevalier 2005a; Bachevalier and Nemanic 2008).

Findings from human functional imaging studies suggest that also the human PHc processes spatial and navigational information

(Köhler et al. 2002, 2005; Buffalo et al. 2006; Staresina et al. 2011). For example, Pihlajamäki et al. (Pihlajamäki et al. 2004) demonstrated heightened PHc (and posterior hippocampal) activation when participants processed novel spatial arrangements of familiar objects, in contrast with the processing of novel objects in the same spatial arrangement. Evidence for a role of the PHc in landmark processing in healthy participants was provided by Maguire et al. (1998), who found heightened PHc metabolism when participants navigated in virtual environments with salient objects and textures compared to when they navigated in empty environments. Similarly, Burgess and colleagues (Burgess et al. 2001) showed increased BOLD activation in the PHc when participants recalled landmarks from memory and in the absence of spatial scene information. Moreover, Epstein and Kanwisher (Epstein and Kanwisher 1998) observed that posterior parts of the bilateral parahippocampal gyri extending into the lingual gyri were preferentially activated when participants observed real or artificial visual scenes, with attenuated activity during the viewing of objects, faces, or scrambled scenes. These relationships prompted Kanwisher and colleagues to label an area in the posterior PHc displaying these characteristics as the parahippocampal place area (PPA; Epstein and Kanwisher 1998; Epstein et al. 1999; see also Grill-Spector and Malach 2004). These studies suggest that PHc processes both perceptual and mnemonic features of its preferred stimuli, that is, the spatial arrangement of objects or landmarks, which underpin our ability to navigate in the environment.

Other authors have suggested that the PHc processes not just spatial landmark or scenic stimuli and memories but more abstract information related to these stimuli (Diana et al. 2007). For example, BOLD activity in the PHc was stronger in response to strongly semantically related object-scene pairs (e.g., a driving wheel inside a car) compared to weakly semantically related object-scene pairs (e.g., a purse on a table; Bar et al. 2008). Bar and colleagues also found heightened PHc activity in response to objects which were strongly associated with a particular environment (e.g., a roulette wheel or beach chair as opposed to a cherry or basket), in the absence of an explicit spatial stimulus (Bar and Aminoff 2003). The sensitivity of the PHc to the meaningfulness of the visuospatial stimuli resembles the PRc's ability to code for the meaning of its preferred stimulus, that is, objects (see above).

Damage to the human PHc results in a pattern of deficits consistent with the functional imaging studies reported above, specifically in the syndrome of topographical disorientation. Two variants of topographical disorientation are recognized: landmark agnosia and anterograde topographic disorientation (Paterson and Zancwill 1945; Whiteley and Warrington 1978; De Renzi 1982; Barrash 1998). Damage to the posterior PHc is associated with landmark agnosia, in which patients are unable to recognize famous or familiar environmental stimuli such as buildings, statues, or scenes (Epstein et al. 1999; Takahashi et al. 2002). These agnostic impairments lead to difficulties navigating the environment despite normal topographical memory and spatial processing ability (Aguirre and D'Esposito 1999). Patients with anterograde topographic disorientation (also known as topographical amnesia; De Renzi et al. 1977) following unilateral or bilateral PHc lesions have difficulties forming representations of new environments, with otherwise intact visuospatial functioning (Barrash 1998; Barrash et al. 2000; Bohbot et al. 2000). These patients are, therefore, also unable to orient and navigate in new environments but may successfully navigate in premorbidly familiar environments. Thus, these findings further support the view that the PHc is primarily involved in the perceptual and mnemonic processing of scenes, that is, the visuospatial arrangement of landmarks, and potentially their meaning, functions which enable orientation and navigation in the world.

The PRc and PHc send afferents to the *entorhinal cortex*, which receives less dense inputs from the amygdala, olfactory structures (e.g., piriform cortex, olfactory bulb), insula and frontal cortex, basal forebrain, thalamus, basal ganglia, and brainstem (Insausti et al. 1987; Suzuki and Amaral 1994b; Canto et al. 2008). A striking feature of the PRc and PHc afferents in the rodent and nonhuman primate ERc is the topographical segregation of their terminations: the anterolateral aspects of the nonhuman primate ERc receive highly integrated visual information via the PRc (Suzuki and Amaral 1994a, 1994b), whereas the posteromedial aspects of the ERc receive information primarily from the parieto-medial temporal visuospatial pathway via the PHc (Suzuki and Amaral 1994a, 1994b; Canto et al. 2008; Kravitz et al. 2011). Notably, in rodents and nonhuman primates, the segregation of inputs is largely preserved in the intrinsic connectivity of the ERc (Dolorfo and Amaral 1998; Chrobak and Amaral 2007).

The afferent and intrinsic pattern of ERc connectivity suggests a relative segregation of object and spatial information processing in the anterolateral and posteromedial ERc, respectively. While largely unexplored in nonhuman and human primates, rodent research partly supports this functional-neuroanatomic division of labor. For example, cells in the rodent ERc receiving prominent visuospatial inputs show high spatial tuning, whereas cells in other ERc regions are only weakly modulated by spatial changes (Fyhn et al. 2004). Furthermore, lesions specifically in this spatially tuned area in the rodent ERc have been associated with spatial, navigational impairments (Steffenach et al. 2005). Perhaps most strikingly, a subgroup of cells in this region shows a high degree of spatial sensitivity when rats run freely in an open environment: these "grid cells" fire regularly as the rat traverses vertices of an imaginary grid of tessellated triangles mapped onto allocentric physical space (Hafting et al. 2005).[3] The dynamics of the population of grid cells may support "path integration," that is, the ability to determine one's current position relative to a starting point based on self-generated movement, as opposed to environmental cues (Witter and Moser 2006; Hasselmo and Brandon 2008). A potential segregation of ERc function has not yet been explicitly tested in primates (but see Suzuki et al. 1997).

A specific role of the anterolateral ERc in object processing, as implied by its prominent PRc inputs, has not been definitively established. However, the entire ERc has been strongly implicated in object recognition memory. Animal lesion studies show that object recognition impairments, albeit mild, can follow selective ERc lesions (Leonard et al. 1995; Meunier et al. 1993) and that concomittant lesions of the PRc and ERc exacerbate the object recognition impairments found with selective PRc lesions (Meunier et al. 1993). A functional imaging study with healthy human participants demonstrated greater ERc activation during rote learning of words compared to the relational processing of words, supporting the role of human ERc in processing of single items (Davachi and Wagner 2002). Given the resolution of common fMRI studies, and the additional effects of Gaussian smoothing enabling group analyses, future human studies addressing this question will require high-resolution fMRI (Carr et al. 2010) in conjunction with refined behavioral tasks.

The most striking impairment following damage to the entire human ERc is episodic memory dysfunction (Eustache et al. 2001; Di Paola et al. 2007; Coutureau and Di Scala 2009). These lesions typically extend beyond the ERc into the hippocampus, such that it is not known whether isolated ERc lesions are sufficient to impair episodic memory functioning. Rather than focusing on the types of information processed or integrated in the ERc, recent studies of episodic memory functioning and the ERc focus on the electrophysiological properties of its neurons, which provide key information about how episodic memories, are formed in downstream hippocampus. Specifically, in computational models, persistent firing upon depolarization and the oscillations of the dendritic membrane

[3]It is tempting to hypothesize similar grid cell properties for human ERc neurons. To our knowledge, a single human fMRI study has found evidence consistent with this hypothesis. Doeller and colleagues (Doeller et al. 2010) found that BOLD activity in the human ERc had a sixfold sinusoidal relationship with "running" direction in a circular-shaped virtual environment. This pattern of activation corresponds to the symmetry of grid cell firing in rodent ERc and putatively reflects whether the participants ran in alignment or misalignment with the grid axes. The ERc was activated as part of a larger network showing these properties, which included the posterior and medial parietal, lateral temporal, and medial prefrontal cortices (Doeller et al. 2010; see also Jacobs et al. 2010).

potential of some ERc neurons may give rise to cyclical and graded firing patterns which support information binding in downstream hippocampus (Hasselmo and Brandon 2008; Wallenstein et al. 1998; see also Fyhn et al. 2007; Lipton and Eichenbaum 2008). In summary, the ERc appears to be involved in both object and spatial processing, although evidence for the anatomical segregation of these processes within the human ERc remains elusive. More evidence from lesion studies exists to suggest that ERc, together with the hippocampus, is critical for the formation of episodic memories, that is, the binding together of contextual and associative information with an object or scene. The ERc's specialized role in episodic memory formation may be reflected not only in the information content delivered by its afferent connections but also by the electrophysiological properties of its neurons.

The perforant pathway connects the ERc with the *hippocampus proper*, with primary projections to the dentate gyrus and weaker projections to the CA1 and CA3 subfields and the subiculum (Witter 2007). Nonhuman primate studies demonstrate that the pathway between the ERc and dentate gyrus has two main components: one set of connections links anterolateral ERc (which receives its primary input from the visual object-processing system via the PRc) with the intermediate and posterior parts of the hippocampus and a second set links posteromedial ERc (the primary termination of PHc efferents coding spatial information) primarily with the posterior hippocampus (e.g., Witter and Amaral 1991; Witter 2007; see also Dolorfo and Amaral 1998). The most anterior parts of the hippocampus receive afferents from forebrain structures such as the amygdala and hypothalamus via the ERc and have been hypothesized potentially mediate endocrinological functions including stress-related physiological responses (Moser and Moser 1998).

Evidence of an anterior-posterior gradient of functional specialization implied by this connectivity pattern has indeed been demonstrated in several animal and human studies. Activation in the anterior extent of the hippocampal body has been demonstrated in response to judging object novelty (Pihlajamäki et al. 2004) and during a crossmodal object-processing task (e.g., Taylor et al. 2006). Similarly, lesions including the anterior hippocampi are associated with object-processing impairments (Barense et al. 2005; Acres et al. 2009; Taylor et al. 2009). Conversely, research on rats suggests relative specialization of the rodent homologue of posterior hippocampus to spatial processing. For example, the highly spatially tuned "place cells" (for reviews, see Eichenbaum et al. 1999; Burgess et al. 2002) are more prevalent in the rodent homologue of posterior compared to anterior primate hippocampus (Jung et al. 1994).[4] Correspondingly, lesions of the rodent homologue of the posterior hippocampus disrupt spatial learning (Colombo et al. 1998; for a review, see Moser and Moser 1998). Although subsequent research has failed to demonstrate place-like cells in the primate hippocampus, the posterior hippocampus nevertheless appears to contribute to spatial processing in primates (Alvarado and Bachevalier 2005b). For example, in human functional imaging studies, spatial tasks elicited activity in the posterior parts of the human hippocampus (e.g., Pihlajamäki et al. 2004), and a morphometric MR study demonstrated more voluminous posterior hippocampi in London taxi drivers with a highly developed spatial abilities (Maguire et al. 1998).

A higher-order anatomical characteristic of the hippocampus, beyond the hypothesized anterior-posterior gradient of functional specialization, is its location at the top of the MTL processing hierarchy (Lavenex and Amaral 2000). This position confers the ultimate integration ability on the hippocampus, functions presumably supported by intrinsic connectivity both longitudinally and mediolaterally (Witter 2007). Thus, the hippocampus has been suggested to bind multisensory object and spatial, contextual, and associational information together to repre-

[4]The original discovery of "place cells" demonstrated that these cells selectively fired according to the animal's location in the environment (O'Keefe and Dostrovsky 1971), while later studies showed that firing patterns were also modulated by other factors such as motivational factors and environmental cues (Lipton and Eichenbaum 2008; see Eichenbaum et al. 1999 for a review).

sent our semantic and episodic memories, also more generally known as "relational memories" (Henke et al. 1997; Eichenbaum et al. 1999; Burgess et al. 2002; Davachi and Wagner 2002; Davachi 2006). In its basic form, these memories bind both spatial and context information from the dorsal stream, transmitted via PHc-ERc connections (Kravitz et al. 2011), together with object information received via PRc-ERc connections (Suzuki and Amaral 1994a). Critically, the primate hippocampus additionally integrates higher-order, more abstract information related to objects and episodes together. For example, the nonhuman primate hippocampus was shown to be involved in a transverse patterning task which requires the formation of indirect associations between items (e.g., A is rewarded with B, B is rewarded with C, but A is not rewarded with C or B with A; Alvarado et al. 2002; Alvarado and Bachevalier 2005b). In human functional imaging studies, the hippocampus was activated during the formation of higher-order, semantic associations (Henke et al. 1997, 1999b; Davachi and Wagner 2002), upon presentation of novel spatial organization of objects or novel combination of familiar objects and familiar locations (i.e., Köhler et al. 2005) and object-space relationships (Hannula and Ranganath 2008). These findings are consistent with the clinical sequelae of isolated hippocampal lesions, that is, the classic amnesic syndrome. Such lesions may occur following carbon monoxide poisoning (Zola-Morgan et al. 1986; Vargha-Khadem et al. 1997; Henke et al. 1999a; Gadian et al. 2000), which causes cellular damage in the CA1 subfield of the hippocampus through hypoxic and histotoxic mechanisms (O'Donnell et al. 2000; Gale and Hopkins 2004). Patients with isolated hippocampal lesions display an anterograde amnesia for episodic memories with otherwise relatively normal cognitive functioning, similar to H.M. (see above; Vargha-Khadem et al. 1997; Zola-Morgan et al. 1986), although the magnitude of the impairment may be milder than that following more widespread MTL lesions (Zola-Morgan et al. 1986).

Recent models of hippocampal functioning emphasize its pattern separation and pattern completion abilities (Rolls 2007; Yassa and Stark 2011). Pattern separation is the appreciation of slight differences between sensory input and existing representations, a function which presumably enables the acquisition of distinct and complex representations corresponding to human episodic memories. The dentate gyrus and the CA3 of the hippocampus proper appear to be critically involved in rodent pattern separation (Leutgeb et al. 2007; Rolls 2007; see Yassa and Stark 2011 for a review), and this process is thought to be modulated by neurogenesis in the dentate gyrus (Deng et al. 2010). Tentative evidence for pattern separation functions in the human dentate gyrus and CA3 was provided by a high-resolution fMRI study by Bakker and colleagues (Bakker et al. 2008). These investigators presented participants with pictures of objects that were either novel, repeated, or slightly modified pictures of the repeated objects (lures). An area encompassing the DG and CA3 showed enhanced patterns of activity to novel and lure objects and weaker responses to object repetitions, suggesting that human DG and CA3 detect subtle differences between sensory input and existing representations. The process of pattern separation is hypothesized to be balanced by pattern completion, that is, the ability to recollect an existing representation on the basis of an incomplete set of cues (O'Reilly and McClelland 1994). This process is thought to be supported by ERc afferents bypassing the dentate gyrus, which may introduce the cue to CA3 to reactivate an existing representation, as well as auto-associative recurrent connectivity in CA3 (Leutgeb et al. 2007; Rolls 2007; Yassa and Stark 2011). The complementary processes of pattern separation and pattern completion may give rise to the capacity of human memory to treat highly similar episodes, such as events in the office on last Monday and Tuesday, as distinct from one another (pattern separation) while enabling the retrieval of a memory based on incomplete information, for example, remembering what took place on Monday based on knowing that a chocolate cake was available during the coffee break (pattern completion).

Taken together, animal and human studies demonstrate that the hippocampus, together with the ERc, binds information across spatial and temporal intervals, ultimately giving rise to complex, multicomponential semantic and episodic memories. These processes take place extremely rapidly and may even proceed in the absence of conscious awareness (Henke 2010). Pattern separation and completion processes in the hippocampus may represent fundamental processes supporting memory formation and retrieval, enabling the prerequisite disambiguation of phenomena and successful retrieval based on fragmentary cues, respectively.

24.3 Alzheimer's Disease and Other Dementias Associated with the MTL

AD is a debilitating neurodegenerative condition which globally affects 3.9% of the individuals over 60 years of age (Qiu et al. 2009). Since the risk of developing AD is strongly linked with increasing age, and given our increasing life expectancies, the prevalence of AD is expected to exponentially increase in the upcoming decades, tripling between 2010 and 2050 (Alzheimer's Association 2011). The clinical diagnosis of probable AD requires the presence of a memory impairment in addition to an impairment in one other domain of cognitive functioning (i.e., language, praxis, gnosis, and executive functions), which is severe enough to affect everyday functioning (American Psychiatric Association 1994). The definite diagnosis of AD is made upon autopsy, where it is characterized by two neuropathological hallmarks: the accumulation of amyloid β-peptide (Aβ) as plaques in the extracellular space in widespread regions of the brain and the formation of insoluble aggregates of hyperphosphorylated isoforms of microtubule-associated tau-proteins (Mattson 2004; Ewers et al. 2011). These abnormal isoforms of tau form neurofibrillary tangles in the nerve cells.

The distribution of neurofibrillary tangle deposition typically follows a sequential progression in the cerebral cortex (Braak and Braak 1991). Correspondingly, the stage of neurofibrillary pathology correlates with cognitive dysfunction, whereas the relationship between Aβ plaques and cognition is less clear (Ghoshal et al. 2002; Guillozet et al. 2003). Neurofibrillary tangles first affect the transentorhinal cortex (TR) of the PRc, from where they spread to the ERc and hippocampus proper and then to the neocortex (Braak and Braak 1985, 1991). Notable exceptions to this pattern exist, for example, a rare "frontal variant" of AD in which the frontal cortex is heavily affected by neurofibrillary tangles potentially early in the course of the disease (Taylor et al. 2008) and posterior cortical atrophy, where neurofibrillary tangles and plaques predominantly accumulate in the parietal and occipital cortices in most cases (Crutch et al. 2012). Typically, however, reduced volumes (Juottonen et al. 1998) and cortical thinning are observed in the PRc and ERc early in the course of disease (Dickerson et al. 2009), and these changes appear to be related to the accumulation of neurofibrillary tangles and consequent neuronal loss (Silbert et al. 2003). MTL atrophy is accompanied by a progressive episodic memory impairment characterized by poor learning and rapid forgetting, as well as semantic memory impairments (Taylor and Monsch 2007; Salmon and Bondi 2009; Salmon 2011). Cortical thinning throughout the neocortex can be observed at later stages of the disease (Lerch et al. 2005) and is associated with progressive impairments in other cognitive domains such as language and visuospatial processing.

The predicted exponential increase in the incidence of AD (Qiu et al. 2009) has refocused dementia research more strongly on identifying the earliest possible markers of neurofibrillary pathology. The discovery of early or "preclinical" markers would enable the initiation of therapies at a point in the disease process when they are expected to be maximally beneficial. One strand of research investigates the utility of fMRI imaging of memory functioning for the early detection of AD. These studies demonstrate that AD patients show decreased activation in the hippocampus during episodic memory tasks relative to controls (Rombouts et al. 2000; Machulda et al.

2003; for a review, see Dickerson and Sperling 2008). However, patients with aMCI, a putative prodromal stage of AD, tend to show the opposite effect, that is, increased MTL BOLD responses during memory tasks compared to normal control participants (Dickerson et al. 2004). In a similar vein, increased functional activity in the MTL was observed in healthy participants carrying one or two apoE ε4 alleles associated with an increased risk for AD (Bondi et al. 2005). Heightened MTL activity in preclinical stages and reduced MTL activity in early AD may reflect compensatory hyperactivation in the early stages of the disease and a breakdown of these compensatory mechanisms as the disease progresses (see, e.g., Dickerson et al. 2004). Thus, the development of preclinical BOLD markers of AD faces the challenging task of discriminating normal from pathologically enhanced or pathologically reduced levels of MTL activity, that is, of defining what "normal" BOLD responses during memory formation are.

A potentially fruitful approach to the identification of very early AD is to combine knowledge about the spatiotemporal sequence of neurofibrillary tangle formation and MTL functional specialization described above (Barbeau et al. 2004; Taylor and Probst 2008). Specifically, since the tau pathology associated with the cognitive dysfunction in AD typically begins in the PRc (Braak and Braak 1991), PRc dysfunction as revealed by neuropsychological testing may signal very early and still preclinical AD changes. Preliminary evidence from cross-sectional studies provides proof of this principle: crossmodal integration and complex perceptual and semantic analyses of individual objects, functions associated with the PRc (see above), are indeed impaired in individuals with amnestic MCI and early AD, and these impairments were shown to be related to the integrity of the PRc as estimated by voxel-based morphometry, cortical thickness, and fractional anisotropy MR measures (Hirni et al. 2011; Kivisaari et al. 2012; Taylor et al. 2011b). We note that the neuropsychological changes associated with PRc dysfunction may be subtle in nature, that is, not necessarily detectable in daily life (viz., episodic memory impairments), but demonstrable upon directed neuropsychological testing. Future interdisciplinary research combining neuropsychological and imaging with genetic and cerebrospinal fluid measures will undoubtedly reveal more specific and valid preclinical markers of AD which will be of great utility in the upcoming decades.

24.4 Anatomy of the MTL

The accurate identification of the MTL subregions is the prerequisite for understanding and studying their functional relevance. Further, we provide an overview of the gross anatomy of the MTL and a segmentation protocol for the reliable identification of these regions on anatomic MR scans. This parcellation scheme is based primarily on cytoarchitecture (Insausti et al. 1998; Suzuki and Amaral 2003a; Blaizot et al. 2010), myeloarchitecture (Hopf 1956), and patterns of white matter connectivity (Suzuki and Amaral 1994a; Saleem et al. 2007; Zilles and Amunts 2009).

24.4.1 Overview of the Gyral and Sulcal Characteristics of the MTL

The MTL region is characterized by three major gyri, the uncus (U, Fig. 24.1), the parahippocampal gyrus (PHg, Figs. 24.1 and 24.2), and the fusiform gyrus (Fg, Fig. 24.2), and two major sulci, the hippocampal fissure (Hf, Fig. 24.2), which is located superior to the parahippocampal gyrus, and the collateral sulcus (Cs, Figs. 24.1 and 24.2), which separates the parahippocampal gyrus from the fusiform gyrus (Fg, Fig. 24.2). Together, these gyral and sulcal landmarks are key to identifying the hippocampus proper, ERc, PRc, and PHc.

The uncus is the most medial and superior gyrus in the MTL, and its characteristic bulges are visible on a surface view (Fig. 24.1). From anterior to posterior sections, these bulges correspond to the gyrus ambiens (gA, Figs. 24.1 and 24.2; part of the ERc), the uncinate gyrus

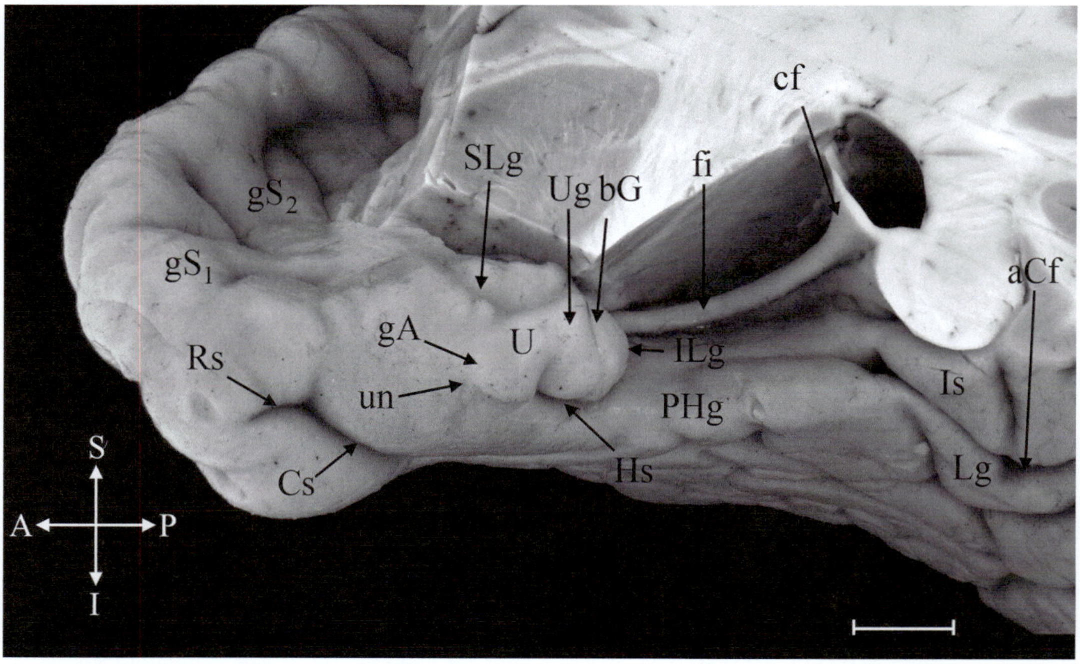

Fig. 24.1 A superomedial view of the right MTL. *Abbreviations*: *aCf* anterior calcarine fissure, *bG* band of Giacomini, *Cs* collateral sulcus, *cf* crus of the fornix, *fi* fimbria, *gA* gyrus ambiens, *gS* gyrus of Schwalbe (this brain has two gyri of Schwalbe, indicated by subscripts), *Hs* hippocampal sulcus, *ILg* intralimbic gyrus, *Is* isthmus, *Lg* lingual gyrus, *PHg* parahippocampal gyrus, *Rs* rhinal sulcus, *SLg* semilunar gyrus, *U* uncus *Ug* uncinate gyrus, and *un* uncal notch. The temporal lobe is viewed from slightly oblique angle medially. Crosshairs indicate *S* superior, *A* anterior, *I* inferior, and *P* posterior. The bar represents circa 1 cm

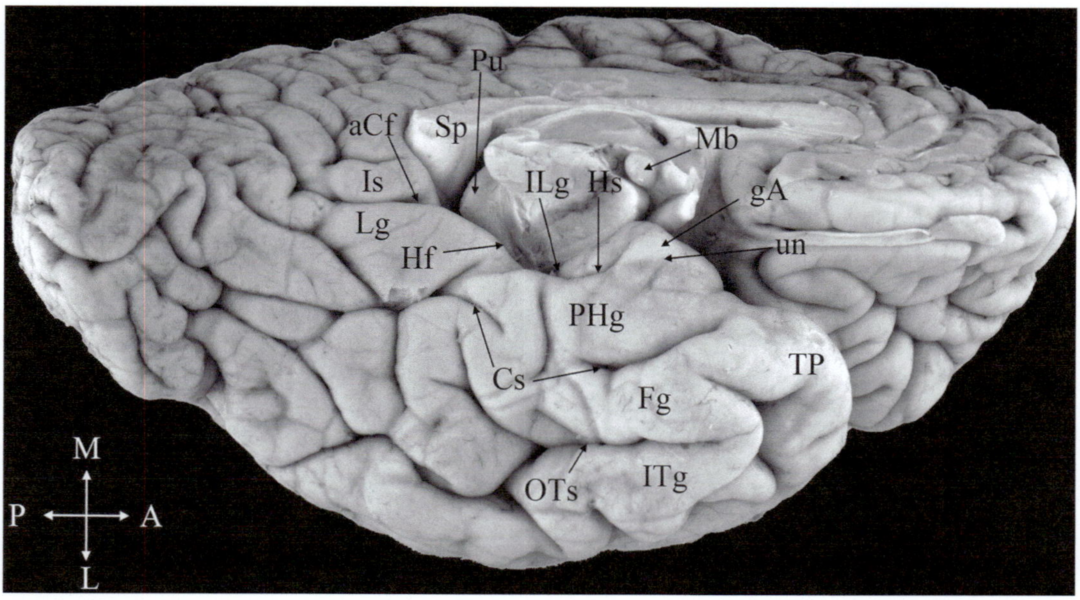

Fig. 24.2 An inferior view of the left cerebral hemisphere. In this brain, the collateral sulcus has an interrupted trajectory. *Abbreviations*: *aCf* anterior calcarine fissure, *Cs* collateral sulcus, *Fg* fusiform gyrus, *gA* gyrus ambiens, *Hf* hippocampal fissure, *Hs* hippocampal sulcus, *ILg* intralimbic gyrus, *Is* isthmus, *ITg* inferotemporal gyrus, *Lg* lingual gyrus, *Mb* mamillary body, *OTs* occipitotemporal sulcus, *Pu* pulvinar, *PHg* parahippocampal gyrus, *Sp* splenium of the corpus callosum, *TP* temporal pole, and *un* uncal notch. The approximate anatomical directions are indicated by crosshairs (*M* medial, *A* anterior, *L* lateral, *P* posterior)

(Ug, Fig. 24.1), and the intralimbic gyrus (ILg, Figs. 24.1, 24.2, 24.6, and 24.7), where the band of Giacomini (bG, Fig. 24.1) separates the uncinate from the intralimbic gyrus. The posterior apex of the intralimbic gyrus represents an important anatomical landmark for the separation of the ERc/PRc from the PHc (see below). The uncal notch (un; Figs. 24.1 and 24.2) is an indentation formed mechanically by the free edge of the tentorium cerebelli (Van Hoesen et al. 2000). The parahippocampal gyrus containing most of the ERc, PRc, and PHc lies inferolateral to the uncus (PHg, Figs. 24.1 and 24.2). The parahippocampal gyrus is bordered inferolaterally by the fusiform gyrus. The temporal pole (TP, Fig. 24.2) represents the anterior extreme of the entire MTL, and it typically contains one or two gyri of Schwalbe on its superior surface (gS, Figs. 24.1 and 24.3).

The hippocampal sulcus (Hs, Fig. 24.1; also known as the uncal sulcus) separates the uncus from the adjacent parahippocampal gyrus (Insausti and Amaral 2004). It starts as a shallow sulcus and deepens progressively at more posterior levels. Posterior to the apex of the intralimbic gyrus, that is, after the uncus ends, the hippocampal sulcus continues as the hippocampal fissure (Fig. 24.2). At more lateral and anterior levels, the rhinal sulcus (Rs, Fig. 24.1) separates the parahippocampal gyrus from the temporal pole (Hanke 1997). The collateral sulcus replaces the rhinal sulcus at more posterior levels, where it separates the parahippocampal gyrus from the fusiform gyrus (Fig. 24.2). The rhinal and collateral sulci are anatomically variable across individuals, for example, the collateral sulcus may be deep or shallow, may bifurcate, or may be interrupted along its anterior-posterior extent. The occipitotemporal sulcus (OTs; Fig. 24.2) is the most lateral sulcus on the ventral surface of the temporal lobe (Fig. 24.2) and separates the fusiform gyrus from the inferior temporal gyrus (ITg, Fig. 24.2; Van Hoesen et al. 2000). At its most posterior levels, the parahippocampal gyrus is longitudinally divided into two gyri by the anterior calcarine fissure (aCf; Figs. 24.1, 24.2, and 24.9): the superior part forms the isthmus of the retrosplenial cortex (Is, Fig. 24.1), while the inferior part forms the lingual gyrus (Lg; Figs. 24.1 and 24.9).

24.4.2 A Segmentation Protocol for the MTL

A protocol for identifying the anatomical borders of the MTL substructures is described below. The protocol begins with the most anterior and lateral structure – the PRc – and continues medially to the ERc, posteriorly to the PHc before describing the most medial structure, the hippocampus proper. All landmarks are based on anatomical studies of the MTL in humans and nonhuman primates (e.g., von Economo and Koskinas 1925; Hopf 1956; Watson et al. 1992; Insausti et al. 1998; Pruessner et al. 2000, 2002; Malykhin et al. 2007; Taylor and Probst 2008) and were

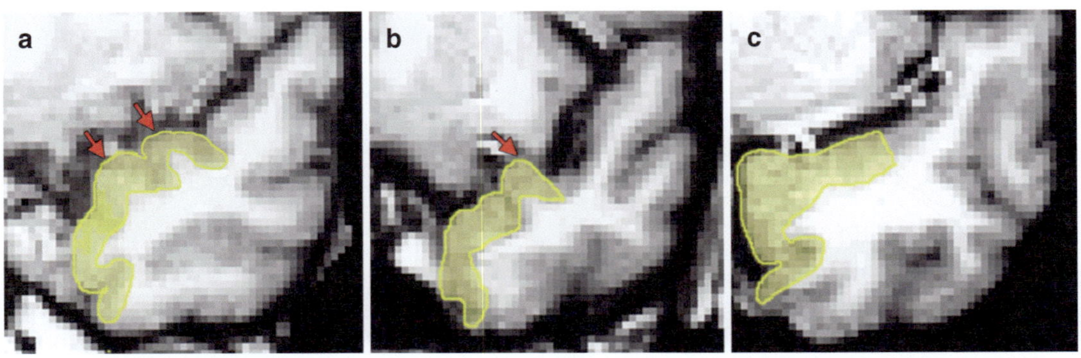

Fig. 24.3 Native space coronal slices of the right hemisphere temporal pole area 1–2 mm anterior to the limen insulae. The figure illustrates the three variants of the gyri of Schwalbe (*red arrows*) and corresponding locations of the PRc (*yellow outlines*): (**a**) a case with two gyri of Schwalbe, (**b**) a case with one gyrus of Schwalbe, and (**c**) a case whose superior aspect of the temporal pole is relatively flat, indicating no gyri of Schwalbe

selected such that they can be readily identified on structural MR images. All landmarks refer to coronal views of volumes of 1 cubic mm resolution reoriented along the AC-PC axis and assume that the contrast is set to optimize the differentiation of gray from white matter.

24.4.2.1 Borders of the Perirhinal Cortex

The PRc lies folded inside the collateral sulcus such that only a small part is visible from the cortical surface (Fig. 24.4). The PRc is bordered anteriorly by the temporal pole, posteriorly by the PHc, medially mainly by the ERc, and laterally by the fusiform gyrus. The medial portion of the PRc, that is, the TR, is a cytoarchitectonically distinct transition region between the PRc and ERc and notable as the site of incipient cortical neurofibrillary pathology in AD (Fig. 24.4; Braak and Braak 1985). The anteriorly situated temporal pole is a heterogenous cortex which shares some commonalities with the PRc (Suzuki and Amaral 2003a; Blaizot et al. 2010). According to some authors, the PRc extends into temporopolar cortex (Suzuki and Amaral 2003a; Insausti et al. 1998; Ding et al. 2009; but see also Brodmann 1909; von Bonin and Bailey 1947). However, since the precise extension of the PRc into the temporal pole and the corresponding anatomical borders are under debate (*cf.* Insausti et al. 1998; Ding et al. 2009; Ding and Van Hoesen 2010), the tempopolar cortex is excluded from this protocol.

The PRc is one of the most challenging structures to identify, in part because the boundaries of this structure have been redefined over time (Suzuki and Amaral 2003b) and because of the variability of its key anatomical landmark – the collateral sulcus (Hanke 1997; Pruessner et al. 2002). The medial and posterior PRc landmarks described below apply to the whole PRc including the TR, its medial extent. After a description of the anatomical borders of the PRc, the anatomical borders of the TR are defined. All landmarks take into account the dependence of the PRc and TR location on the shape and depth of the collateral sulcus (Insausti et al. 1998; Taylor and Probst 2008).

Perirhinal Cortex

Anterior Border

A cytoarchitectonic study of the human MTL demonstrated that the anterior portion of the

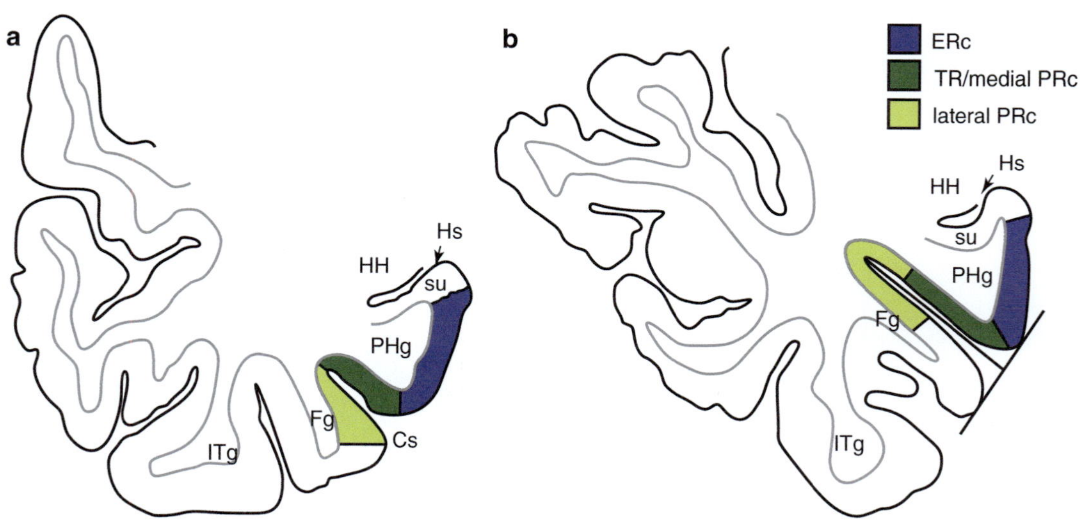

Fig. 24.4 Coronal view of the medial temporal lobe at the level of the hippocampal sulcus (similar coronal level as Fig. 24.8). The locations of the PRc and TR depend on the depth of the collateral sulcus (*Cs*; see text): (**a**) borders when the collateral sulcus is of regular depth (i.e., 1–1.5 cm) and (**b**) when the collateral sulcus is deep (i.e., > 1.5 cm). Abbreviations: *Fg* fusiform gyrus, *HH* hippocampal head, *Hs* hippocampal sulcus, *ITg* inferotemporal gyrus, *PHg* parahippocampal gyrus, *su* subiculum of the hippocampus

PRc wraps around the anterior end of the ERc (Insausti et al. 1998). The anterior border of the PRc is located circa 24 mm posterior to the apex of the temporal pole or a few millimeters anterior to the most anterior appearance of gray matter of the limen insulae (i.e., frontotemporal junction; Fig. 24.8; Insausti et al. 1998). Since the length of the temporal pole is more variable than the appearance of the limen insulae gray matter, the anterior PRc border is defined as 2 mm anterior to the most anterior coronal slice containing gray matter in the limen insulae, which corresponds to approximately $y = 9$ in MNI coordinates (Fig. 24.8). The collateral sulcus is typically visible at this level. As noted above, the cytoarchitectonic similarities between the temporopolar region and the PRc indicate that this border may underestimate the true anterior extent of the PRc; however, the resolution of this issue requires additional research (see, e.g., Insausti et al. 1998; Suzuki and Amaral 2003b).

Superolateral/Medial Border

At levels anterior to the limen insulae, the superolateral border is defined with respect to the number and position of the gyri of Schwalbe, which are considered part of the PRc (see Figs. 24.1, 24.3, and 24.8). In the presence of two gyri of Schwalbe, each laterally bordered by a temporopolar sulcus (prevalence ca. 80%; Insausti et al. 1998), the superolateral border is the fundus of the most lateral temporopolar sulcus (Figs. 24.3a and 24.8). When there is one gyrus of Schwalbe (prevalence ca. 12%; Insausti et al. 1998), the superolateral border of the PRc is defined as the fundus of the temporopolar sulcus (see Fig. 24.3b). If the gyrus of Schwalbe is not visible (prevalence ca. 8%; Insausti et al. 1998), the superolateral border is defined as the midpoint between the medial and lateral corners of the superior surface of the temporal pole (Fig. 24.3c; Insausti et al. 1998).

At the level of the gray matter of the limen insulae and posterior to this landmark, the medial border of the PRc is the shoulder of the medial bank of the collateral sulcus (Fig. 24.8; Insausti et al. 1998; Taylor and Probst 2008). This also serves as the medial border of the entire TR (see below). If the collateral sulcus is not yet present, or is discontinuous, the medial PRc border is estimated by approximating the angle of the trajectory of the shoulder of the medial bank of the collateral sulcus from more posterior slices.[5] If the collateral sulcus is bifurcated, the criteria described above are applied to the most medial sulcus (Taylor and Probst 2008). Posteriorly, the PRc wraps medially around the ERc and extends 2–4 mm posterior to the last slice containing the apex of the intralimbic gyrus (i.e., the posterior border of the ERc). At this level, the medial border of the PRc extends to the most medial aspect of the parahippocampal gyrus (*cf.* medial ERc border below).

Lateral Border

The lateral border of the PRc depends on the length and shape of the collateral sulcus (Insausti et al. 1998). If the collateral sulcus is of regular depth between 1 and 1.5 cm deep (82% of cases; Insausti et al. 1998), the lateral boundary is the shoulder of the lateral bank of the collateral sulcus (Fig. 24.4a). If the collateral sulcus is shallow, that is, less than 1 cm deep (16% of cases; Insausti et al. 1998), the lateral border is the midpoint of the fusiform gyrus. We note that this criterion is not applied to the most anterior sections where the collateral sulcus begins to appear; in these anterior sections, the criteria for the regular collateral sulcus are applied or the border is estimated from more posterior slices with an obvious collateral sulcus (*cf.* (Insausti et al. 1998), Fig. 24.5). Finally, if the collateral sulcus is deeper than 1.5 cm (2% of cases), the lateral border is the midpoint between the fundus and the shoulder of the lateral bank of the collateral sulcus (Fig. 24.4b).

Posterior Border

As in its anterior aspect, the PRc wraps around the posterior end of the ERc forming a border averaging 3 mm wide (range, 2–4 mm; Insausti et al. 1998; see also Krimer et al. 1997). The

[5]The protocol assumes that in cases where the collateral sulcus cannot be visualized or is discontinuous, the lateral and medial PRc borders are determined on coronal slices anterior and posterior to the interrupted section, and that imaginary lines are drawn from these anterior and posterior levels to connect the lateral borders and the medial borders of the PRc.

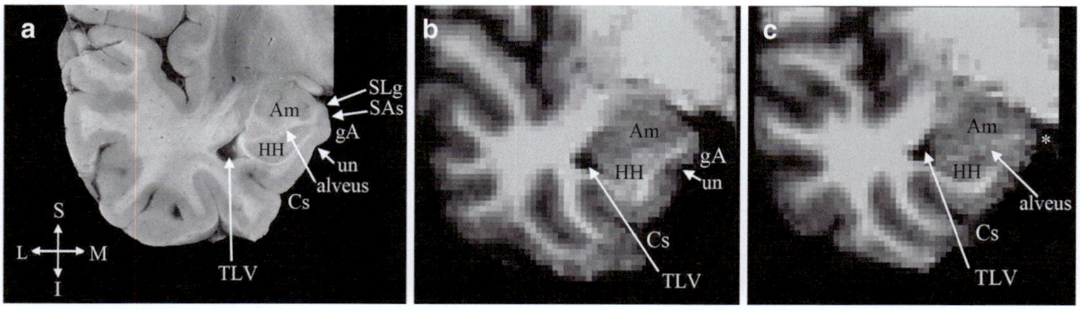

Fig. 24.5 Sections of the temporal lobe at the level of the uncus (approximate MNI $y = -5$): (**a**) a histological section and (**b**) an MRI slice at a similar coronal level where the gyrus ambiens (*gA*) and uncal notch (*un*) are visible. (**c**) An MRI slice at a similar coronal level where the gA and un are not visible. In these instances, the medial apex of the parahippocampal gyrus (*asterisk*) is defined as the medial ERc border. Abbreviations: *Am* amygdala, *Cs* collateral sulcus, *gA* gyrus ambiens, *HH* hippocampal head, *SAs* semiannular sulcus, *SLg* semilunar gyrus and *TLV* temporal horn of the lateral ventricle, *un* uncal notch. Anatomical directions: *S* superior, *M* medial, *I* inferior, *L* lateral

posterior border is therefore set at 3 mm posterior to the last coronal slice still containing the apex of the intralimbic gyrus, that is, the posterior border of the ERc (e.g., if the last coronal slice containing the intralimbic gyrus is MNI $y = -18$, the last posterior slice with the PRc is MNI $y = -21$, see Fig. 24.8).

Transentorhinal Area

Anterior Border

The medial aspect of the PRc, the TR, is defined as an area of transition between the ERc and PRc (Braak and Braak 1985). Therefore, its anterior border is defined as the first slice where the ERc is present, that is, 2 mm posterior to the first anterior slice where the white matter of the limen insulae is visible (Fig. 24.8; see Sect. 19.4.2.2).

Medial Border

The medial border of the TR is identical to the medial border of the PRc described above, that is, the shoulder of the medial bank of the collateral sulcus (Insausti et al. 1998; Taylor and Probst 2008; Fig. 24.4 and 24.8.

Lateral Border

If the depth of the collateral sulcus equals or is less than 1.5 cm, the lateral border of the TR is defined as the fundus of the collateral sulcus (Fig. 24.4a; Taylor and Probst 2008). If the collateral sulcus is deeper than 1.5 cm, the lateral border is the midpoint between (i) the shoulder of the medial bank of the collateral sulcus and (ii) the midpoint of the lateral bank of the collateral sulcus (Fig. 24.4b; Insausti et al. 1998; Taylor and Probst 2008). If the collateral sulcus is bifurcated, these criteria are applied to the most medial sulcus (Taylor and Probst 2008).

Posterior Border

The posterior border of the TR is identical to the posterior border of the ERc, that is, 1 mm posterior to the last slice containing the apex of the intralimbic gyrus (see below).

24.4.2.2 Borders of the Entorhinal Cortex

The ERc is the largest cortical field on the parahippocampal gyrus and is entirely visible from the medial surface view. Macroscopically, the anterior portion of the ERc is characterized by small bumps on the cortical surface called *verrucae hippocampi* (Klingler 1948). The ERc encompasses the gyrus ambiens at anterior levels (Figs. 24.1, 24.2, 24.5, and 24.8). The gyrus ambiens is superomedially neighbored by the semiannular sulcus, beyond which lies the semilunar gyrus of the periamygdaloid cortex. At more posterior levels, the subiculum of the hippocampus proper neighbors the ERc superomedially. The PRc surrounds the anterior, inferior, and lateral sides of the ERc (Insausti et al. 1998).

Anterior Border

Cytoarchitectonic studies have demonstrated that the PRc surrounds the anterior end of the ERc (Insausti et al. 1998). However, because the oblique orientation of the anterior end of the ERc is difficult to delineate, a conservative anterior border is defined corresponding to the most anterior coronal slice with the full extent of the ERc (but see Insausti et al. 1998). This level corresponds approximately to a coronal slice 2 mm posterior to the first anterior slice where the white matter of the limen insulae is visible. Note that because of this conservative border, a segment of the MTL is left uncategorized (Fig. 24.8).

Medial Border

At anterior levels, the medial border of the ERc is the semiannular sulcus (Fig. 24.5). However, because this sulcus is very shallow and seldom identifiable on MR images, the medial border of the anterior ERc is defined here as the midpoint (i.e., medial apex) of the gyrus ambiens (Figs. 24.5b, 24.8). If the gyrus ambiens is not visible, the medial border is the shoulder (i.e., medial apex) of the superomedial bank of the parahippocampal gyrus (see Fig. 24.5c, 24.8). The medial ERc border moves slightly inferiorly when the hippocampal sulcus emerges (Fig. 24.8). However, because this transition is difficult to detect on MR images, an arbitrary landmark is defined as 1 mm anterior to first anterior slice where the hippocampal sulcus can be visualized (see Fig. 24.8). At this and more posterior levels, the most medial extent of the parahippocampal gyrus, that is, its medial apex, is the medial border of the ERc.

Lateral Border

The lateral border of the ERc is identical to the medial border of the PRc/TR (see above and Figs. 24.4 and 24.8; Taylor and Probst 2008; Krimer et al. 1997).

Posterior Border

The posterior border of the ERc is defined as 1 mm posterior to the last slice containing the apex of the intralimbic gyrus (Fig. 24.6; note that the apex is located in between slices Fig. 24.8, $y = -18$, which is not shown).

24.4.2.3 Borders of the Parahippocampal Cortex

The PHc is located in the posterior portion of the parahippocampal gyrus posterior to the PRc and ERc (Van Hoesen 1982; Sewards 2011). However, disagreement exists regarding the precise cytoarchitectonic features of the PHc, and correspondingly, the anatomical boundaries of the PHc are inconsistently defined in the literature (see, e.g., von Economo and Koskinas 1925; Hopf 1956; Saleem et al. 2007; Thangavel et al. 2008). Here, we draw upon the conceptualizations of the PHc as a proisocortical region, that is, a transitional zone between allocortex and neocortex, and as the posterior continuation of the PRc and ERc

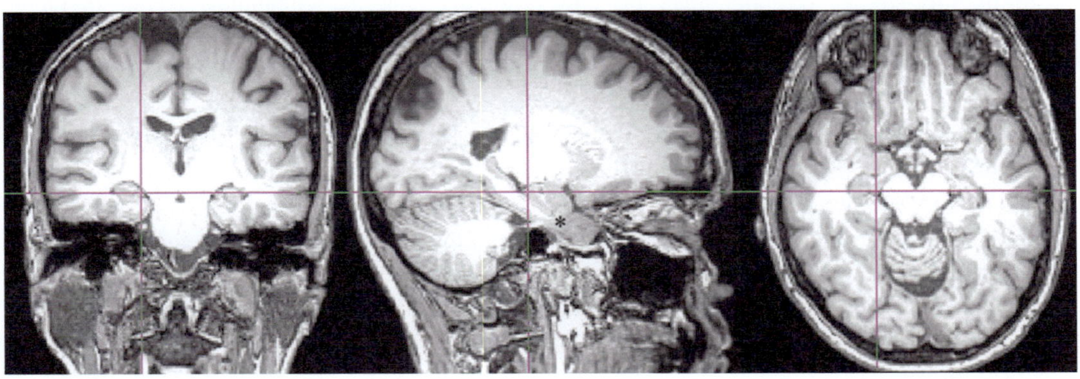

Fig. 24.6 Coronal, sagittal, and axial views of one participant with the crosshair position indicating the location of the apex of the intralimbic gyrus. The *asterisk* in the sagittal view indicates the cone-shaped crossing of the alveus and parahippocampal gyrus white matter, which marks the anterior limit of the hippocampal head

(Suzuki and Amaral 2003a; Saleem et al. 2007). Thus, the definition of the lateral border of the PHc described below is consistent with Hopf (1956; see also Sewards 2011) and corresponds closely to anatomical descriptions in nonhuman primates (Suzuki and Amaral 2003a; Saleem et al. 2007).

As noted above, the PHc is defined as the posterior continuation of the PRc and ERc, located inferolateral to the subiculum of the hippocampal body and tail. Posteriorly, the anterior calcarine fissure divides the PHc longitudinally into the inferiorly situated lingual gyrus and the superiorly situated isthmus of the retrosplenial cortex (Figs. 24.1, 24.2, and 24.9). The PHc occupies parts of the lingual gyrus and merges without clear anatomical landmarks with the infra- and retrosplenial cortices (Vogt et al. 2006). For this reason, the posterior limit of the PHc is conservatively restricted to levels anterior to the emergence of the calcarine fissure.

Anterior Border

The anterior boundary of the PHc is defined as the first slice after the posterior border of PRc, that is, 4 mm posterior to the last slice containing the apex of the intralimbic gyrus (Fig. 24.9).

Medial Border

The subiculum of the hippocampus proper neighbors the PHc medially (*cf.* Figure 24.4). Thus, the medial border is the medial apex of the parahippocampal gyrus (Fig. 24.9).

Lateral Border

According to studies on nonhuman primates (Suzuki and Amaral 2003a; Saleem et al. 2007) and the myeloarchitectonic study by Hopf (1956; see Sewards 2011), the PHc represents the posterior extension of the PRc and ERc (but see von Economo and Koskinas 1925). Thus, the lateral border of the PHc is adjusted according to the depth of the collateral sulcus in the same manner as for the lateral border of the PRc (see Section "Perirhinal Cortex"; Figs. 24.4 and 24.9).

Posterior Border

The posterior end of the PHc is funnel-shaped and progressively merges with the retrosplenial region. According to Vogt et al. (2006), the PHc extends posteriorly several millimeters past the posterior limit of the splenium. However, because the medial and lateral PHc borders at these posterior levels are unclear, a conservative posterior border is defined as the first posterior slice where the pulvinar is no longer visible (Figs. 24.2 and 24.9). Anterior to this level, the lateral and medial landmarks described above can be used.

24.4.2.4 Borders of the Hippocampus Proper

This chapter focuses on the retrocommissural part of the hippocampus proper, extending from the inferior and medial side of the amygdala at the uncinate gyrus to an area posterior and inferior to the splenium of the corpus callosum (Fig. 24.7). This part of the hippocampus is entirely situated inferior to the corpus callosum and appears as a C-shaped structure when viewed from above (Fig. 24.7). Posterior to the apex of the uncus, the hippocampus proper arches laterally around the upper midbrain and curves medially and superiorly, continuing as a thin strip of gray matter of vestigial hippocampus (*indusium griseum*) on the superior surface of the corpus callosum (supracommissural hippocampus) before descending at anterior levels to the subcallosal area (precommissural hippocampus). The supra- and precommissural hippocampi are excluded from this segmentation. The alveus is made of the fibers emanating from the pyramidal cells of the hippocampus. It covers the Ammon's horn superiorly and laterally (Fig. 24.5), and its fibers converge to form the fimbria, oriented roughly along the longitudinal axis of the hippocampus (Duvernoy 1998). The fimbria is continuous with a prominent, flattened white matter tract, the crus of the fornix (Figs. 24.1 and 24.9), which begins at posterior levels of the hippocampus and curves superomedially below the corpus callosum. These white matter tracts likewise are excluded from the segmentation (Hogan et al. 2000; Pantel et al. 2000, but see also Pruessner et al. 2000; Malykhin et al. 2007).

Because different anterior to posterior areas of the hippocampus exhibit different patterns of connectivity (Witter and Amaral 1991), which presumably corresponds to functional specializa-

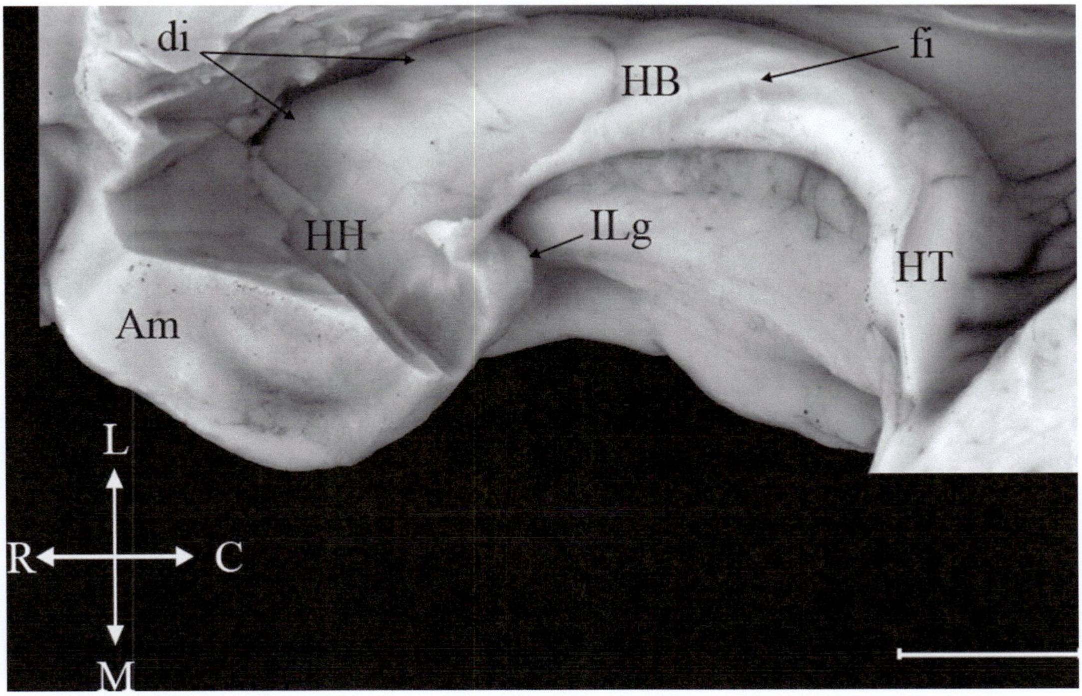

Fig. 24.7 Superior view of the C-shaped hippocampal formation on the right hemisphere after removing the roof of the temporal horn and parts of the amygdala. This view thereby reveals the intra- and extraventricular aspects of the hippocampal formation. Abbreviations: *Am* amygdala, *di* hippocampal digitations, *fi* fimbria, *HB* hippocampal body, *HH* hippocampal head, *HT* hippocampal tail, and *ILg* intralimbic gyrus. *Anatomical directions*: *L* lateral, *P* posterior, *M* medial, and *A* anterior. The bar represents circa 1 cm

tion along its longitudinal axis (see Sect. 19.2; Colombo et al. 1998; Moser and Moser 1998; Giovanello et al. 2004), we describe anatomical landmarks for the hippocampal head, body, and tail separately (see also Watson et al. 1992; Pantel et al. 2000; Pruessner et al. 2000; Maller et al. 2006; Malykhin et al. 2007). Anatomical tracing typically starts at the anterior border of the hippocampal body and continues to the posterior end of the hippocampal tail. The most anterior aspect, the hippocampal head, lies adjacent to the amygdala and is the most challenging hippocampal structure to trace. This protocol, therefore, starts with the body of the hippocampus and then discusses the tail and finally the head of the hippocampus.

Hippocampal Body

The hippocampal body consists of subfields CA1–3 and the subiculum which is located on the superior bank of the parahippocampal gyrus. The fimbria is located on the superomedial side of the hippocampus and has a slightly curved trajectory toward the hippocampal tail, where it leaves the hippocampus and continues its path superomedially as the crus of the fornix (Fig. 24.1). For a graphical illustration of the segmentation of the hippocampal body, see Figs. 24.8 and 24.9.

Anterior Border

The anterior border of the hippocampal body is defined as one slice posterior to the posterior apex of the intralimbic gyrus (i.e., the last slice containing the intralimbic gyrus; Fig. 24.8; Malykhin et al. 2007).

Medial Border

The subiculum of the hippocampus proper extends to the medial apex of the parahippocampal gyrus, which represents the medial border of the hippocampus proper (Figs. 24.8 and 24.9; Watson et al. 1992).

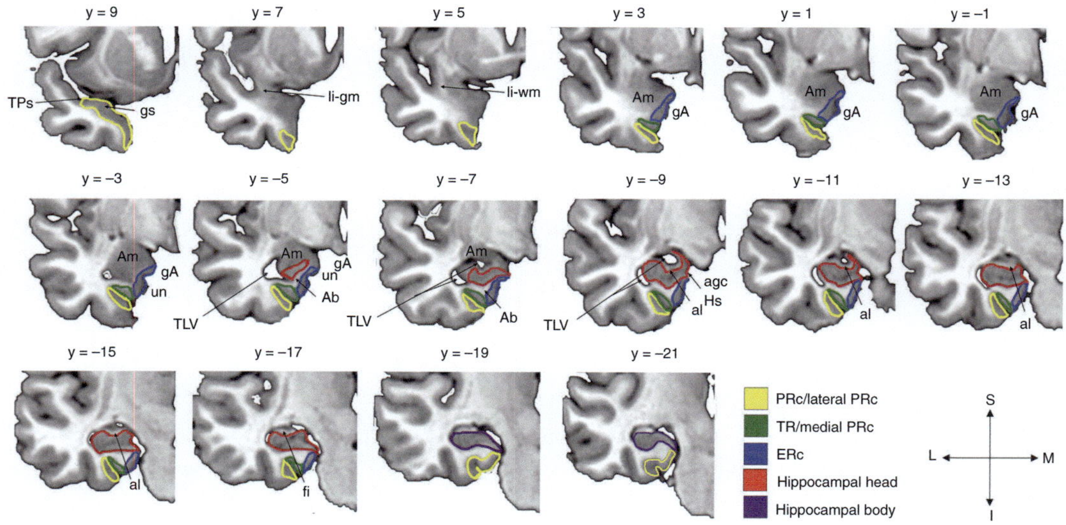

Fig. 24.8 Coronal sections of the temporal lobe at anterior to posterior levels every 2 mm. The coronal level is identified in MNI coordinates. The asterisk represents the most anterior slice where the TLV is continuous with the quadrigeminal cistern (i.e., where ventricular slit is present). The structures are drawn on an MriCron template (http://www.mccauslandcenter.sc.edu/mricro/mricron/). Note that a part of the medical surface is unsegmented due to the unreliability of tracing the oblique anterior end of the ERc (see text). The fimbria begins only at the level of posterior hippocampal head. *Abbreviations*: *Ab* angular bundle (parahippocampal gyrus white matter), *al* alveus, *Am* amygdala, *fi* fimbria, *gA* gyrus ambiens, *Hs* hippocampal sulcus, *ILg* intralimbic gyrus (the apex is located at y = −18), *qgc* quadrigeminal cistern, li-*gm* limen insulae gray matter, *li-wm* limen insulae white matter, *TLV* temporal horn of the lateral ventricle, and *un* uncal notch. Anatomical directions: *S* superior, *M* medial, *I* inferior, and *L* lateral

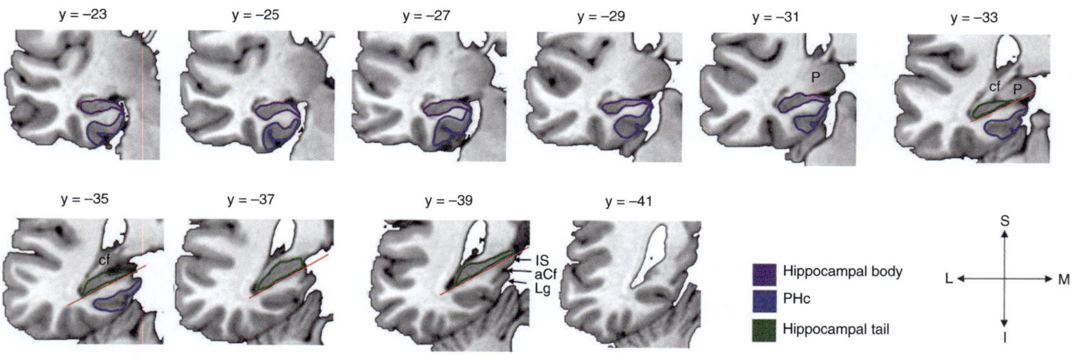

Fig. 24.9 Coronal sections of the temporal lobe at anterior to posterior levels every 2 mm. The numbers represent different coronal levels in MNI (*y*) coordinates. The structures are drawn on an MriCron template (http://www.mccauslandcenter.sc.edu/mricro/mricron/). The red line illustrates the arbitrary border used as the inferomedial limit of the hippocampal tail. *Abbreviations*: *aCf* anterior calcarine fissure, *cf* crus of the fornix, *Is* isthmus, *Lg* lingual gyrus, and *P* pulvinar. Anatomical directions: *S* superior, *M* medial, *I* inferior, and *L* lateral

Lateral Border

The body of the hippocampus extends laterally to the temporal horn of the lateral ventricle (Figs. 24.8 and 24.9; Pantel et al. 2000; Pruessner et al. 2000; Malykhin et al. 2007).

Inferior Border

Inferiorly and inferomedially, the body of the hippocampus is bordered by the white matter of the angular bundle of the parahippocampal gyrus (Figs. 24.8 and 24.9; Pantel et al. 2000; Malykhin et al. 2007).

Superior Border

The temporal horn of the lateral ventricle forms the superior boundary of the hippocampal body. Care should be taken to exclude the white matter of the fimbria (Hogan et al. 2000; Pantel et al. 2000 but see also Pruessner et al. 2000; Malykhin et al. 2007). Sagittal views may aid the visualization of the continuous border between the hippocampus proper and the cerebrospinal fluid of the lateral ventricle. Care must also be taken to exclude the voluminous choroid plexus, which fills the temporal horn of the lateral ventricle on the superior aspect of the hippocampus.

Posterior Border

The posterior border of the body of the hippocampus is one slice posterior to the first coronal slice where the crus of the fornix is clearly separated from the wall of the lateral ventricle or where its full profile is visible in columnar form, even if it is still attached to the lateral ventricle (Fig. 24.9; Maller et al. 2006; Malykhin et al. 2007).

Hippocampal Tail

The tail of the hippocampus proper funnels slightly and turns medially before steeply ascending around the splenium of the corpus callosum (Fig. 24.7). The CA1 subfield occupies a progressively more medial position and forms the gyrus of Andreas Retzius on the surface of the parahippocampal gyrus, while the CA3 subfield forms the gyrus fasciolaris on the superior aspect of the hippocampal fissure (Duvernoy 1998). The location of the hippocampal tail is illustrated in Fig. 24.9.

Anterior Border

The anterior border of the hippocampal tail is defined as the first slice posterior to the posterior limit of the hippocampal body (Fig. 24.9; Maller et al. 2006; Malykhin et al. 2007).

Medial Border

The isthmus is located on the medial aspect of the hippocampus in an area which had been occupied by the subiculum at more anterior levels (Fig. 24.9). To ensure the exclusion of the isthmus, an arbitrary medial border for the hippocampal tail is defined: an oblique, straight line drawn from the inside inferolateral corner of the angular bundle along the white matter of the parahippocampal gyrus to the quadrigeminal cistern (see Fig. 24.9). The hippocampal tail is defined as the gray matter superolateral to this line.

Lateral Border

The lateral border of the hippocampal tail is the white matter of the ascending crus of the fornix and the temporal horn of the lateral ventricle (Fig. 24.9; Pantel et al. 2000; Maller et al. 2006).

Superior Border

The tail of the hippocampus proper is superiorly bordered by the crus of the fornix and the white matter of the splenium of the corpus callosum (Fig. 24.9). The pulvinar should be carefully avoided; toward this end, the sagittal plane is helpful in distinguishing the gray matter of the hippocampal tail from the gray matter of the thalamus (Pantel et al. 2000; Malykhin et al. 2007).

Inferior Border

The inferior border is the white matter of the parahippocampal gyrus (Pantel et al. 2000; Malykhin et al. 2007).

Posterior Border

The posterior portion of the hippocampal tail appears as an ovoid-shaped mass of gray matter (Fig. 24.9). The complete disappearance of this shape marks the posterior limit of the hippocampal formation (Fig. 24.9).

Hippocampal Head

The hippocampal head (CA1–3, dentate gyrus, subiculum) abutting the temporal horn of the lateral ventricle bends medially and again posteriorly to become part of the uncus (Insausti and Amaral 2004). Anteriorly, the head of the hippocampus is located inferior to the amygdala (Fig. 24.7), which occupies a progressively larger superolateral area of the hippocampal-amygdaloid complex at more anterior levels (Fig. 24.8). Segmentation begins at posterior levels.

Posterior Border

The posterior border of the hippocampal head is the apex of the intralimbic gyrus, that is, the last slice containing this structure (Figs. 24.6 and 24.8; Duvernoy 1998; Malykhin et al. 2007).

This point may best be identified by navigating through sagittal slices.

Medial Border

At posterior levels, the hippocampal head is segmented up to the most medial apex of the parahippocampal gyrus (Fig. 24.8), whereas at anterior levels, the medial border is limited by the white matter of the parahippocampal gyrus (Fig. 24.8). The transition between the two landmarks takes place one slice anterior to the most anterior slice where the uncal sulcus is last visible, corresponding approximately to the level where the semilunar gyrus and anterior cortical nucleus of the amygdala appear.

Lateral Border

The lateral border is the medial wall of the temporal horn of the lateral ventricle (Pantel et al. 2000; Pruessner et al. 2000). If the white matter of the alveus is visible next to the wall of the lateral ventricle, it is excluded (Hogan et al. 2000; Pantel et al. 2000).

Superior Border

At posterior levels, the superior border can be identified as the temporal horn of the lateral ventricle or the white matter of the alveus if visible (Fig. 24.8). At more anterior levels where the amygdala is no longer separated from the hippocampus by a ventricular slit (transition approximately at Fig. 24.8), the hippocampus is delimited from the amygdala using the white matter of the alveus surrounding the superior aspect of the hippocampal head (Watson et al. 1992). If the alveus is not visible, especially at the most anterior levels, the location of the alveus and thus superior border is estimated from sagittal slices, where the alveus is usually easier to identify. The uncal recess of the inferior horn of the lateral ventricle may additionally aid delineation of the superomedial border of the hippocampal head (Watson et al. 1992; Hogan et al. 2000; Pruessner et al. 2000).

Inferior Border

The hippocampal head is inferiorly bordered by the white matter of the parahippocampal gyrus (Malykhin et al. 2007; Pruessner et al. 2000).

Anterior Border

The anterior border is defined as the most anterior corner of the conical profile formed by the parahippocampal gyrus white matter and the alveus, as visualized on sagittal views (see Fig. 24.6; Pantel et al. 2000; Pruessner et al. 2000). When this point is selected on the sagittal slice, the view is changed to coronal, where the medial, lateral, superior, and inferior borders can be identified.

24.5 fMRI in Alzheimer's Disease

Several techniques have been used to study AD-related disruptions of brain function. These include fMRI during cognitive tasks and during rest. Studies focusing on task-related activity in AD have found patterns of relative BOLD activation and deactivation depending on disease stage and the specific task used (e.g., Bondi et al. 2005; Gould et al. 2006; Rémy et al. 2005; Rombouts et al. 2005). However, the use of task-related fMRI may be impractical in the context of AD, particularly in clinical settings. The data may be difficult to obtain as the tasks more often than not require a significant amount of effort from the participant. The interpretation of these data may also prove challenging as patients with AD pathology may differ considerably in the levels of cognitive performance and the ability to sustain attention. In comparison, resting-state measurements do not require the participant to engage in a task, and they are, therefore, less strenuous for the patient. The interpretation of data may also be more straightforward as individual levels of task performance do not need to be taken into account.

Resting-state fMRI is based on fluctuations of spontaneous metabolic activity during rest, and it is most often used to test functional coupling or connectivity of different brain regions (for reviews, see Dennis and Thompson 2014; Liu et al. 2008). Several studies have reported decreases in hippocampal connectivity during rest in subjects with AD-related pathology (e.g., Allen et al. 2007; Wang et al. 2006). Specifically, AD has been shown to be associated with reduced hippocampal connectivity with multiple areas in the brain, including the medial prefrontal cortex and anterior cingulate cortex. These regions are associated with episodic memory and may, therefore, play a role in the memory dysfunction in AD.

Independent component analysis has revealed disruptions in resting-state networks in AD. Most prominently, AD is associated with reductions in the default mode network connectivity, particularly in the hippocampus and posterior cingulate (Agosta et al. 2012; Binnewijzend et al. 2012; Damoiseaux et al. 2012; Greicius et al. 2004; Petrella et al. 2011). Several authors have also found increases particularly in the prefrontal cortex resting-state connectivity (Agosta et al. 2012; Supekar et al. 2008; Wang et al. 2006). In one study, the connectivity in the executive network in AD was associated with performance in tasks of executive functioning and language (Agosta et al. 2012) with increase in activity associated with better cognitive score. Therefore, the authors interpreted the findings as reflecting a compensatory mechanism in response to the pathological changes taking place in the brain.

The studies indicate that there are typical patterns of fMRI resting-state connectivity in AD. In the future, these measures may help in the detection of AD and may predict the conversion of AD longitudinally. However, to date, these measures have not been shown to be better predictors of AD pathology than cognitive scores (Petrella et al. 2011).

24.6 Summary

This chapter skimmed the surface of research on the functional neuroanatomy of the MTL. The most influential model of MTL functioning today emphasizes the role of the entire MTL in the formation of conscious memories. This view is supported by numerous patient findings as well as the dense interconnectivity within the MTL, enabling the subregions to work in concert, acting as a unified region. Animal and more recently human neuroscientific research, using ever more sophisticated methods and neuropsychological paradigms, indicates additional levels of processing in the MTL beyond declarative memory formation. Hierarchical, connectivity-based approaches provide a framework within which to study these multidimensional aspects of cognitive functioning in which each MTL subregion is also functionally specialized for a particular kind of information processing. This work not only furthers our basic understanding of the functional neuroanatomy of this complex system but also has obvious clinical implications for patients with acquired brain damage and neurodegenerative disorders, most notably AD. Thus, concerted activity among all MTL structures appears to take place in parallel with functionally specialized processing in each substructure, enabling successful memory encoding and retrieval of complex events, concepts, and scenes.

The prerequisite for advancements in MTL research is the use of well-defined and reliable anatomic landmarks, such as those reported in this chapter. Moreover, the use of different methodologies, tasks, and populations is essential to increase our understanding of human MTL function. Case or patient studies remain a cornerstone in MTL research, providing valuable information about the functions that are lost as a consequence of different kinds and locations of brain damage (e.g., Squire and Wixted 2011). However, this approach is limited by the fact that lesions typically encompass more than one cytoarchitectonic area, that is, that selective lesions of PRc, ERc, or PHc are rare. Thus, voxel-based volumetric methods (e.g., Tyler et al. 2005; Ashburner 2007) and surface-based methods offer increasingly reliable anatomical precision in patient studies (Dale et al. 1999; Fischl et al. 1999; Klein et al. 2010; Kivisaari et al. 2012). FMRI in healthy individuals, in particular, high-resolution imaging, has become increasingly important as it provides high spatial information on the systems normally engaged during a particular task (e.g., Henson 2005), although it does not provide information about whether the activated regions are *necessary* for the particular function. Finally, resting-state fMRI and diffusion-tensor imaging, among others, can increase our knowledge about the functional and structural connectivity of these areas in vivo, respectively, which is fundamental to our understanding of how the MTL areas work as a network and interact with other brain areas (e.g., Wang et al. 2006; Catani and Thiebaut de Schotten 2008). Converging evidence from diverse neuroscientific approaches using valid anatomic guidelines is expected to significantly increase our functional-neuroanatomic understanding of the MTL.

Acknowledgments The authors thank Dr. Daniela Hirni and Dr. Mia Liljeström for comments and helpful discussions. The authors also thank photographer Martin Portmann and the Departments of Neuropathology and Neuroradiology, University Hospital Basel, for providing the postmortem and MRI brain data, respectively. This research was supported by a Swiss National Science Foundation Ambizione Fellowship (KIT), a grant from the Alzheimer's Association of Both Basels (KIT), Academy of Finland (grant #286070 to SLK), the Finnish Concordia Fund (SLK), the Finnish Cultural Foundation (SLK), and the Swiss Federal Commission for Scholarships for Foreign Students (Berne) (SLK).

References

Acres K, Taylor KI et al (2009) Complementary hemispheric asymmetries in object naming and recognition: a voxel-based correlational study. Neuropsychologia 47:1836–1843

Aggleton JP, Brown MW (1999) Episodic memory, amnesia, and the hippocampal-anterior thalamic axis. Behav Brain Sci 22:425–489

Aggleton JP, Brown MW (2006) Interleaving brain systems for episodic and recognition memory. Trends Cogn Sci 10:455–463

Aggleton JP, Mishkin M (1985) Mamillary-body lesions and visual recognition in monkeys. Exp Brain Res 58:190–197

Agosta F, Pievani M, Geroldi C, Copetti M, Frisoni GB, Filippi M (2012) Resting state fMRI in Alzheimer's disease: beyond the default mode network. Neurobiol Aging 33:1564–1578

Aguirre GK, D'Esposito M (1999) Topographical dis-orientation: a synthesis and taxonomy. Brain 122:1613–1628

Allen G, Barnard H, McColl R et al (2007) Reduced hippocampal functional connectivity in Alzheimer disease. Arch Neurol 64:1482–1487

Alvarado MC, Bachevalier J (2005a) Comparison of the effects of damage to the perirhinal and parahippocampal cortex on transverse patterning and location memory in rhesus macaques. J Neurosci 25:1599–1609

Alvarado MC, Bachevalier J (2005b) Selective neurotoxic damage to the hippocampal formation impairs performance of the transverse patterning and location memory tasks in rhesus macaques. Hippocampus 15:118–131

Alvarado MC, Wright AA et al (2002) Object and spatial relational memory in adult rhesus monkeys is impaired by neonatal lesions of the hippocampal formation but not the amygdaloid complex. Hippocampus 12:421–433

Alzheimer's Association (2011) 2011 Alzheimer's disease facts and figures. Alzheimers Dement 7: 208–244

American Psychiatric Association (ed) (1994) Diagnostic and statistical manual of mental disorders, 4th edn. American Psychiatric Association, Washington, DC

Ashburner J (2007) A fast diffeomorphic image registration algorithm. NeuroImage 38:95–113

Bachevalier J, Nemanic S (2008) Memory for spatial location and object-place associations are differently processed by the hippocampal formation, parahippocampal areas TH/TF and perirhinal cortex. Hippocampus 18:64–80

Bakker A, Kirwan CB et al (2008) Pattern separation in the human hippocampal CA3 and dentate gyrus. Science 319:1640–1642

Bar M, Aminoff E (2003) Cortical analysis of visual context. Neuron 38:347–358

Bar M, Aminoff E et al (2008) Scenes unseen: the parahippocampal cortex intrinsically subserves contextual associations, not scenes or places per se. J Neurosci 28:8539–8544

Barbeau E, Didic M et al (2004) Evaluation of visual recognition memory in MCI patients. Neurology 62:1317–1322

Barense MD, Bussey TJ et al (2005) Functional specialization in the human medial temporal lobe. J Neurosci 25:10239–10246

Barense MD, Gaffan D et al (2007) The human medial temporal lobe processes online representations of complex objects. Neuropsychologia 45: 2963–2974

Barense MD, Henson RNA et al (2010) Medial temporal lobe activity during complex discrimination of faces, objects, and scenes: effects of viewpoint. Hippocampus 20:389–401

Barrash J (1998) A historical review of topographical disorientation and its neuroanatomical correlates. J Clin Exp Neuropsychol 20:807–827

Barrash J, Damasio H et al (2000) The neuroanatomical correlates of route learning impairment. Neuropsychologia 38:820–836

Bellgowan PSF, Bandettini PA et al (2006) Improved BOLD detection in the medial temporal region using parallel imaging and voxel volume reduction. NeuroImage 29:1244–1251

Binnewijzend MAA, Schoonheim MM, Sanz-Arigita E et al (2012) Resting-state fMRI changes in Alzheimer's disease and mild cognitive impairment. Neurobiol Aging 33:2018–2028

Blaizot X, Mansilla F et al (2010) The human parahippocampal region: I. Temporal pole cytoarchitectonic and MRI correlation. Cereb Cortex 20:2198–2212

Bohbot VD, Allen JJB et al (2000) Memory deficits characterized by patterns of lesions to the hippocampus and parahippocampal cortex. Ann N Y Acad Sci 911:355–368

Bondi MW, Houston WS et al (2005) FMRI evidence of compensatory mechanisms in older adults at genetic risk for Alzheimer disease. Neurology 64: 501–508

Braak H, Braak E (1985) On areas of transition between entorhinal allocortex and temporal isocortex in the human brain. Normal morphology and lamina-specific pathology in Alzheimer's disease. Acta Neuropathol 68:325–332

Braak H, Braak E (1991) Neuropathological stageing of Alzheimer-related changes. Acta Neuropathol 82:239–259

Brodmann K (1909) Vergleichende Lokalisationlehre der Grosshirnrinde. Barth, Leipzig

Brown MW, Aggleton JP (2001) Recognition memory: what are the roles of the perirhinal cortex and hippocampus? Nat Rev Neurosci 2:51–61

Buffalo EA, Bellgowan PSF et al (2006) Distinct roles for medial temporal lobe structures in memory for objects and their locations. Learn Mem 13:638–643

Burgess N, Maguire EA et al (2001) A temporoparietal and prefrontal network for retrieving the spatial context of lifelike events. NeuroImage 14:439–453

Burgess N, Maguire EA et al (2002) The human hippocampus and spatial and episodic memory. Neuron 35:625–641

Bussey TJ, Saksida LM (2002) The organization of visual object representations: a connectionist model of effects of lesions in perirhinal cortex. Eur J Neurosci 15:355–364

Bussey TJ, Saksida LM et al (2002) Perirhinal cortex resolves feature ambiguity in complex visual discriminations. Eur J Neurosci 15(2):365–374

Bussey TJ, Saksida LM et al (2005) The perceptual-mnemonic/feature conjunction model of perirhinal cortex function. Q J Exp Psychol B 58:269–282

Canto CB, Wouterlood FG et al (2008) What does anatomical organization of entorhinal cortex tell us? Neural Plast 2008:1–18

Carr VA, Rissman J et al (2010) Imaging the human medial temporal lobe with high-resolution fMRI. Neuron 65:298–308

Catani M, Thiebaut de Schotten M (2008) A diffusion tensor imaging tractography atlas for virtual in vivo dissections. Cortex 44:1105–1132

Chrobak JJ, Amaral DG (2007) Entorhinal cortex of the monkey: VII. Intrinsic connections. J Comp Neurol 500:612–633

Colombo M, Fernandez T et al (1998) Functional differentiation along the anterior-posterior axis of the hippocampus in monkeys. J Neurophysiol 80:1002–1005

Corkin S (1984) Lasting consequences of bilateral medial temporal lobectomy: clinical course and experimental findings in H.M. Semin Neurol 4:249–259

Corkin S, Amaral DG et al (1997) H. M'.s medial temporal lobe lesion: findings from magnetic resonance imaging. J Neurosci 17:3964–3979

Coutureau E, Di Scala G (2009) Entorhinal cortex and cognition. Prog Neuro-Psychopharmacol Biol Psychiatry 33:753–761

Crutch SJ, Lehmann M et al (2012) Posterior cortical atrophy. Lancet Neurol 11:170–178

Cusack R, Russell B et al (2005) An evaluation of the use of passive shimming to improve frontal sensitivity in fMRI. NeuroImage 24:82–91

Dale AM, Fischl B et al (1999) Cortical surface-based analysis—I. Segmentation and surface reconstruction. Neuroimage 9:179–194

Damoiseaux JS, Prater KE, Miller BL et al (2012) Functional connectivity tracks clinical deterioration in Alzheimer's disease. Neurobiol Aging 33:828.e19–828.e30

Davachi L (2006) Item, context and relational episodic encoding in humans. Curr Opin Neurobiol 16:693–700

Davachi L, Wagner AD (2002) Hippocampal contributions to episodic encoding: insights from relational and item-based learning. J Neurophysiol 88: 982–990

De Renzi E (1982) Disorders of space exploration and cognition. Wiley, New York

De Renzi E, Faglioni P et al (1977) Topographical amnesia. J Neurol Neurosurg Psychiatry 40:498–505

Deng W, Aimone JB et al (2010) New neurons and new memories: how does adult hippocampal neurogenesis affect learning and memory? Nat Rev Neurosci 11:339–350

Dennis EL, Thompson PM (2014) Functional brain connectivity using fMRI in aging and Alzheimer's disease. Neuropsychol Rev 24:49–62

Di Paola M, Macaluso E et al (2007) Episodic memory impairment in patients with Alzheimer's disease is correlated with entorhinal cortex atrophy a voxel-based morphometry study. J Neurol 254:774–781

Diana RA, Yonelinas AP et al (2007) Imaging recollection and familiarity in the medial temporal lobe: a three-component model. Trends Cogn Sci 11:379–386

Dickerson BC, Sperling RA (2008) Functional abnormalities of the medial temporal lobe memory system in mild cognitive impairment and Alzheimer's disease: insights from functional MRI studies. Neuropsychologia 46:1624–1635

Dickerson BC, Salat DH et al (2004) Medial temporal lobe function and structure in mild cognitive impairment. Ann Neurol 56:27–35

Dickerson BC, Feczko E et al (2009) Differential effects of aging and Alzheimer's disease on medial temporal lobe cortical thickness and surface area. Neurobiol Aging 30(3):432–440

Ding S-L, Van Hoesen GW (2010) Borders, extent, and topography of human perirhinal cortex as revealed using multiple modern neuroanatomical and pathological markers. Hum Brain Mapp 31:1359–1379

Ding S-L, Van Hoesen GW et al (2009) Parcellation of human temporal polar cortex: a combined analysis of multiple cytoarchitectonic, chemoarchitectonic, and pathological markers. J Comp Neurol 514:595–623

Doeller CF, Barry C et al (2010) Evidence for grid cells in a human memory network. Nature 463:657–661

Dolorfo CL, Amaral DG (1998) Entorhinal cortex of the rat: topographic organization of the cells of origin of the perforant path projection to the dentate gyrus. J Comp Neurol 398:25–48

Duvernoy HM (1998) The human hippocampus, 2nd edn. Springer, Belin

Eichenbaum H, Dudchenko P et al (1999) The hippocampus, memory and place cells: is it spatial memory or a memory space? Neuron 23:209–226

Eichenbaum H, Yonelinas AP et al (2007) The medial temporal lobe and recognition memory. Annu Rev Neurosci 30:123–152

Epstein R, Kanwisher N (1998) A cortical representation of the local visual environment. Nature 392: 598–601

Epstein R, Harris A et al (1999) The parahippocampal place area: recognition, navigation, or encoding? Neuron 23:115–125

Eustache F, Desgranges B et al (2001) Entorhinal cortex disruption causes memory deficit in early Alzheimer's disease as shown by PET. Neuroreport 12:683–685

Ewers M, Sperling RA et al (2011) Neuroimaging markers for the prediction and early diagnosis of Alzheimer's disease dementia. Trends Neurosci 34:430–442

Fischl B, Sereno MI et al (1999) Cortical surface-based analysis—II: inflation, flattening, and a surface-based coordinate system. NeuroImage 9:195–207

Fyhn M, Molden S et al (2004) Spatial representation in the entorhinal cortex. Science 305:1258–1264

Fyhn M, Hafting T et al (2007) Hippocampal remapping and grid realignment in entorhinal cortex. Nature 446:190–194

Gadian DG, Aicardi J et al (2000) Developmental amnesia associated with early hypoxic–ischaemic injury. Brain 123:499–507

Gale SD, Hopkins RO (2004) Effects of hypoxia on the brain: neuroimaging and neuropsychological findings following carbon monoxide poisoning and obstructive sleep apnea. J Int Neuropsychol Soc 10:60–71

Ghoshal N, García-Sierra F et al (2002) Tau conformational changes correspond to impairments of episodic memory in mild cognitive impairment and Alzheimer's disease. Exp Neurol 177:475–493

Giovanello KS, Schnyer DM et al (2004) A critical role for the anterior hippocampus in relational memory: evidence from an fMRI study comparing associative and item recognition. Hippocampus 14:5–8

Gould RL, Brown RG, Owen AM et al (2006) Task-induced deactivations during successful paired associates learning: an effect of age but not Alzheimer's disease. NeuroImage 31:818–831

Greicius MD, Srivastava G, Reiss AL et al (2004) Default-mode network activity distinguishes Alzheimer's disease from healthy aging: evidence from functional MRI. Proc Natl Acad Sci 101:4637–4642

Grill-Spector K, Malach R (2004) The human visual cortex. Annu Rev Neurosci 27:649–677

Guillozet AL, Weintraub S et al (2003) Neurofibrillary tangles, amyloid, and memory in aging and mild cognitive impairment. Arch Neurol 60:729–736

Hafting T, Fyhn M et al (2005) Microstructure of a spatial map in the entorhinal cortex. Nature 436:801–806

Hanke J (1997) Sulcal pattern of the anterior parahippocampal gyrus in the human adult. Ann Anat 179:335–339

Hannula DE, Ranganath C (2008) Medial temporal lobe activity predicts successful relational memory binding. J Neurosci 28:116–124

Hasselmo ME, Brandon MP (2008) Linking cellular mechanisms to behavior: entorhinal persistent spiking and membrane potential oscillations may underlie path integration, grid cell firing, and episodic memory. Neural Plast 2008:1–12

Henke K (2010) A model for memory systems based on processing modes rather than consciousness. Nat Rev Neurosci 11:523–532

Henke K, Buck A et al (1997) Human hippocampus establishes associations in memory. Hippocampus 7:249–256

Henke K, Kroll NEA et al (1999a) Memory lost and regained following bilateral hippocampal damage. J Cogn Neurosci 11:682–697

Henke K, Weber B et al (1999b) Human hippocampus associates information in memory. Proc Natl Acad Sci U S A 96:5884–5889

Henson R (2005) A mini-review of fMRI studies of human medial temporal lobe activity associated with recognition memory. Q J Exp Psychol B 58:340–360

Hirni D, Monsch AU et al (2011) Relative association of perirhinal and entorhinal cortex integrity with semantic and episodic memory performance: implications for early detection of Alzheimer's disease. In: 288.0 Neuroscience meeting planner. Society for Neuroscience, Washington, DC

Hogan RE, Mark KE et al (2000) Mesial temporal sclerosis and temporal lobe epilepsy: MR imaging deformation-based segmentation of the hippocampus in five patients. Radiology 216:291–297

Hopf A (1956) Über die Verteilung myeloarchitektonischer Merkmale in der Stirnhirnrinde beim Menschen. J Hirnforsch 2:311–333

Insausti R, Amaral DG (2004) Hippocampal formation. In: Paxinos G, Mai JK (eds) The human nervous system. Elsevier, Amsterdam, pp 871–914

Insausti R, Amaral DG et al (1987) The entorhinal cortex of the monkey: II. Cortical afferents. J Comp Neurol 264:356–395

Insausti R, Juottonen K et al (1998) MR volumetric analysis of the human entorhinal, perirhinal, and temporopolar cortices. AJNR Am J Neuroradiol 19: 659–671

Jacobs J, Kahana MJ et al (2010) A sense of direction in human entorhinal cortex. Proc Natl Acad Sci U S A 107:6487–6492

Jung MW, Wiener SI et al (1994) Comparison of spatial firing characteristics of units in dorsal and ventral hippocampus of the rat. J Neurosci 14:7347–7356

Juottonen K, Laakso MP et al (1998) Volumes of the entorhinal and perirhinal cortices in Alzheimer's disease. Neurobiol Aging 19(1):15–22

Kivisaari SL, Tyler LK et al (2012) Medial perirhinal cortex disambiguates confusable objects. Brain 135:3757–3769

Klein A, Ghosh SS et al (2010) Evaluation of volume-based and surface-based brain image registration methods. NeuroImage 51:214–220

Klingler J (1948) Die makroskopische Anatomie der Ammonsformation. Kommissionsverlag von Gebrüder Fretz A.G, Zürich

Köhler S, Crane J et al (2002) Differential contributions of the parahippocampal place area and the anterior hippocampus to human memory for scenes. Hippocampus 12:718–723

Köhler S, Danckert S et al (2005) Novelty responses to relational and non-relational information in the hippocampus and the parahippocampal region: a comparison based on event-related fMRI. Hippocampus 15:763–774

Kravitz DJ, Saleem KS et al (2011) A new neural framework for visuospatial processing. Nat Rev Neurosci 12:217–230

Krimer LS, Hyde TM et al (1997) The entorhinal cortex: an examination of cyto- and myeloarchitectonic organization in humans. Cereb Cortex 7:722–731

Lashley KS (1929) Brain mechanisms and intelligence: a quantitative study of injuries to the brain. University of Chicago Press, Chicago

Lavenex P, Amaral DG (2000) Hippocampal-neocortical interaction: a hierarchy of associativity. Hippocampus 10:420–430

Lavenex P, Suzuki WA et al (2004) Perirhinal and parahippocampal cortices of the macaque monkey: intrinsic projections and interconnections. J Comp Neurol 472:371–394

Lee ACH, Barense MD et al (2005) The contribution of the human medial temporal lobe to perception: bridging the gap between animal and human studies. Q J Exp Psychol B 58:300–325

Lee ACH, Scahill VL et al (2008) Activating the medial temporal lobe during oddity judgment for faces and scenes. Cereb Cortex 18:683–696

Leonard BW, Amaral DG et al (1995) Transient memory impairment in monkeys with bilateral lesions of the entorhinal cortex. J Neurosci 15:5637–5659

Lerch JP, Pruessner JC et al (2005) Focal decline of cortical thickness in Alzheimer's disease identified by computational neuroanatomy. Cereb Cortex 15:995–1001

Leutgeb JK, Leutgeb S et al (2007) Pattern separation in the dentate gyrus and CA3 of the hippocampus. Science 315:961–966

Lipton PA, Eichenbaum H (2008) Complementary roles of hippocampus and medial entorhinal cortex in episodic memory. Neural Plast 2008:1–8

Liu Z, Murray EA et al (2000) Learning motivational significance of visual cues for reward schedules requires rhinal cortex. Nat Neurosci 3:1307–1315

Liu Y, Wang K, Yu C et al (2008) Regional homogeneity, functional connectivity and imaging markers of Alzheimer's disease: a review of resting-state fMRI studies. Neuropsychologia 46:1648–1656

Machulda MM, Ward HA et al (2003) Comparison of memory fMRI response among normal, MCI, and Alzheimer's patients. Neurology 61:500–506

Maguire EA, Frith CD et al (1998) Knowing where things are: parahippocampal involvement in encoding object locations in virtual large-scale space. J Cogn Neurosci 10:61–76

Mahut H, Zola-Morgan S et al (1982) Hippocampal resections impair associative learning and recognition memory in the monkey. J Neurosci 2:1214–1220

Maller JJ, Réglade-Meslin C et al (2006) Sex and symmetry differences in hippocampal volumetrics: before and beyond the opening of the crus of the fornix. Hippocampus 16:80–90

Malykhin NV, Bouchard TP et al (2007) Three-dimensional volumetric analysis and reconstruction of amygdala and hippocampal head, body and tail. Psychiatry Res 155:155–165

Mattson MP (2004) Pathways towards and away from Alzheimer's disease. Nature 430:631–639

Meunier M, Bachevalier J et al (1993) Effects on visual recognition of combined and separate ablations of the entorhinal and perirhinal cortex in rhesus monkeys. J Neurosci 13:5418–5432

Mishkin M (1978) Memory in monkeys severely impaired by combined but not by separate removal of amygdala and hippocampus. Nature 273:297–298

Mishkin M, Ungerleider LG et al (1983) Object vision and spatial vision: two cortical pathways. Trends Neurosci 6:414–417

Mishkin M, Suzuki WA et al (1997) Hierarchical organization of cognitive memory. Philos Trans R Soc Lond B Boil Sci 352:1461–1467

Montaldi D, Mayes AR (2010) The role of recollection and familiarity in the functional differentiation of the medial temporal lobes. Hippocampus 20:1291–1314

Montaldi D, Mayes AR (2011) Familiarity, recollection and medial temporal lobe function: an unresolved issue. Trends Cogn Sci 15:339–340

Moscovitch M, Rosenbaum RS et al (2005) Functional neuroanatomy of remote episodic, semantic and spatial memory: a unified account based on multiple trace theory. J Anat 207:35–66

Moser M-B, Moser EI (1998) Functional differentiation in the hippocampus. Hippocampus 8:608–619

Moss HE, Rodd JM et al (2005) Anteromedial temporal cortex supports fine-grained differentiation among objects. Cereb Cortex 15:616–627

Murray EA, Mishkin M (1998) Object recognition and location memory in monkeys with excitotoxic lesions of the amygdala and hippocampus. J Neurosci 18:6568–6582

Murray EA, Richmond BJ (2001) Role of perirhinal cortex in object perception, memory, and associations. Curr Opin Neurobiol 11:188–193

Murray EA, Malkova L et al (1998) Crossmodal associations, intramodal associations, and object identification in macaque monkeys. In: Milner AD (ed) Comparative neuropsychology. Oxford University Press, Oxford, pp 51–69

O'Donnell P, Buxton PJ et al (2000) The magnetic resonance imaging appearances of the brain in acute carbon monoxide poisoning. Clin Radiol 55:273–280

O'Kane G, Kensinger EA et al (2004) Evidence for semantic learning in profound amnesia: an investigation with patient H.M. Hippocampus 14:417–425

O'Keefe J, Dostrovsky J (1971) The hippocampus as a spatial map: preliminary evidence from unit activity in the freely-moving rat. Brain Res 34:171–175

O'Neil EB, Cate AD et al (2009) Perirhinal cortex contributes to accuracy in recognition memory and perceptual discriminations. J Neurosci 29:8329–8334

O'Reilly RC, McClelland JL (1994) Hippocampal conjunctive encoding, storage, and recall: avoiding a trade-off. Hippocampus 4:661–682

Pantel J, O'Leary DS et al (2000) A new method for the in vivo volumetric measurement of the human hippocampus with high neuroanatomical accuracy. Hippocampus 10:752–758

Paterson A, Zancwill OL (1945) A case of topographical disorientation associated with a unilateral cerebral lesion. Brain 68:188–212

Petrella JR, Sheldon FC, Prince SE (2011) Default mode network connectivity in stable vs progressive mild cognitive impairment. Neurology 76:511–517

Pihlajamäki M, Tanila H et al (2004) Visual presentation of novel objects and new spatial arrangements of objects differentially activates the medial temporal lobe subareas in humans. Eur J Neurosci 19:1939–1949

Pruessner JC, Li LM et al (2000) Volumetry of hippocampus and amygdala with high-resolution MRI and three-dimensional analysis software: minimizing the discrepancies between laboratories. Cereb Cortex 10:433–442

Pruessner JC, Köhler S et al (2002) Volumetry of temporopolar, perirhinal, entorhinal and parahippocampal cortex from high-resolution MR images: considering the variability of the collateral sulcus. Cereb Cortex 12:1342–1353

Qiu C, Kivipelto M et al (2009) Epidemiology of Alzheimer's disease: occurrence, determinants, and strategies toward intervention. Dialogues Clin Neurosci 11:111–128

Ranganath C (2010) A unified framework for the functional organization of the medial temporal lobes and the phenomenology of episodic memory. Hippocampus 20:1263–1290

Rémy F, Mirrashed F, Campbell B et al (2005) Verbal episodic memory impairment in Alzheimer's disease: a combined structural and functional MRI study. NeuroImage 25:253–266

Rolls ET (2007) An attractor network in the hippocampus: theory and neurophysiology. Learn Mem 14:714–731

Rombouts SARB, Barkhof F et al (2000) Functional MR imaging in Alzheimer's disease during memory encoding. AJNR Am J Neuroradiol 21:1869–1875

Rombouts SARB, Goekoop R, Stam CJ et al (2005) Delayed rather than decreased BOLD response as a marker for early Alzheimer's disease. NeuroImage 26:1078–1085

Saleem KS, Price JL et al (2007) Cytoarchitectonic and chemoarchitectonic subdivisions of the perirhinal and parahippocampal cortices in macaque monkeys. J Comp Neurol 500:973–1006

Salmon DP (2011) Neuropsychological features of mild cognitive impairment and preclinical Alzheimer's disease. Curr Top Behav Neurosci 179:34–41

Salmon DP, Bondi MW (2009) Neuropsychological assessment of dementia. Annu Rev Psychol 60:257–282

Schmidt CF, Degonda N et al (2005) Sensitivity-encoded (SENSE) echo planar fMRI at 3T in the medial temporal lobe. NeuroImage 25:625–641

Schwarzbauer C, Mildner T et al (2010) Dual echo EPI – the method of choice for fMRI in the presence of magnetic field inhomogeneities? NeuroImage 49:316–326

Scoville WB, Milner B (1957) Loss of recent memory after bilateral hippocampal lesions. J Neurol Neurosurg Psychiatry 20:11–21

Sewards TV (2011) Adolf Hopf's 1954 myeloarchitectonic parcellation of the human temporal lobe: a review and assessment. Brain Res Bull 86:298–313

Silbert LC, Quinn JF et al (2003) Changes in premorbid brain volume predict Alzheimer's disease pathology. Neurology 61:487–492

Skotko BG, Rubin DC et al (2008) H.M'.s personal crossword puzzles: understanding memory and language. Memory 16:89–96

Squire LR, Wixted JT (2011) The cognitive neuroscience of human memory since H.M. Annu Rev Neurosci 34:259–288

Squire LR, Zola SM (1998) Episodic memory, semantic memory and amnesia. Hippocampus 8:205–211

Squire LR, Zola-Morgan S (1988) Memory: brain systems and behavior. Trends Neurosci 11:170–175

Squire LR, Stark CEL et al (2004) The medial temporal lobe. Annu Rev Neurosci 27:279–306

Staresina BP, Duncan KD et al (2011) Perirhinal and parahippocampal cortices differentially contribute to later recollection of object- and scene-related event details. J Neurosci 31:8739–8747

Steffenach H-A, Witter M et al (2005) Spatial memory in the rat requires the dorsolateral band of the entorhinal cortex. Neuron 45(2):301–313

Supekar K, Menon V, Rubin D et al (2008) Network analysis of intrinsic functional brain connectivity in Alzheimer's disease. PLoS Comput Biol 4:e1000100

Suzuki WA, Amaral DG (1994a) Perirhinal and parahippocampal cortices of the macaque monkey: cortical afferents. J Comp Neurol 350:497–533

Suzuki WA, Amaral DG (1994b) Topographic organization of the reciprocal connections between the monkey entorhinal cortex and the perirhinal and parahippocampal cortices. J Neurosci 14:1856–1877

Suzuki WA, Amaral DG (2003a) Perirhinal and parahippocampal cortices of the macaque monkey: cytoarchitectonic and chemoarchitectonic organization. J Comp Neurol 463:67–91

Suzuki WA, Amaral DG (2003b) Where are the perirhinal and parahippocampal cortices? A historical overview of the nomenclature and boundaries applied to the primate medial temporal lobe. Neuroscience 120:893–906

Suzuki WA, Miller EK et al (1997) Object and place memory in the macaque entorhinal cortex. J Neurophysiol 78:1062–1081

Takahashi S, Yonezawa H et al (2002) Selective reduction of diffusion anisotropy in white matter of Alzheimer disease brains measured by 3.0 Tesla magnetic resonance imaging. Neurosci Lett 332:45–48

Taylor KI, Monsch AU (2007) The neuropsychology of Alzheimer's disease. In: Richter RW, Richter BZ (eds) Alzheimer's disease? The basics. A physician's guide to the practical management. The Humana Press Inc., Totowa

Taylor KI, Probst A (2008) Anatomic localization of the transentorhinal region of the perirhinal cortex. Neurobiol Aging 29:1591–1596

Taylor KI, Moss HE et al (2006) Binding crossmodal object features in perirhinal cortex. Proc Natl Acad Sci U S A 103:8239–8244

Taylor KI, Probst A et al (2008) Clinical course of neuropathologically confirmed frontal-variant Alzheimer's disease. Nat Clin Pract Neurol 4:226–232

Taylor KI, Stamatakis EA et al (2009) Crossmodal integration of object features: voxel-based correlations in brain-damaged patients. Brain 132:671–683

Taylor KI, Devereux BJ et al (2011a) Conceptual structure: towards an integrated neuro-cognitive account. Lang Cogn Proc 26:1368–1401

Taylor KI, Kivisaari S et al (2011b) Crossmodal integration of audiovisual objects is related to anteromedial temporal lobe integrity in patients with very early Alzheimer's disease. In: 287.20 Neuroscience meeting planner. Society for Neuroscience, Washington, D.C.

Thangavel R, Van Hoesen GW et al (2008) Posterior parahippocampal gyrus pathology in Alzheimer's disease. Neuroscience 154:667–676

Tyler LK, Stamatakis EA et al (2004) Processing objects at different levels of specificity. J Cogn Neurosci 16(3):351–362

Tyler LK, Marslen-Wilson W et al (2005) Dissociating neuro-cognitive component processes: voxel-based correlational methodology. Neuropsychologia 43:771–778

Van Hoesen GW (1982) The parahippocampal gyrus: new observations regarding its cortical connections in the monkey. Trends Neurosci 5:345–350

Van Hoesen GW (1995) Anatomy of the medial temporal lobe. Magn Reson Imaging 13:1047–1055

Van Hoesen GW, Augustinak JC et al (2000) The parahippocampal gyrus in Alzheimer's disease: clinical and preclinical neuroanatomical correlates. Ann N Y Acad Sci 911:254–274

Vargha-Khadem F, Gadian DG et al (1997) Differential effects of early hippocampal pathology on episodic and semantic memory. Science 277:376–380

Victor M, Adams RD et al (1989) The Wernicke-Korsakoff syndrome and related neurologic disorders due to alcoholism and malnutrition, 2nd edn. F.A. Davis Co, Philadelphia

Vogt BA, Vogt L et al (2006) Cytology and functionally correlated circuits of human posterior cingulate areas. NeuroImage 29:452–466

von Bonin G, Bailey P (1947) The neocortex of *Macaca mulatta*. University of Illinois Press, Urbana

von Economo C, Koskinas GN (1925) Die Cytoarchitecktonik der Grosshirnrinde des erwachsenen Menschen. Springer, Berlin

Wallenstein GV, Hasselmo ME et al (1998) The hippocampus as an associator of discontiguous events. Trends Neurosci 21:317–323

Wang L, Zang Y et al (2006) Changes in hippocampal connectivity in the early stages of Alzheimer's disease: evidence from resting state fMRI. NeuroImage 31:496–504

Wang W-C, Lazzara MM et al (2010) The medial temporal lobe supports conceptual implicit memory. Neuron 68:835–842

Watson C, Andermann F et al (1992) Anatomic basis of amygdaloid and hippocampal volume measurement by magnetic resonance imaging. Neurology 42:1743–1750

Whiteley AM, Warrington EK (1978) Selective impairment of topographical memory: a single case study. J Neurol Neurosurg Psychiatry 41:575–578

Winblad B, Palmer K et al (2004) Mild cognitive impairment—beyond controversies, towards a consensus: report of the International Working Group on Mild Cognitive Impairment. J Intern Med 256:240–246

Witter MP (2007) The perforant path: projections from the entorhinal cortex to the dentate gyrus. In: Scharfman HE (ed) The dentate gyrus: a comprehensive guide to structure, function, and clinical implications. Elsevier, Boston, pp 43–61

Witter MP, Amaral DG (1991) Entorhinal cortex of the monkey: V. Projections to the dentate gyrus, hippocampus, and subicular complex. J Comp Neurol 307:437–459

Witter MP, Moser EI (2006) Spatial representation and the architecture of the entorhinal cortex. Trends Neurosci 29:671–678

Yassa MA, Stark CEL (2011) Pattern separation in the hippocampus. Trends Neurosci 34:515–525

Yonelinas AP (2002) The nature of recollection and familiarity: a review of 30 years of research. J Mem Lang 46:441–517

Zilles K, Amunts K (2009) Receptor mapping: architecture of the human cerebral cortex. Curr Opin Neurol 22:331–339

Zola-Morgan S, Squire LR et al (1986) Human amnesia and the medial temporal region: enduring memory impairment following a bilateral lesion limited to field CA1 of the hippocampus. J Neurosci 6: 2950–2967

Zola-Morgan S, Squire LR et al (1989a) Lesions of the hippocampal formation but not lesions of the fornix or the mammillary nuclei produce long-lasting memory impairment in monkeys. J Neurosci 9:898–913

Zola-Morgan S, Squire LR et al (1989b) Lesions of the amygdala that spare adjacent cortical regions do not impair memory or exacerbate the impairment following lesions of the hippocampal formation. J Neurosci 9:1922–1936

Zola-Morgan S, Squire LR et al (1989c) Lesions of perirhinal and parahippocampal cortex that spare the amygdala and hippocampal formation produce severe memory impairment. J Neurosci 9:4355–4370

Brain Network Functional Connectivity in Alzheimer's Disease and Frontotemporal Dementia

25

Juan Helen Zhou, Kwun Kei Ng, and Siwei Liu

25.1 Introduction

Neurodegeneration is marked by a gradual and selective brain network breakdown, leading to specific behavioral and cognitive dysfunctions. Alzheimer's disease (AD) and frontotemporal dementia (FTD) are the two most common neurodegenerative diseases among patients less than 65 years of age (Ratnavalli et al. 2002; Ikeda et al. 2004), while AD is more common among patients older than 65 years of age (see clinical and pathological characteristics in Box 25.1). Based on neuropathology studies (Braak and Braak 1991) and transgenic animal models (Palop et al. 2007), the network-based neurodegeneration hypothesis was proposed more than two decades ago and suggests that each disease targets a specific large-scale neuronal network. As effective, disease-specific and personalized treatments are emerging for neurodegenerative diseases, an objective, noninvasive, biologically based network-sensitive neuroimaging assay is needed to predict risk, diagnose early stages, and monitor the course and treatment of neurodegenerative diseases. Unlike traditional region-based fMRI approaches, the resting-state fMRI-based (rsfMRI) functional connectivity approach can map large-scale brain networks in vivo and detect specific network dysfunction in disease. To date, rsfMRI has been widely used to chart normal human functional connectivity architecture (Greicius et al. 2003; Damoiseaux et al. 2006; Biswal et al. 2010) and predict individual differences in human behavior and cognition (Di Martino et al. 2009; Hampson et al. 2006; Seeley et al. 2007). In this chapter, we will focus on the converging findings of rsfMRI-based functional connectivity alterations in neurodegenerative diseases (Bokde et al. 2009; Pievani et al. 2011; Sperling et al. 2010; Sorg et al. 2009; Dickerson and Sperling 2009; Guye et al. 2010; Di Biasio et al. 2011; Firbank et al. 2011), especially AD and FTD, as well as preclinical and prodromal populations (Zhou and Seeley 2014)

Box 25.1 Alzheimer's Disease (AD) and Frontotemporal Dementia (FTD)

AD is a chronic neurodegenerative disease that usually starts slowly and worsens over time. AD typically begins with episodic memory loss with prominent medial temporal, posterior cingulate/precuneus, and lateral temporoparietal atrophy (Hyman et al. 1984; Mitchell et al. 2002) and progresses to other cognitive deficits such as language

J. H. Zhou (✉) · K. K. Ng · S. Liu
Center for Sleep and Cognition, Yong Loo Lin School of Medicine, National University of Singapore, Singapore, Singapore
e-mail: helen.zhou@nus.edu.sg; eric.ng@nus.edu.sg; cisy.liu@nus.edu.sg

S. Ulmer, O. Jansen (eds.), *fMRI*, https://doi.org/10.1007/978-3-030-41874-8_25

and visuospatial functions and functional decline. The AD clinical syndrome strongly predicts underlying AD neuropathology, identified by beta-amyloid-rich neuritic plaques and tau-immunoreactive neurofibrillary tangles. The presence of apolipoprotein E (APOE) ε4 is the strongest genetic risk factor of sporadic AD (Dubois et al. 2007).

The clinical FTD spectrum consists of three behavioral or language-related subtypes: behavioral variant (BvFTD) (Seeley et al. 2011), semantic variant primary progressive aphasia (svPPA), and nonfluent/agrammatic variant of primary progressive aphasia (nfvPPA) (Gorno-Tempini et al. 2011). BvFTD features prominent social misconduct and emotional deficits, with anterior cingulate, fronto-insular, striatal, and frontopolar degeneration. SvPPA results in loss of word and object meaning accompanied by left predominant temporal pole and subgenual cingulate involvement. NfvPPA presents with nonfluent, effortful, and agrammatic speech and is associated with left frontal operculum, dorsal anterior insula, and precentral gyrus atrophy.

FTD syndromes result from a group of distinct underlying molecular pathological entities referred to collectively as frontotemporal lobar degeneration (FTLD). FTLD is further divided into three major molecular classes, including tau (FTLD-tau), transactive response DNA binding protein of 43 kDa (TDP-43, FTLD-TDP), and, the least common, fused in sarcoma (FUS) protein (FTLD-FUS) (Mackenzie et al. 2010). Although most patients have sporadic disease, several autosomal-dominant culprit genes have been identified, with mutations in the genes encoding microtubule-associated protein tau (*MAPT*), progranulin (*GRN*), and *C9orf72* accounting for the majority of known genetic causes (Whitwell et al. 2012).

25.2 Mapping Brain Networks Using Resting-State Functional Magnetic Resonance Imaging

During the resting-state fMRI recording, subjects are instructed to remain still and stay awake (often with eyes fixated on a cross) without any specific stimuli. Since only compliance with staying awake is needed, rsfMRI can be easily acquired from diseased populations, including AD patients (Teipel et al. 2016). In the absence of changes evoked by external stimuli as in task-based fMRI, rsfMRI captures the spontaneous macroscopic hemodynamic blood oxygenation level-dependent (BOLD) fluctuations at slow frequencies (<0.1 Hz). Regions that often coactivate or deactivate to perform specific cognitive functions during tasks show a high temporal correlation in their BOLD fluctuations (Biswal et al. 2010; Smith et al. 2009), as first observed between bilateral motor cortices (Biswal et al. 1995). This suggests that the temporal synchrony reveals the intrinsic functional connectivity between brain regions (Wig et al. 2011). The functional relevance of rsfMRI-based connectivity is further validated when functional connectivity patterns in the visual cortex consistent with the topographical hierarchy of its polysynaptic anatomical pathways were reported in anaesthetized monkeys (Vincent et al. 2007). The multiregion intrinsic connectivity networks (ICNs) (Sporns and Betzel 2016; Menon 2011) recapitulated by rsfMRI FCs have homologues across species (Vincent et al. 2007) and are systematically altered by psychophysiological conditions, such as wakefulness (Samann et al. 2011) and developmental stages (Gao et al. 2015), pointing to their fundamental role in cognition. Critically, impaired cognitive performance and behavior are associated with the disrupted interactions among these brain networks (Cole et al. 2014; Spronk et al. 2018), which can potentially explain symptom manifestation and pathological mechanisms of many neurodegenerative diseases.

RsfMRI FC is most commonly defined as the Pearson's correlation between the BOLD time series of spatially distributed brain regions, although many other temporal synchronization indices exist (Pedersen et al. 2018). A number of popular approaches can be used to derive rsfMRI FC (Fig. 25.1). Here, we summarize the current four major methods in the field.

Seed-based analysis (Fig. 25.1a) extracts ICNs by correlating the BOLD signals of a seed region to all other voxels of the brain (Biswal et al. 1995). The representativeness and utility of the connectivity pattern are thus seed-dependent. Every voxel in the resulting ICN map represents connectivity with the seed region. Using five characteristic seeds of five distinctive neurodegenerative syndromes, including AD and variants of FTD, Seeley and colleagues (2009) performed seed-based FC mapping in healthy rsfMRI data and demonstrated close correspondence between syndrome-specific degeneration patterns and healthy ICNs, supporting the network-based neurodegeneration hypothesis (Fig. 25.2).

Other approaches consider multiple brain regions simultaneously. In **independent component analysis (ICA)** (Fig. 25.1b), spontaneous BOLD signals from all brain voxels are decomposed into spatially nonoverlapping and temporally coherent networks (McKeown et al. 2003; Erhardt et al. 2011). The resulting ICN maps represent connectivity to the specific network. For example, Qian and colleagues (2015) used ICA to extract the default mode network, dorsal attention network, and ventral attention network and showed divergent changes in these networks in AD and amnestic MCI patients. We note that while seed-based and ICA approaches have been mainly used for extracting within-network connectivity (usually at the voxel level), they are also sensitive to between-network connectivity (e.g., between a DMN seed and non-DMN voxels (Chen et al. 2017a) and internetwork connectivity using ICA (Bos et al. 2014); see below).

Seed-based functional connectivity (one to many) can be extended to the whole brain (many to many) by analyzing **parcellation-based connectivity matrices** (Fig. 25.1c). Based on a set of predefined regions of interest (ROI) covering the whole brain using brain parcellation techniques (Wig et al. 2014; Arslan et al. 2018), the functional connectivity between all ROI pairs is computed and arranged into an adjacency matrix. The synchrony between different independent components (i.e., spatial maps) derived from ICA can also be treated similarly (Allen et al. 2014). With the spatial resolution appropriate for the research question, this approach concisely summarizes the complex connectivity patterns between and within multiple brain regions or networks.

Once measures of functional connectivity are obtained, univariate or multivariate statistical analysis can be performed to identify discernible differences between groups or conditions. For high-dimensional matrices, the **graph theoretical approach** (Fig. 25.1d) is highly useful to capture and visualize complex brain interactions and the network topology embedded therein. A brain graph comprises nodes (ROIs) connected by edges (functional connectivity). Nodes can be clustered according to their edge strength to form networks or communities characterized by stronger within-network connectivity and weaker between-network connectivity. To capture topological properties, graph theoretical measures can be calculated at nodal, network, and whole-brain levels (Sporns 2013; Fornito et al. 2013). These measures have been proven to be highly useful for revealing disease mechanisms. As detailed in Sect. 25.6 of this chapter, Zhou and colleagues (2012) derived functional connectivity matrices among 1128 ROIs (635,628 ROI pairs); graph theoretical topological parameters were computed to contrast the network-based neurodegenerative hypothesis against alternative disease-spreading mechanisms.

Beyond these static functional connectivity methods (synchrony over several minutes), recent advances in **dynamic, time-varying functional connectivity** (synchrony over tens of seconds) may provide a more refined spatiotemporal profile of the functional network organizational changes (Fig. 25.1e). For example, a seed-, ICA-, or parcellation-based approach can be combined with a sliding window approach, followed by a clustering algorithm (Allen et al. 2014) to identify representative "dynamic connectivity states", which can then be subject to graph theoretical analysis to contrast their topo-

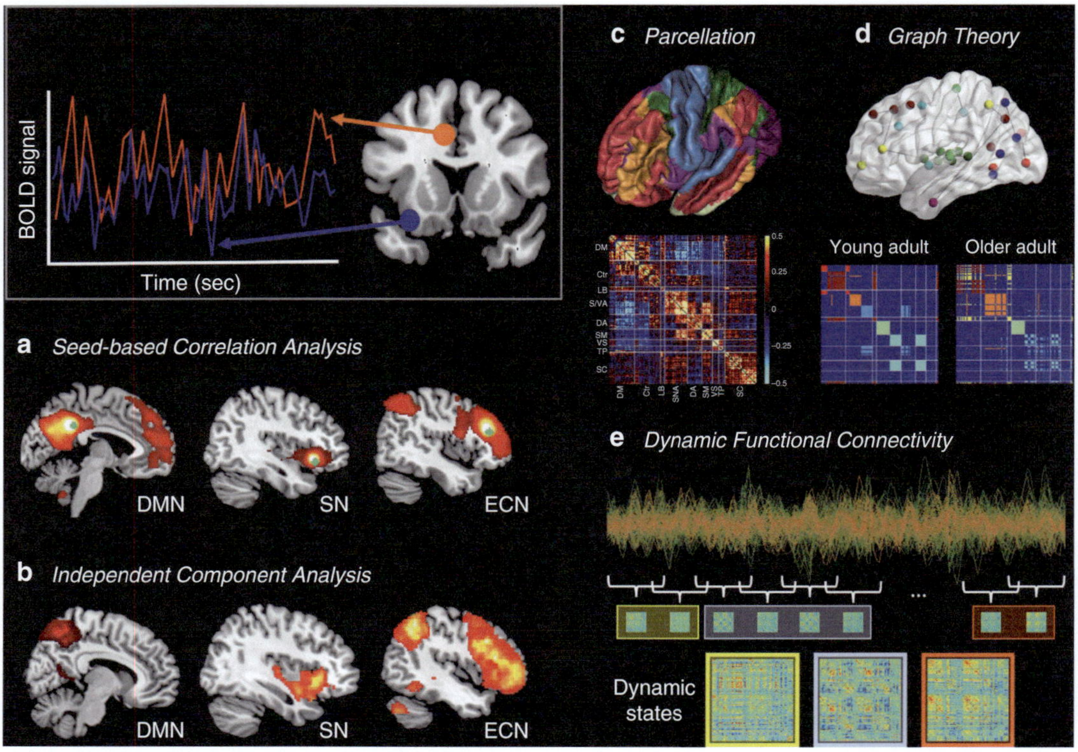

Fig. 25.1 Resting-state fMRI-based functional connectivity derivation and analytical methods. Top left: The most common definition of functional connectivity (FC) is the temporal synchrony of the slow oscillation of the blood-oxygen-level-dependent (BOLD) signals between two brain regions of interest (ROIs), quantified by Pearson's correlation. (**a**) Three high-level intrinsic connectivity networks (ICNs; hot color) were derived using a seed-based approach, taking representative ROIs within each network as seeds (green dots): the default mode network (DMN), the salience network (SN), and the executive control network (ECN). (**b**) The same three ICNs were derived using independent component analysis (ICA) without the need for predefined seeds, showing high correspondence with their seed-based counterparts. (**c**) The parcellation approach is akin to a multiple-seed approach, capturing FC between all possible ROI pairs in an FC matrix. Besides spheres, ROIs can be functionally homogenous patches following anatomical/cytoarchitectural constraints. They also do not have to always include the whole brain. ROIs are often ordered to show major network structure (apparent hot colored squares along the diagonal) and the interrelations between networks (hot and cool colored off-diagonal cells). (**d**) A brain graph abstracts brain networks into nodes (spheres of different colors representing brain regions in different ICNs) and edges (thin lines representing FC). Methods such as community detection can be applied to this abstraction to highlight key network architecture, for instance, the differences in ICN ("community") membership of brain regions between healthy young and older adults: brain regions belonging to the same ICN in the more optimal young brain are more scattered into different ICNs in the older brain. (E) FC among parcellated ROIs can be derived from much shorter data (e.g., 20–40 s instead of 8 min), resulting in multiple FC matrices across time. These matrices can be clustered according to their spatial similarities to give a more discrete view of time-varying FC dynamics. Each cluster centroid represents a "dynamic connectivity state," and its occurrence may be associated with cognition and behavior. The rendering of the FreeSurfer parcellation in (C) (Yeo et al. 2011) is created using the open-source software 3D Slicer (https://www.slicer.org/)

logical differences. Additional parameters such as the time spent in a certain state and the transition probabilities between states can be further evaluated for their sensitivity to diseases (Quevenco et al. 2017). Brenner and colleagues (2018) identified four states in a group of amnestic mild cognitive impairment (aMCI) and healthy older adults and observed that individuals with aMCI spent significantly more time in a putative costly state. Combining these methods with careful data preprocessing and parameter setting (Box 25.2), rsfMRI provides a network-sensitive, immediately repeatable, noninvasive tool to examine human functional connectome in health and disease.

25.3 Dementia Subtypes Featuring Distinct Functional Connectivity Network Changes

Previous studies have confirmed the network-based neurodegeneration hypothesis in humans by demonstrating that spatial atrophy patterns in five distinct neurodegenerative syndromes, including AD and variants of FTD, mirror normal human ICNs derived from rsfMRI (Seeley et al. 2009) (Fig. 25.2). The next question is whether different dementia subtypes feature syndrome-specific functional connectivity changes in these large-scale brain networks. In the following subsections, we provide neuroimaging evidence in AD versus FTD and their variants.

AD and bvFTD feature divergent network changes: AD causes atrophy within a posterior hippocampal-cingulo-temporal-parietal network, which resembles the "default mode network" (DMN) (Greicius et al. 2003; Buckner et al. 2005; Toussaint et al. 2014). The pioneer work by Greicius and colleagues found reduced DMN functional connectivity in AD patients compared to age-matched healthy controls (Greicius et al. 2004), and these findings have been replicated by many other studies (Zhou and Seeley 2014). BvFTD, in contrast, features atrophy in anterior insula, anterior cingulate cortex (ACC), and striatal and thalamic regions, mirroring the "salience network" (SN) (Seeley et al. 2007; Boccardi et al. 2005; Seeley et al. 2008a). The role of this network in salience processing was emphasized because its key hubs, the ACC and frontoinsular, activate in response to diverse emotionally significant internal and external stimuli or conditions (Craig 2009; Craig 2002). Elements of the DMN are usually involved in episodic memory, mental-state attribution, and visuospatial imagery (Buckner et al. 2005; Zysset et al. 2003; Cavanna and Trimble 2006) despite the fact that part of the DMN often deactivates in response to diverse cognitive tasks (Raichle et al. 2001; Shulman et al. 1997). Notably, while the anterior SN degenerates in bvFTD, posterior cortical functions survive or even thrive and are, at times,

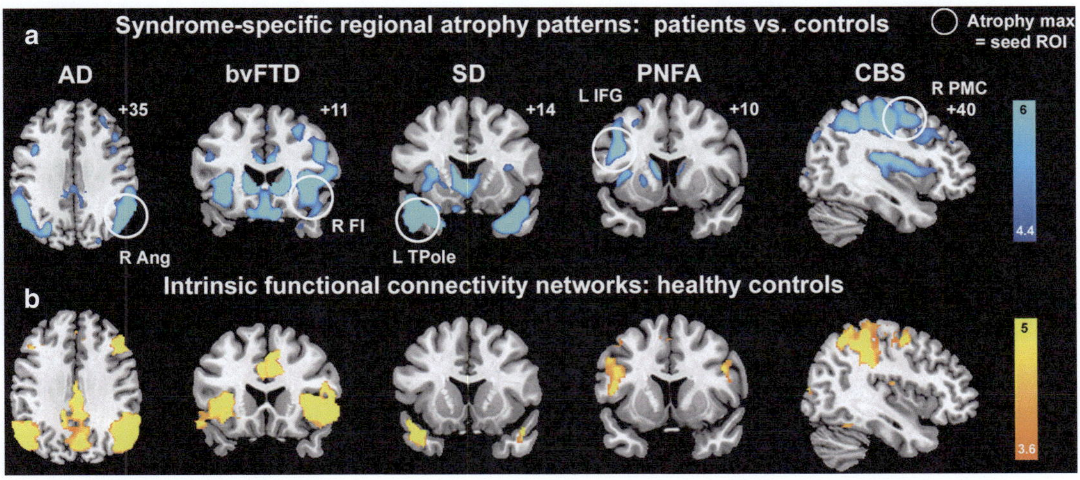

Fig. 25.2 Convergent syndromic atrophy in neurodegenerative diseases and intrinsic connectivity networks in health. (**a**) Five distinct clinical syndromes showed dissociable atrophy patterns, whose cortical maxima (circled) provided seed ROIs for ICN and structural covariance analyses. (**b**) ICN mapping experiments identified five distinct networks anchored by the five syndromic atrophy seeds. Color bars indicate *t*-scores. In coronal and axial images, the left side of the image corresponds to the left side of the brain. Abbreviations: *ANG* angular gyrus, *FI* frontoinsula, *IFGoper* inferior frontal gyrus, pars opercularis, *PMC* premotor cortex, *TPole* temporal pole. (Figure is adapted from Seeley et al. (2009) with permission)

associated with emergent visual creativity (Miller et al. 1998; Seeley et al. 2008b). By comparison, AD maintains socioemotional functions while losing episodic memory and visuospatial function. Based on the inversely correlated relationship between the salience and default mode networks in the healthy brain (Greicius and Menon 2004; Fox et al. 2005) and the opposing symptom-deficit profiles of AD and bvFTD, Zhou and colleagues found divergent functional connectivity changes of the DMN and SN in AD and bvFTD using ICA-based rsfMRI ICN mapping (Zhou et al. 2010). Specifically, the SN connectivity was disrupted in bvFTD but was enhanced in AD, while the DMN connectivity was disrupted in AD but enhanced in bvFTD (Fig. 25.3). The SN dysconnectivity at the right frontoinsular also tracks disease severity in bvFTD patients. Such divergent network profiles in AD and bvFTD have been substantiated by a host of convergent findings obtained with complementary task-free fMRI and other imaging

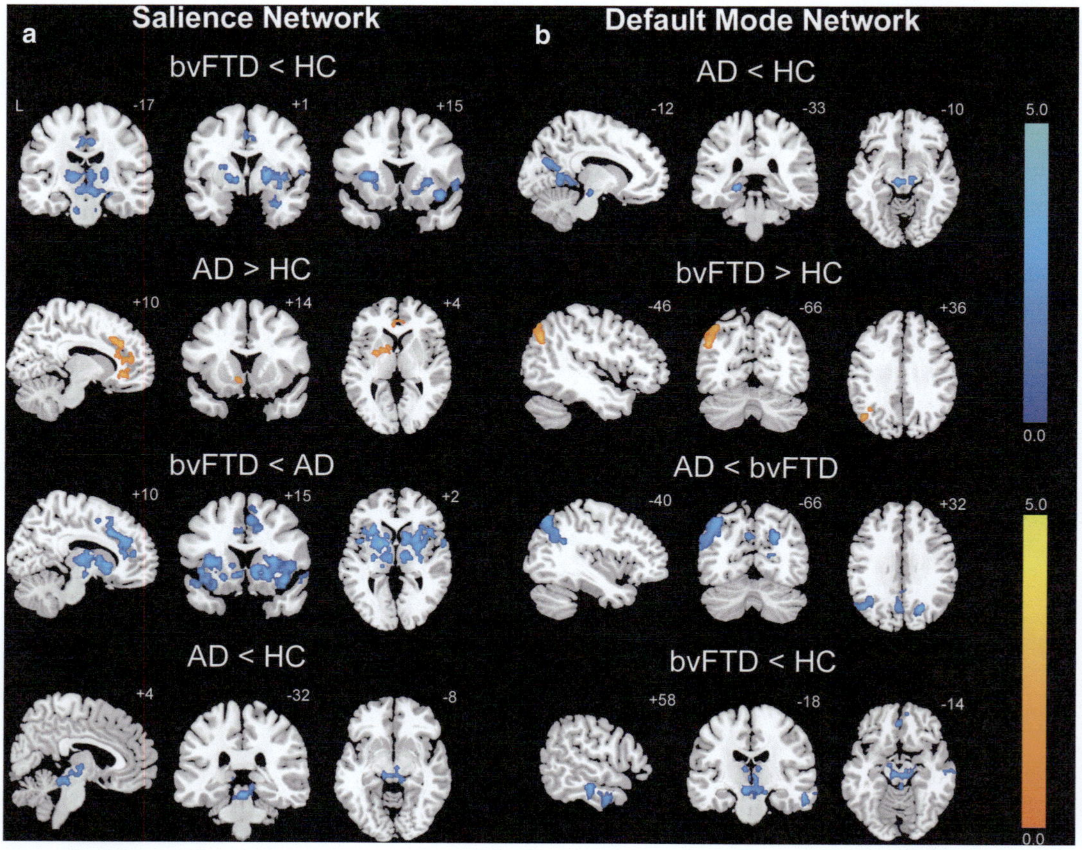

Fig. 25.3 BvFTD and Alzheimer's disease feature divergent salience network and DMN dynamics. Group difference maps illustrate clusters of significantly reduced or increased connectivity for each ICN. In the salience network (**a**), patients with bvFTD showed distributed connectivity reductions compared to healthy controls (HC) and patients with Alzheimer's disease (AD), whereas patients with Alzheimer's disease showed increased connectivity in anterior cingulate cortex and ventral striatum compared to healthy controls. In the DMN (**b**), patients with Alzheimer's disease showed several connectivity impairments compared to healthy controls and patients with bvFTD, whereas patients with bvFTD showed increased left angular gyrus connectivity. Patients with bvFTD and Alzheimer's disease further showed focal brainstem connectivity disruptions within their "released" network (DMN for bvFTD, salience network for Alzheimer's disease). Results are displayed at a joint height and extent probability threshold of $p < 0.05$, corrected at the whole brain level. Color bars represent t-scores, and statistical maps are superimposed on the Montreal Neurological Institute template brain. (Figure is adapted from Zhou et al. (2010) with permission)

methods (de Haan et al. 2012; Machulda et al. 2011; Bai et al. 2009; Brier et al. 2012; Whitwell et al. 2011; Farb et al. 2013; Filippi et al. 2013).

AD variants feature differential network changes: A significant number of AD patients exhibit non-memory deficits such as language, executive function, and higher visual functions (Snowden et al. 2007). Three major types of AD variants include logopenic variant of primary progressive aphasia (lvPPA), posterior cortical atrophy (PCA), and early-onset Alzheimer's disease (EOAD). In addition to common atrophy in the posterior DMN (Lehmann et al. 2010; Migliaccio et al. 2009), AD variants suffer from atrophy and hypometabolism in distinct brain regions related to executive function, language, or visual functions (Lehmann et al. 2013). In parallel, evidence from rsfMRI studies has highlighted that similar local pathological changes, together with variant-specific aggregate spread along different brain networks, could underlie the clinico-anatomical variations of AD. Using a seed-based approach, Lehmann and colleagues (2013) demonstrated the topographic similarity between the variant-specific atrophy in AD and the deficit-related functional networks in healthy controls (Fig. 25.4). Specifically, besides common involvement of the posterior DMN, this study identified intrinsic functional networks related to variant-specific cognitive deficits by seeding variant-specific atrophy regions in healthy controls. Atrophy specific to the lvPPA was seated in the language network (Lehmann et al. 2013). Similarly findings were reported in another study comparing lvPPA and amnesic AD patients matched on amyloid deposition (Whitwell et al. 2015). Atrophy regions specific to the PCA were linked with the higher visual network (Lehmann et al. 2013). Disrupted functional connectivity was also reported in a later study examining dorsal and ventral visual networks separately in PCA (Migliaccio et al. 2016). For EOAD whose clinical symptom onset takes place before 65 years of age, the anterior SN and right ECN are specifically targeted (Lehmann et al. 2013; Gour et al. 2014), in parallel with impairments in visuoconstruction, executive function, and language (Joubert et al. 2016). Indeed, compared to healthy controls, EOAD showed extensive FC network alterations (Filippi et al. 2017), including longer functional path length, lower mean nodal strength, lower local efficiency, and a lower clustering coefficient. Interestingly, in contrast with late-onset AD, EOAD did not show more FC impairment in the DMN (Gour et al. 2014; Lehmann et al. 2015; Adriaanse et al. 2014a); instead, it had more disruptions outside the DMN (Gour et al. 2014; Adriaanse et al. 2014a). Compared to bvFTD, network disruption was more global in EOAD; in particular, there was more breakdown over the posterior networks, including the parietal regions (Filippi et al. 2017).

Moreover, AD frequently co-occurs with cerebrovascular disease (CeVD) (Toledo et al. 2013), which has emerged as the leading cause of age-related cognitive impairment (Schneider et al. 2009; Chen et al. 2016). On its own, CeVD is associated with declines in executive function (Prins et al. 2005), reduced frontal lobe metabolism (Kuczynski et al. 2009), and disrupted functional connectivity in frontoparietal regions (Schaefer et al. 2014). Together, AD and CeVD are proposed to have additive effects on cognitive decline (Zekry et al. 2002a; Iadecola 2010; Attems and Jellinger 2014; Kalheim et al. 2017). For the same clinical severity of dementia, patients with pure AD exhibited more severe AD pathology (amyloid β and tau) than those comorbid with CeVD (Toledo et al. 2013; Goulding et al. 1999; Zekry et al. 2002b). One recent rsfMRI study from Chong and colleagues (2017) demonstrated divergent network changes in AD with and without CeVD. AD patients without CeVD, but not AD patients with CeVD, showed reductions in posterior DMN functional connectivity. By comparison, while both groups exhibited parietal reductions in executive control network functional connectivity, only AD patients with CeVD showed increases in frontal executive control network connectivity. Importantly, these distinct executive control network changes were recapitulated in prodromal AD patients with and without CeVD. Higher DMN functional connectivity correlated with greater hippocampal volumes, while

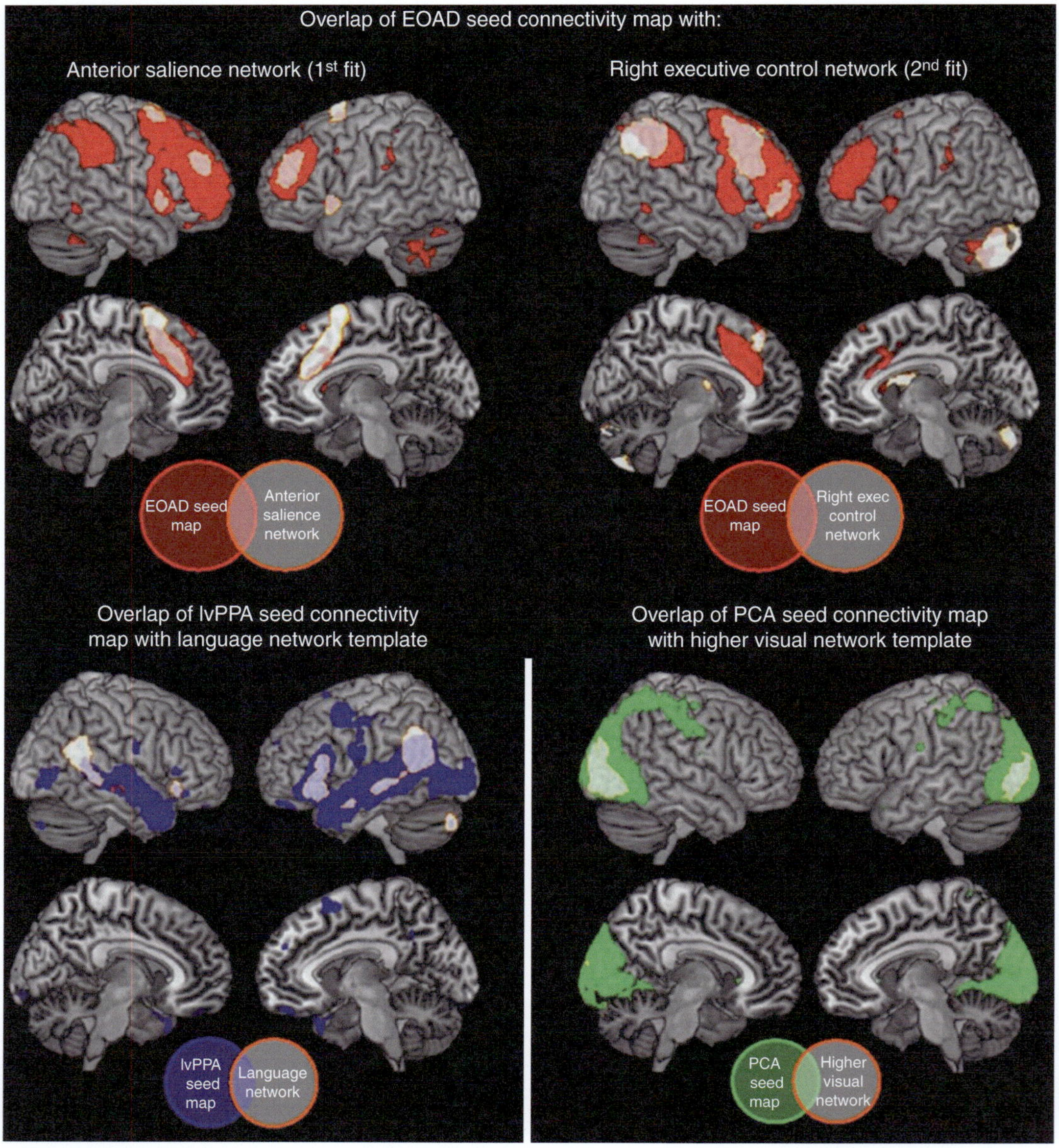

Fig. 25.4 Overlapping between seed-based FC networks based on specific atrophied ROIs and the best-fitting functional network templates. The EOAD seed FC map showed two strong fits: the anterior SN showed the best fit with the left hemisphere FC map, and the right ECN showed the best fit with the right hemisphere FC map. The lvPPA seed and PCA seed FC maps showed the best fit with the language and higher visual networks, respectively. Abbreviations: *FC* functional connectivity, *ECN* executive control network, *PCC* posterior cingulate cortex, *EOAD* early-onset Alzheimer's disease, *lvPPA* the logopenic variant of primary progressive aphasia, *PCA* the posterior cortical atrophy. (Figure is adapted from Lehmann et al. (2013) with permission)

higher executive control network functional connectivity correlated with more severe white matter hyperintensity across all AD patients (Fig. 25.5). These differential neural network functional changes reflect a combination of more severe CeVD and less severe AD network degeneration phenotype in AD patients with CeVD, which is closely associated with pathology.

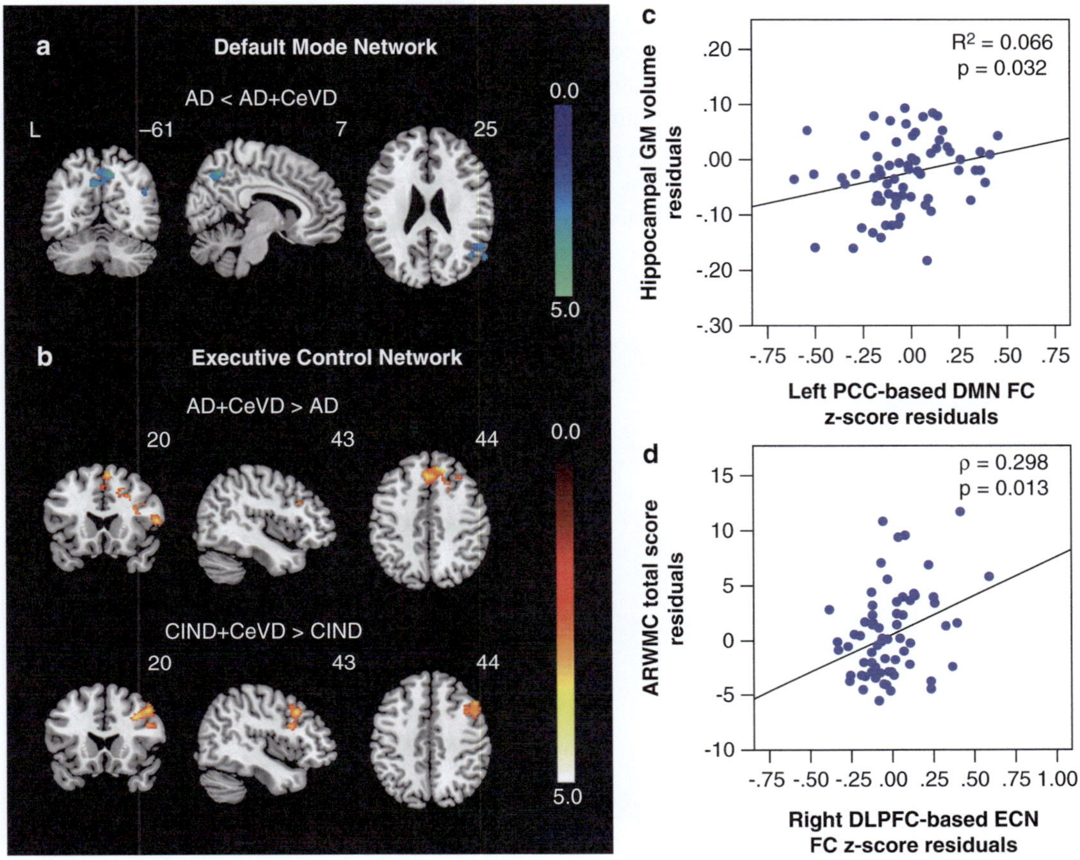

Fig. 25.5 Divergent functional connectivity changes in Alzheimer's disease (AD) patients with and without cerebrovascular disease (CeVD). (**a**) Compared to AD with CeVD patients, AD without CeVD patients showed reduced (cold color) FC in the key posterior DMN regions, including precuneus, PCC, and angular gyrus. (**b**) Compared to AD without CeVD patients, AD with CeVD patient showed increase (hot color) in the frontal regions of the ECN. Similar increase in frontal ECN was also seen in the CIND with CeVD patients compared to the CIND without CeVD patients. Results are shown at a height threshold of $p < 0.01$ and a cluster-extent threshold of $p < 0.05$. Color bars indicate *t*-scores. (**c**) Across AD with and without CeVD patients, higher DMN FC (*z*-score residuals) based on the left PCC was related to larger gray matter volumes (*z*-score residuals). (**d**) Higher ECN FC based on the right DLPFC (*z*-score residuals) correlated with more severe white matter hyperintensity (measured by age-related white matter changes total score residuals). Residuals were calculated after controlling for age, gender, education, handedness, and ethnicity. Abbreviations: *CeVD* cerebrovascular disease, *FC* functional connectivity, *AD* Alzheimer's disease, *CIND* cognitive impaired but no dementia, *DMN* default mode network, *ECN* executive control network, *PCC* posterior cingulate cortex, *DLPFC* dorsolateral prefrontal cortex. (Figure is adapted from Chong et al. (2017) with permission)

Emerging evidence on network changes in FTD variants: Although relatively scarce compared to AD, distinct rsfMRI-based network disruptions have been found in FTD variants. SvPPA was associated with extensive functional dysconnectivity between the anterior temporal lobe and multiple speech processing areas (Guo et al. 2013). NfvPPA is related to the network anchored by the inferior frontal gyrus (Wilson et al. 2012). Although the functional connectivity patterns in nfvPPA have not been examined directly, one recent rsfMRI study in patients with primary progressive apraxia of speech revealed reduced functional connectivity between the supplementary motor area and speech and language regions, including the left lateral prefrontal cortex (Botha et al. 2018). More importantly, specific functional connectivity changes relate to behavioral impairment in FTD variants. Both bvFTD and scPPA patients had reduced frontolimbic connectivity that was associated with lower disinhibition scores and elevated local connectivity within the prefrontal cortex that was associated with apathy scores (Farb et al. 2013). Recent studies using graph theoretical analyses on the whole-brain functional connectome revealed distinct abnormal network topology in bvFTD and svPPA. Notably, bvFTD patients featured a loss of hubs in frontal lobes involving the ACC, orbitofrontal cortex, and caudate nucleus, which were associated with executive dysfunction (Filippi et al. 2017; Agosta et al. 2013) (Fig. 25.6a), while svPPA patients had a loss of hubs and reduced nodal degree in the inferior and ventral temporal

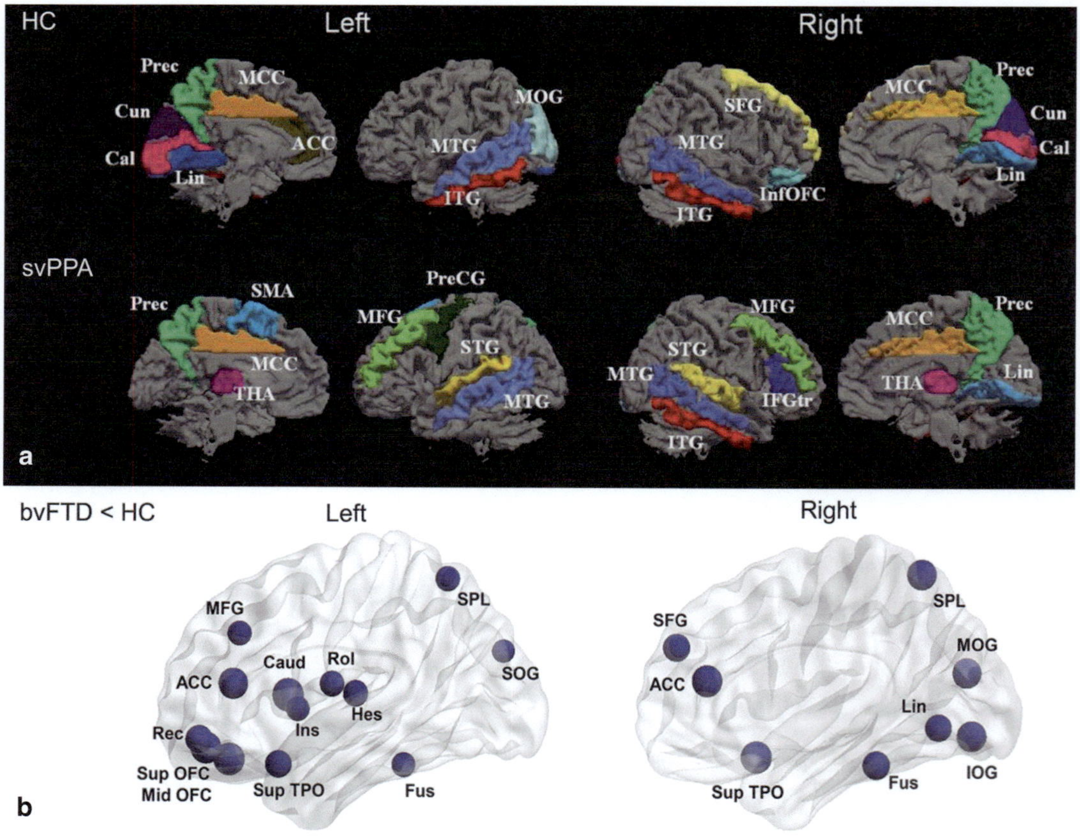

Fig. 25.6 Graph theoretical analysis revealed brain functional hub changes in FTD patients. (**a**) Hubs identified in svPPA patients and healthy controls based on either integrated nodal degree or betweenness centrality (>1 standard deviation above the network average). Regions including the left ITG, ACC, Lin, MOG, right SFG, InfOFC, Cal, and Cun were specific to the controls, while regions including STG, MFG, THA, right IFG, left PreCG, and SMA were only found in the svPPA patients. (**b**) Decreased degree centrality in cortical hubs was found in bvFTD patients compared to the controls. Node size is proportional to the value difference of the integrated nodal parameters between bvFTD patients and controls. Abbreviations: *ACC* anterior cingulate cortex, *Cal* calcarine cortex, *Caud* caudate nucleus, *Cun* cuneus, *Fus* fusiform gyrus, *Hes* Heschl gyrus, *IFGtr* inferior frontal gyrs (pars triangularis), *InfOFC* inferior orbitofrontal cortex, *Ins* insula, *IOG* inferior occipital gyrus, *ITG* inferior temporal gyrus, *Lin* lingual gyrus, *MCC* middle cingulate cortex, *MFG* middle frontal gyrus, *MOG* middle occipital gyrus, *MTG* middle temporal gyrus, *OFC* orbitofrontal cortex, *Prec* precuneus, *PoCG* postcentral gyrus, *PreCG* precentral gyrus, *Rec* gyrus rectus, *Rol* rolandic operculum, *SFG* superior frontal gyrus, *SMA* supplementary motor cortex, *SOG* superior occipital gyrus, *SPL* t superior parietal lobule, *STG* superior temporal gyrus, THA, thalamus, *TPO* temporal pole, *HC* healthy controls, *bvFTD* the behavioral variant of frontotemporal dementia, svPPA, semantic variant of primary progressive aphasia. (Figure is adapted from Agosta et al. (2013, 2014) with permission)

regions and occipital cortices (Agosta et al. 2014) (Fig. 25.6b). Additionally, the network centrality combined with social-executive behavioral measures had been applied to distinguish bvFTD patients from healthy controls and frontoinsular stroke with a high classification rate (Sedeno et al. 2016).

Taken together, brain functional deterioration is driven by specific symptom-associated networks, supporting the selective network breakdown model in neurodegeneration.

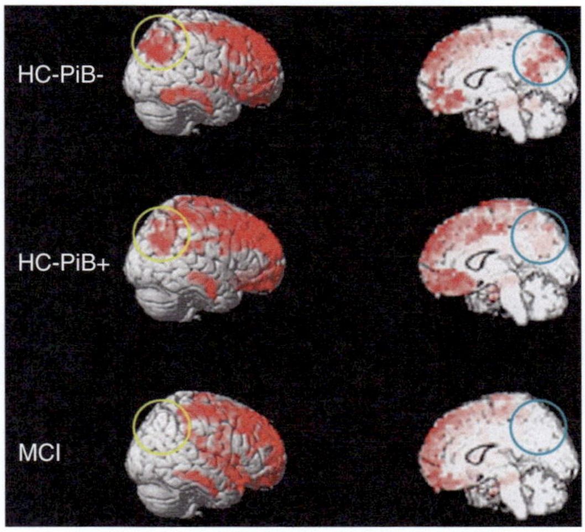

Fig. 25.7 Loss of cortical hubs in prodromal stage of dementia. Whole-brain connectivity in PCC was largely reduced among MCI patients, compared to being a hub region of the DMN in the PiB-negative healthy elderly. Loss of cortical hubs in MCI were both found in the medial (blue) and the lateral (yellow) part of the hemisphere, while similar but subtle changes were found in PiB-positive healthy elderly. Abbreviations: *HC-PiB−* PiB-negative healthy controls, *HC-PiB+* PiB-positive healthy controls, and *MCI* PiB-positive patients with mild cognitive impairment. (Figure is adapted from Drzezga et al. (2011) with permission)

25.4 Detecting Early Network Changes and Predicting Conversion in the Prodromal Stage of Dementia

By the time patients arrive at the clinical AD stage, neuronal loss and structural disconnection have become substantial. Increasing attention in the field of aging and dementia research is devoted to characterizing the prodromal stage of the disease, hoping for more fruitful interventions to slow down or halt disease progression. **Mild cognitive impairment** (MCI) is an intermediate stage between the expected cognitive decline of normal aging and clinically diagnosed dementia. RsfMRI-based functional connectivity mapping is improving our understanding in brain network changes, both during the long windy journey of AD development and at the tipping point of disease conversion.

MCI stage: Network alterations that characterize the AD stage can be observed in patients with MCI. Functional disconnections of the DMN hubs, including the posterior cingulate cortex (PCC), were detected in MCI patients, even when brain gray matter atrophy was barely detectable (Drzezga et al. 2011; Sorg et al. 2007; Qi et al. 2010; Zhan et al. 2016; Gili et al. 2011). In particular, cortical hubs as defined by the degree of whole-brain connectivity to the seed region (i.e., high degree centrality) were largely reduced in the PCC/precuneus and angular and lateral temporal gyrus among MCI patients compared to the Pittsburg compound B (*PiB*)-negative healthy elderly. Subtle connectivity disruptions were already present in *PiB*-positive asymptomatic individuals (Fig. 25.7) (Drzezga et al. 2011). Moreover, consistent with the hippocampus disconnection hypothesis (Yassa et al. 2011; Das et al. 2013), disruption of the FC with hippocampus in the key DMN regions, such as the precuneus, PCC, and medial prefrontal regions, was implicated in aMCI (Brueggen et al. 2016; de Flores et al. 2017; Tahmasian et al. 2015). Lower hippocampal FC (with PCC/precuneus and middle temporal regions) was also associated with poor performance in primacy recall task (Brueggen et al. 2016) and lower Mini-Mental State Examination scores (Liu et al. 2016a). Applying graph theory on whole-brain functional connectomes, aMCI patients had higher characteristic functional path lengths in aMCI compared to healthy controls, indicating reduced network efficiency (i.e., information transfer across distant brain regions) (Wang et al. 2013a).

Conversion: While more than half of MCI patients convert to dementia within 5 years, with an annual conversion rate at approximately 25%, others remained at the stage of MCI for a long period of time (Petersen et al. 2001). Looking at disease progression, resting-stage FC differentiates aMCI patients who progressed to AD from those who did not. Similar to AD patients having lower within-DMN (precuneus and PCC) connectivity, aMCI patients exhibited an intermediate intra-DMN FC level between the AD patients and healthy controls. More importantly, only the aMCI patients who were stable over the following 2 years, and not the aMCI patients later converting to AD, had significantly higher DMN FC than the AD patients (Binnewijzend et al. 2012). In parallel, Serra and colleagues reported that a lower baseline FC of the precuneus within the DMN predicted disease conversion at 2-year follow-up (Serra et al. 2016). Interestingly, Petrella and colleagues used ICA to identify the DMN and calculated the goodness-of-fit score to represent the similarity of each individual's DMN to those of the normal controls. They found that DMN similarity between the MCI non-converters and controls was significantly higher than the similarity between the MCI converters and the normal controls (Petrella et al. 2011). However, more longitudinal studies with independent validation and inclusion of other risk factors, such as the presence of genetic risk factors, are needed for a better prediction of conversion to dementia.

Heterogeneity: MCI has several clinical etiologies and includes two main subtypes: amnestic and non-amnestic MCI. aMCI is typically considered a symptomatic predementia stage of AD. In contrast, non-amnestic MCI is often characterized by preserved memory function and a greater degree of deficits in attention, language, visuospatial, and executive function, which might be more related to other neurodegenerative or nondegenerative conditions such as vascular or psychiatric disorders (Petersen et al. 1999; Petersen 2011). Emerging studies have begun to shed light onto the differential network changes in these two subtypes of MCI. For example, Dunn and colleagues found both subtypes had similar levels of intra-DMN connectivity, but the impaired FC between the PCC and hippocampus was related to poor performance in episodic memory retrieval only in aMCI patients (not in non-amnestic MCI) (Dunn et al. 2014). Furthermore, heterogeneity in MCI also stems from the comorbidity of other pathologies such as cerebrovascular disease (CeVD) and different subtypes of dementia. Mirroring the differences at the dementia stage, rsfMRI studies demonstrated a divergent functional network disruption of the DMN and ECN in patients with cognitive impairment, but no dementia, with and without CeVD (Chong et al. 2017) (Fig. 25.5b).

Subjective memory complaints: Subjective memory complaints (SMC) represent a type of complaint made by individuals with no clear impairment on objective psychometric testing. There is rapidly increasing evidence that this subjectively experienced cognitive decline, even at the stage of normal performance on cognitive tests (i.e., pre-MCI and preprodromal), is associated with increased likelihood of biomarker abnormalities consistent with AD pathology and an increased risk for future cognitive decline and AD dementia (Jessen et al. 2014; Rabin et al. 2017). A recent study by Rönnlund and colleagues (2015) studied 2043 elderly persons over 60 years old and found that SMC individuals were more likely to develop dementia in their 10-year follow-up. Postmortem brain autopsies showed that individuals with SMC had more neuritic amyloid plaques in regions that are vulnerable to AD (Kryscio et al. 2014). For rsfMRI, one study reported increased DMN FC in SMC compared to healthy controls without SMC (Hafkemeijer et al. 2013), while another study suggested that the right hippocampal FC in SMC was lower than that of controls but higher than in the MCI group (Wang et al. 2013b). Considering the nonlinear dynamics in rsfMRI time series with larger sample sizes, Jiang and colleagues (2018) revealed more dynamic network changes in SMC involving distributed regions such as the PCC, the medial parahippocampus, and the lateral and inferior temporal regions, which parallel the lower DMN FC in SMC indicated in one MEG study (López-Sanz et al. 2017). Moreover, older adults with cognitive complaints showed brain atrophy similar to that of aMCI or AD patients (Saykin et al. 2006; Peter et al. 2014) and was associated with episodic memory decline over time (Peter et al. 2014). Mirroring functional connectivity changes, one recent study also demonstrated lower global efficiency and weaker rich club connections based on white matter structural connectivity in SMC (Shu et al. 2017). However, inconsistency in the research findings mainly due to different strategies in measuring subjective cognitive decline and heterogeneity in samples (Snitz et al. 2015) still needs to be resolved. It is crucial to examine the early structural and functional brain changes in SMC and its associations with biomarkers to predict risk for conversion to dementia.

25.5 Characterizing Preclinical Changes in Functional Network Organization

Based on decades of AD research, Jack and colleagues proposed the AD pathological cascade model (Jack Jr et al. 2013), hypothesizing that insidious changes in brain function and structure have already been accumulating when an individual shows minimal or even no cognitive or behavioral decline at a much younger age, well before irreversible damages are observed (Yang et al. 2014; Fouquet et al. 2014). Not only may this presymptomatic period mark the "true" disease onset, making it an important phase for the complete understanding of AD pathology, but it is also believed to be a time window for more effective intervention and preventative strategies (Papenberg et al. 2015; Sperling et al. 2014). Therefore, much rsfMRI research has targeted brain functional network changes in preclinical individuals. For instance, Chhatwal and colleagues found dissociable functional connectivity changes related to normal ageing and AD (Chhatwal et al. 2018). Comparing the brain parcellation-based FC between preclinical adults at risk for autosomal-dominant AD and their age-matched healthy counterparts, AD-related changes were more restricted to the within-network FC of major ICNs. Comparing the FC between a separate group of young adults and older adults free of AD biomarkers, age-related changes were more diffused across networks and affected "anticorrelations" between networks (Fig. 25.8). A similar divergence in diffused and specific network FC changes has been reported elsewhere (Klaassens et al. 2017). What contributes to such deviation of the AD effect from the normal aging effect on brain connectivity patterns in asymptomatic individuals remains to be fully elucidated. However, among the myriad of potential risk factors and biomarkers for AD, the apolipoprotein ε4 (APOE ε4) allele, beta amyloid (Aβ), and tau have received the most attention.

APOE genotype: The APOE ε4 allele unequivocally increases the risk of early- and late-onset AD (Strittmatter et al. 1993; Mahley et al. 2006) and is hypothesized to do so by altering lipid generation, Aβ clearance, and inflammation processes (Yu et al. 2014; Kanekiyo et al. 2014). Possession of the APOE ε4 allele has been associated with both decreased and increased connectivity in the DMN regions (Fleisher et al. 2009; Filippini et al. 2009; Damoiseaux et al. 2012) and other high-level cognitive ICNs. For instance, using seed-based FC, one study revealed lower connectivity between a PCC seed and the posterior DMN regions, which was accompanied by higher connectivity between an ACC seed and the SN regions in the APOE ε4 carriers relative to non-carriers (Machulda et al. 2011). In addition to within-network connectivity, between-network connectivity, which is often negative ("anticorrelations") between the task-negative DMN and task-positive ICNs, is also altered by ε4 possession. Anticorrelation is generally interpreted as the competing and regulatory operations between internal and external mentation (Fox et al. 2005; Menon and Uddin 2010); networks showing suboptimal anticorrelation are suggestive of losing functional segregation and are a hallmark finding in healthy aging (Ferreira et al. 2016; Ng et al. 2016). Chen and colleagues (2017b) observed overlapping atrophy and decreased functional deactivation in the right precuneus during a memory task in healthy ε4 carriers compared to non-carriers. By deriving the FC seeding at this region, ε4 carriers had less negative FC between the precuneus and superior temporal gyrus and less posi-

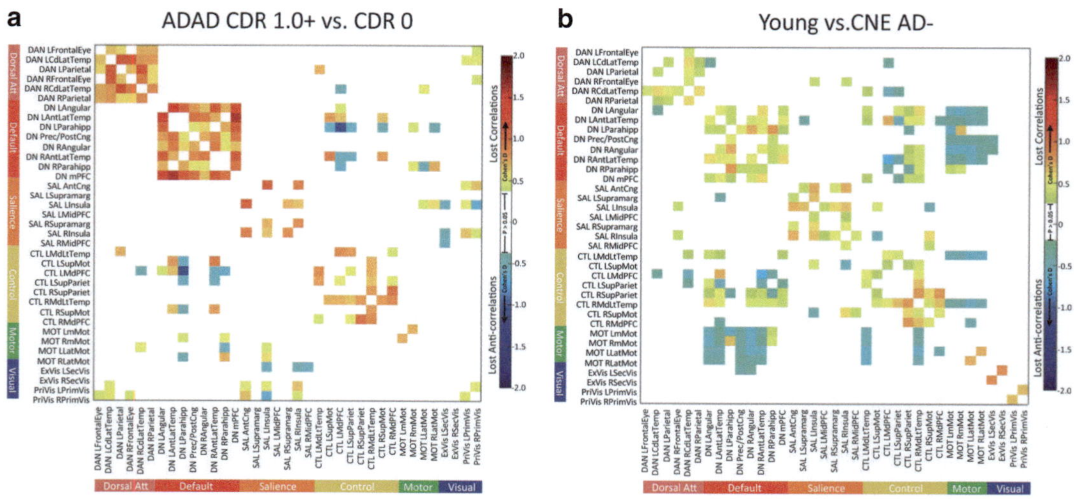

Fig. 25.8 Divergent changes in functional connectivity (FC) characterize AD and healthy aging. (**a**) Using young adults with autosomal-dominant AD risk as a proxy of late-onset sporadic AD, aberrant changes in resting-state FC due to AD pathology (relative to healthy young adult) were more restricted to be within intrinsic connectivity networks (hot-colored cells along the diagonal). (**b**) In contrast, aberrant changes in FC due to normative aging (between healthy young adults and older adults without AD biomarkers) were present in most networks but with much smaller effect sizes and featured disproportionally more negative FC (anticorrelations) between networks (cool colors off-diagonal). Abbreviations: *ADAD* Autosomal dominant Alzheimer's disease, *CDR* Cognitive Dementia Rating Scale, *CNE* Cognitively normal elderly. (Figure is adapted from Chhatwal et al. (2018) with permission)

tive FC between the precuneus and anterior cingulate cortex, superior frontal gyrus, and middle frontal gyrus. These regions encompassed the DMN and attention/executive control networks (Fig. 25.9a–c), suggesting a disrupted balance between these networks at rest, which in turn affects their interactions under cognitive demand, as reflected in the (de)activation differences. Consistent with this DMN-executive control network relationship, Ng and colleagues used parcellation-based FC to demonstrate that ε4 carriers had a more rapid increase in the FC between the DMN and the executive control network over time, indicating a faster loss of functional segregation between the two networks with opposing dynamics (Fig. 25.9d). This change in network segregation was further associated with decline in processing speed performance (Ng et al. 2016, 2018). Across these reviewed studies, the key involvement of the DMN and the other high-level cognitive networks, whose complementary dynamics often match with syndrome differences among different neurodegenerative diseases (Zhou and Seeley 2014), may point to a genetic moderation of network-based neurodegeneration.

FTD genetic risk: In parallel to studying individuals with genetic risk for AD, recent rsfMRI work has moved toward characterizing the early functional connectivity changes in individuals at risk for FTD. Abnormal salience network (SN) functional connectivity was found in presymptomatic C90rf72, GRN, and MAPT carriers (Dopper et al. 2014; Borroni et al. 2012). These genes were consistently involved in bvFTD, demonstrating that ICN changes exist decades before disease onset (Premi et al. 2014). However, no agreement on the specific pattern of changes has yet been reached (Dopper et al. 2014; Borroni et al. 2012; Pievani et al. 2014). To date, researchers have started to investigate the issue by considering technical factors (Gordon et al. 2016), the possible influence of different pathologies (Ahmed et al. 2016), and distinct temporal and spatial profiles (Gordon et al. 2016).

Aβ and tau burden: Aβ is a peptide fragment of the amyloid precursor protein that often accu-

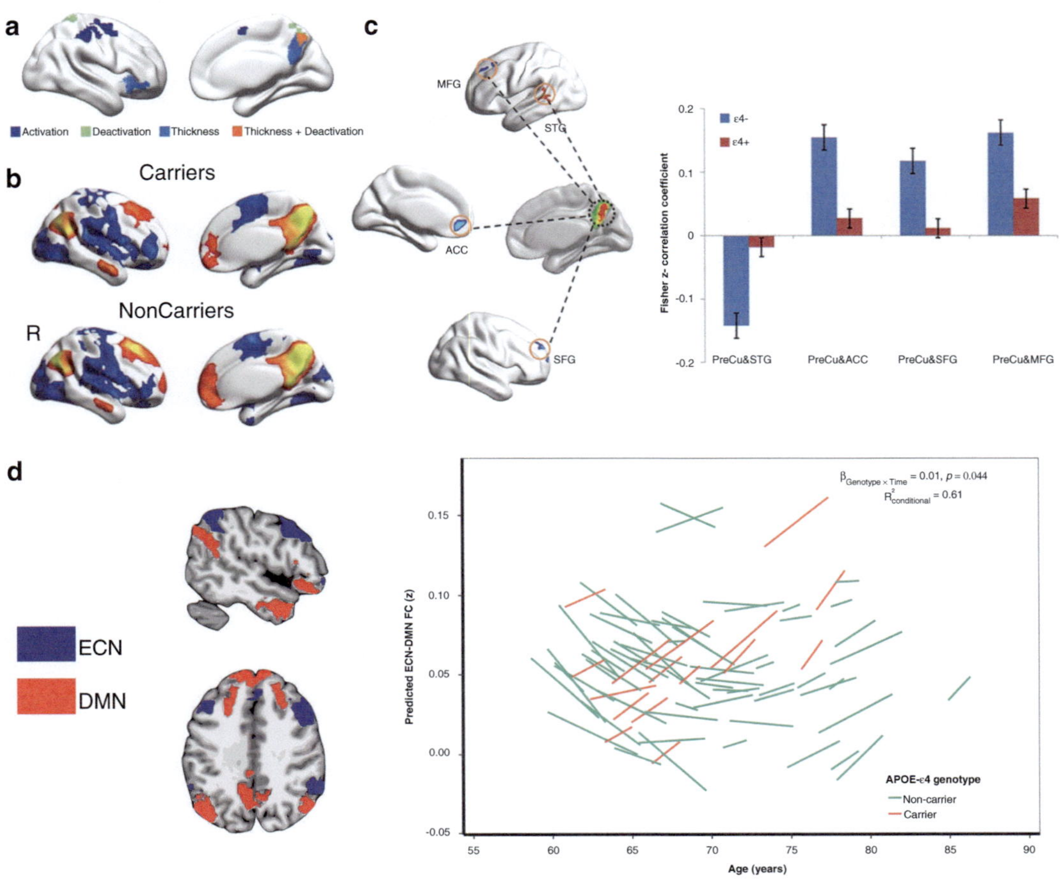

Fig. 25.9 APOE genotype influences brain functional connectivity in healthy older adults. Healthy older adults who were APOE ε4 carriers had more atrophy and deactivations in a memory task in the precuneus (orange regions in **a**; showing only the right hemisphere). Whole-brain functional connectivity based on this precuneus seed yielded similar connectivity topography regardless of genotype (**b**; positive connectivity in hot color, negative connectivity in cool color; showing only the right hemispheres), but carriers evidenced weaker anticorrelations between the default mode network regions and the control/attention network regions (negatively signed bar in **c**) and weaker correlations within these networks (positively signed bars in **c**). This difference in internetwork connectivity between the default mode network (DMN) and high-level cognitive networks (showing example regions of the DMN in red and executive control network in blue (Yeo et al. 2011)) was also observed longitudinally (**d**), where ε4 carriers (orange lines) showed faster loss of segregation (increased connectivity) over a span of 4 years than non-carriers (green lines), i.e., genotype × time interaction. Abbreviations: *ACC* anterior cingulate cortex, *PreCu* precunues, *MFG* medial frontal gyrus, *SFG* superior frontal gyrus, *STG* superior temporal gyrus, *FC* functional connectivity, *DMN* default mode network, *ECN* executive control network. (Figures are modified from Chen et al. (2017b) and Ng et al. (2018) with permission)

mulates extracellularly as plaques when misfolded. It is proposed to be a neurotoxin causing synaptic damage and is key to AD progression (Jack Jr et al. 2013; Gouras et al. 2015). Excessive hyper-phosphorylated tau protein accumulates intracellularly, forming neurofibrillary tangles that lead to neuronal dysfunction (Iqbal et al. 2010). Compared to Aβ, tau accumulation progression is more systematic and more closely related to cognitive decline and clinical symptoms (Tosun et al. 2017; Hoenig et al. 2018; Lewis and Dickson 2016). Because of the temporal antecedence of Aβ, tau is often examined with Aβ deposition concurrently in healthy and preclinical populations.

While far from clear (Herrup 2015), the influence of Aβ on functional connectivity has been consistently demonstrated. Two studies have indicated that the amount of Aβ deposits was negatively correlated with the DMN connectivity (ventral medial prefrontal cortex, angular gyrus, and medial posterior regions), and the lower connectivity was associated with poorer working memory performance in normal aging (Kikuchi et al. 2011; Mormino et al. 2011). As described in Sect. 25.4 above, using a whole-brain, voxel-wise, seed-based FC method, Drzezga and colleagues (2011) observed a general decrease in FC at cortical "hubs" (contiguous voxels showing strong FC to the rest of the brain) in the right angular and posterior cingulate cortex/precuneus (PCC) cortices across healthy older adults with low Aβ, healthy older adults with high Aβ, and individuals with mild cognitive impairment. This and other studies have also shown that hypometabolism was highly associated with the distribution of Aβ deposition and FC changes, suggesting that Aβ may compromise synaptic functioning, leading to "disconnections" (Forster et al. 2012; Brier et al. 2014).

Such disconnection may occur quite early in the AD pathological process. Gili and colleagues (2011) found that DMN connectivity disruption in the PCC resulted in reduced connectivity in MCI patients in the absence of gray matter atrophy compared to controls. Using seed-based FC restricted to the medial temporal lobe regions, Song (2015) and colleagues reported that the cortical Aβ load was related to disrupted FC of the perirhinal cortex but not to cognition or atrophy. Since perirhinal cortex is the earliest region affected by tau in AD (Braak et al. 2011), their results may suggest that the influence of Aβ deposition on brain function occurs in the very early stages of the disease progression evidenced by aberrant FC changes, which may be linked to later tau accumulation and subsequent memory loss.

Other studies have suggested that Aβ deposition can impact the brain-cognition relationship. Looking at the major intrinsic networks for high-level cognition using ICA-based FC, Lim and colleagues (2014) found that Aβ-positive individuals had higher DMN (PCC and hippocampal) FC and lower ECN FC than individuals low in Aβ. They attributed the higher DMN FC, which contrasted with past studies (Drzezga et al. 2011; Sheline et al. 2010), to compensatory or reserve processes. Within the Aβ-positive group, higher Aβ deposition (in the anterior cingulate cortex) was associated with higher ECN FC, lower posterior DMN FC, and weaker ECN-DMN anticorrelations. These differences in FC were related to episodic memory performance, suggesting that Aβ deposition can mediate or moderate the connectivity-memory associations in a fashion that resembles the neuronal spread pattern, i.e., the "epicenter" of the DMN propagating pathological attributes to other high-level networks (e.g., ECN) through its key functional connections (Fig. 25.10). Moreover, using seed-based FC, Buckley and colleagues (2017) reported that not only baseline connectivity in the associative functional networks (default, salience, and executive control) predicted longitudinal composite cognitive decline, but Aβ burden moderated this connectivity-cognition relationship. Specifically, persons with higher Aβ and lower baseline connectivity had the worst decline in cognitive performance over 6 years, as measured by their preclinical Alzheimer cognitive composite scores. These findings highlight the devastating effects brought about by the Aβ burden when brain functional networks lack resiliency and can occur as early as the preclinical stage (Jack Jr et al. 2013).

When probed simultaneously, Wang and colleagues (2013c) observed that presence of cerebrospinal fluid (CSF) Aβ biomarker or CSF tau biomarker was associated with lower DMN FC and, to a lesser extent, anticorrelations. In a recent study, Sepulcre and coworkers (2017a) reported tau and Aβ to be associated with hypo- and hyperfunctional connectivity in a group of cognitively normal older adults, respectively. Extracting parcellation-based FC from four associative ICNs and applying multiple regression analysis, with global cortical amyloid, regional tau, and amyloid-tau interaction as covariates of interest, Schultz and colleagues (2017) revealed the interaction between tau and Aβ on network functional connectivity to be nonlinear. For individuals with low levels of tau in the inferior temporal and inferior parietal regions, indicating better preserved neuronal

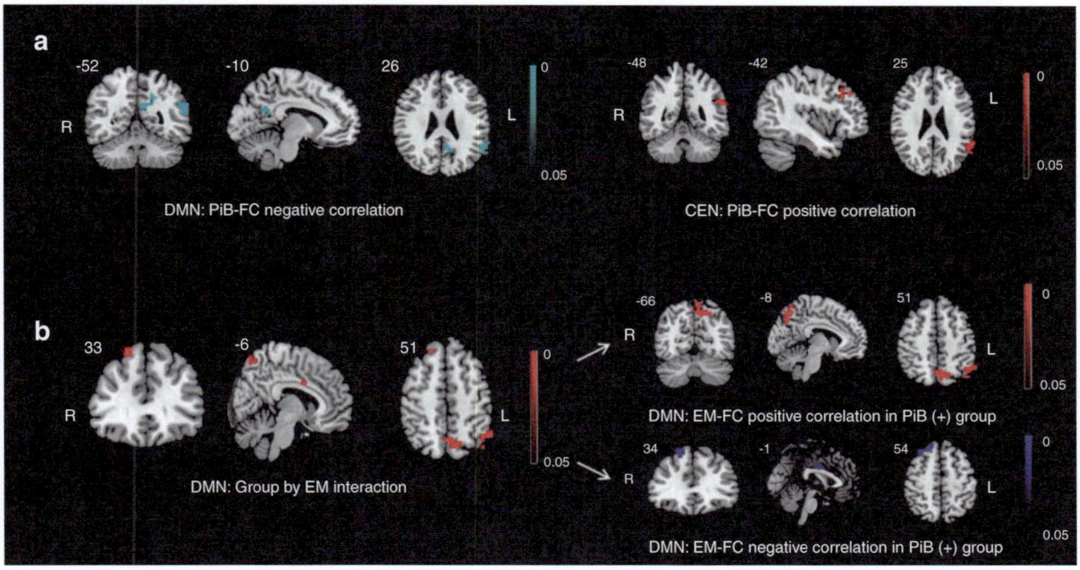

Fig. 25.10 Amyloid and tau deposition moderate functional connectivity in healthy elderly with amyloid burden. Within the group of cognitive normal older adults with amyloid burden (PiB(+)), higher regional (anterior cingulate cortex) Aβ deposition was associated with lower DMN FC (A left) and higher ECN FC (A right). Changes in DMN connectivity had functional implication, as significant group × episodic memory interactions were observed in the posterior and frontal DMN FC (B left). Specifically, poorer episodic memory was associated with higher FC in frontal DMN (B upper arrow) and lower FC in posterior DMN (B lower arrow), consistent with the critical involvement of the posterior DMN in AD. Abbreviations: *DMN* default mode network, *ECN* executive control network, *EM* episodic memory, *FC* functional connectivity, *PiB* Pittsburgh compound B. (Figure is modified from Lim et al. (2014) with permission)

function, those who were Aβ-positive showed higher connectivity in the DMN and the salience network (SN). By contrast, for individuals with high tau levels, those who were Aβ-positive showed *lower* connectivity in these networks. The authors postulated a hyperconnectivity-hypoconnectivity transition, in which hyperconnectivity may represent a response to the pathological markers (e.g., promote tau spread) (Keller and Christopher 2017) or compensation against them, and the subsequent hypoconnectivity is a reflection of network functionality loss. Finally, such distinct effects of tau and Aβ on functional connectivity were also found using a whole-brain computational model, with Aβ having a greater influence on connectivity strength and tau having a greater influence on whole-brain integration (metastability) (Demirtas et al. 2017). While this is a promising topic due to the high fidelity of these biomarkers to AD, many properties regarding such divergence, such as their reproducibility, regional specificity, and tau-Aβ interdependence (Sepulcre et al. 2017b), remain to be clarified and confirmed.

Despite their individual potency, the possession of a particular risk factor is often a necessary but not sufficient condition for developing neurodegenerative diseases (Snowdon and Study 2003). Risk factors not only exert unique effects (e.g., ε4-related changes in DMN functional connectivity in the absence of Aβ deposition) (Sheline et al. 2010; Lim et al. 2015) but also synergize to aggravate AD risk, such as the Aβ pathology promoted by ε4 (Reinvang et al. 2013; Liu et al. 2016b; Liu et al. 2017) and the tau-Aβ interaction (Tosun et al. 2017; Schultz et al. 2017). They may also interact with other fundamental individual attributes such as sex (Riedel et al. 2016; Heise et al. 2014). Furthermore, the brain may possess protective mechanisms, such as compensatory processes (Scheller et al. 2018; Luo et al. 2017; Ye et al. 2016) and cognitive reserves (Franzmeier et al. 2017), to be resilient against pathological aging (Damoiseaux 2012). For instance, the left frontal hubs have recently been argued to represent brain reserve in healthy and MCI individuals: higher left frontal connectivity was associated with better education, better residual memory performance (accounting for age and hippocampal atrophy), and delayed cognitive decline (Franzmeier et al. 2018). A more thorough understanding of these intricate associations is needed for the discovery of more sensitive biomarkers and individualized intervention schemes.

In conclusion, even in preclinical settings, functional connectivity is a highly viable tool to unravel the complex "scaffolding" process of normal and pathological aging. It will remain an exciting research topic, likely resulting in important interventional and treatment insights for dementia in the near future (Reuter-Lorenz and Park 2014).

25.6 Uncovering Disease Mechanisms and the Underlying Neuropathology

Network breakdown modeling: Intrinsic functional connectivity derived from rsfMRI data provides insights into how disease progresses to target a specific large-scale network. At least four disease-general hypotheses have been put forth and can be summarized: (1) "nodal stress," in which regions subject to heavy network traffic (i.e., "hubs") undergo activity-related "wear and tear" that gives rise to or worsens disease (Buckner et al. 2009; Saxena and Caroni 2011); (2) "transneuronal spread," in which some toxic agent propagates along network connections, perhaps through "prion-like" templated conformational changes (Baker et al. 1994; Frost and Diamond 2010; Frost et al. 2009; Jucker and Walker 2011; Lee et al. 2010; Ridley et al. 2006; Walker et al. 2006; Prusiner 1984); (3) "trophic failure," in which network connectivity disruption undermines internodal trophic factor support, accelerating disease within nodes lacking collateral trophic sources (Salehi et al. 2006; Appel 1981; Klupp et al. 2015); and (4) "shared vulnerability," in which networked regions feature a common gene or protein expression signature (Richiardi et al. 2015) that confers disease-specific susceptibility, evenly distributed throughout the network. These non-mutually exclusive candidate network degeneration mechanisms make competing predictions about how healthy network architecture should influence disease-associated regional vulnerability.

To test these competing predictions using rsfMRI data from healthy populations, Zhou and co-workers identified critical network epicenters in each of the five neurodegenerative syndromes whose normal connectivity profiles most resembled the syndrome-associated atrophy patterns. Using graph theoretical analyses, regions with higher total connectional flow and, more consistently, shorter functional paths to the epicenters in a healthy brain functional connectome, showed greater syndrome-associated vulnerability (Fig. 25.11) (Zhou et al. 2012). This observation raised the possibility that activity-dependent mechanisms, such as oxidative stress, local extracellular milieu fluctuations, or glia-dependent phenomena, influence regional vulnerability. This influence might be a key factor in determining sites of initial onset or secondary onset (i.e., progression). Second, nodes with shorter connectional paths to an epicenter showed greater vulnerability, suggesting that transneuronal spread represents one of the key factors driving early-target network degeneration, most likely by the physical transmission of toxic disease proteins or other agents along axons. In other words, epicenter infiltration by disease may provide privileged but graded access across the network that determines where the disease will arrive next. Overwhelmingly, the transneuronal spread model fits to both the target and off-target networks across the whole brain. In summary, the findings best fit a model in which initial vulnerability may reflect a node's centrality (i.e., "hubness") within the target network, whereas downstream vulnerability is more closely related to a node's connectional proximity to the most vulnerable "epicenter" regions. Further longitudinal studies are needed to investigate the network-based neurodegeneration hypothesis to account for how

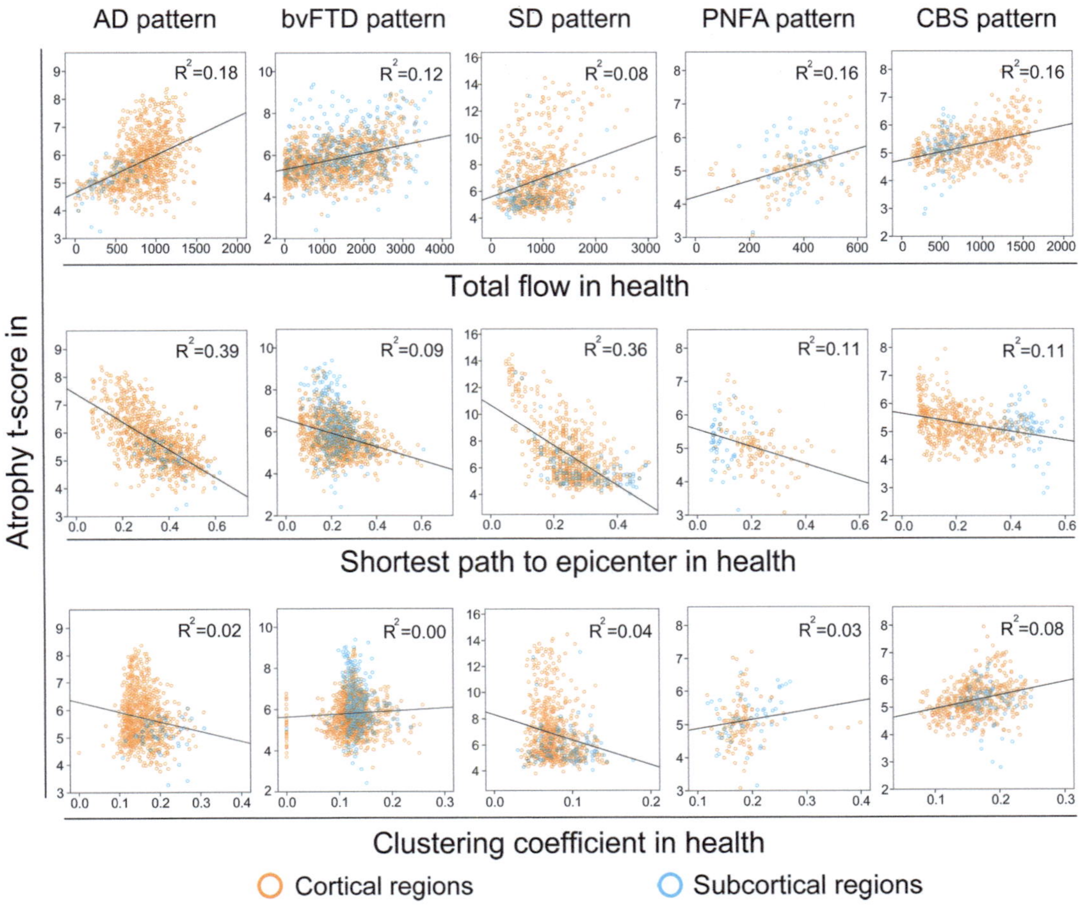

Fig. 25.11 Intranetwork graph theoretical connectivity measures in health predict atrophy severity in disease. Regions with high total connectional flow (row 1) and shorter functional paths to the epicenters (row 2) showed significantly greater disease vulnerability ($p < 0.05$ family-wise error corrected for multiple comparisons in AD, bvFTD, SD, PNFA, and CBS), whereas inconsistent weaker or nonsignificant relationships were observed between clustering coefficient and atrophy (row 3). Cortical regions = blue circles; subcortical regions = orange circles. (Figure is adapted from (Zhou et al. 2012) with permission)

these changes "outside" of the epicenters may arise and whether or how they are differentially associated with symptoms.

Relationship with pathophysiology: Maps of functional connectivity also provide a means to understand why certain lesions and connectional abnormalities are particularly disruptive and even predict the underlying pathology. For example, by mapping in vivo Aβ deposition with Pittsburg compound B (*PiB*) *PET* in patients with AD and controls, Buckner and colleagues found that the DMN cortical hubs in healthy controls resembled the high Aβ burden in AD (Buckner et al. 2009). This finding suggested that hubs, while acting as critical relay stations for information processing, may also augment the underlying pathological cascade in AD. Alterations of the resting-state functional network relates to the underlying disease pathophysiology. Within the DMN, Marchitelli and colleagues (2018) found association between glucose uptake and network activities in AD-targeting regions (e.g., PCC) among MCI patients. Moreover, precuneus-hippocampus FC was correlated with metabolism within the hippocampus in both aMCI and AD (Tahmasian et al. 2015), supporting the hippocampus disconnection hypothesis (Yassa et al. 2011; Das et al. 2013). Voxel-wise correlation showed that precuneus-based FC was associated with the ratio of Aβ42/P-tau181p in CSF among MCI patients (Li et al. 2013). Similarly, across MCI patients and controls, an increased β-amyloid burden was correlated with lower whole-brain FC in the PCC after controlling for gray matter density (Drzezga et al. 2011). In contrast, results from AD patients are rather mixed. Adriaanse and colleagues did not find an association between the average DMN FC and the average amyloid burden within the DMN (Adriaanse et al. 2014b). However, Malpas and colleagues reported that both CSF p-tau and CSF Aβ were related to functional networks in AD (Malpas et al. 2016). Specifically, while CSF p-tau was linked to an FC network with right anterior entorhinal cortex as a hub, CSF Aβ was associated with the anterior DMN. Taken together, resting-state FC networks have divergent associations with pathological biomarkers, and such relationships may vary with disease progression.

Differential diagnosis: Based on the divergent functional connectivity patterns among dementia patients and healthy controls, researchers have begun to develop functional connectivity-based biomarkers to distinguish among dementia subtypes and controls. Using rsfMRI, Greicius and colleagues calculated the goodness-of-fit score to the DMN at the individual level and achieved 85% sensitivity and 75% specificity differentiating AD from controls (Greicius et al. 2004). The clustering coefficient derived from graph theoretical analyses of rsfMRI distinguished AD participants from the controls with a sensitivity of 72% and a specificity of 78% (Supekar et al. 2008). A recent study computed whole-brain correlation-based connectivity among 116 region of interests and achieved 85% sensitivity and 80% specificity between the AD group and the non-AD group (MCI and controls) (Chen et al. 2011). Using graph theoretical measures, Khazaee and colleagues (2017) were able to classify AD, MCI, and control individuals with 93.3% accuracy; furthermore, hub counting showed a progressive decrease from control to AD, suggesting that AD is characterized by aberrant network communication. Such classification success and implications to hub disruption is consistent with the findings of Dai and colleagues (2015), which demonstrated hub-oriented impairment, in addition to disrupted internetwork connectivity, in AD compared to controls. Based on the observations that bvFTD and AD feature divergent connectivity effects on the SN and DMN, Zhou and colleagues (2010) illustrated that a summary score incorporating both networks might better differentiate bvFTD from AD and each patient group from healthy controls, achieving a sensitivity of 92% and specificity of 96% in a three-group classification and 100% differentiation between AD and bvFTD. This suggested that brain network functional connectivity, including both hyper- and hypo-connectivity changes, might prove more specific to predict disease diagnoses and prognosis. However, replication in multiple independent datasets and validation in pathologically verified clinical samples are needed.

25.7 Conclusion and Future Directions

In conclusion, under the umbrella of the network-based degeneration principle, network-sensitive rsfMRI-based functional connectivity mapping has begun to shed light on group-level functional brain network changes across a host of neurodegenerative disease syndromes (Greicius and Kimmel 2012), vulnerable patterns in preclinical and prodromal stages, prediction of disease progression, selective network breakdown mechanisms in disease, and associations with endophenotypes of molecular pathological changes (amyloid and tau accumulation). Increasingly, researchers hope to utilize rsfMRI-based functional connectivity to evaluate intervention efficacy and help the screening and stratification of patients for individualized treatment. For instance, after 12 weeks of donepezil treatment in mild AD, stronger recovery in the network connectivity with hippocampus was associated with cognitive improvement measured by Mini-Mental State Examination scores (Goveas et al. 2011). However, complex preprocessing and data analytical steps are involved in rsfMRI-based FC mapping to be able to make scientifically and clinically useful inferences on brain network dysfunction in dementia. As the field is moving toward open science, with transparent and reproducible research and data sharing across multiple sites, it is important to ensure good practices in collection, analysis, and inference of rsfMRI data (Smith and Nichols 2018). Here, we highlight several methodological considerations and provide important tips for functional connectivity mapping in dementia (see Box 25.2).

Box 25.2 Methodological Considerations for rsfMRI-Based Functional Connectivity Mapping

1. *General guidelines:*
   - Each method has its pros and cons. Choose the right study design based on the research question and whether it is hypothesis-driven (i.e., specific seed or network) or data-driven (i.e., whole-brain) study. For instance, seed choices (e.g., shape, location, and size) can alter conclusions (Chen et al. 2017a). It is encouraged to use a functional localizer or to select seeds based on previous meta-analysis or brain parcellation studies. The parcellation-based FC approach may give more consistent observations under some conditions, but vary in sensitivity for other analyses due to multiple comparison correction. ICA automatically extracts multiple networks, but decisions such as the number of components and generalization to out-sample (Schultz et al. 2014) still need to be made.
   - Global signal regression remains a topic of debate. It minimizes physiological noise with the potential risk of losing neural signals and interpretability of connectivity strength (Murphy and Fox 2017). The current consensus states that its use is affected by research questions, populations of interest, and sometimes the analytical method (e.g., ICA is suggested not to be paired with global signal regression).
   - Always look at the raw and intermediate data and functional connectivity maps at the individual level before moving on to group-level analysis.
   - Carefully control for scanner-related artifacts, sleepiness, motion, and registration error during data collection and analysis.
   - Static and dynamic connectivity measures may be sensitive to different attributes, thus which to use (or both) depends on the research questions (Córdova-Palomera et al. 2017). Of note, dynamic connectivity is still in its infancy at the time of writing, and a few critical theoretical and analytical issues remain to be addressed (Laumann et al. 2017).
   - To control false-positive inferences, multiple comparison correction needs to be incorporated (Gong et al. 2018). This concern may be more prominent in some methods (e.g., seed based) than in others.
2. *Tips for functional connectivity mapping in dementia:*
   - Inaccuracies in the registration step due to atrophy or white matter lesions could be more severe in dementia and aging populations (Razlighi et al. 2014) and may require additional treatment during analysis, such as native-space analysis or the use of age-specific or group-specific templates. The potential influence of atrophy on functional connectivity should also be taken into account.
   - Motion, whose impact on functional connectivity is well documented (Power et al. 2015; Satterthwaite et al. 2017), may differ considerably

between healthy and dementia participants. Perform rigorous motion quality controls to select good participants and use motion-censoring steps (Ciric et al. 2017).

- Vigilance fluctuation induces changes in functional connectivity (Falahpour et al. 2018; Wang et al. 2016). Since the elderly are more likely to fall asleep, we encourage concurrent eye tracking with rsfMRI recording to ensure comparable vigilance between groups.

encephalopathy. Mol Neurobiol 8(1):25–39. https://doi.org/10.1007/BF02778005

Binnewijzend MA, Schoonheim MM, Sanz-Arigita E, Wink AM, van der Flier WM, Tolboom N et al (2012) Resting-state fMRI changes in Alzheimer's disease and mild cognitive impairment. Neurobiol Aging 33(9):2018–2028. https://doi.org/10.1016/j.neurobiolaging.2011.07.003

Biswal B, Yetkin FZ, Haughton VM, Hyde JS (1995) Functional connectivity in the motor cortex of resting human brain using echo-planar MRI. Magn Reson Med 34(4):537–541

Biswal BB, Mennes M, Zuo X-N, Gohel S, Kelly C, Smith SM et al (2010) Toward discovery science of human brain function. Proc Natl Acad Sci U S A 107(10):4734–4739. https://doi.org/10.1073/pnas.0911855107

Boccardi M, Sabattoli F, Laakso MP, Testa C, Rossi R, Beltramello A et al (2005) Frontotemporal dementia as a neural system disease. Neurobiol Aging 26(1):37–44

Bokde AL, Ewers M, Hampel H (2009) Assessing neuronal networks: understanding Alzheimer's disease. Prog Neurobiol 89(2):125–133. https://doi.org/10.1016/j.pneurobio.2009.06.004

Borroni B, Alberici A, Cercignani M, Premi E, Serra L, Cerini C et al (2012) Granulin mutation drives brain damage and reorganization from preclinical to symptomatic FTLD. Neurobiol Aging 33(10):2506–2520. https://doi.org/10.1016/j.neurobiolaging.2011.10.031

Bos DJ, van Raalten TR, Oranje B, Smits AR, Kobussen NA, Belle J et al (2014) Developmental differences in higher-order resting-state networks in Autism Spectrum Disorder. Neuroimage Clin 4:820–827. https://doi.org/10.1016/j.nicl.2014.05.007

Botha H, Utianski RL, Whitwell JL, Duffy JR, Clark HM, Strand EA et al (2018) Disrupted functional connectivity in primary progressive apraxia of speech. Neuroimage Clin. 18:617–629. https://doi.org/10.1016/j.nicl.2018.02.036

Braak H, Braak E (1991) Neuropathological staging of Alzheimer-related changes. Acta Neuropathol (Berl) 82(4):239–259

Braak H, Thal DR, Ghebremedhin E, Del Tredici K (2011) Stages of the pathologic process in Alzheimer disease: age categories from 1 to 100 years. J Neuropathol Exp Neurol 70(11):960–969. https://doi.org/10.1097/NEN.0b013e318232a379

Brenner EK, Hillary FG, Grossner EC, Bernier RA, Gilbert N, Sathian K et al (2018) Diminished neural network dynamics in amnestic mild cognitive impairment. Int J Psychophysiol 130:63–72. https://doi.org/10.1016/j.ijpsycho.2018.05.001

Brier MR, Thomas JB, Snyder AZ, Benzinger TL, Zhang D, Raichle ME et al (2012) Loss of intranetwork and internetwork resting state functional connections with Alzheimer's disease progression. J Neurosci 32(26):8890–8899. https://doi.org/10.1523/JNEUROSCI.5698-11.2012

Brier MR, Thomas JB, Ances BM (2014) Network dysfunction in Alzheimer's disease: refining the disconnection hypothesis. Brain Connect 4(5):299–311. https://doi.org/10.1089/brain.2014.0236

Brueggen K, Kasper E, Dyrba M, Bruno D, Pomara N, Ewers M et al (2016) The primacy effect in amnestic mild cognitive impairment: associations with hippocampal functional connectivity. Front Aging Neurosci 8:244. https://doi.org/10.3389/fnagi.2016.00244

Buckley RF, Schultz AP, Hedden T, Papp KV, Hanseeuw BJ, Marshall G et al (2017) Functional network integrity presages cognitive decline in preclinical Alzheimer disease. Neurology 89(1):29–37. https://doi.org/10.1212/WNL.0000000000004059

Buckner RL, Snyder AZ, Shannon BJ, LaRossa G, Sachs R, Fotenos AF et al (2005) Molecular, structural, and functional characterization of Alzheimer's disease: evidence for a relationship between default activity, amyloid, and memory. J Neurosci 25(34):7709–7717

Buckner RL, Sepulcre J, Talukdar T, Krienen FM, Liu H, Hedden T et al (2009) Cortical hubs revealed by intrinsic functional connectivity: mapping, assessment of stability, and relation to Alzheimer's disease. J Neurosci 29(6):1860–1873

Cavanna AE, Trimble MR (2006) The precuneus: a review of its functional anatomy and behavioural correlates. Brain 129(3):564–583

Chen G, Ward BD, Xie C, Li W, Wu Z, Jones JL et al (2011) Classification of Alzheimer disease, mild cognitive impairment, and normal cognitive status with large-scale network analysis based on resting-state functional MR imaging. Radiology 259(1):213–221. https://doi.org/10.1148/radiol.10100734

Chen C, Homma A, Mok VC, Krishnamoorthy E, Alladi S, Meguro K et al (2016) Alzheimer's disease with cerebrovascular disease: current status in the Asia-Pacific region. J Intern Med 280(4):359–374. https://doi.org/10.1111/joim.12495

Chen JE, Glover GH, Greicius MD, Chang C (2017a) Dissociated patterns of anti-correlations with dorsal and ventral default-mode networks at rest. Hum Brain

Mapp 38(5):2454–2465. https://doi.org/10.1002/hbm.23532

Chen Y, Liu Z, Zhang J, Chen K, Yao L, Li X et al (2017b) Precuneus degeneration in nondemented elderly individuals with APOE ε4: evidence from structural and functional MRI analyses. Hum Brain Mapp 38(1):271–282. https://doi.org/10.1002/hbm.23359

Chhatwal JP, Schultz AP, Johnson KA, Hedden T, Jaimes S, Benzinger TLS et al (2018) Preferential degradation of cognitive networks differentiates Alzheimer's disease from ageing. Brain 141(5):1486–1500. https://doi.org/10.1093/brain/awy053

Chong JSX, Liu S, Loke YM, Hilal S, Ikram MK, Xu X et al (2017) Influence of cerebrovascular disease on brain networks in prodromal and clinical Alzheimer's disease. Brain 140(11):3012–3022. https://doi.org/10.1093/brain/awx224

Ciric R, Wolf DH, Power JD, Roalf DR, Baum GL, Ruparel K et al (2017) Benchmarking of participant-level confound regression strategies for the control of motion artifact in studies of functional connectivity. NeuroImage 154:174–187. https://doi.org/10.1016/j.neuroimage.2017.03.020

Cole MW, Repovš G, Anticevic A (2014) The frontoparietal control system: a central role in mental health. Neuroscientist 20(6):652–664. https://doi.org/10.1177/1073858414525995

Córdova-Palomera A, Kaufmann T, Persson K, Alnæs D, Doan NT, Moberget T et al (2017) Disrupted global metastability and static and dynamic brain connectivity across individuals in the Alzheimer's disease continuum. Sci Rep 7:40268. https://doi.org/10.1038/srep40268

Craig AD (2002) How do you feel? Interoception: the sense of the physiological condition of the body. Nat Rev Neurosci 3(8):655–666

Craig AD (2009) How do you feel--now? The anterior insula and human awareness. Nat Rev Neurosci 10(1):59–70

Dai Z, Yan C, Li K, Wang Z, Wang J, Cao M et al (2015) Identifying and mapping connectivity patterns of brain network hubs in Alzheimer's disease. Cereb Cortex 25(10):3723–3742. https://doi.org/10.1093/cercor/bhu246

Damoiseaux JS (2012) Resting-state fMRI as a biomarker for Alzheimer's disease? Alzheimers Res Ther 4(2):8. https://doi.org/10.1186/alzrt106

Damoiseaux JS, Rombouts SARB, Barkhof F, Scheltens P, Stam CJ, Smith SM et al (2006) Consistent resting-state networks across healthy subjects. Proc Natl Acad Sci U S A 103(37):13848–13853

Damoiseaux JS, Seeley WW, Zhou J, Shirer WR, Coppola G, Karydas A et al (2012) Gender modulates the APOE ε4 effect in healthy older adults: convergent evidence from functional brain connectivity and spinal fluid Tau levels. J Neurosci 32(24):8254–8262. https://doi.org/10.1523/JNEUROSCI.0305-12.2012

Das SR, Pluta J, Mancuso L, Kliot D, Orozco S, Dickerson BC et al (2013) Increased functional connectivity within medial temporal lobe in mild cognitive impairment. Hippocampus 23(1):1–6. https://doi.org/10.1002/hipo.22051

de Flores R, Mutlu J, Bejanin A, Gonneaud J, Landeau B, Tomadesso C et al (2017) Intrinsic connectivity of hippocampal subfields in normal elderly and mild cognitive impairment patients. Hum Brain Mapp 38(10):4922–4932. https://doi.org/10.1002/hbm.23704

de Haan W, van der Flier WM, Koene T, Smits LL, Scheltens P, Stam CJ (2012) Disrupted modular brain dynamics reflect cognitive dysfunction in Alzheimer's disease. NeuroImage 59(4):3085–3093. https://doi.org/10.1016/j.neuroimage.2011.11.055

Demirtas M, Falcon C, Tucholka A, Gispert JD, Molinuevo JL, Deco G (2017) A whole-brain computational modeling approach to explain the alterations in resting-state functional connectivity during progression of Alzheimer's disease. Neuroimage Clin 16:343–354. https://doi.org/10.1016/j.nicl.2017.08.006

Di Biasio F, Vanacore N, Fasano A, Modugno N, Gandolfi B, Lena F et al (2011) Neuropsychology, neuroimaging or motor phenotype in diagnosis of Parkinson's disease-dementia: which matters most? J Neural Transm 119(5):597–604. https://doi.org/10.1007/s00702-011-0733-3

Di Martino A, Shehzad Z, Kelly C, Roy AK, Gee DG, Uddin LQ et al (2009) Relationship between cingulo-insular functional connectivity and autistic traits in neurotypical adults. Am J Psychiatry 166(8):891–899

Dickerson BC, Sperling RA (2009) Large-scale functional brain network abnormalities in Alzheimer's disease: insights from functional neuroimaging. Behav Neurol 21(1):63–75. https://doi.org/10.3233/BEN-2009-0227

Dopper EG, Rombouts SA, Jiskoot LC, den Heijer T, de Graaf JR, de Koning I et al (2014) Structural and functional brain connectivity in presymptomatic familial frontotemporal dementia. Neurology 83(2):e19–e26. https://doi.org/10.1212/wnl.0000000000000583

Drzezga A, Becker JA, Van Dijk KRA, Sreenivasan A, Talukdar T, Sullivan C et al (2011) Neuronal dysfunction and disconnection of cortical hubs in non-demented subjects with elevated amyloid burden. Brain 134(6):1635–1646. https://doi.org/10.1093/brain/awr066

Dubois B, Feldman HH, Jacova C, Dekosky ST, Barberger-Gateau P, Cummings J et al (2007) Research criteria for the diagnosis of Alzheimer's disease: revising the NINCDS-ADRDA criteria. Lancet Neurol 6(8):734–746. https://doi.org/10.1016/S1474-4422(07)70178-3

Dunn CJ, Duffy SL, Hickie IB, Lagopoulos J, Lewis SJ, Naismith SL et al (2014) Deficits in episodic memory retrieval reveal impaired default mode network connectivity in amnestic mild cognitive impairment. Neuroimage Clin 4:473–480. https://doi.org/10.1016/j.nicl.2014.02.010

Erhardt EB, Rachakonda S, Bedrick EJ, Allen EA, Adali T, Calhoun VD (2011) Comparison of multi-subject ICA methods for analysis of fMRI data. Hum Brain Mapp 32(12):2075–2095. https://doi.org/10.1002/hbm.21170

Falahpour M, Chang C, Wong CW, Liu TT (2018) Template-based prediction of vigilance fluctuations in resting-state fMRI. NeuroImage 174:317–327. https://doi.org/10.1016/j.neuroimage.2018.03.012

Farb NA, Grady CL, Strother S, Tang-Wai DF, Masellis M, Black S et al (2013) Abnormal network connectivity in frontotemporal dementia: evidence for prefrontal isolation. Cortex 49(7):1856–1873. https://doi.org/10.1016/j.cortex.2012.09.008

Ferreira LK, Regina AC, Kovacevic N, Martin Mda G, Santos PP, Carneiro Cde G et al (2016) Aging effects on whole-brain functional connectivity in adults free of cognitive and psychiatric disorders. Cereb Cortex 26(9):3851–3865. https://doi.org/10.1093/cercor/bhv190

Filippi M, Agosta F, Scola E, Canu E, Magnani G, Marcone A et al (2013) Functional network connectivity in the behavioral variant of frontotemporal dementia. Cortex 49(9):2389–2401. https://doi.org/10.1016/j.cortex.2012.09.017

Filippi M, Basaia S, Canu E, Imperiale F, Meani A, Caso F et al (2017) Brain network connectivity differs in early-onset neurodegenerative dementia. Neurology 89(17):1764–1772. https://doi.org/10.1212/WNL.0000000000004577

Filippini N, MacIntosh BJ, Hough MG, Goodwin GM, Frisoni GB, Smith SM et al (2009) Distinct patterns of brain activity in young carriers of the APOE-epsilon4 allele. Proc Natl Acad Sci U S A 106(17):7209–7214

Firbank MJ, Allan LM, Burton EJ, Barber R, O'Brien JT, Kalaria RN (2011) Neuroimaging predictors of death and dementia in a cohort of older stroke survivors. J Neurol Neurosurg Psychiatry 83(3):263–367. https://doi.org/10.1136/jnnp-2011-300873

Fleisher AS, Sherzai A, Taylor C, Langbaum JBS, Chen K, Buxton RB (2009) Resting-state BOLD networks versus task-associated functional MRI for distinguishing Alzheimer's disease risk groups. NeuroImage 47(4):1678–1690

Fornito A, Zalesky A, Breakspear M (2013) Graph analysis of the human connectome: promise, progress, and pitfalls. NeuroImage 80:426–444. https://doi.org/10.1016/j.neuroimage.2013.04.087

Forster S, Grimmer T, Miederer I, Henriksen G, Yousefi BH, Graner P et al (2012) Regional expansion of hypometabolism in Alzheimer's disease follows amyloid deposition with temporal delay. Biol Psychiatry 71(9):792–797. https://doi.org/10.1016/j.biopsych.2011.04.023

Fouquet M, Besson FL, Gonneaud J, Joie RL, Chételat G (2014) Imaging brain effects of APOE4 in cognitively normal individuals across the lifespan. Neuropsychol Rev 24(3):290–299. https://doi.org/10.1007/s11065-014-9263-8

Fox MD, Snyder AZ, Vincent JL, Corbetta M, Van Essen DC, Raichle ME (2005) The human brain is intrinsically organized into dynamic, anticorrelated functional networks. Proc Natl Acad Sci U S A 102(27):9673–9678

Franzmeier N, Duering M, Weiner M, Dichgans M, Ewers M (2017) Alzheimer's Disease Neuroimaging Initiative. Left frontal cortex connectivity underlies cognitive reserve in prodromal Alzheimer disease. Neurology 88(11):1054–1061. https://doi.org/10.1212/WNL.0000000000003711

Franzmeier N, Hartmann J, Taylor ANW, Araque-Caballero MA, Simon-Vermot L, Kambeitz-Ilankovic L et al (2018) The left frontal cortex supports reserve in aging by enhancing functional network efficiency. Alzheimers Res Ther 10(1):28. https://doi.org/10.1186/s13195-018-0358-y

Frost B, Diamond MI (2010) Prion-like mechanisms in neurodegenerative diseases. Nat Rev Neurosci 11(3):155–159

Frost B, Ollesch J, Wille H, Diamond MI (2009) Conformational diversity of wild-type Tau fibrils specified by templated conformation change. J Biol Chem 284(6):3546–3551

Gao W, Alcauter S, Elton A, Hernandez-Castillo CR, Smith JK, Ramirez J et al (2015) Functional network development during the first year: relative sequence and socioeconomic correlations. Cereb Cortex 25(9):2919–2928. https://doi.org/10.1093/cercor/bhu088

Gili T, Cercignani M, Serra L, Perri R, Giove F, Maraviglia B et al (2011) Regional brain atrophy and functional disconnection across Alzheimer's disease evolution. J Neurol Neurosurg Psychiatry 82(1):58–66. https://doi.org/10.1136/jnnp.2009.199935

Gong W, Wan L, Lu W, Ma L, Cheng F, Cheng W et al (2018) Statistical testing and power analysis for brain-wide association study. Med Image Anal 47:15–30. https://doi.org/10.1016/j.media.2018.03.014

Gordon E, Rohrer JD, Fox NC (2016) Advances in neuroimaging in frontotemporal dementia. J Neurochem 138(S1):193–210. https://doi.org/10.1111/jnc.13656

Gorno-Tempini ML, Hillis AE, Weintraub S, Kertesz A, Mendez M, Cappa SF et al (2011) Classification of primary progressive aphasia and its variants. Neurology 76(11):1006–1014. https://doi.org/10.1212/WNL.0b013e31821103e6

Goulding J, Signorini D, Chatterjee S, Nicoll J, Stewart J, Morris R et al (1999) Inverse relation between Braak stage and cerebrovascular pathology in Alzheimer predominant dementia. J Neurol Neurosurg Psychiatry 67(5):654–657

Gour N, Felician O, Didic M, Koric L, Gueriot C, Chanoine V et al (2014) Functional connectivity changes differ in early and late-onset alzheimer's disease. Hum Brain Mapp 35(7):2978–2994. https://doi.org/10.1002/hbm.22379

Gouras GK, Olsson TT, Hansson O (2015) beta-Amyloid peptides and amyloid plaques in Alzheimer's disease. Neurotherapeutics 12(1):3–11. https://doi.org/10.1007/s13311-014-0313-y

Goveas JS, Xie C, Ward BD, Wu Z, Li W, Franczak M et al (2011) Recovery of hippocampal network connectivity correlates with cognitive improvement in mild Alzheimer's disease patients treated with done-

pezil assessed by resting-state fMRI. J Magn Reson Imaging 34(4):764–773. https://doi.org/10.1002/jmri.22662
Greicius MD, Kimmel DL (2012) Neuroimaging insights into network-based neurodegeneration. Curr Opin Neurol 25(6):727–734. https://doi.org/10.1097/Wco.0b013e32835a26b3
Greicius MD, Menon V (2004) Default-mode activity during a passive sensory task: uncoupled from deactivation but impacting activation. J Cogn Neurosci 16(9):1484–1492
Greicius MD, Krasnow B, Reiss AL, Menon V (2003) Functional connectivity in the resting brain: a network analysis of the default mode hypothesis. Proc Natl Acad Sci U S A 100(1):253–258
Greicius MD, Srivastava G, Reiss AL, Menon V (2004) Default-mode network activity distinguishes Alzheimer's disease from healthy aging: evidence from functional MRI. Proc Natl Acad Sci U S A 101(13):4637–4642
Guo CC, Gorno-Tempini ML, Gesierich B, Henry M, Trujillo A, Shany-Ur T et al (2013) Anterior temporal lobe degeneration produces widespread network-driven dysfunction. Brain 136(Pt 10):2979–2991. https://doi.org/10.1093/brain/awt222
Guye M, Bettus G, Bartolomei F, Cozzone PJ (2010) Graph theoretical analysis of structural and functional connectivity MRI in normal and pathological brain networks. MAGMA 23(5-6):409–421. https://doi.org/10.1007/s10334-010-0205-z
Hafkemeijer A, Altmann-Schneider I, Oleksik AM, van de Wiel L, Middelkoop HAM, van Buchem MA et al (2013) Increased functional connectivity and brain atrophy in elderly with subjective memory complaints. Brain Connect 3(4):353–362. https://doi.org/10.1089/brain.2013.0144
Hampson M, Driesen NR, Skudlarski P, Gore JC, Constable RT (2006) Brain connectivity related to working memory performance. J Neurosci 26(51):13338–13343
Heise V, Filippini N, Trachtenberg AJ, Suri S, Ebmeier KP, Mackay CE (2014) Apolipoprotein E genotype, gender and age modulate connectivity of the hippocampus in healthy adults. NeuroImage 98:23–30. https://doi.org/10.1016/j.neuroimage.2014.04.081
Herrup K (2015) The case for rejecting the amyloid cascade hypothesis. Nat Neurosci 18(6):794–799. https://doi.org/10.1038/nn.4017
Hoenig MC, Bischof GN, Seemiller J, Hammes J, Kukolja J, Onur OA et al (2018) Networks of tau distribution in Alzheimer's disease. Brain 141(2):568–581. https://doi.org/10.1093/brain/awx353
Hyman BT, Damasio AR, Van Hoesen GW, Barnes CL (1984) Alzheimer's disease: cell-specific pathology isolates the hippocampal formation. Science 298:83–95
Iadecola C (2010) The overlap between neurodegenerative and vascular factors in the pathogenesis of dementia. Acta Neuropathol (Berl) 120(3):287–296. https://doi.org/10.1007/s00401-010-0718-6
Ikeda M, Ishikawa T, Tanabe H (2004) Epidemiology of frontotemporal lobar degeneration. Dement Geriatr Cogn Disord 17(4):265–268. https://doi.org/10.1159/000077151
Iqbal K, Liu F, Gong CX, Grundke-Iqbal I (2010) Tau in Alzheimer disease and related tauopathies. Curr Alzheimer Res 7(8):656–664
Jack CR Jr, Knopman DS, Jagust WJ, Petersen RC, Weiner MW, Aisen PS et al (2013) Tracking pathophysiological processes in Alzheimer's disease: an updated hypothetical model of dynamic biomarkers. Lancet Neurol 12(2):207–216. https://doi.org/10.1016/S1474-4422(12)70291-0
Jessen F, Wolfsgruber S, Wiese B, Bickel H, Mosch E, Kaduszkiewicz H et al (2014) AD dementia risk in late MCI, in early MCI, and in subjective memory impairment. Alzheimers Dement 10(1):76–83. https://doi.org/10.1016/j.jalz.2012.09.017
Jiang L, Sui D, Qiao K, Dong H-M, Chen L, Han Y (2018) Impaired functional criticality of human brain during Alzheimer's disease progression. Sci Rep 8(1):1324. https://doi.org/10.1038/s41598-018-19674-7
Joubert S, Gour N, Guedj E, Didic M, Guériot C, Koric L et al (2016) Early-onset and late-onset Alzheimer's disease are associated with distinct patterns of memory impairment. Cortex 74:217–232. https://doi.org/10.1016/j.cortex.2015.10.014
Jucker M, Walker LC (2011) Pathogenic protein seeding in Alzheimer disease and other neurodegenerative disorders. Ann Neurol 70(4):532–540. https://doi.org/10.1002/ana.22615
Kalheim LF, Bjornerud A, Fladby T, Vegge K, Selnes P (2017) White matter hyperintensity microstructure in amyloid dysmetabolism. J Cereb Blood Flow Metab 37(1):356–365. https://doi.org/10.1177/0271678X15627465
Kanekiyo T, Xu H, Bu G (2014) ApoE and Aβ in Alzheimer's disease: accidental encounters or partners? Neuron 81(4):740–754. https://doi.org/10.1016/j.neuron.2014.01.045
Keller AS, Christopher L (2017) Distinct phases of tau, amyloid, and functional connectivity in healthy older adults. J Neurosci 37(37):8857–8859. https://doi.org/10.1523/JNEUROSCI.1687-17.2017
Khazaee A, Ebrahimzadeh A, Babajani-Feremi A, Alzheimer's Disease Neuroimaging Initiative (2017) Classification of patients with MCI and AD from healthy controls using directed graph measures of resting-state fMRI. Behav Brain Res 322(Pt B):339–350. https://doi.org/10.1016/j.bbr.2016.06.043
Kikuchi M, Hirosawa T, Yokokura M, Yagi S, Mori N, Yoshikawa E et al (2011) Effects of brain amyloid deposition and reduced glucose metabolism on the default mode of brain function in normal aging. J Neurosci 31(31):11193–11199. https://doi.org/10.1523/JNEUROSCI.2535-11.2011
Klaassens BL, van Gerven JMA, van der Grond J, de Vos F, Möller C, Rombouts SARB (2017) Diminished posterior precuneus connectivity with the default mode network differentiates normal aging from Alzheimer's

disease. Front Aging Neurosci 9:97. https://doi.org/10.3389/fnagi.2017.00097

Klupp E, Grimmer T, Tahmasian M, Sorg C, Yakushev I, Yousefi BH et al (2015) Prefrontal hypometabolism in Alzheimer disease is related to longitudinal amyloid accumulation in remote brain regions. J Nucl Med 56(3):399–404. https://doi.org/10.2967/jnumed.114.149302

Kryscio RJ, Abner EL, Cooper GE, Fardo DW, Jicha GA, Nelson PT et al (2014) Self-reported memory complaints: implications from a longitudinal cohort with autopsies. Neurology 83(15):1359–1365. https://doi.org/10.1212/WNL.0000000000000856

Kuczynski B, Jagust W, Chui HC, Reed B (2009) An inverse association of cardiovascular risk and frontal lobe glucose metabolism. Neurology 72(8):738–743. https://doi.org/10.1212/01.wnl.0000343005.35498.e5

Laumann TO, Snyder AZ, Mitra A, Gordon EM, Gratton C, Adeyemo B et al (2017) On the stability of BOLD fMRI correlations. Cereb Cortex 27(10):4719–4732. https://doi.org/10.1093/cercor/bhw265

Lee JK, Jin HK, Endo S, Schuchman EH, Carter JE, Bae JS (2010) Intracerebral transplantation of bone marrow-derived mesenchymal stem cells reduces amyloid-beta deposition and rescues memory deficits in Alzheimer's disease mice by modulation of immune responses. Stem Cells 28(2):329–343. https://doi.org/10.1002/stem.277

Lehmann M, Rohrer JD, Clarkson MJ, Ridgway GR, Scahill RI, Modat M et al (2010) Reduced cortical thickness in the posterior cingulate gyrus is characteristic of both typical and atypical Alzheimer's disease. J Alzheimers Dis 20(2):587–598. https://doi.org/10.3233/jad-2010-1401

Lehmann M, Madison CM, Ghosh PM, Seeley WW, Mormino E, Greicius MD et al (2013) Intrinsic connectivity networks in healthy subjects explain clinical variability in Alzheimer's disease. Proc Natl Acad Sci U S A 110(28):11606–11611. https://doi.org/10.1073/pnas.1221536110

Lehmann M, Madison C, Ghosh PM, Miller ZA, Greicius MD, Kramer JH et al (2015) Loss of functional connectivity is greater outside the default mode network in nonfamilial early-onset Alzheimer's disease variants. Neurobiol Aging 36(10):2678–2686. https://doi.org/10.1016/j.neurobiolaging.2015.06.029

Lewis J, Dickson DW (2016) Propagation of tau pathology: hypotheses, discoveries, and yet unresolved questions from experimental and human brain studies. Acta Neuropathol (Berl) 131(1):27–48. https://doi.org/10.1007/s00401-015-1507-z

Li X, Li T-Q, Andreasen N, Wiberg MK, Westman E, Wahlund L-O (2013) Ratio of Aβ42/P-tau181p in CSF is associated with aberrant default mode network in AD. Sci Rep 3:1339. https://doi.org/10.1038/srep01339

Lim HK, Nebes R, Snitz B, Cohen A, Mathis C, Price J et al (2014) Regional amyloid burden and intrinsic connectivity networks in cognitively normal elderly subjects. Brain 137(12):3327–3338. https://doi.org/10.1093/brain/awu271

Lim YY, Villemagne VL, Laws SM, Pietrzak RH, Snyder PJ, Ames D et al (2015) APOE and BDNF polymorphisms moderate amyloid β-related cognitive decline in preclinical Alzheimer's disease. Mol Psychiatry 20(11):1322–1328. https://doi.org/10.1038/mp.2014.123

Liu J, Zhang X, Yu C, Duan Y, Zhuo J, Cui Y et al (2016a) Impaired parahippocampus connectivity in mild cognitive impairment and Alzheimer's disease. J Alzheimers Dis 49(4):1051–1064. https://doi.org/10.3233/JAD-150727

Liu Y, Tan L, Wang H-F, Liu Y, Hao X-K, Tan C-C et al (2016b) Multiple effect of APOE genotype on clinical and neuroimaging biomarkers across Alzheimer's disease spectrum. Mol Neurobiol 53(7):4539–4547. https://doi.org/10.1007/s12035-015-9388-7

Liu CC, Zhao N, Fu Y, Wang N, Linares C, Tsai CW et al (2017) ApoE4 accelerates early seeding of amyloid pathology. Neuron 96(5):1024–1032. e3. https://doi.org/10.1016/j.neuron.2017.11.013

López-Sanz D, Bruña R, Garcés P, Martín-Buro MC, Walter S, Delgado ML et al (2017) Functional connectivity disruption in subjective cognitive decline and mild cognitive impairment: a common pattern of alterations. Front Aging Neurosci 9:109. https://doi.org/10.3389/fnagi.2017.00109

Luo X, Qiu T, Jia Y, Huang P, Xu X, Yu X et al (2017) Intrinsic functional connectivity alterations in cognitively intact elderly APOE ε4 carriers measured by eigenvector centrality mapping are related to cognition and CSF biomarkers: a preliminary study. Brain Imaging Behav 11(5):1290–1301. https://doi.org/10.1007/s11682-016-9600-z

Machulda MM, Jones DT, Vemuri P, McDade E, Avula R, Przybelski S et al (2011) Effect of APOE epsilon4 status on intrinsic network connectivity in cognitively normal elderly subjects. Arch Neurol 68(9):1131–1136. https://doi.org/10.1001/archneurol.2011.108

Mackenzie IR, Neumann M, Bigio EH, Cairns NJ, Alafuzoff I, Kril J et al (2010) Nomenclature and nosology for neuropathologic subtypes of frontotemporal lobar degeneration: an update. Acta Neuropathol (Berl) 119(1):1–4. https://doi.org/10.1007/s00401-009-0612-2

Mahley RW, Weisgraber KH, Huang Y (2006) Apolipoprotein E4: A causative factor and therapeutic target in neuropathology, including Alzheimer's disease. Proc Natl Acad Sci U S A 103(15):5644–5651. https://doi.org/10.1073/pnas.0600549103

Malpas CB, Saling MM, Velakoulis D, Desmond P, O'Brien TJ (2016) Differential functional connectivity correlates of cerebrospinal fluid biomarkers in dementia of the Alzheimer's type. Neurodegener Dis 16(3-4):147–151. https://doi.org/10.1159/000438924

Marchitelli R, Aiello M, Cachia A, Quarantelli M, Cavaliere C, Postiglione A et al (2018) Simultaneous resting-state FDG-PET/fMRI in Alzheimer disease: relationship between glucose metabolism and intrinsic activity. NeuroImage 176:246–258. https://doi.org/10.1016/j.neuroimage.2018.04.048

McKeown MJ, Hansen LK, Sejnowski TJ (2003) Independent component analysis of functional MRI: what is signal and what is noise? Curr Opin Neurobiol 13(5):620–629

Menon V (2011) Large-scale brain networks and psychopathology: a unifying triple network model. Trends Cogn Sci 15(10):483–506. https://doi.org/10.1016/j.tics.2011.08.003

Menon V, Uddin LQ (2010) Saliency, switching, attention and control: a network model of insula function. Brain Struct Funct 214(5-6):655–667. https://doi.org/10.1007/s00429-010-0262-0

Migliaccio R, Agosta F, Rascovsky K, Karydas A, Bonasera S, Rabinovici GD et al (2009) Clinical syndromes associated with posterior atrophy: early age at onset AD spectrum. Neurology 73(19):1571–1578. https://doi.org/10.1212/WNL.0b013e3181c0d427

Migliaccio R, Gallea C, Kas A, Perlbarg V, Samri D, Trotta L et al (2016) Functional connectivity of ventral and dorsal visual streams in posterior cortical atrophy. J Alzheimers Dis 51(4):1119–1130. https://doi.org/10.3233/jad-150934

Miller BL, Cummings J, Mishkin F, Boone K, Prince F, Ponton M et al (1998) Emergence of artistic talent in frontotemporal dementia. Neurology 51(4):978–982

Mitchell TW, Mufson EJ, Schneider JA, Cochran EJ, Nissanov J, Han LY et al (2002) Parahippocampal tau pathology in healthy aging, mild cognitive impairment, and early Alzheimer's disease. Ann Neurol 51(2):182–189

Mormino EC, Smiljic A, Hayenga AO, Onami SH, Greicius MD, Rabinovici GD et al (2011) Relationships between beta-amyloid and functional connectivity in different components of the default mode network in aging. Cereb Cortex 21(10):2399–2407. https://doi.org/10.1093/cercor/bhr025

Murphy K, Fox MD (2017) Towards a consensus regarding global signal regression for resting state functional connectivity MRI. NeuroImage 154:169–173. https://doi.org/10.1016/j.neuroimage.2016.11.052

Ng KK, Lo JC, Lim JKW, Chee MWL, Zhou J (2016) Reduced functional segregation between the default mode network and the executive control network in healthy older adults: a longitudinal study. NeuroImage 133:321–330. https://doi.org/10.1016/j.neuroimage.2016.03.029

Ng KK, Qiu Y, Lo JC-Y, Koay ES-C, Koh W-P, Chee MW-L et al (2018) Functional segregation loss over time is moderated by APOE genotype in healthy elderly. Hum Brain Mapp 39(7):2742–2752. https://doi.org/10.1002/hbm.24036

Palop JJ, Chin J, Roberson ED, Wang J, Thwin MT, Bien-Ly N et al (2007) Aberrant excitatory neuronal activity and compensatory remodeling of inhibitory hippocampal circuits in mouse models of Alzheimer's disease. Neuron 55(5):697–711

Papenberg G, Salami A, Persson J, Lindenberger U, Bäckman L (2015) Genetics and functional imaging: effects of APOE, BDNF, COMT, and KIBRA in aging. Neuropsychol Rev 25(1):47–62. https://doi.org/10.1007/s11065-015-9279-8

Pedersen M, Omidvarnia A, Zalesky A, Jackson GD (2018) On the relationship between instantaneous phase synchrony and correlation-based sliding windows for time-resolved fMRI connectivity analysis. NeuroImage 2018(181):85–94. https://doi.org/10.1016/j.neuroimage.2018.06.020

Peter J, Scheef L, Abdulkadir A, Boecker H, Heneka M, Wagner M et al (2014) Gray matter atrophy pattern in elderly with subjective memory impairment. Alzheimers Dement 10(1):99–108. https://doi.org/10.1016/j.jalz.2013.05.1764

Petersen RC (2011) Clinical practice. Mild cognitive impairment. N Engl J Med 364(23):2227–2234. https://doi.org/10.1056/NEJMcp0910237

Petersen RC, Smith GE, Waring SC, Ivnik RJ, Tangalos EG, Kokmen E (1999) Mild cognitive impairment: clinical characterization and outcome. Arch Neurol 56(3):303–308

Petersen RC, Doody R, Kurz A, Mohs RC, Morris JC, Rabins PV et al (2001) Current concepts in mild cognitive impairment. Arch Neurol 58(12):1985–1992. https://doi.org/10.1001/archneur.58.12.1985

Petrella JR, Sheldon FC, Prince SE, Calhoun VD, Doraiswamy PM (2011) Default mode network connectivity in stable vs progressive mild cognitive impairment. Neurology 76(6):511–517. https://doi.org/10.1212/WNL.0b013e31820af94e

Pievani M, de Haan W, Wu T, Seeley WW, Frisoni GB (2011) Functional network disruption in the degenerative dementias. Lancet Neurol 10(9):829–843. https://doi.org/10.1016/S1474-4422(11)70158-2

Pievani M, Filippini N, van den Heuvel MP, Cappa SF, Frisoni GB (2014) Brain connectivity in neurodegenerative diseases--from phenotype to proteinopathy. Nat Rev Neurol 10(11):620–633. https://doi.org/10.1038/nrneurol.2014.178

Power JD, Schlaggar BL, Petersen SE (2015) Recent progress and outstanding issues in motion correction in resting state fMRI. NeuroImage 105:536–551. https://doi.org/10.1016/j.neuroimage.2014.10.044

Premi E, Cauda F, Gasparotti R, Diano M, Archetti S, Padovani A et al (2014) Multimodal fMRI resting-state functional connectivity in granulin mutations: the case of fronto-parietal dementia. PLoS One 9(9):e106500. https://doi.org/10.1371/journal.pone.0106500

Prins ND, van Dijk EJ, den Heijer T, Vermeer SE, Jolles J, Koudstaal PJ et al (2005) Cerebral small-vessel disease and decline in information processing speed, executive function and memory. Brain 128(Pt 9):2034–2041. https://doi.org/10.1093/brain/awh553

Prusiner SB (1984) Some speculations about prions, amyloid, and Alzheimer's disease. N Engl J Med 310(10):661–663. https://doi.org/10.1056/NEJM198403083101021

Qi Z, Wu X, Wang Z, Zhang N, Dong H, Yao L et al (2010) Impairment and compensation coexist in amnestic

MCI default mode network. NeuroImage 50(1):48–55. https://doi.org/10.1016/j.neuroimage.2009.12.025

Qian S, Zhang Z, Li B, Sun G (2015) Functional-structural degeneration in dorsal and ventral attention systems for Alzheimer's disease, amnestic mild cognitive impairment. Brain Imaging Behav 9(4):790–800. https://doi.org/10.1007/s11682-014-9336-6

Quevenco FC, Preti MG, van Bergen JM, Hua J, Wyss M, Li X et al (2017) Memory performance-related dynamic brain connectivity indicates pathological burden and genetic risk for Alzheimer's disease. Alzheimers Res Ther 9(1):24. https://doi.org/10.1186/s13195-017-0249-7

Rabin LA, Smart CM, Amariglio RE (2017) Subjective cognitive decline in preclinical Alzheimer's disease. Annu Rev Clin Psychol 13:369–396. https://doi.org/10.1146/annurev-clinpsy-032816-045136

Raichle ME, MacLeod AM, Snyder AZ, Powers WJ, Gusnard DA, Shulman GL (2001) A default mode of brain function. Proc Natl Acad Sci U S A 98(2):676–682

Ratnavalli E, Brayne C, Dawson K, Hodges JR (2002) The prevalence of frontotemporal dementia. Neurology 58(11):1615–1621

Razlighi QR, Habeck C, Steffener J, Gazes Y, Zahodne LB, Mackay-Brandt A et al (2014) Unilateral disruptions in the default network with aging in native space. Brain Behav 4(2):143–157. https://doi.org/10.1002/brb3.202

Reinvang I, Espeseth T, Westlye LT (2013) APOE-related biomarker profiles in non-pathological aging and early phases of Alzheimer's disease. Neurosci Biobehav Rev 37(8):1322–1335. https://doi.org/10.1016/j.neubiorev.2013.05.006

Reuter-Lorenz PA, Park DC (2014) How does it STAC up? Revisiting the scaffolding theory of aging and cognition. Neuropsychol Rev 24(3):355–370. https://doi.org/10.1007/s11065-014-9270-9

Richiardi J, Altmann A, Milazzo AC, Chang C, Chakravarty MM, Banaschewski T et al (2015) BRAIN NETWORKS. Correlated gene expression supports synchronous activity in brain networks. Science 348(6240):1241–1244. https://doi.org/10.1126/science.1255905

Ridley RM, Baker HF, Windle CP, Cummings RM (2006) Very long term studies of the seeding of beta-amyloidosis in primates. J Neural Transm 113(9):1243–1251. https://doi.org/10.1007/s00702-005-0385-2

Riedel BC, Thompson PM, Brinton RD (2016) Age, APOE and sex: triad of risk of Alzheimer's disease. J Steroid Biochem Mol Biol 160:134–147. https://doi.org/10.1016/j.jsbmb.2016.03.012

Ronnlund M, Sundstrom A, Adolfsson R, Nilsson LG (2015) Subjective memory impairment in older adults predicts future dementia independent of baseline memory performance: evidence from the Betula prospective cohort study. Alzheimers Dement 11(11):1385–1392. https://doi.org/10.1016/j.jalz.2014.11.006

Salehi A, Delcroix JD, Belichenko PV, Zhan K, Wu C, Valletta JS et al (2006) Increased App expression in a mouse model of Down's syndrome disrupts NGF transport and causes cholinergic neuron degeneration. Neuron 51(1):29–42

Samann PG, Wehrle R, Hoehn D, Spoormaker VI, Peters H, Tully C et al (2011) Development of the brain's default mode network from wakefulness to slow wave sleep. Cereb Cortex 21(9):2082–2093. https://doi.org/10.1093/cercor/bhq295

Satterthwaite TD, Ciric R, Roalf DR, Davatzikos C, Bassett DS, Wolf DH (2017) Motion artifact in studies of functional connectivity: characteristics and mitigation strategies. Hum Brain Mapp. https://doi.org/10.1002/hbm.23665

Saxena S, Caroni P (2011) Selective neuronal vulnerability in neurodegenerative diseases: from stressor thresholds to degeneration. Neuron 71(1):35–48. https://doi.org/10.1016/j.neuron.2011.06.031

Saykin AJ, Wishart HA, Rabin LA, Santulli RB, Flashman LA, West JD et al (2006) Older adults with cognitive complaints show brain atrophy similar to that of amnestic MCI. Neurology 67(5):834–842. https://doi.org/10.1212/01.wnl.0000234032.77541.a2

Schaefer A, Quinque EM, Kipping JA, Arelin K, Roggenhofer E, Frisch S et al (2014) Early small vessel disease affects frontoparietal and cerebellar hubs in close correlation with clinical symptoms--a resting-state fMRI study. J Cereb Blood Flow Metab 34(7):1091–1095. https://doi.org/10.1038/jcbfm.2014.70

Scheller E, Schumacher LV, Peter J, Lahr J, Wehrle J, Kaller CP et al (2018) Brain aging and APOE epsilon4 interact to reveal potential neuronal compensation in healthy older adults. Front Aging Neurosci 10:74. https://doi.org/10.3389/fnagi.2018.00074

Schneider JA, Arvanitakis Z, Leurgans SE, Bennett DA (2009) The neuropathology of probable Alzheimer disease and mild cognitive impairment. Ann Neurol 66(2):200–208. https://doi.org/10.1002/ana.21706

Schultz AP, Chhatwal JP, Huijbers W, Hedden T, van Dijk KR, McLaren DG et al (2014) Template based rotation: a method for functional connectivity analysis with a priori templates. NeuroImage 102(Pt 2):620–636. https://doi.org/10.1016/j.neuroimage.2014.08.022

Schultz AP, Chhatwal JP, Hedden T, Mormino EC, Hanseeuw BJ, Sepulcre J et al (2017) Phases of hyperconnectivity and hypoconnectivity in the default mode and salience networks track with amyloid and tau in clinically normal individuals. J Neurosci 37(16):4323–4331. https://doi.org/10.1523/JNEUROSCI.3263-16.2017

Sedeno L, Couto B, Garcia-Cordero I, Melloni M, Baez S, Morales Sepulveda JP et al (2016) Brain network organization and social executive performance in frontotemporal dementia. J Int Neuropsychol Soc 22(2):250–262. https://doi.org/10.1017/s1355617715000703

Seeley WW, Menon V, Schatzberg AF, Keller J, Glover GH, Kenna H et al (2007) Dissociable intrinsic connectivity networks for salience processing and executive control. J Neurosci 27(9):2349–2356. https://doi.org/10.1523/jneurosci.5587-06.2007

Seeley WW, Crawford R, Rascovsky K, Kramer JH, Weiner M, Miller BL et al (2008a) Frontal paralimbic network atrophy in very mild behavioral variant frontotemporal dementia. Arch Neurol 65(2):249–255

Seeley WW, Matthews BR, Crawford RK, Gorno-Tempini ML, Foti D, Mackenzie IR et al (2008b) Unravelling Bolero: progressive aphasia, transmodal creativity and the right posterior neocortex. Brain 131(Pt 1):39–49

Seeley WW, Crawford RK, Zhou J, Miller BL, Greicius MD (2009) Neurodegenerative diseases target large-scale human brain networks. Neuron 62(1):42–52. https://doi.org/10.1016/j.neuron.2009.03.024

Seeley WW, Zhou J, Kim EJ (2011) Frontotemporal dementia: what can the behavioral variant teach us about human brain organization? Neuroscientist 18(4):373–385. https://doi.org/10.1177/1073858411410354

Sepulcre J, Sabuncu MR, Li Q, El Fakhri G, Sperling R, Johnson KA (2017a) Tau and amyloid beta proteins distinctively associate to functional network changes in the aging brain. Alzheimers Dement 13(11):1261–1269. https://doi.org/10.1016/j.jalz.2017.02.011

Sepulcre J, Grothe MJ, Sabuncu M, Chhatwal J, Schultz AP, Hanseeuw B et al (2017b) Hierarchical organization of tau and amyloid deposits in the cerebral cortex. JAMA Neurol 74(7):813–820. https://doi.org/10.1001/jamaneurol.2017.0263

Serra L, Cercignani M, Mastropasqua C, Torso M, Spanò B, Makovac E et al (2016) Longitudinal changes in functional brain connectivity predicts conversion to Alzheimer's disease. J Alzheimers Dis 51(2):377–389. https://doi.org/10.3233/JAD-150961

Sheline YI, Raichle ME, Snyder AZ, Morris JC, Head D, Wang S et al (2010) Amyloid plaques disrupt resting state default mode network connectivity in cognitively normal elderly. Biol Psychiatry 67(6):584–587. https://doi.org/10.1016/j.biopsych.2009.08.024

Shu N, Wang X, Bi Q, Zhao T, Han Y (2017) Disrupted topologic efficiency of white matter structural connectome in individuals with subjective cognitive decline. Radiology 286(1):229–238. https://doi.org/10.1148/radiol.2017162696

Shulman GL, Corbetta M, Fiez JA, Buckner RL, Miezin FM, Raichle ME et al (1997) Searching for activations that generalize over tasks. Hum Brain Mapp 5(4):317–322. https://doi.org/10.1002/(SICI)1097-0193(1997)5:4<317::AID-HBM19>3.0.CO;2-A

Smith SM, Nichols TE (2018) Statistical challenges in "big data" human neuroimaging. Neuron 97(2):263–268. https://doi.org/10.1016/j.neuron.2017.12.018

Smith SM, Fox PT, Miller KL, Glahn DC, Fox PM, Mackay CE et al (2009) Correspondence of the brain's functional architecture during activation and rest. Proc Natl Acad Sci U S A 106(31):13040–13045. https://doi.org/10.1073/pnas.0905267106

Snitz BE, Lopez OL, McDade E, Becker JT, Cohen AD, Price JC et al (2015) Amyloid-beta imaging in older adults presenting to a memory clinic with subjective cognitive decline. J Alzheimers Dis 48(Suppl 1):S151–S1S9. https://doi.org/10.3233/JAD-150113

Snowden JS, Stopford CL, Julien CL, Thompson JC, Davidson Y, Gibbons L et al (2007) Cognitive phenotypes in Alzheimer's disease and genetic risk. Cortex 43(7):835–845

Snowdon DA, Study N (2003) Healthy aging and dementia: findings from the Nun Study. Ann Intern Med 139(5 Pt 2):450–454

Song Z, Insel PS, Buckley S, Yohannes S, Mezher A, Simonson A et al (2015) Brain amyloid-β burden is associated with disruption of intrinsic functional connectivity within the medial temporal lobe in cognitively normal elderly. J Neurosci 35(7):3240–3247. https://doi.org/10.1523/JNEUROSCI.2092-14.2015

Sorg C, Riedl V, Mühlau M, Calhoun VD, Eichele T, Läer L et al (2007) Selective changes of resting-state networks in individuals at risk for Alzheimer's disease. Proc Natl Acad Sci U S A 104(47):18760–18765. https://doi.org/10.1073/pnas.0708803104

Sorg C, Riedl V, Perneczky R, Kurz A, Wohlschlager AM (2009) Impact of Alzheimer's disease on the functional connectivity of spontaneous brain activity. Curr Alzheimer Res 6(6):541–553

Sperling RA, Dickerson BC, Pihlajamaki M, Vannini P, LaViolette PS, Vitolo OV et al (2010) Functional alterations in memory networks in early Alzheimer's disease. NeuroMolecular Med 12(1):27–43. https://doi.org/10.1007/s12017-009-8109-7

Sperling R, Mormino E, Johnson K (2014) The evolution of preclinical Alzheimer's disease: implications for prevention trials. Neuron 84(3):608–622. https://doi.org/10.1016/j.neuron.2014.10.038

Sporns O (2013) Network attributes for segregation and integration in the human brain. Curr Opin Neurobiol 23(2):162–171. https://doi.org/10.1016/j.conb.2012.11.015

Sporns O, Betzel RF (2016) Modular brain networks. Annu Rev Psychol 67(1):613–640. https://doi.org/10.1146/annurev-psych-122414-033634

Spronk M, Kulkarni K, Ji JL, Keane B, Anticevic A, Cole MW (2018) A whole-brain and cross-diagnostic perspective on functional brain network dysfunction. bioRxiv. https://doi.org/10.1101/326728

Strittmatter WJ, Saunders AM, Schmechel D, Pericak-Vance M, Enghild J, Salvesen GS et al (1993) Apolipoprotein E: high-avidity binding to beta-amyloid and increased frequency of type 4 allele in late-onset familial Alzheimer disease. Proc Natl Acad Sci U S A 90(5):1977–1981

Supekar K, Menon V, Rubin D, Musen M, Greicius MD (2008) Network analysis of intrinsic functional brain connectivity in Alzheimer's disease. PLoS Comput Biol 4(6):e1000100

Tahmasian M, Pasquini L, Scherr M, Meng C, Förster S, Mulej Bratec S et al (2015) The lower hippocampus global connectivity, the higher its local metabolism in Alzheimer disease. Neurology 84(19):1956–1963. https://doi.org/10.1212/WNL.0000000000001575

Teipel S, Grothe MJ, Zhou J, Sepulcre J, Dyrba M, Sorg C et al (2016) Measuring cortical connectivity in Alzheimer's disease as a brain neural network pathology: toward clinical applications. J Int Neuropsychol Soc 22(2):138–163. https://doi.org/10.1017/S1355617715000995

Toledo JB, Arnold SE, Raible K, Brettschneider J, Xie SX, Grossman M et al (2013) Contribution of cerebrovascular disease in autopsy confirmed neurodegenerative disease cases in the National Alzheimer's Coordinating Centre. Brain 136(Pt 9):2697–2706. https://doi.org/10.1093/brain/awt188

Tosun D, Landau S, Aisen PS, Petersen RC, Mintun M, Jagust W et al (2017) Association between tau deposition and antecedent amyloid-beta accumulation rates in normal and early symptomatic individuals. Brain 140(5):1499–1512. https://doi.org/10.1093/brain/awx046

Toussaint PJ, Maiz S, Coynel D, Doyon J, Messe A, de Souza LC et al (2014) Characteristics of the default mode functional connectivity in normal ageing and Alzheimer's disease using resting state fMRI with a combined approach of entropy-based and graph theoretical measurements. NeuroImage 101:778–786. https://doi.org/10.1016/j.neuroimage.2014.08.003

Vincent JL, Patel GH, Fox MD, Snyder AZ, Baker JT, Van Essen DC et al (2007) Intrinsic functional architecture in the anaesthetized monkey brain. Nature 447(7140):83–86. https://doi.org/10.1038/nature05758

Walker LC, Levine H 3rd, Mattson MP, Jucker M (2006) Inducible proteopathies. Trends Neurosci 29(8):438–443. https://doi.org/10.1016/j.tins.2006.06.010

Wang J, Zuo X, Dai Z, Xia M, Zhao Z, Zhao X et al (2013a) Disrupted functional brain connectome in individuals at risk for Alzheimer's disease. Biol Psychiatry 73(5):472–481. https://doi.org/10.1016/j.biopsych.2012.03.026

Wang Y, Risacher SL, West JD, McDonald BC, Magee TR, Farlow MR et al (2013b) Altered default mode network connectivity in older adults with cognitive complaints and amnestic mild cognitive impairment. J Alzheimers Dis 35(4):751–760. https://doi.org/10.3233/JAD-130080

Wang L, Brier MR, Snyder AZ, Thomas JB, Fagan AM, Xiong C et al (2013c) Cerebrospinal fluid Abeta42, phosphorylated Tau181, and resting-state functional connectivity. JAMA Neurol 70(10):1242–1248. https://doi.org/10.1001/jamaneurol.2013.3253

Wang C, Ong J, Patanaik A, Zhou J, Chee MWL (2016) Spontaneous eyelid closures link vigilance fluctuation with fMRI dynamic connectivity states. Proc Natl Acad Sci U S A 113(34):9653–9658. https://doi.org/10.1073/pnas.1523980113

Whitwell JL, Josephs KA, Avula R, Tosakulwong N, Weigand SD, Senjem ML et al (2011) Altered functional connectivity in asymptomatic MAPT subjects: a comparison to bvFTD. Neurology 77(9): 866–874. https://doi.org/10.1212/WNL.0b013e31822c61f2

Whitwell JL, Weigand SD, Boeve BF, Senjem ML, Gunter JL, DeJesus-Hernandez M et al (2012) Neuroimaging signatures of frontotemporal dementia genetics: C9ORF72, tau, progranulin and sporadics. Brain 135(Pt 3):794–806. https://doi.org/10.1093/brain/aws001

Whitwell JL, Jones DT, Duffy JR, Strand EA, Machulda MM, Przybelski SA et al (2015) Working memory and language network dysfunctions in logopenic aphasia: a task-free fMRI comparison with Alzheimer's dementia. Neurobiol Aging 36(3):1245–1252. https://doi.org/10.1016/j.neurobiolaging.2014.12.013

Wig GS, Schlaggar BL, Petersen SE (2011) Concepts and principles in the analysis of brain networks. Ann N Y Acad Sci 1224:126–146. https://doi.org/10.1111/j.1749-6632.2010.05947.x

Wig GS, Laumann TO, Petersen SE (2014) An approach for parcellating human cortical areas using resting-state correlations. Neuroimage 93(Part 2):276–291. https://doi.org/10.1016/j.neuroimage.2013.07.035

Wilson SM, Galantucci S, Tartaglia MC, Gorno-Tempini ML (2012) The neural basis of syntactic deficits in primary progressive aphasia. Brain Lang 122(3):190–198. https://doi.org/10.1016/j.bandl.2012.04.005

Yang AC, Huang C-C, Liu M-E, Liou Y-J, Hong C-J, Lo M-T et al (2014) The APOE ε4 allele affects complexity and functional connectivity of resting brain activity in healthy adults. Hum Brain Mapp 35(7):3238–3248. https://doi.org/10.1002/hbm.22398

Yassa MA, Mattfeld AT, Stark SM, Stark CEL (2011) Age-related memory deficits linked to circuit-specific disruptions in the hippocampus. Proc Natl Acad Sci U S A 108(21):8873–8878. https://doi.org/10.1073/pnas.1101567108

Ye Q, Su F, Shu H, Gong L, Xie C, Zhang Z et al (2016) The apolipoprotein E gene affects the three-year trajectories of compensatory neural processes in the left-lateralized hippocampal network. Brain Imaging Behav 11(5):1446–1458. https://doi.org/10.1007/s11682-016-9623-5

Yeo BTT, Krienen FM, Sepulcre J, Sabuncu MR, Lashkari D, Hollinshead M et al (2011) The organization of the human cerebral cortex estimated by intrinsic functional connectivity. J Neurophysiol 106(3):1125–1165. https://doi.org/10.1152/jn.00338.2011

Yu J-T, Tan L, Hardy J (2014) Apolipoprotein E in Alzheimer's disease: an update. Annu Rev Neurosci 37(1):79–100. https://doi.org/10.1146/annurev-neuro-071013-014300

Zekry D, Duyckaerts C, Moulias R, Belmin J, Geoffre C, Herrmann F et al (2002a) Degenerative and vascular lesions of the brain have synergistic effects in dementia of the elderly. Acta Neuropathol (Berl) 103(5):481–487. https://doi.org/10.1007/s00401-001-0493-5

Zekry D, Hauw JJ, Gold G (2002b) Mixed dementia: epidemiology, diagnosis, and treatment. J Am Geriatr Soc 50(8):1431–1438

Zhan Y, Ma J, Alexander-Bloch AF, Xu K, Cui Y, Feng Q et al (2016) Longitudinal study of impaired intra- and inter-network brain connectivity in subjects at high risk for Alzheimer's disease. J Alzheimers Dis 52(3):913–927. https://doi.org/10.3233/JAD-160008

Zhou J, Seeley WW (2014) Network dysfunction in Alzheimer's disease and frontotemporal dementia: implications for psychiatry. Biol Psychiatry 75(7):565–573. https://doi.org/10.1016/j.biopsych.2014.01.020

Zhou J, Greicius MD, Gennatas ED, Growdon ME, Jang JY, Rabinovici GD et al (2010) Divergent network connectivity changes in behavioural variant frontotemporal dementia and Alzheimer's disease. Brain 133(5):1352–1367

Zhou J, Gennatas ED, Kramer JH, Miller BL, Seeley WW (2012) Predicting regional neurodegeneration from the healthy brain functional connectome. Neuron 73(6):1216–1227. https://doi.org/10.1016/j.neuron.2012.03.004

Zysset S, Huber O, Samson A, Ferstl EC, von Cramon DY (2003) Functional specialization within the anterior medial prefrontal cortex: a functional magnetic resonance imaging study with human subjects. Neurosci Lett 335(3):183–186

fMRI in Parkinson's Disease

26

Hartwig R. Siebner, David Meder,
and Damian M. Herz

Abbreviations

ACC	Anterior cingulate cortex
BA	Brodmann area
BG	Basal ganglia
BOLD	Blood-oxygenation-level-dependent
CMA	Cingulate motor area
COMT	Catechol O-methyltransferase
DCM	Dynamic causal modeling
DLPFC	Dorsolateral prefrontal cortex
fMRI	Functional magnetic resonance imaging
GPe	External globus pallidus
GPi	Internal globus pallidus
HC	Healthy control subjects
ICD	Impulse control disorder
IFG	Inferior frontal gyrus
IPC	Inferior parietal cortex
LEDD	Levodopa-equivalent daily dose
LID	Levodopa-induced dyskinesia
M1	Primary motor cortex
MCI	Mild cognitive impairment
MFC	Middle frontal cortex
MFG	Middle frontal gyrus
OFC	Orbitofrontal cortex
PC	Parietal cortex
PD	Parkinson's disease
PDCP	Parkinson's disease–related cognitive pattern
PDRP	Parkinson's disease–related pattern
PET	Positron-emission tomography
PFC	Prefrontal cortex
PM	Premotor cortex
PPI	Psychophysiological interaction
Pre-SMA	Pre-supplementary motor area
RS-fMRI	Resting-state functional magnetic resonance imaging
SEM	Structural equation modeling
SMA	Supplementary motor area
SNc	Substantia nigra pars compacta
SNr	Substantia nigra pars reticulata
SPC	Superior parietal cortex
SPECT	Single-photon emission computed tomography
STN	Subthalamic nucleus
VS	Ventral striatum
VTA	Ventral tegmental area

H. R. Siebner
Danish Research Centre for Magnetic Resonance, Copenhagen University Hospital Hvidovre, Hvidovre, Denmark

Department of Neurology, Copenhagen University Hospital Bispebjerg, Copenhagen, Denmark
e-mail: hartwig.siebner@drcmr.dk

D. Meder (✉)
Danish Research Centre for Magnetic Resonance, Copenhagen University Hospital Hvidovre, Hvidovre, Denmark
e-mail: davidm@drcmr.dk

D. M. Herz
Department of Neurology, Copenhagen University Hospital Bispebjerg, Copenhagen, Denmark
e-mail: damianh@drcmr.dk

S. Ulmer, O. Jansen (eds.), *fMRI*, https://doi.org/10.1007/978-3-030-41874-8_26

26.1 Clinical Features and Pathophysiology of Parkinson's Disease

Parkinson's disease (PD) is a progressive neurodegenerative disorder of unknown cause characterized by the cardinal features slowness of movement (akinesia), rigidity, and tremor at rest (Postuma et al. 2015).

However, non-motor features are common and involve disorders of cognitive, autonomic, and sensory function (Schapira et al. 2017). Motor impairment in PD has been linked to degeneration of dopaminergic neurons in substantia nigra pars compacta (SNc), leading to abnormal neural processing in the loops connecting cortex and basal ganglia (BG). These loops are thought to subserve action selection, i.e., execution of a selected movement while competing motor programs are inhibited (Mink 1996). This function is implemented by three distinct pathways in the BG (see Fig. 26.1 for a simplified model). According to this model, the activation of the direct pathway leads to a focused disinhibition of thalamocortical connections, while the indirect pathway broadly inhibits surrounding connections (Albin et al. 1989; DeLong 1990). Additionally, a hyperdirect pathway connecting cortex and the subthalamic nucleus (STN) can serve as a global stop signal for any movement (Nambu et al. 2000). The activation of the hyperdirect pathway can cancel previous or impulsive movements. The consecutive activation of the direct and indirect pathway facilitates the execution of the selected movement while inhibiting competing motor programs. Since dopamine activates the direct pathway via D1 receptors and inhibits the indirect pathway via D2 receptors, dopamine depletion can lead to an increased inhibition of thalamocortical connections via the indirect pathway and thereby cause akinesia. Although this original model is very helpful to explain this cardinal motor feature in PD, it has limitations. Therefore, complex properties such as changes in synaptic plasticity and neural discharge patterns are implemented in current models (Obeso et al. 2017), which are beyond the scope of this book chapter.

Importantly, it needs to be recalled that the cortico-basal ganglia-thalamo-cortical loops do not merely involve motor networks but consist of additional loops, which subserve cognitive or limbic functions (Fig. 26.2; Alexander et al. 1986). Neurodegeneration in PD affects more prominently the caudally localized sensorimotor basal ganglia loops, while the more rostrally localized associative and limbic loops are relatively spared (Rinne et al. 2001).

26.2 Neuroimaging in Parkinson's Disease

Functional neuroimaging techniques, such as positron-emission tomography (PET), single-photon emission computed tomography (SPECT), and functional magnetic resonance imaging (fMRI), have been widely used to study the function and dysfunction of neural networks. Early neuroimaging studies of patients with PD mainly involved PET measurements of regional cerebral blood flow (e.g., Jahanshahi et al. 1995; Playford et al. 1992). With the exception of PD patients treated with deep brain stimulation, fMRI has largely replaced PET as the imaging method of choice to study disease-related changes in neural activity and connectivity. In contrast to PET, fMRI does not involve exposure to radiation, which restricts the number of blood flow measurements with PET. Further, fMRI is widely available and has better spatial and temporal resolution, the latter allowing for the analysis of event-related activity. This makes PET and fMRI valuable complementary tools for studying changes in neural networks in PD. In the following sections, we will mainly focus on studies using fMRI. We report a selection of studies that were conducted at rest as well as during motor tasks and non-motor tasks. We do not cover all studies but highlight selected studies that are especially relevant for the given topic. Additionally, we included a section about preclinical compensation of dopaminergic degeneration, an exciting research field studying asymptomatic carriers of PD-related mutations. An overview of the selected publications is given in Table 26.1.

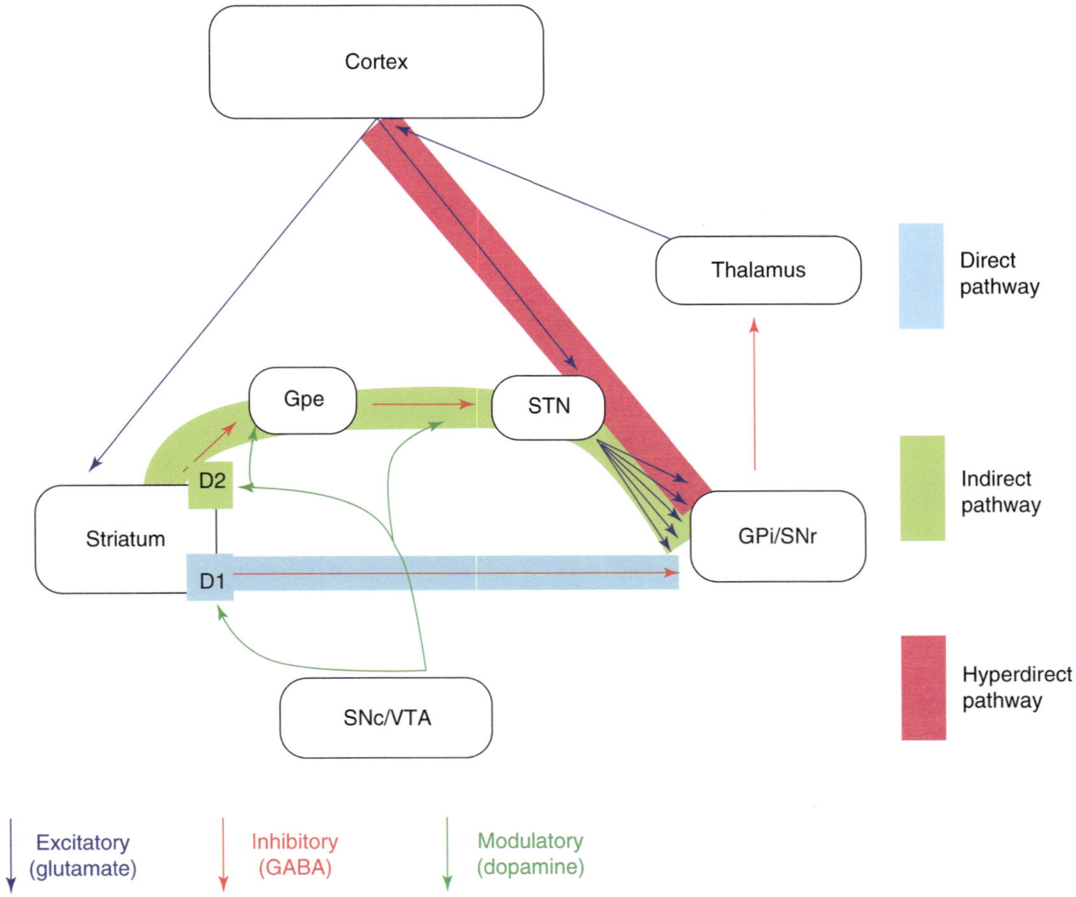

Fig. 26.1 A simplified model of cortico-subcortical pathways. Efferent connections from the cortex are processed in the BG and projected back to the cortex via the thalamus in closed feedback loops. The direct pathway connects the striatum, comprising putamen and caudate nucleus, with the internal globus pallidus (*GPi*)/substantia nigra pars reticulata (*SNr*). Since this connection as well as the connection between *GPi*/*SNr* and thalamus both are inhibitory, the activation of the direct pathway leads to a disinhibition of thalamocortical connections. On the other hand, the activation of the indirect pathway leads to a disinhibition of the *STN* via the external globus pallidus (*GPe*). The *STN* has diverging excitatory efferent connections to *GPi/SNr*, which consecutively leads to an inhibition of thalamocortical connections. The dopaminergic innervation of the striatum leads to an activation of the direct pathway via *D1* receptors and an inhibition of the indirect pathway via *D2* receptors and has therefore an excitatory influence on movements. In the case of motor loops, dopamine modulates mainly connections from substantia nigra pars compacta (*SNc*) to dorsal striatum while modulating connections from ventral tegmental area (*VTA*) to ventral striatum in the case of limbic loops. The hyperdirect pathway consists of a connection from the cortex to subthalamic nucleus (*STN*) bypassing the striatum. This connection can exert a fast global stop signal over the motor system. For simplicity reasons, feedback connections within the BG are omitted

26.2.1 Functional Connectivity Assessed with Resting-State fMRI

Resting-state fMRI (RS-fMRI) measures spontaneous low-frequency (<0.1 Hz) fluctuations in the blood-oxygen-level-dependent (BOLD) signal in the whole brain while participants are at rest. These regional BOLD signal fluctuations are temporally correlated within functional brain networks and thus provide an index of functional connectivity (Biswal et al. 1995; Raichle 2015). RS-fMRI is particularly suited for functional connectivity studies of the motor system in PD patients with motor disability. Since RS-fMRI does not require patients to engage in a motor

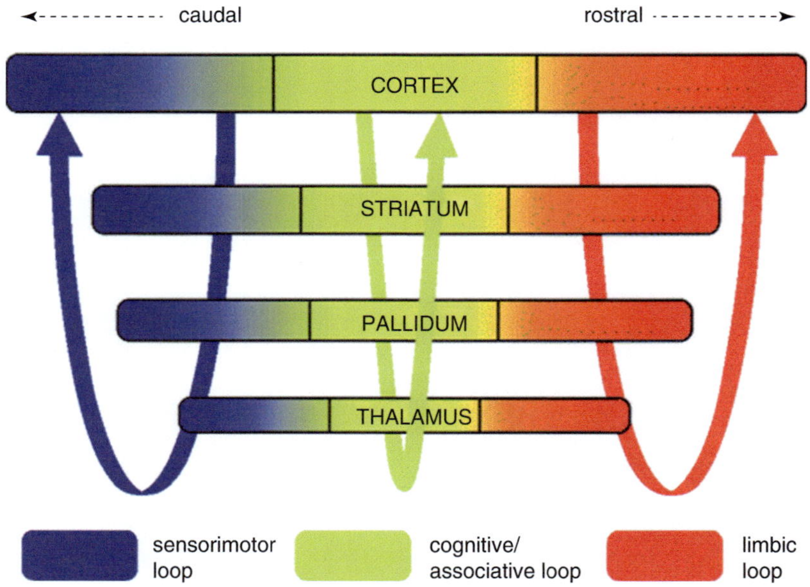

Fig. 26.2 Spatially and functionally distinct cortico-subcortical feedback loops. Each of the loops has its origin in the cortex and is processed via the input (*striatum*) and output structure of the BG (*pallidum*) to the thalamus and back to the cortex. This organization is thought to underlie action selection and reinforcement (Redgrave et al. 2008)

Table 26.1 Selected publications studying patients with PD during rest, motor paradigms, and non-motor paradigms as well as studies of asymptomatic carriers of PD-related mutations

Authors	Year	*Participants*	OFF/ ON	Paradigm	Main findings in patients with Parkinson's disease
Resting-state fMRI studies					
Helmich et al.	2010	41 PD & 36 HC	OFF	Resting state	Reduced spatial segregation of connections between the cortex and putamen
Luo et al.	2014	52 PD & HC	OFF (drug-naïve)	Resting state	Reduced connectivity between entire striatum and mesolimbic regions. Reduced connectivity between posterior putamen and sensorimotor regions.
Rolinski et al.	2015	32 PD, 19 HC	OFF/ ON (28 only)	Resting state	In the OFF state, PD patients have reduced BG connectivity, especially in posterior putamen. BG activity in the OFF state could distinguish PD patients with 81% accuracy.
Skidmore et al.	2013	15 PD & HC	OFF	Resting state	Decreased activity in SMA, PFC, right MFG, and left cerebellum and increased activity in right cerebellum. Based on this activity pattern, PD patients can be distinguished from controls with 92% sensitivity and 87% specificity
Vo et al.	2017	20 PD & HC. 14 PD & HC as validation sample	OFF/ ON (9 only)	Resting state	PD-related pattern (PDRP) found with fMRI similar to PDRP in PET, validated in independent sample. PDRP diminished ON. PDRP expression correlating with motor disability
Activation fMRI during motor tasks					
Buhmann et al.	2003	8 (drug-naive)	OFF/ ON	Simple paced finger opposition task	Decreased activity in SMA and M1 in the OFF state. L-Dopa increases activity in SMA and M1

Table 26.1 (continued)

Authors	Year	*Participants*	OFF/ ON	Paradigm	Main findings in patients with Parkinson's disease
Haslinger et al.	2001	8	OFF/ ON	Paced single joystick movements in a freely chosen direction	Decreased activity in pre-SMA and increased activity in M1 and lateral PM in the OFF state. L-Dopa increases activity in SMA and decreases activity in M1, lateral PM, and SPC
Herz et al.	2014	13 LID, 13 non-LID	OFF/ OFF to ON	GoNogo task	During NoGo trials, levodopa led to stronger activity increase in pre-SMA and putamen in LID patients, pre-SMA increase correlated with LID severity.
Kraft et al.	2009	12	OFF/ ON	Simple uni- and bimanual power grip	Decreased activity in putamen in OFF state compared to healthy controls, no difference in ON state.
Rowe et al.	2002	12	OFF	Simple paced overlearned motor sequence task, with and without an additional attentional task	Increased SMA activity during a simple task but less attention-related augmentation of SMA activity due to an impaired connectivity between PFC and both SMA and lateral PM
Rowe et al.	2010	16	OFF/ ON	Simple visually paced finger-tapping task	In the ON state selection of action is associated with enhanced coupling between PFC and pre-SMA. In the OFF state action, selection is linked to coupling between PFC and lateral PM
Sabatini et al.	2000	6	OFF	Complex sequential motor task	Decreased activity in pre-SMA and right DLPFC, and increased activity in M1, lateral PM, IPC, SMA, and ACC
Wu et al.	2010	15	OFF	Unimanual, bimanual in-phase and bimanual anti-phase movements	Decreased activity in SMA and BG and increased activity in M1, PM, IFG, precuneus, and cerebellum during anti-phase movements. SMA has decreased connectivity to BG and dorsolateral PFC and increased connectivity to M1, PC, precuneus, and cerebellum
Wu et al.	2011	18	OFF/ ON	Self-initiated tapping task	PD patients in the OFF state show a decreased connectivity between BG and cortical areas (M1, pre-SMA, PM) as well as the cerebellum. In contrast, connections between cortico-cerebellar regions are strengthened
Activation fMRI studies of non-motor functions					
Ekman et al.	2014	28 PD without MCI, 11 PD with MCI	OFF (drug-naïve) & ON	Working memory (2-back) task	Longitudinal study testing drug-naïve patients and 12 months later ON medication. PD patients with MCI had lower MFC activation and lower connectivity between caudate and fusiform gyrus at both time points.
Lewis et al.	2003	21 (cognitively impaired and unimpaired)	ON	Working-memory task	Impairment in working memory is associated with decreased activity in the striatum and PFC
MacDonald et al.	2011	20	OFF/ ON	Simple selection task	L-Dopa enhances interference control but impairs encoding and facilitation of consistent stimulus–stimulus relations

(continued)

Table 26.1 (continued)

Authors	Year	*Participants*	OFF/ ON	Paradigm	Main findings in patients with Parkinson's disease
Marklund et al.	2009	20 (drug-naive)	OFF	Working-memory (2-back) task	PD patients show a transient (phasic) underactivation in caudate nuclei, putamen, and globus pallidus and sustained (tonic) underactivation in anterior putamen
Nombela et al.	2014	168 PD, 85 HC	ON	Executive planning, visuospatial function, and memory task	In executive planning task (tower of London), met/met carriers (higher PFC DA levels) showed highest activity in PFC areas and caudate with lower LEDD, Val/Val carriers (low DA levels in PFC) showed highest activity with higher LEDD.
Politis et al.	2013	12 hypersexuality-ICD, 12 non-ICD	OFF/ ON	Passive viewing of reward cues (including sexually themed) and neutral cues	No interaction between medication and ICD status, but increased activity in several brain regions, including VS, to sexual cues independent of medication.
Rowe et al.	2008	19	OFF/ ON	Bimodality continuous performance task	Lateral PFC and caudate nucleus activation show a nonlinear U-shaped relationship to motor disease severity. L-Dopa leads to a shift in this U-shaped function, indicating differential neurodegeneration in distinct connections between cortex and BG
Voon et al.	2010	22 (with and without impulse control disorder)	OFF/ ON	Probabilistic learning task	Dopamine agonists increase the rate of learning from gain outcomes in susceptible PD patients and lead to an increased prediction error in the striatum
Voon et al.	2011	28 (with and without impulse control disorder)	OFF/ ON	Risk-taking task	Patients with impulse control disorders make more risky choices and show decreased activation in OFC and ACC. Dopamine agonists enhance sensitivity to risk along with decreased activation in the VS. the opposite is observed in patients without impulse control disorders
Williams-Gray et al.	2008	29 (high- and low-COMT-activity genotype)	ON	Cognitive task probing the ability to form attentional "sets"	PD patients with low-COMT-activity genotype fail to form an attentional "set." this is associated with an underactivation across frontoparietal attentional networks
Genetically informed pre-clinical fMRI studies					
Buhmann et al.	2005	12 (asymptomatic carriers of a Parkin mutation)	–	Internally selected and externally determined finger movements	Asymptomatic Parkin-mutation carriers show increased activity in right rostral CMA and left dorsal PM during internally selected movements
Van Nuenen et al.	2009	22 (asymptomatic carriers of a Parkin or a Pink1 mutation)	–	Simple sequences of three thumb-to-finger opposition movements	In contrast to healthy controls, asymptomatic Parkin- and Pink1-mutation carriers show activation of pre-SMA and right rostral dorsal PM during simple movements

Studies are listed in alphabetical order in each section

Abbreviations: *ACC* anterior cingulate cortex, *BG* basal ganglia, *CMA* cingulate motor area, *COMT* catechol O-methyltransferase, *DA* Dopamine, *DLPFC* dorsolateral prefrontal cortex, *HC* healthy control subjects, *ICD* impulse control disorders, *IFG* inferior frontal gyrus, *IPC* inferior parietal cortex, *LEDD* Levodopa-equivalent daily dose, LID levodopa-induced dyskinesia, *M1* primary motor cortex, *MCI* mild cognitive impairment, *MFC* middle frontal cortex, *MFG* middle frontal gyrus, *OFC* orbitofrontal cortex, *PD* Parkinson's disease, *PDRP* Parkinson's disease–related pattern, *PFC* prefrontal cortex, *PM* premotor cortex, *Pre-SMA* pre-supplementary motor area, *SMA* supplementary motor area, *SPC* superior parietal cortex, VS Ventral striatum task, the connectivity patterns are not confounded by task performance. However, when comparing PD patients with healthy controls, PD patients can have excessive head movements, especially in the OFF state. This reduces the BOLD signal and can lead to ostensible differences between groups that are not due to actual differences in brain connectivity.

Two recent reviews provide a thorough overview over RS-fMRI in PD (Tahmasian et al. 2017; Hohenfeld et al. 2018). Here we present some core concepts and selected studies. RS data can be analyzed with independent component analysis to reveal separate intrinsic neural networks. RS-PET studies have consistently shown a so-called PD-related pattern (PDRP) of RS activity with increased pallido-thalamic and pontine activity, in combination with reduced premotor (PM), supplementary motor area (SMA), and posterior parietal cortex activation compared to healthy subjects. Another pattern with decreased medial frontal and parietal as well as increased cerebellar and nucleus dentatus activity is related to cognitive decline (PD-related cognitive pattern, PDCP) (Eidelberg 2009). These patterns are prominent in PD patients, but not in healthy controls, and have recently been replicated with fMRI (Vo et al. 2017).

Besides the above network-based approach, RS-fMRI can also be used to study the connectivity profile of predefined regions of interest. Using this approach, most studies find reduced activity between the sensorimotor areas in the cortex, thalamus, and striatum (Tahmasian et al. 2015; Hohenfeld et al. 2018). In line with the known anatomical progression of the neurodegeneration, anterior and posterior putamen seem to have different functional connectivity changes. For example, one study showed decreased connectivity between inferior parietal cortex (IPC) and posterior putamen and an increased connectivity between IPC and anterior putamen on PD patients in the OFF state (i.e., at least 12 h after withdrawal from dopaminergic medication) relative to healthy controls (Helmich et al. 2010). Another study comparing drug-naïve PD patients with healthy controls found reduced cortico-striatal connectivity for both anterior and posterior putamen, but more prominently in the latter (Luo et al. 2014). RS-fMRI studies have also confirmed the increase in coupling between STN and sensorimotor cortex that had been suggested in animal studies (Baudrexel et al. 2011; Kurani et al. 2015; see also Jia et al. 2018 during self-initiated movements).

Other groups have examined whether RS-fMRI can be used as a biomarker to distinguish between PD patients and healthy controls. For example, Skidmore et al. (Skidmore et al. 2013) found that PD patients showed decreased activity in SMA, prefrontal cortex (PFC), right middle frontal gyrus (MFG), and the left cerebellum as well as increased activity in the right cerebellum. Based on this distributed pattern of activity changes, it was possible to distinguish between PD patients and healthy controls with 92% sensitivity and 87% specificity. Focusing on the BG network, Rolinski found generally reduced BG connectivity, especially with posterior putamen, and achieved 81% accuracy in classifying PD patients (Rolinski et al. 2015). Generally, sensitivity and specificity of classification between PD and healthy controls with RS-fMRI seem to be around 90%, but somewhat lower when applying the same analysis on independent validation samples (Szewczyk-Krolikowski et al. 2014; Chen et al. 2015; e.g. Badea et al. 2017; Pläschke et al. 2017). These results suggest that RS-fMRI might play an important role as a biomarker for PD in the future.

26.2.2 Functional MRI Studies of Motor Control

Given the prominent motor symptoms of PD, numerous fMRI studies have investigated the associated neural correlates. Herz et al. performed an activation-likelihood estimation meta-analysis (Eickhoff et al. 2012) of the literature, revealing a consistent decrease of activity in posterior putamen during motor tasks (Herz et al. 2014a). Studying patients with a stronger motor impairment increased the likelihood of detecting this decrease. A fronto-parietal network comprising pre-supplementary motor area (pre-SMA), primary motor cortex (M1), and IPC as well as superior parietal lobule was differently activated in PD patients compared to healthy controls. However, the direction of change (increase or decrease of activation) was inconsistent across studies. For example, Haslinger et al. (2001) performed fMRI during auditory-paced single joystick movements in a freely chosen direction in eight patients OFF and ON medication. The study revealed reduced activation of the pre-SMA along with an increased activation of M1 and lateral PM in the OFF condition compared to control subjects. After the intake of levodopa, patients showed an activation pattern similar to healthy controls. On the other hand, using a grip-force task another study found decreased activity in a large network across the cortex in PD patients both ON and OFF medication compared to healthy controls (Kraft et al. 2009). In the OFF state, activity in posterior putamen was decreased compared to the ON state and compared to healthy controls. Studies finding increased activity of motor areas in the OFF state usually propose a compensational mechanism (e.g., Sabatini et al. 2000; Haslinger et al. 2001), whereas the deficient activation of these areas is attributed to the degeneration of dopaminergic neurons in SNc, leading to decreased excitatory input from BG to cortical motor areas (e.g., Buhmann et al. 2003; Kraft et al. 2009, see also Sect. 18.1). However, the different direction of effects might also be due to differences in task difficulty and performance.

For example, it has been shown that attention is an important factor that determines the cortical activity patterns during motor tasks. Rowe et al. (2002) addressed this issue using a simple paced overlearned sequence task in 12 PD patients in the OFF condition. While patients showed a greater than normal activation in SMA during the simple motor task, they failed to augment SMA activity when they were asked to actively attend to their actions. Connectivity analysis based on structural equation modeling (SEM; Büchel and Friston 1997) revealed that in contrast to healthy controls, patients did not increase effective connectivity between PFC and both lateral PM and SMA when they were asked to attend to their actions. This finding indicates that a disconnection between prefrontal attentional networks and frontoparietal motor networks might underlie the commonly observed underactivation in SMA.

Other studies have not only investigated changes in activity, but also alterations in the connectivity patterns among brain regions forming functional neural networks (Rowe et al. 2010). For example, PD patients in the OFF state have been shown to be impaired during the performance of bimanual anti-phase movements, which was associated with decreased activity in SMA and BG and increased activity in multiple areas such as M1, lateral PM, and cerebellum (Wu et al. 2010). Using the psychophysiological interaction (PPI) method (Friston et al. 1997), connectivity analysis revealed decreased influence of the SMA to prefrontal regions and BG which was paralleled by an increased coupling with M1, cerebellum, parietal areas, and precuneus. The same group found similar results in 18 PD patients during a self-initiated unimanual tapping task (Wu et al. 2011). The increased cortico-cortical and cortico-cerebellar connectivity might compensate for impaired coupling between executive motor areas and BG and explain the observed hyperactivation in M1 in progressed PD (Haslinger et al. 2001; Sabatini et al. 2000). Using a different type of connectivity analysis, dynamic causal modeling (DCM; Friston et al. 2003), Rowe et al. assessed cortico-cortical connectivity during a simple visually paced finger-tapping task in 16 patients with PD both OFF and ON medication (Rowe et al. 2010). In medicated patients as well as healthy controls, action selection was associated with increased coupling between PFC and Pre-SMA. In contrast, patients OFF medication showed enhanced coupling between PFC and lateral PM.

Besides the paucity of movement vigor (bradykinesia), many PD patients start to experience excessive involuntary movements after the intake of levodopa after some years of treatment (Cilia et al. 2014). This phenomenon is termed levodopa-induced dyskinesia (LID), and it is difficult to investigate with fMRI due to the movement artifacts. However, some studies have shed light onto the underlying neurobiology. Herz et al. scanned LID patients in the OFF state and then immediately after levodopa intake until dyskinetic movements appeared (Herz et al. 2014b). LID patients showed a stronger increase in activity in pre-SMA and left putamen following levodopa intake compared to non-LID patients during motor inhibition in a Go-Nogo task. The degree of increase in pre-SMA activity was positively correlated with the severity of motor symptoms.

Taken together, fMRI studies of the motor system in PD have given important insights into the pathophysiology underlying motor impairment and revealed potential compensatory mechanisms. The regions most consistently shown to be affected are SMA, M1, and posterior putamen (Meder et al. 2018). Network analyses have been used to assess abnormal task-related connectivity patterns in PD and highlight the importance of attentional networks in modulating motor loops.

26.2.3 Functional MRI Studies of Non-motor Functions

Even though the motor symptoms of PD are the most prominent, the disease also leads to numerous non-motor symptoms affecting cognition, sleep, mood, autonomic function, and pain (Schapira et al. 2017). First, this can be explained by the prominent involvement of dopamine in cognitive processes such as learning (reward prediction error signaling), effort allocation, and risk taking (e.g., Niv 2007; Christopoulos et al. 2009; Schultz 2017). This is mostly mediated by the other main dopamine nucleus in the brain, the ventral tegmental area (VTA), which is affected by neurodegeneration as well, albeit to a lesser degree (Alberico et al. 2015). Second, PD also leads to neurodegeneration in other neurotransmitter systems, including the noradrenergic, cholinergic, and serotonergic system (Hawkes et al. 2010). Cognitive impairment in PD is commonly described as a disorder of frontal executive function that comprises attentional control, such as working memory, set-switching, and planning, as well as control of reward-related behavior and risk-taking (Meder et al. 2018). The nature of cognitive deficits in PD patients is rather complex, since they depend on disease severity, medication, and genotype (Rowe et al. 2008; Williams-Gray et al. 2008). The optimal dopamine level differs for the motor, cognitive, and limbic loops and is commonly described as an inverted-U-shaped relationship between dopaminergic state and function (Fig. 26.3). However, the optimal dose of levodopa replacement is usually based on motor improvement and can there-

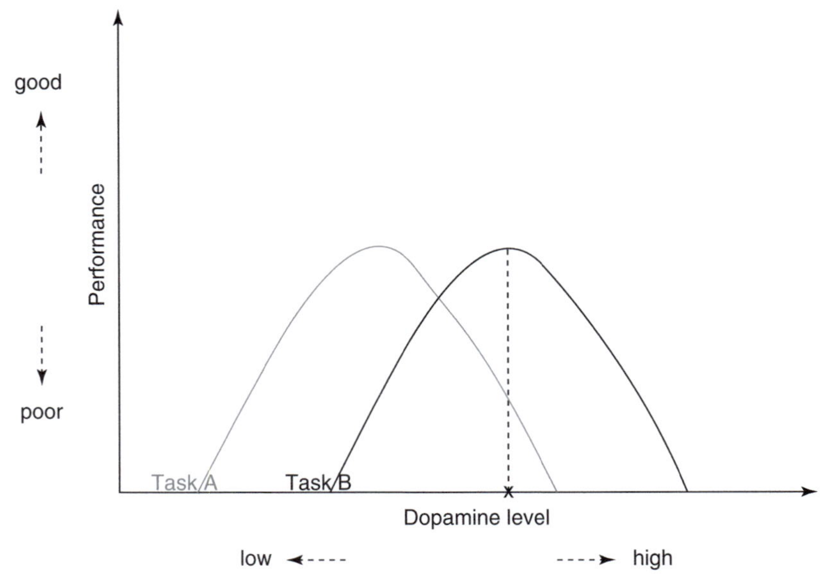

Fig. 26.3 Different optimal dopamine levels for different tasks/functions schematically. While a given dopamine level X optimizes performance on *task B*, it impairs performance on *task A*, which has a lower optimal dopamine level. Such dopamine-dependent differences in performance can be observed in paradigms probing different neural system (e.g., motor vs. cognitive) or different aspects of cognitive control (e.g., stability vs. flexibility)

fore lead to a suboptimal level of dopamine in non-motor loops (Cools and D'Esposito 2011).

To investigate the neural underpinnings of impaired working memory in PD, Lewis and coworkers studied 21 PD patients with and without cognitive deficits in the ON state using a working-memory paradigm (Lewis et al. 2003). They could show that impairments in working memory were associated with decreased activity in local sites in the BG and frontal lobe. Since this hypoactivation was not seen in PD patients without cognitive deficits, the authors concluded that cognitive deficits in PD are linked to cortico-subcortical loops distinct to loops responsible for motor impairment. Marklund et al. (2009) performed fMRI during a 2-back working-memory task in 20 untreated de novo PD patients to assess the distinct processes of working memory. The 2-back task required participants to indicate whether a presented word matched the one presented two times earlier. The results suggested that working-memory dysfunction in early PD is mainly caused by dysregulated phasic dopamine responses in the caudate, even though the initial signs of tonic control impairment were also observed. The important role of the caudate was shown in another study using a similar task where functional connectivity between caudate and fusiform gyrus was reduced in PD patients with mild cognitive impairments (Ekman et al. 2014).

An important theme of recent neuroimaging research was to clarify how dopaminergic medication impacts different brain functions in PD (Rowe et al. 2008). To elucidate the effect of dopamine on different cortico-subcortical loops, MacDonald et al. used a selection paradigm in 20 PD patients before and after the intake of levodopa (MacDonald et al. 2011). During the behavioral experiment, patients had to encode stimulus–stimulus relations, which is thought to be processed in the ventral striatum, and control interference, which is thought to be mediated by the dorsal striatum. While dopamine replacement enhanced dorsal striatum function (interference control), it impaired function mediated by the ventral striatum (encoding of stimulus–stimulus relations). Another study showed complex inverted U-shape relationships in different circuits, interacting with medication and disease severity (Rowe et al. 2008). 19 PD patients performed a bimodality continuous performance task in which letters were shown at one of eight radial locations. Here, a target trial was defined either by the position or type of letter. Subjects were instructed to indicate whether a trial was a target trial and were given a monetary bonus if three sequential targets within a given dimension were detected successfully. Thus, to receive the reward, participants had to identify the relevant stimulus dimension (spatial or verbal) and detect the target trials accordingly. PD patients were able to successfully solve the task but showed interindividual differences in neural activation depending on disease severity as reflected by motor impairment. Both lateral PFC and caudate nucleus showed a nonlinear U-shaped relationship between motor impairment and task-related neural activity. Patients with the most and the least motor impairment showed higher task-related activity, whereas patients with medium disease severity showed lower task-related activity. Dopamine replacement led to a lateral shift of this relationship, improving motor impairment but not cognitive function.

Attentional control in PD patients also critically depends on their catechol O-methyltransferase (COMT) genotype, which affects dopamine levels in PFC (Collins and Williams-Gray 2016). For example, Williams-Gray and colleagues (Williams-Gray et al. 2008) studied 16 patients with high-activity COMT genotypes (val/val) and 13 patients with low-activity COMT genotypes (met/met) with a sophisticated paradigm probing the ability to form an attentional "set" in the ON condition. Patients with low-activity COMT genotypes failed to show a normal approach of shifting attention, which was associated with an underactivation across frontoparietal attentional networks. Another study on a large cohort of PD patients and healthy controls revealed interaction effects between COMT genotype and medication on fronto-striatal regions' activity in an executive planning task (Nombela et al. 2014).

Changes in reward-related behavior have important clinical implications. Impulse control disorders (ICD), such as pathological gambling or compulsive shopping, are frequently observed in PD patients and are associated with the use of dopamine agonists (Weintraub et al. 2015). However, the mechanisms underlying impaired control of reward-related behavior and risk-taking by dopamine agonists are not entirely understood. To address this question, Voon and coworkers studied 22 PD patients with and without excessive gambling and shopping behavior using a probabilistic learning task (Voon et al. 2010). In this task, participants had to learn if a symbol was associated with reward or loss. A third condition included neutral trials. Unpredicted, surprising outcomes, for instance, when a symbol that only has a 20% reward probability leads to an actual reward, give rise to a prediction error signal in the ventral striatum that updates the internal representations of reward predictions (Rushworth and Behrens 2008). Patients with ICDs showed an increased striatal prediction error signal in the gain condition after the intake of dopamine agonists, signaling a better-than-expected outcome. It was argued that this dysregulation might bias PD patients with ICDs toward compulsive reward-seeking behaviors.

The central role of striatum in ICD has also been found in another study by the same group where an alteration in risk control in PD patients ICD after the intake of medication was associated with decreased activity in the ventral striatum (Voon et al. 2011). Also Politis et al. found stronger activity in ventral striatum to sexual cues in PD patients with ICD (Politis et al. 2013). Generally, it seems that ICD patients have a marked imbalance between the beneficial effects of dopaminergic medication in motor circuits and the detrimental effects on cognition and reward processing (Meder et al. 2018). It has been suggested that this pathology leads to an increased uncertainty about the utility of future actions, which is at the basis of many aspects of ICD behaviors (Averbeck et al. 2013).

Taken together, studies investigating non-motor functions in PD have shown that alterations in networks involved in attentional control occur already in early disease stages. Dopaminergic therapy has differential effects on neural functions depending on the task (e.g., motor and cognitive) and disease severity. Additionally, dopamine agonist can alter the control of reward-related behavior and risk-taking by affecting the regulation of dopaminergic signaling in the striatum and thereby lead to serious side effects such as ICDs. A recent overview over neuroimaging studies on cognitive flexibility, learning, and reward processing in PD is provided in Meder et al. (2018).

26.2.4 Preclinical Compensation

Mutations in the Parkin and PINK1 gene are among the most common recessively inherited genes that can cause familial forms of PD (Gasser 2007; Greenland et al. 2018). Non-manifesting heterozygous carriers of Parkin and PINK1 mutations show a subclinical nigrostriatal dopaminergic degeneration (Hilker et al. 2001; Khan et al. 2005) and give the unique opportunity to study preclinical compensational mechanisms of dopaminergic dysfunction. Importantly, asymptomatic carriers do not show motor impairment, allowing for the assessment of motor-related neural activity without a behavioral confound. Buhmann et al. (Buhmann et al. 2005) studied 12 non-manifesting carriers of a Parkin mutation during unimanual simple finger-to-thumb opposition movements. The movements were visually paced at a frequency of 0.33 Hz, and the finger that had to be used was either internally or externally cued. Non-manifesting mutation carriers showed a stronger activation of rostral cingulate motor area (CMA) and left dorsal PM during internally cued compared to externally cued movements. Connectivity analysis using PPI additionally revealed an increased effective connectivity between rostral CMA and the dopamine-deficient left posterior putamen during internally cued movements in Parkin-mutation carriers. A consecutive study by van Nuenen and colleagues included 9 PINK1-mutation carriers and 13 Parkin-mutation carriers (van Nuenen et al. 2009). Participants had to perform visually cued simple sequences of three unimanual thumb-to-finger opposition movements. In contrast to healthy controls, both PINK1- and Parkin-mutation carriers showed an increased activation of Pre-SMA and the right dorsal PM during the motor task.

These two studies show that a preclinical nigrostriatal dopaminergic degeneration leads to a compensatory increase in the activity of motor cortical areas within task-specific networks. Such compensatory mechanisms could explain why patients with sporadic PD first become symptomatic several years after the neurodegeneration of dopaminergic striatonigral neurons has started. The results additionally indicate that it might be possible to detect PD using fMRI even before motor symptoms manifest. Especially the unprecedented detail obtained by ultra-high-field MR scanning is expected to bear high potential (Lehericy et al. 2017). This genetically informed approach could be easily extended to other patient groups carrying mutations in other genes associated with PD. An alternative strategy is to perform fMRI studies in populations with clinical signs such as anosmia or REM sleep disorder that might precede the motor manifestation of PD and, thus, are associated with an increased risk to develop PD during later life (Savica et al. 2010). The insights gained from studying preclinical populations has been reviewed in Barber et al. (2017).

26.3 Perspectives

Studies using fMRI have given important insights into abnormal neural networks underlying motor and non-motor symptoms in PD. An important fact one has to bear in mind when interpreting these results is that the reported studies almost entirely included patients with akinetic-rigid PD, since tremor heavily interferes with data acquisition. Sophisticated devices, such as online monitoring and correction of movements, would allow for studying this large group of PD patients. Additionally, using pharmacologically modulated fMRI, dynamic changes in neural activity can be assessed by scanning patients during a period from the absence until the emergence of involuntary movements (Herz et al. 2014b; Cerasa et al. 2015; Herz et al. 2015). Such studies are necessary to improve our knowledge of pathophysiological changes underlying hyperkinetic movement disorders. Network analyses of resting-state as well as task-related fMRI have been shown to be sensitive to changes caused by PD. Recent advances in the imaging of structural changes in small nuclei with ultra-high-field imaging are promising tools for precision medicine approaches to precise diagnostics and individualized treatment (Lehericy et al. 2017). Longitudinal studies could help to better understand the effect of progressive neurodegeneration on neural networks and to relate activity patterns to emerging symptoms or side effects. Such studies could render detecting patients vulnerable to side effects possible and be used to tailor therapy to the underlying pathology of the individual patient.

References

Alberico SL, Cassell MD, Narayanan NS (2015) The vulnerable ventral tegmental area in Parkinson's disease. Basal Ganglia 5:51–55. https://doi.org/10.1016/j.baga.2015.06.001

Albin RL, Young AB, Penney JB (1989) The functional anatomy of basal ganglia disorders. Trends Neurosci 12:366–375

Alexander GE, DeLong MR, Strick PL (1986) Parallel Organization of Functionally Segregated Circuits Linking Basal Ganglia and Cortex. Annu Rev Neurosci 9:357–381. https://doi.org/10.1146/annurev.ne.09.030186.002041

Averbeck BB, Djamshidian A, O'Sullivan SS et al (2013) Uncertainty about mapping future actions into rewards may underlie performance on multiple measures of impulsivity in behavioral addiction: evidence from Parkinson's disease. Behav Neurosci 127:245–255. https://doi.org/10.1037/a0032079

Badea L, Onu M, Wu T et al (2017) Exploring the reproducibility of functional connectivity alterations in Parkinson's disease. PLoS One 12:e0188196. https://doi.org/10.1371/journal.pone.0188196

Barber TR, Klein JC, Mackay CE, Hu MTM (2017) Neuroimaging in pre-motor Parkinson's disease. Neuroimage Clin 15:215–227. https://doi.org/10.1016/j.nicl.2017.04.011

Baudrexel S, Witte T, Seifried C et al (2011) Resting state fMRI reveals increased subthalamic nucleus-motor cortex connectivity in Parkinson's disease. NeuroImage 55:1728–1738. https://doi.org/10.1016/j.neuroimage.2011.01.017

Biswal B, Yetkin FZ, Haughton VM, Hyde JS (1995) Functional connectivity in the motor cortex of resting human brain using echo-planar MRI. Magn Reson Med 34:537–541

Büchel C, Friston KJ (1997) Modulation of connectivity in visual pathways by attention: cortical interactions evaluated with structural equation modelling and fMRI. Cereb Cortex 7:768–778

Buhmann C, Binkofski F, Klein C et al (2005) Motor reorganization in asymptomatic carriers of a single mutant Parkin allele: a human model for presymptomatic parkinsonism. Brain 128:2281–2290. https://doi.org/10.1093/brain/awh572

Buhmann C, Glauche V, Stürenburg HJ et al (2003) Pharmacologically modulated fMRI---cortical responsiveness to levodopa in drug-naive hemiparkinsonian patients. Brain 126:451–461. https://doi.org/10.1093/brain/awg033

Cerasa A, Koch G, Donzuso G et al (2015) A network centred on the inferior frontal cortex is critically involved in levodopa-induced dyskinesias. Brain 138:414–427. https://doi.org/10.1093/brain/awu329

Chen Y, Yang W, Long J et al (2015) Discriminative analysis of Parkinson's disease based on whole-brain functional connectivity. PLoS One 10:e0124153. https://doi.org/10.1371/journal.pone.0124153

Christopoulos GI, Tobler PN, Bossaerts P et al (2009) Neural correlates of value, risk, and risk aversion contributing to decision making under risk. J Neurosci 29:12574–12583. https://doi.org/10.1523/JNEUROSCI.2614-09.2009

Cilia R, Akpalu A, Sarfo FS et al (2014) The modern pre-levodopa era of Parkinson's disease: insights into motor complications from sub-Saharan Africa. Brain 137:2731–2742. https://doi.org/10.1093/brain/awu195

Collins LM, Williams-Gray CH (2016) The genetic basis of cognitive impairment and dementia in Parkinson's disease. Front Psych 7. https://doi.org/10.3389/fpsyt.2016.00089

Cools R, D'Esposito M (2011) Inverted-U-shaped dopamine actions on human working memory and cognitive control. Biol Psychiatry 69:e113–e125. https://doi.org/10.1016/j.biopsych.2011.03.028

DeLong MR (1990) Primate models of movement disorders of basal ganglia origin. Trends Neurosci 13:281–285

Eickhoff SB, Bzdok D, Laird AR et al (2012) Activation likelihood estimation meta-analysis revisited. NeuroImage 59:2349–2361. https://doi.org/10.1016/j.neuroimage.2011.09.017

Eidelberg D (2009) Metabolic brain networks in neurodegenerative disorders: a functional imaging approach. Trends Neurosci 32:548–557. https://doi.org/10.1016/j.tins.2009.06.003

Ekman U, Eriksson J, Forsgren L et al (2014) Longitudinal changes in task-evoked brain responses in Parkinson's disease patients with and without mild cognitive impairment Front Neurosci 8:8. https://doi.org/10.3389/fnins.2014.00207

Friston KJ, Buechel C, Fink GR et al (1997) Psychophysiological and modulatory interactions in neuroimaging. NeuroImage 6:218–229. https://doi.org/10.1006/nimg.1997.0291

Friston KJ, Harrison L, Penny W (2003) Dynamic causal modelling. NeuroImage 19:1273–1302. https://doi.org/10.1016/S1053-8119(03)00202-7

Gasser T (2007) Update on the genetics of Parkinson's disease. Mov Disord 22(Suppl 17):S343–S350. https://doi.org/10.1002/mds.21676

Greenland JC, Williams-Gray CH, Barker RA (2018) The clinical heterogeneity of Parkinson's disease and its therapeutic implications. European Journal of Neuroscience in press: doi 49:328. https://doi.org/10.1111/ejn.14094

Haslinger B, Erhard P, Kämpfe N et al (2001) Event-related functional magnetic resonance imaging in Parkinson's disease before and after levodopa. Brain 124:558–570

Hawkes CH, Del Tredici K, Braak H (2010) A timeline for Parkinson's disease. Parkinsonism Relat Disord 16:79–84. https://doi.org/10.1016/j.parkreldis.2009.08.007

Helmich RC, Derikx LC, Bakker M et al (2010) Spatial remapping of cortico-striatal connectivity in Parkinson's disease. Cereb Cortex 20:1175–1186. https://doi.org/10.1093/cercor/bhp178

Herz DM, Eickhoff SB, Løkkegaard A, Siebner HR (2014a) Functional neuroimaging of motor control in parkinson's disease: a meta-analysis. Hum Brain Mapp 35:3227–3237. https://doi.org/10.1002/hbm.22397

Herz DM, Haagensen BN, Christensen MS et al (2014b) The acute brain response to levodopa heralds dyskinesias in Parkinson disease. Ann Neurol 75:829–836. https://doi.org/10.1002/ana.24138

Herz DM, Haagensen BN, Christensen MS et al (2015) Abnormal dopaminergic modulation of striato-cortical networks underlies levodopa-induced dyskinesias in humans. Brain 138:1658–1666. https://doi.org/10.1093/brain/awv096

Hilker R, Klein C, Ghaemi M et al (2001) Positron emission tomographic analysis of the nigrostriatal dopaminergic system in familial parkinsonism associated with mutations in the parkin gene. Ann Neurol 49: 367–376

Hohenfeld C, Werner CJ, Reetz K (2018) Resting-state connectivity in neurodegenerative disorders: is there potential for an imaging biomarker? NeuroImage: Clinical 18:849–870. https://doi.org/10.1016/j.nicl.2018.03.013

Jahanshahi M, Jenkins IH, Brown RG et al (1995) Self-initiated versus externally triggered movements. I An investigation using measurement of regional cerebral blood flow with PET and movement-related potentials in normal and Parkinson's disease subjects Brain 118(Pt 4):913–933

Jia Q, Gao L, Zhang J et al (2018) Altered functional connectivity of the subthalamic nucleus during self-initiated movement in Parkinson's disease. J Neuroradiol 45:249–255. https://doi.org/10.1016/j.neurad.2017.11.008

Khan NL, Scherfler C, Graham E et al (2005) Dopaminergic dysfunction in unrelated, asymptomatic carriers of a single parkin mutation. Neurology 64:134–136. https://doi.org/10.1212/01.WNL.0000148725.48740.6D

Kraft E, Loichinger W, Diepers M et al (2009) Levodopa-induced striatal activation in Parkinson's disease: a functional MRI study. Parkinsonism Relat Disord 15:558–563. https://doi.org/10.1016/j.parkreldis.2009.02.005

Kurani AS, Seidler RD, Burciu RG et al (2015) Subthalamic nucleus—sensorimotor cortex functional connectivity in de novo and moderate Parkinson's disease. Neurobiol Aging 36:462–469. https://doi.org/10.1016/j.neurobiolaging.2014.07.004

Lehericy S, Vaillancourt DE, Seppi K et al (2017) The role of high-field magnetic resonance imaging in parkinsonian disorders: pushing the boundaries forward. Mov Disord 32:510–525. https://doi.org/10.1002/mds.26968

Lewis SJG, Dove A, Robbins TW et al (2003) Cognitive impairments in early Parkinson's disease are accompanied by reductions in activity in frontostriatal neural circuitry. J Neurosci 23:6351–6356

Luo C, Song W, Chen Q et al (2014) Reduced functional connectivity in early-stage drug-naive Parkinson's disease: a resting-state fMRI study. Neurobiol Aging 35:431–441. https://doi.org/10.1016/j.neurobiolaging.2013.08.018

MacDonald PA, MacDonald AA, Seergobin KN et al (2011) The effect of dopamine therapy on ventral and dorsal striatum-mediated cognition in Parkinson's disease: support from functional MRI. Brain 134:1447–1463. https://doi.org/10.1093/brain/awr075

Marklund P, Larsson A, Elgh E et al (2009) Temporal dynamics of basal ganglia under-recruitment in Parkinson's disease: transient caudate abnormalities during updating of working memory. Brain 132:336–346. https://doi.org/10.1093/brain/awn309

Meder D, Herz DM, Rowe JB et al (2018) The role of dopamine in the brain - lessons learned from Parkinson's disease. NeuroImage 190:79. https://doi.org/10.1016/j.neuroimage.2018.11.021

Mink JW (1996) The basal ganglia: focused selection and inhibition of competing motor programs. Prog Neurobiol 50:381–425. https://doi.org/10.1016/S0301-0082(96)00042-1

Nambu A, Tokuno H, Hamada I et al (2000) Excitatory cortical inputs to pallidal neurons via the subthalamic nucleus in the monkey. J Neurophysiol 84:289–300. https://doi.org/10.1152/jn.2000.84.1.289

Niv Y (2007) Cost, benefit, tonic, phasic. Ann N Y Acad Sci 1104:357–376. https://doi.org/10.1196/annals.1390.018

Nombela C, Rowe JB, Winder-Rhodes SE et al (2014) Genetic impact on cognition and brain function in newly diagnosed Parkinson's disease: ICICLE-PD study. Brain 137:2743–2758. https://doi.org/10.1093/brain/awu201

Obeso JA, Stamelou M, Goetz CG et al (2017) Past, present, and future of Parkinson's disease: a special essay on the 200th anniversary of the shaking palsy. Mov Disord 32:1264–1310. https://doi.org/10.1002/mds.27115

Pläschke RN, Cieslik EC, Müller VI et al (2017) On the integrity of functional brain networks in schizophrenia, Parkinson's disease, and advanced age: evidence from connectivity-based single-subject classification. Hum Brain Mapp 38:5845–5858. https://doi.org/10.1002/hbm.23763

Playford ED, Jenkins IH, Passingham RE et al (1992) Impaired mesial frontal and putamen activation in Parkinson's disease: a positron emission tomography study. Ann Neurol 32:151–161. https://doi.org/10.1002/ana.410320206

Politis M, Loane C, Wu K et al (2013) Neural response to visual sexual cues in dopamine treatment-linked hypersexuality in Parkinson's disease. Brain 136:400–411. https://doi.org/10.1093/brain/aws326

Postuma RB, Berg D, Stern M et al (2015) MDS clinical diagnostic criteria for Parkinson's disease. Mov Disord 30:1591–1601. https://doi.org/10.1002/mds.26424

Raichle ME (2015) The restless brain: how intrinsic activity organizes brain function. Phil Trans R Soc B 370:20140172. https://doi.org/10.1098/rstb.2014.0172

Redgrave P, Gurney K, Reynolds J (2008) What is reinforced by phasic dopamine signals? Brain Res Rev 58:322–339. https://doi.org/10.1016/j.brainresrev.2007.10.007

Rinne OJ, Nurmi E, Ruottinen HM et al (2001) [(18)F]FDOPA and [(18)F]CFT are both sensitive PET markers to detect presynaptic dopaminergic hypofunction in early Parkinson's disease. Synapse 40:193–200. https://doi.org/10.1002/syn.1042

Rolinski M, Griffanti L, Szewczyk-Krolikowski K et al (2015) Aberrant functional connectivity within the basal ganglia of patients with Parkinson's disease. NeuroImage: Clinical 8:126–132. https://doi.org/10.1016/j.nicl.2015.04.003

Rowe J, Stephan KE, Friston K et al (2002) Attention to action in Parkinson's disease: impaired effective connectivity among frontal cortical regions. Brain 125:276–289

Rowe JB, Hughes L, Ghosh BCP et al (2008) Parkinson's disease and dopaminergic therapy—differential effects on movement, reward and cognition. Brain 131:2094–2105. https://doi.org/10.1093/brain/awn112

Rowe JB, Hughes LE, Barker RA, Owen AM (2010) Dynamic causal modelling of effective connectivity from fMRI: are results reproducible and sensitive to Parkinson's disease and its treatment? NeuroImage 52:1015–1026. https://doi.org/10.1016/j.neuroimage.2009.12.080

Rushworth MFS, Behrens TEJ (2008) Choice, uncertainty and value in prefrontal and cingulate cortex. Nat Neurosci 11:389–397. https://doi.org/10.1038/nn2066

Sabatini U, Boulanouar K, Fabre N et al (2000) Cortical motor reorganization in akinetic patients with

Parkinson's disease: a functional MRI study. Brain 123(Pt 2):394–403

Savica R, Rocca WA, Ahlskog JE (2010) When does Parkinson disease start? Arch Neurol 67:798–801. https://doi.org/10.1001/archneurol.2010.135

Schapira AHV, Chaudhuri KR, Jenner P (2017) Non-motor features of Parkinson disease. Nat Rev Neurosci 18:435–450. https://doi.org/10.1038/nrn.2017.62

Schultz W (2017) Reward prediction error. Curr Biol 27:R369–R371. https://doi.org/10.1016/j.cub.2017.02.064

Skidmore FM, Yang M, Baxter L et al (2013) Apathy, depression, and motor symptoms have distinct and separable resting activity patterns in idiopathic Parkinson disease. NeuroImage 81:484–495. https://doi.org/10.1016/j.neuroimage.2011.07.012

Szewczyk-Krolikowski K, Menke RAL, Rolinski M et al (2014) Functional connectivity in the basal ganglia network differentiates PD patients from controls. Neurology 83:208–214. https://doi.org/10.1212/WNL.0000000000000592

Tahmasian M, Bettray LM, van Eimeren T et al (2015) A systematic review on the applications of resting-state fMRI in Parkinson's disease: does dopamine replacement therapy play a role? Cortex 73:80–105. https://doi.org/10.1016/j.cortex.2015.08.005

Tahmasian M, Eickhoff SB, Giehl K et al (2017) Resting-state functional reorganization in Parkinson's disease: an activation likelihood estimation meta-analysis. Cortex 92:119–138. https://doi.org/10.1016/j.cortex.2017.03.016

van Nuenen BFL, Weiss MM, Bloem BR et al (2009) Heterozygous carriers of a Parkin or PINK1 mutation share a common functional endophenotype. Neurology 72:1041–1047. https://doi.org/10.1212/01.wnl.0000338699.56379.11

Vo A, Sako W, Fujita K et al (2017) Parkinson's disease-related network topographies characterized with resting state functional MRI. Hum Brain Mapp 38:617–630. https://doi.org/10.1002/hbm.23260

Voon V, Gao J, Brezing C et al (2011) Dopamine agonists and risk: impulse control disorders in Parkinson's; disease. Brain 134:1438–1446. https://doi.org/10.1093/brain/awr080

Voon V, Pessiglione M, Brezing C et al (2010) Mechanisms underlying dopamine-mediated reward Bias in compulsive behaviors. Neuron 65:135–142. https://doi.org/10.1016/j.neuron.2009.12.027

Weintraub D, David AS, Evans AH et al (2015) Clinical spectrum of impulse control disorders in Parkinson's disease. Mov Disord 30:121–127. https://doi.org/10.1002/mds.26016

Williams-Gray CH, Hampshire A, Barker RA, Owen AM (2008) Attentional control in Parkinson's disease is dependent on COMT val 158 met genotype. Brain 131:397–408. https://doi.org/10.1093/brain/awm313

Wu T, Wang L, Hallett M et al (2010) Neural correlates of bimanual anti-phase and in-phase movements in Parkinson's disease. Brain 133:2394–2409. https://doi.org/10.1093/brain/awq151

Wu T, Wang L, Hallett M et al (2011) Effective connectivity of brain networks during self-initiated movement in Parkinson's disease. NeuroImage 55:204–215. https://doi.org/10.1016/j.neuroimage.2010.11.074

Incidental Findings in Neuroimaging Research: Ethical Considerations

27

Stephan Ulmer, Thomas C. Booth, Guy Widdershoven, Olav Jansen, Gunther Fesl, Rüdiger von Kummer, and Stella Reiter-Theil

27.1 Introduction

Neuroimaging—especially functional MR imaging (fMRI)—opens the door to non-invasively map cortical processing and to understand how our brain works. fMRI evolved from basic (Ogawa et al. 1990, 1993; Kwong et al. 1992) and clinical applications in the 1990s (Yousry et al. 1995) to become a powerful and ubiquitous tool in neurocognitive research. Because fMRI can be used to answer clinical questions, the more the research conducted, the greater the potential for clinical translation and subsequent patient benefit. This book focuses on the clinical applications of fMRI; however, prior to any routine clinical use, there is a need to test its reliability in healthy controls. The focus of this chapter is on ethical questions raised by incidental findings (IF) in fMRI in healthy volunteers and the conclusions to be drawn. Considering ethical issues is important in patient care but should be taken even more serious in healthy volunteers. Ethical issues relevant to fMRI concern how the requirements of voluntary participation and privacy are handled

S. Ulmer (✉)
Department of Radiology and Nuclear Medicine, Kantonsspital Winterthur, Winterthur, Switzerland

neurorad.ch, Zurich, Switzerland

Department of Radiology and Neuroradiology, University Hospital Schleswig-Holstein, Kiel, Germany

T. C. Booth
School of Biomedical Engineering & Imaging Sciences, King's College, London, UK

Department of Neuroradiology, King's College Hospital NHS Foundation Trust, London, UK
e-mail: tombooth@doctors.org.uk

G. Widdershoven
Netherlands School of Primary Care Research (CaRe), VU Medical Center, Amsterdam, The Netherlands
e-mail: g.widdershoven@vumc.nl

O. Jansen
Department of Radiology and Neuroradiology, University Hospital Schleswig-Holstein, Kiel, Germany
e-mail: o.jansen@neurorad.uni-kiel.de

G. Fesl
Radiologie Augsburg Friedberg ÜBAG, Augsburg, Germany

Abteilung für Neuroradiologie, Klinikum Grosshadern, Ludwig-Maximilians-Universität München, Munich, Germany
e-mail: gunther.fesl@med.uni-muenchen.de

R. von Kummer
Abteilung Neuroradiologie, Universitätsklinikum Carl Gustav Carus, Dresden, Germany
e-mail: ruediger.vonkummer@uniklinikum-dresden.de

S. Reiter-Theil
Clinical Ethics University Hospital Basel/Psychiatric Hospitals of the University Basel, Basel, Switzerland
e-mail: s.reiter-theil@unibas.ch

S. Ulmer, O. Jansen (eds.), *fMRI*, https://doi.org/10.1007/978-3-030-41874-8_27

by the researchers (Carli et al. 2012), how harm is prevented and whether appropriate information and decisional aids are offered to the subjects or patients before obtaining informed consent (Reiter-Theil and Stingelin Giles 2007). Because an IF can have a major impact on the subject's life, the management pertaining to such a discovery should be analysed thoroughly (Ulmer et al. 2009).

27.2 Incidental Finding Prevalence

An IF is defined as a previously undetected abnormality of potential clinical relevance that is unrelated to the purpose of the examination (Illes et al. 2006). Within the last decade, IF were increasingly recognised as a new problem to deal within neuroimaging research (Garnett et al. 2011). The wider use of neuroimaging in research results in a higher prevalence of IF (Booth et al. 2012), and recent publications have emphasised the need for improved management (Woodward and Toms 2009; Ulmer et al. 2009; Hartwigsen et al. 2010). IF are frequent; the prevalence of recognisable and clinically significant neuropathologies ranges between 2% and 9% in the general population. All 'deviations from normal' (i.e. clinically significant, insignificant and indeterminate findings) are even more frequent (Katzman et al. 1999; Weber and Knopf 2006; Vernooij et al. 2007; Brown and Hasso 2008; Illes and Chin 2008; Hartwigsen et al. 2010; Ulmer et al. 2012). The prevalence of IF can be considerably higher in certain populations, i.e. the elderly (e.g. Alphs et al. 2006; Gupta and Belay 2008). In a recent meta-analysis (Morris et al. 2009) of 16 studies with a total of 19,559 people, IF were found in only 2.7% of the cases. This study, however, clearly underestimates their actual prevalence as findings such as small white matter lesions, lacunar infarcts or microhaemorrhages were excluded. It is noteworthy that MR image resolution varied between studies; furthermore, in some studies, scans were not read by neuroradiologists; thus, a considerable amount of IF might have been missed.

27.3 Consequences Arising from Incidental Findings

An IF may impact the subject's life in a multitude of ways. Tumours (ranging between 0.2% and 1.6% in the general population) or vascular abnormalities (ranging from 0.5% to 1.8%; Katzman et al. 1999; Weber and Knopf 2006; Vernooij et al. 2007) may require immediate neurosurgical, endovascular or medical therapy or, at the very least, require follow-up (Morris et al. 2009; Illes and Chin 2008; Hartwigsen et al. 2010). Other findings may herald the onset of disease (such as multiple sclerosis) even in the absence of clinical symptoms at the time of diagnosis (Okuda et al. 2009; Ulmer et al. 2012). Many findings may require medical treatment and have a profound impact on the subject's life, especially in planning a family, choosing a career, obtaining insurance and engaging in recreational activities. A volunteer who is informed that he/she has brain abnormality may decide to change some aspects of his/her daily routine and also formulate new goals in life.

Besides the consequences of discovering an IF for the individual, there may be implications for the wider community. For example, many brain lesions can cause clinical symptoms such as seizures, which can put the surrounding population at substantial risk (e.g. from a subsequent motor vehicle accident). Detection of such lesions is clearly of societal benefit—indeed the disclosure of an IF in this scenario is mandatory according to the World Medical Association, which represents approximately 80 national medical associations despite the usual right of a subject 'not to know' (see below; World Medical Association 2008).

There are also financial implications. Some lesions never become symptomatic, yet follow-up imaging of such lesions often incurs considerable costs for the individual, the state or insurance companies depending on the national health-care system (Machaalany et al. 2009). On the other hand, an early identification of an IF might be of unequivocal benefit to the patient if the condition is treatable and early diagnosis improves outcome. The prevention, as well as a reduction, of the risk of death or long-term disability may even reduce overall health costs.

27.4 Consent

Although it is widely agreed amongst researchers that consent should be obtained from the volunteer prior to neuroimaging research, in practice, the information provided at the time differs widely between research groups. In the UK, for example, over 10% of participants are not apprised of contingency plans, potential benefits and harms should any IF be found, despite an expectation from the National Research Ethics Service (2007; Booth et al. 2012). Radiologists are more likely than non-radiologists to discuss the potential implications of IF, which likely reflect greater familiarity with common IF and the issues that they raise. About 20% of researchers discuss whether any IF are likely to be treatable, which is a European 'Additional Protocol' requirement (Council of Europe Steering Committee on Bioethics 2004). This practice is, not surprisingly, more common amongst medical (i.e. medically qualified) than nonmedical researchers. The WHO/UNESCO also recommend discussion prior to the consent of 'the extent of the investigator's responsibility to provide medical services to the participant' should an IF be discovered (The Council for International Organizations of Medical Sciences (CIOMS) 2002). This ethical guideline is followed by 42% of researchers in the UK. Practice also differs between countries. For example, just over one-third of UK researchers warn volunteers that the reanalysis of the data in the future may lead to recontact after the study has finished. This compares to only 4% in the USA (Lawrenz and Sobotka 2008), despite the recommendation that such information is routinely given (Wolf et al. 2008). In the UK, medical researchers are more likely than nonmedical researchers to discuss recontact, which may again reflect differences in the perception of the wider implications and limits of researchers' responsibilities.

27.5 Detection of Incidental Findings

Even if an unexpected finding may be of no clinical concern to the volunteer, the research data may be confounded, for example, if an arachnoid cyst is discovered during an fMRI study. In this example, normalising brains (e.g. to the Montreal Neurological Institute (MNI) space) may lead to incorrect topographical localisation of functional areas. For most fMRI research groups, anatomical images consist of high-resolution T_1-weighted sequences (such as a MPRage or SPGR) which are used for an overlay. Nonetheless, although these sequences differentiate grey and white matter well, they are likely to be inadequate for clinical screening purposes where additional T_2-weighted sequences (TSE or FLAIR), contrast agents and additional orthogonal acquisitions may be required.

In neuroimaging research, there is no universally agreed approach to acquiring and reporting scans in the anticipation of IF (Booth et al. 2010). In terms of reporting strategies, UK and US studies show wide variation amongst researchers (Booth et al. 2012; Illes et al. 2004). This ranges from no radiological review of images to 'reactive' strategies (where radiological advice is sought only if an abnormality is noticed by a researcher or radiographer) to 'proactive' (all images are reviewed by a radiologist) and 'very proactive' (where additional anatomical imaging is performed routinely to better identify and characterise any IF) reporting (Ulmer et al. 2009; Booth et al. 2010). There may also be variation as to whether a specialist radiologist reports a study (e.g. a neuroradiologist reviewing a brain MRI) as opposed to a non-specialist.

'Proactive' radiological review of research images is likely to provide more sensitive and specific detection of significant IF (Royal and Peterson 2008). Furthermore, the IF prevalence meta-analysis mentioned above (Morris et al. 2009) demonstrates that the detection of IF almost doubles if a 'very proactive' strategy is adopted. In the UK, the 'reactive' strategy is the most common reporting method (26%), although few researchers (16%) consider this ideal practice (defined as without funding or time constraints; Booth et al. 2012). On the other hand, the most popular ideal reporting strategy is 'proactive' reporting by specialist radiologists (29%) but is the current practice for only 14% of researchers. Medical researchers, especially radiologists, tend toward more 'proactive' reporting strategies compared with nonmedical investigators.

The reasons for researchers not undertaking 'proactive' reporting may reflect no or little access to a radiological opinion, cost limitations, limited awareness of the frequency and implications of IF and opinions as to the extent of responsibility of the researcher with regard to detection of such abnormalities (Royal and Peterson 2008). Additionally, policies of 'reactive' reporting are sometimes justified on the grounds that the detection of IF lies outside the remit of the research study (Miller et al. 2008).

27.6 Disclosure of Incidental Findings

There are few publications relating to the disclosure of IF. Regardless of the reporting method, research groups must decide how to manage an IF once it is discovered. In the same UK study mentioned above, IF disclosure management is shown to vary and be influenced by the background of the principal investigator. Here, researchers most commonly disclose IF to volunteers when judged 'relevant' (47%), and a similar percentage considers this ideal (46%). Face-to-face disclosure is the most common method of communication (41%) and is thought by many to be ideal (70%). Disclosure is performed most commonly by the volunteer's family practitioner (43%), which is also thought to be ideal practice by one-third of the responders (32%).

Nonmedical researchers are more likely never to disclose IF to the volunteer. The two common reasons given for this are that non-clinicians process the images, which makes subsequent disclosure appear inappropriate, and that disclosure is harmful and causes stress to the volunteer.

Those who have been researchers for a shorter period of time are more likely to disclose IF 'routinely' to the volunteer than those who have been researchers for a longer period, but more experienced investigators are more likely than less experienced researchers to disclose IF to the volunteer if this is felt to be 'relevant'. Medical researchers are more likely to use a research team physician to disclose IFs than nonmedical researchers, as are radiologists compared with non-radiologists. Nonmedical researchers are more likely to use the volunteer's own family practitioner but also feel this is ideal practice.

Neuroimaging studies, however, are not designed to screen for IF. In research, there is rarely a traditional physician–patient relationship, and in many research groups, there are no neuroradiologists reading brain MRI scans. Furthermore, additional high-resolution anatomical MR imaging is not performed to reduce scanning time and cost, yet adequate image resolution is required to enable the detection of IF.

27.7 Ethical Considerations

Ethical standards for conducting research with human beings were formulated several decades ago in the Declaration of Helsinki in 1975 as well as in the Belmont Report in 1979, which relied on earlier documents such as the Nuremberg Code from 1947 (Declaration of Helsinki 1975; The National Commission for the Protection of Human Subjects of Biomedical and Behavioral Research 1979; Tröhler and Reiter-Theil 1998). Basic principles of research ethics include the respect of the volunteers and their autonomy, avoiding harm (non-maleficence), promoting the well-being of subjects participating in research studies (beneficence) and fairness (Beauchamp and Childress 2009).

There are a variety of ethical arguments in favour of different management strategies. On one hand, the aim in research is not to detect IF, and therefore it can be argued that this is not the researcher's responsibility. On the other hand, if an IF could be detected easily by the researcher and if that could help to avoid harm to the volunteer in the future, it could be considered the researcher's responsibility not to miss it.

The ability of detecting IF obviously varies amongst professional groups performing research, largely dependent upon the training of the researcher in reading and interpreting MR images. Because a lesion not detected by a doctoral student is more likely to be detected by a radiologist, the question arises as to who should perform or read the scan.

We hold the view that, if resources allow it, an acceptable image quality should be used during imaging and that trained neuroradiologists should read the scans. Potentially this reduces the likelihood of missing IF and allows the clinical significance of such lesions to be determined by fuller characterisation. This might have a major impact on the subject's life, and although evidence is lacking, the net effect is likely to be one of beneficence. For example, this approach may allow treatable pathologies to be detected early before they may become symptomatic and cause problems for the individual (respecting the individual voluntarily participating in research) or others.

One basic question is whether IF should be communicated to the volunteers at all. Kirschen et al. (2006) published data from a survey on subjects' expectations regarding the detection and management of IF in neuroimaging research which suggests that IF should be communicated to the volunteers. In that study, 54% of the subjects expected abnormalities to be detected should they be present and >90% preferred IF to be communicated to them. This was despite the researchers obtaining written informed consent without the mention of the disclosure of findings. Furthermore, the subjects of research studies expect that their images are read by a trained person regardless of the information given during the process of consent. The authors underline that clarity about procedures for handling IF is essential to ensure that the subjects' expectations are consistent with, or adjusted to, the purpose of the study.

The PI's responsibility does not end with detecting IF. Indeed, it becomes more complex after that. Once IF are detected, a standardised management protocol needs to be followed to take care of any further diagnostic tests or treatment that may result from these findings (Illes et al. 2006; Gupta and Belay 2008; Ulmer et al. 2009; Hartwigsen et al. 2010). Cooperation between research groups and clinicians has been suggested (Ulmer et al. 2009; Hartwigsen et al. 2010), including an outpatient service, to take care of these volunteers. Consistent with the ethical principle of respecting the autonomy of the volunteers, if such management was to be offered, each subject could decide whether they prefer to use this service or their primary care physician or want to ignore such findings altogether or until they become symptomatic. In our local (Germany) experience, however, all volunteers used the outpatient service. Respecting the autonomy of a research participant is important should volunteers not want to be told of any unexpected scan findings. In these cases, the principal investigator (PI) may face a dilemma when detecting an IF: on the one hand, the wishes of the individual subject 'not to know' should be respected; on the other hand, it could be argued that it is problematic if researchers acquire information relevant for future health which they are not allowed to share with the volunteer. Furthermore, the IF may put the community at risk as discussed above. A possible solution is to exclude volunteers who explicitly state they do not want any information about IF to be disclosed to them.

In genetics, there are also published papers dealing with similar principles. Most research studies are not carried out under the Clinical Laboratory Improvement Amendments (CLIA)–certified laboratory testing guidelines of quality assurance (Clinical Laboratory Improvement Amendments, CLIA, n.d.; http://www.cms.hhs.gov/CLIA), and often researchers are not clinically certified to evaluate the clinical significance of genetic or genomic IF (Van Ness 2008). In 2004, the National Heart, Lung, and Blood Institute (NHLBI) of the US National Institutes of Health developed a set of recommendations where genetic results should be reported to the research participant depending on whether there was a significant risk of disease and whether the disease would have important health implications (i.e. fatal consequences or substantial morbidity); moreover, the recommendations suggested that this should be made explicit in the study design and Institutional Review Board (IRB) approval (National Heart, Lung, and Blood Institute 2004). Furthermore, only CLIA-certified tests should be reported as clinically valid. Knoppers et al. (2006) concluded that at the international level, an ethical duty exists to return individual genetic research results to the subject after proof of validity, significance and benefit. Even where these criteria are met, the right of the research participant 'not to know' also has to be taken into consideration. In 1991, the Council for International Organizations of Medical Sciences (CIOMS) International Guidelines for Ethical Review of Epidemiological Studies maintain that being informed of findings 'that pertain to their health' is one of the 'reasonable' benefits of participation for 'communities, groups and individuals' in research (The Council for International Organizations of Medical Sciences (CIOMS) 1991). A similar position was also expressed by the Council of Europe (Council of Europe, n.d. http://www.coe.int/T/E/Legal_affairs/Legal_cooperation/Bioethics/Activities/Biomedical_research/Protocol_Biomedical_research.pdf and http://conventions.coe.int/treaty/en/Treaties/Html/164.htm).

At-risk family members also should be considered in the discussion as to whether there is a need or requirement for the disclosure of IF (Knoppers et al. 2006).

An international recommendation on handling theses complex issues has yet to be produced. Researchers should be aware of the problem of IF; in the absence of general guidelines, they have to come up with local and individual solutions to ensure responsible management of their volunteers even in the absence of international recommendations. However, there are useful sources of information available from various imaging centres, for example, in the appendix of a UK summary of an international meeting on IF (Royal College of Radiologists (RCR) 2011).

27.8 Recommendations

The management of IF varies between institutions and countries (Booth et al. 2010). International or European guidelines would—as in other fields—be prudent but are not yet established. In our opinion, volunteers who enable research to be performed should be offered the following:

- Initially informed consent will be obtained from the participant, which should include information about the possibility of detecting IF with a thorough explanation as to what the consequences might be. The exact requirements of informed consent depend on national regulations, but it might be pragmatic to explain to the participant that IF, if discovered, have to be documented from this point forward, and that they may require immediate treatment and further imaging or follow-up exams. Furthermore, IF might have a major impact on the individual's life and therefore should be disclosed to the participant.
- If the person performing the research is not medically qualified, a medical professional should be incorporated into the team in order to obtain informed consent from the volunteer. Although dependent on the nation's healthcare system, it appears sensible for any subsequent costs of discovering an IF—if not covered by the volunteer's insurance company—to be underwritten by the research institution. As discussed earlier, the right 'not to know' can be problematic. A possible solution is to exclude volunteers who explicitly state that they do not want to know any information about IF. It remains a matter of debate what scans, if any, should be obtained in addition to those required for the research. Additional T_2-weighted sequences and additional orthogonal acquisitions appear judicious.

If no neuroradiologist is part of the research group, it would be sensible for the scanning protocol to be discussed with an external expert. We do not recommend an intravenous contrast agent as this is intrusive to the volunteer. As in standard clinical practice, the neuroradiologist reading the scans should take responsibility for detecting abnormalities. There are several options to compensate for costs that arise from professional reading of these images, the suitability of which depends on the local institution (Booth et al. 2010; Hartwigsen et al. 2010). As discussed earlier, in our opinion, professional reading of the images is an ethical requirement, not only to enable the detection of IF but also to depict deviations from normal that might hamper further post-processing of the data, that is, for the topographical location of functional areas.

- In our opinion, further steps need to be in place should an IF be discovered. These include a medical professional being able to explain the consequences of the IF. Questions from the volunteer, who might have become a patient, should be answered professionally. An outpatient service, taking care of further steps including additional screening or treatment, has proven to be useful (Hartwigsen et al. 2010; Ulmer et al. 2009, 2012). Some patients prefer to see their primary care physician, so this option should also be available. Again, costs that might arise could be covered by either the volunteers' insurance or a dedicated institutional insurance policy for volunteers in general.

References

Alphs HH, Schwartz BS et al (2006) Findings on brain MRI from research studies of occupational exposure to known neurotoxicants. AJR Am J Roentgenol 187:1043–1047

Beauchamp TL, Childress JF (eds) (2009) Principles of biomedical ethics, 6th edn. Oxford University Press, Oxford. ISBN-13: 978-0-19-533570-5

Booth TC, Jackson A et al (2010) Incidental findings discovered in 'healthy' volunteers during research imaging; legal and ethical lessons from UK and overseas. Br J Radiol 83:456–465

Booth TC, Jackson A et al (2012) Management of incidental findings during imaging research in 'healthy' volunteers; current UK practice. Br J Radiol 85:11–21

Brown DA, Hasso AN (2008) Toward a uniform policy for handling incidental findings in neuroimaging research. AJNR Am J Neuroradiol 29:1425–1427

Carli V, Hadlaczky G et al (2012) Maintaining confidentiality in prospective studies: anonymous repeated measurements via email procedure (ARME). J Med Ethics 38:127–129

Clinical Laboratory Improvement Amendments, CLIA; Centers for Medicare and Medicaid Services. Clinical Laboratory Improvement Amendments. http://www.cms.hhs.gov/CLIA

Council of Europe. http://www.coe.int/T/E/Legal_affairs/Legal_cooperation/Bioethics/Activities/Biomedical_research/Protocol_Biomedical_research.pdf and http://conventions.coe.int/treaty/en/Treaties/Html/164.htm

Council of Europe Steering Committee on Bioethics (2004) Additional protocol to the convention on human rights and biomedicine concerning biomedical research. http://conventions.coe.int

Declaration of Helsinki (1975) WMA declaration of Helsinki – ethical principles for medical research involving human subjects. www.wma.net/en/30publications/10policies/b3/

Garnett A, Whiteley L et al (2011) Neuroethics and fMRI: mapping a fledgling relationship. PLoS One 6:e18537

Gupta SN, Belay B (2008) Intracranial incidental findings on brain MR images in a pediatric neurology practice: a retrospective study. J Neurol Sci 264:34–37

Hartwigsen G, Siebner HR et al (2010) Incidental findings are frequent in young healthy individuals undergoing magnetic resonance imaging in brain research imaging studies: a prospective single-center study. J Comput Assist Tomogr 34:596–600

Illes J, Chin VN (2008) Bridging philosophical and practical implications of incidental findings in brain research. J Law Med Ethics 36(298–304):212

Illes J, Kirschen MP et al (2004) Discovery and disclosure of incidental findings in neuroimaging research. J Magn Reson Imaging 20:743–747

Illes J, Kirschen MP et al (2006) Ethics. Incidental findings in brain imaging research. Science 311:783–784

Katzman GL, Dagher AP et al (1999) Incidental findings on brain magnetic resonance imaging from 1000 asymptomatic volunteers. JAMA 282:36–39

Kirschen MP, Jaworska A et al (2006) Subjects' expectations in neuroimaging research. J Magn Reson Imaging 23:205–209

Knoppers BM, Joly Y et al (2006) The emergence of an ethical duty to disclose genetic research results: international perspectives. Eur J Hum Genet 14:1170–1178

Kwong KK, Belliveau JW et al (1992) Dynamic magnetic resonance imaging of human brain activity during primary sensory stimulation. Proc Natl Acad Sci U S A 89:5675–5679

Lawrenz F, Sobotka S (2008) Empirical analysis of current approaches to incidental findings. J Law Med Ethics 36:249–255

Machaalany J, Yam Y et al (2009) Potential clinical and economic consequences of noncardiac incidental findings on cardiac computed tomography. J Am Coll Cardiol 54:1533–1541

Miller FG, Mello MM et al (2008) Incidental findings in human research: what do investigators owe research participants? J Law Med Ethics 36:271–279

Morris Z, Whiteley WN et al (2009) Incidental findings on brain magnetic resonance imaging: systematic review and meta-analysis. BMJ 339:b3016

National Heart, Lung, and Blood Institute (NHLBI) of the US National Institutes of Health (2004). http://www.nhlbi.nih.gov/meetings/workshops/gene-results.htm

National Research Ethics Service (2007) National Patient Safety Agency information sheets and consent forms. Guidance for researchers and reviewers. http://www.nres.npsa.nhs.uk/EasySiteWeb/GatewayLink.aspx?alld

Ogawa S, Lee TM et al (1990) Brain magnetic resonance imaging with contrast dependent on blood oxygenation. Proc Natl Acad Sci U S A 87:9868–9872

Ogawa S, Menon RS et al (1993) Functional brain mapping by blood oxygenation level-dependent contrast magnetic resonance imaging. A comparison of signal characteristics with a biophysical model. Biophys J 64:803–812

Okuda DT, Mowry EM et al (2009) Incidental MRI anomalies suggestive of multiple sclerosis: the radiologically isolated syndrome. Neurology 72:800–805

Reiter-Theil S, Stingelin Giles N (2007) Ethical aspects of screening and preventive diagnosis with radiological imaging. In: Reiser MF, van Kaick G, Fink C, Schoenberg SO (eds) Screening and preventive diagnosis with radiological imaging. Springer, Berlin, pp 137–146

Royal College of Radiologists (RCR) (2011) Management of incidental findings detected during research imaging. www.rcr.ac.uk/docs/radiology/pdf/BFCR(11)8_Ethics.pdf

Royal JM, Peterson BS (2008) The risks and benefits of searching for incidental findings in MRI research scans. J Law Med Ethics 36:305–314

The Council for International Organizations of Medical Sciences (CIOMS) (1991) International Guidelines for Ethical Review of Epidemiological, European Federation of the International Epidemiologist Association (IEA). http://www.dundee.ac.uk/iea/GoodPract.htm

The Council for International Organizations of Medical Sciences (CIOMS) (2002) International ethical guidelines for biomedical research involving human subjects. http://www.cioms.ch

The National Commission for the Protection of Human Subjects of Biomedical and Behavioral Research (1979) Belmont report. http://ohsr.od.nih.gov/guidelines/belmont.html

Tröhler U, Reiter-Theil S (eds) (1998) Ethics codes in medicine: foundations and achievements 1947–1997. Ashgate, Aldershot

Ulmer S, Jensen UR et al (2009) Impact of incidental findings on neuroimaging research using functional MR imaging. AJNR Am J Neuroradiol 30(4):E55

Ulmer S, Stippich C et al (2012) Incidence and responsible management of incidental findings (IF) in neuroimaging research. Nervenheilkunde 31(4):246–249

Van Ness B (2008) Genomic research and incidental findings. J Law Med Ethics 36(2):292–297, 212

Vernooij MW, Ikram MA et al (2007) Incidental findings on brain MRI in the general population. N Engl J Med 357:1821–1828

Weber F, Knopf H (2006) Incidental findings in magnetic resonance imaging of the brains of healthy young men. J Neurol Sci 240:81–84

Wolf SM, Lawrenz FP et al (2008) Managing incidental findings in human subjects research: analysis and recommendations. J Law Med Ethics 36:219–248

Woodward CI, Toms AP (2009) Incidental findings in "normal" volunteers. Clin Radiol 64:951–953

World Medical Association (2008) World Medical Association declaration on the Rights of the Patient. http://www.wma.net

Yousry TA, Schmid UD et al (1995) Topography of the cortical motor hand area: prospective study with functional MR imaging and direct cortical mapping at surgery. Radiology 195:23–29

Index

A

Aβ, 398
Absence-seizure model, 205, 207
Activation likelihood estimation (ALE), 120–122
Activation patterns, 229, 230
Activation studies, principle of, 225, 226
Activity dependent synaptic plasticity, 288
Alternative modelling approaches, 178
Alzheimer's disease (AD), 3, 364, 365, 385, 386
  dementia, network changes and predicting conversion, 395–397
  dementia subtypes, 389–391, 393, 395
  fMRI in, 376, 377
  mapping brain networks, 386–389
Amore data-driven approach, 199
Amplitude of Low Frequency Fluctuations (ALFF), 336
Amyloid, 401
Analysis of covariance (ANCOVA), 105
Anatomical connectivity, 324, 325
Anatomo-functional brain imaging methods
  BOLD signal, 134
  brain maturation, 134
  clinical research applications
    language, 141–142
    memory functions, 143
    motor cortex, 141
    reading, 142
    short- and long-range connectivity, 140
  data analysis, 139–140
  experimental design
    activation and reference tasks choice, 135, 136
    age *vs*. performance, 137
    group studies, 136–137
    monitoring of task performance, 136
    paradigm design, 134–135
  feasibility, 138, 139
  fMRI during rest, 134
  focal anatomical/functional abnormality, 133
  motor plasticity, 133
  multimodal imaging, 140
  resting-state fMRI, 143–145
  technical issues, 137, 138
Anterior temporal lobe (ATL), 241
Aphasia, 228
Apolipoprotein E (APOE), 386, 399
Arterial spin labeling (ASL), 69
  accurate CBF quantification, 77
  background suppression, 78, 79
  blood flow-related parameters, 73
  CASL and PASL, 77
  imaging readouts, 79–83
  inter-subject differences, 74
  low spatial resolution, 75
  noninvasive nature, 74
  PASL labeling methods, 77
  pCASL, 75, 76
  perfusion-weighted signal, 74
  tSNR, 75
  UHF, 83, 84
  VSASL, 78
Arteriovenous malformation (AVM), 4
Awake craniotomy, 313, 314
Axonal connectivity, 322

B

BA 44, 324
Background suppression, 78, 79
Balanced-steady-state free precession (b-SSFP) fMRI, 33
Between-network RS fMRI abnormalities, 342, 343
Blood oxygen level-dependent (BOLD), 16, 19–25, 31, 65, 67–69, 158, 226, 242, 267–270, 280
Boltzmann equation, 29
Brain
  specialized modules in, 321, 322
  structure-function relationships in, 322–324
Brain-computer-interface (BCI) technology, 37
Brain connectivity, 324
BrainMap, 119
Brain maturation, 134
Brain network functional connectivity
  dementia, network changes and predicting conversion, 395–397
  dementia subtypes, 389–393, 395
  differential diagnosis, 404
  functional network organization, characterizing preclinical changes, 397–402
  mapping brain networks, 386–388
  methodological considerations, 405
  relationship with pathophysiology, 403, 404
  uncovering disease mechanisms and neuropathology, 402

S. Ulmer, O. Jansen (eds.), *fMRI*, https://doi.org/10.1007/978-3-030-41874-8

Brain organization, 321
Brain oxygen level-dependent (BOLD), 102
Brain parcellation techniques, 387
Brain plasticity, 335
Brain shift, 316, 317
Brain tumors, 234, 235
Broca's area, 12

C

Cat's layer model, 70
Central sulcus (CS), 5
Cerebellar RS FC, 341
Cerebral blood flow (CBF), 15, 65, 73
Cerebral blood volume (CBV), 65, 232
Childhood absence epilepsy (CAE), 206
Clinical Laboratory Improvement Amendment (CLIA), 437
Clinical motor, 272–274
Cognitive impairment, 345
Cognitive networks, 340
Cognitive rehabilitation, 347, 348
Combined TMS-fMRI approach, 162
Condition-and-map approach, 168
Connectivity matrix, 246
Connectivity models, 321, 322
Continuous ASL (CASL), 75
Convergent syndromic atrophy, 389
Coordinate-based meta-analysis (CBMA), 118, 120, 126, 127
Coregistration, 97, 98
Cortical dysplasia, 149
Cortical structural lesion, 197
Cortico-subcortical pathways, 419

D

Deep brain stimulation (DBS), 41
Deep gray matter RS FC, 340, 341
Default mode network (DMN), 144, 201, 289, 338, 339, 389
Dementia subtypes, 389–393, 395
Depression, 345
Deterministic and stochastic models, 331
Diagnostic Statistical Manual of Mental Disorders, Fifth Edition (DSM-V), 59
Diffusion tensor imaging (DTI), 150, 265, 306
Direct cortical stimulation (DCS)
  indications for, 312
    clinical condition, 312
    tumor localization and function, 312, 313
  intraoperative MRI, 316
  methods
    awake craniotomy, 313, 314
    intraoperative MRI, 316
    stimulation, 315, 316
  practical considerations, 316
Discrete cosine transform (DCT), 106
Divergent functional connectivity, 393
Dorsal anterior cingulate cortex/supplementary motor cortex (dACC/SMA), 122
Double-acquisition background suppressed (DABS), 82
Dynamic causal modelling (DCM), 127, 328–330
  application, 331–333
  comparison, 331
  deterministic and stochastic models, 331
  model estimation, 330, 331
Dynamic connectivity states, 387
Dynamic imaging of coherent sources (DICS), 185
DYNAmic Multi-coIl TEchnique (DYNAMITE), 32
Dysplasia, 149

E

Echo planar imaging (EPI), 5, 30, 91, 97
EEG and fMRI recordings (EEG-fMRI)
  focal epilepsy
    interictal activity, 179, 180
    localisation-related epilepsy, 182
    mesial temporal lobe epilepsy, 180
    noninvasive tool, 180
    seizures, 182
  IGE
    absences and cognitive impairment, 184
    BOLD signal changes, 183, 184
    functional connectivity, 184–185
    PPR, 185
    SEEG exploration, 182
    short GSW paroxysms, 182
  local epilepsy, 179–182
  methods
    artefact correction, 177
    equipment, 176–177
    noninvasive tool, 180
    methodological refinements, 178–179
    spike-triggered manner, 175, 176
    statistical analysis, 177, 178
  paediatric EEG-fMRI studies
    epileptic encephalopathy, 186
    self-limited focal epilepsies, 185–186
    spike-related BOLD changes, 185
EEG band-power regressor, 200
Effective connectivity, DCM, 328–330
  application, 331–333
  deterministic and stochastic models, 331
  model comparison, 331
  model estimation, 330, 331
Electrophysiological methods
  CBF, 15, 24, 25
  blood oxygenation, 15
  compound neural signal, 16–18
  coupling of synaptic activity, 23–25
  functional imaging, 15
  neural correlate of BOLD signal, 19–23
  passive electric properties, 18, 19
Eloquent areas, 4, 311, 317
Entorhinal cortex, 360, 370, 371
Epilepsy, 297
Epileptic dip, 196

Epileptic encephalopathy, 186
Episodic memory, 361, 364, 377
Experience dependent synaptic plasticity, 288
Extracellular field potentials (EFP), 16
Extracellular recording, 16

F

Family-wise error rate (FWER), 110
Fatigue, 345
Fiber tracking methods (DTI), 40
Fixed-effects (FFX) analysis, 113
Flow-sensitive alternating inversion recovery (FAIR), 77
Focal motor seizures, 195
Focal seizures, 194
Frameless neuronavigation systems, 304
Frequency-dependent behaviour, 18
Frontotemporal dementia (FTD), 385, 386
  dementia, network changes and predicting conversion, 395–397
  dementia subtypes, 389–391, 393, 395
  mapping brain networks, 386–389
Full width at half maximum (FWHM), 100
Functional brain networks, 419
Functional connectivity, 325
  analysis, 184
  resting-state, 325–327, 419, 423
  task-based functional connectivity, 326, 328
Functional integration, 321
Functional magnetic resonance imaging (fMRI), 29, 90, 117, 149, 226, 270, 271
Functional network organization, 397–402
Functional segregation, 321

G

Generalised spike-wave discharges (GSW), 182
Generalized paroxysmal fast activity (GPFA), 209
Generalized tonic-clonic seizures (GTCS), 203, 208, 209
General linear model (GLM), 90, 102, 196
  ANOVA, 105
  BOLD signal, 102, 105
  canonical HRF, 104, 106
  design matrix, 105
  event-related fMRI, 108
  Gaussian kernel, 104
  generative model, 102
  multiple regressors, 108
  OLS equation, 106
  short-range serial or temporal correlations, 106
  slice-timing correction, 106
GingerALE software, 122
Glial tumors, 311
Glioblastoma, 303
Global signal regression (GSR), 295
Gradient echo (GRE) techniques, 80
Granger causality, 200
Granger causality mapping (GCM), 127, 328
Graph analysis, 343
Graph theoretical analysis, 394
Graph theoretical approach, 387
Graph theoretical metrics, 144

H

Haemodynamic response function (HRF), 102
Hahn spin-echo (HSE)-based BOLD contrast, 32
Hamilton Depression Rating Scale (HAM-D), 60
Head motion, 139
Hemodynamic-based fMRI, 66
Hemodynamic response function (HRF), 41
Heschl's gyrus, 12, 13, 217
Heschl's sulcus, 12
Heterogeneity, 396
Hippocampal sulcus, 367
Hippocampus
  higher-order anatomical characteristic of, 362
  MTL, 372
    body, 373–375
    head, 374–376
    tail, 375
Human Connectome Project, 247
Hypoconnectivity, 332

I

Ideal practice, 435
Idiopathic generalised epilepsy (IGE)
  absences and cognitive impairment, 184
  BOLD signal changes, 183, 184
  functional connectivity, 184–185
  PPR, 185
  SEEG exploration, 182
  short GSW paroxysms, 182
Imaging epileptic seizures
  focal epilepsy, 202
  focal seizures, 194
    BOLD activation, 197, 198
    decreased BOLD, 201, 202
    hemodynamic and metabolic responses, 196
    identifying primary region, 198–200
    pre-ictal period, 202, 203
    propagation of epileptic seizures, 200, 201
    reflex epilepsies, 203, 204
    statistical modeling, 196, 197
  generalized seizures
    absence seizures, 204–206
    EEG spike-wave discharge, 207
    GTCS, 208, 209
    loss of consciousness, 207
    negative BOLD signal, 206–207
    neurovascular coupling, 206–207
    photosensitive epilepsy, 208
    tonic seizures, 209–211
  identifying primary region, 199
  interictal discharges, 194
  language and motor-task paradigms, 193
  pharmaco-fMRI, 193
  pre-ictal period, 203
  stereotyped events, 194

Impulse control disorders (ICD), 426
Incidental finding (IF), 434
  consent, 434, 435
  consequences, 434
  detection of, 435, 436
  disclosure of, 436
  ethical considerations, 436–438
  management, 438
Independent component analysis (ICA), 144, 387
Inferior frontal gyrus, 229, 230, 232, 234
Information theory, 98
Intermittent theta burst stimulation (iTBS), 347
International League Against Epilepsy (ILAE), 193
Internetwork connectivity, 342
Intra-axial brain tumors
  brain tumor resection, resting-state fMRIi in, 306, 307
  DTI, 306
  resection within language areas, 305
Intracarotid amobarbital (Wada) test, 241
Intracortical stimulation (ICS), 267
Intracranial space-occupying lesions, 311
Intrinsic connectivity networks (ICNs), 386
ISI Web of Knowledge, 119

J
Jacksonian march, 200
Juvenile myoclonic epilepsy (JME), 206

L
Lagged-regressor approach, 200
Laminar surface-based analysis method, 35
Language activation, 226, 228
Language dominance, 235, 236
Language function
  activation patterns vs. recovery of, 229, 230
  in brain tumors, 234, 235
Language lateralization
  TLE, 241–244
  as verbal memory outcome predictor, 253–256
Language system, 297, 298
Large-scale network connectivity, 343
Laterality index (LI), 244
Lateral premotor cortex (PMC), 331
Left temporal lobe epilepsy (LTLE), 141, 143
Lennox-Gastaut syndrome, 186, 209, 211
Lesion-based research, 217
Local field potentials (LFPs), 17, 322
Localisation-related epilepsy, 182
Lorentzian forces, 137

M
Magnetic-resonance-encephalography (MREG) sequence, 179
Magnetoencephalography (MEG), 149
Mapping brain networks, 386–388
Mass-univariate approach, 102
MATLAB software, 91
Matrix similarity metric, 246
Maximum intensity projection (MIP), 111
Maximum likelihood method, 102
Medial temporal lobe (MTL), 249, 250, 356
  anatomy, 365–367
  functional neuroanatomy, 356–364
  memory outcome predictor, 250, 252
  segmentation protocol, 367, 368
    entorhinal cortex, 370, 371
    hippocampus proper, borders, 372–376
    parahippocampal cortex, 371, 372
    perirhinal cortex, borders of, 368, 369
    transentorhinal area, 370
Medical researchers, 435
Meta-analytic connectivity mapping (MACM), 326
Middle cerebral artery (MCA), 150
Mild cognitive impairment (MCI), 395, 400
Monkey auditory cortex, 217
Motor control, functional MRI studies of, 423–425
Motor cortex mapping, 270
Motor rehabilitation, 347
Motor system modeling effective connectivity in, 331–333
MRI-compatible EEG recording system, 176
Multichannel coils, 32
Multimodal brain mapping
  congenital right hemiparesis, 150, 152, 153
  hemispheric right polymicrogyria, 154, 155
  non-paretic hand, 152
  pharmaco-refractory seizures, 152
  polymicrogyric cortex harbours, 150
  therapy-refractory focal seizures, 149
Multiple sclerosis (MS), 335
  between-network RS fMRI abnormalities, 342, 343
  cerebellar RS FC, 341
  clinical disability, ambulation and balance, 344
  cognitive impairment, depression and fatigue, 345, 346
  cognitive networks, 340
  cognitive rehabilitation, 347, 348
  deep gray matter RS FC, 340, 341
  diagnosis and differential diagnosis, 343, 344
  DMN, 338, 339
  graph analysis, large-scale network connectivity by, 343
  methodological issues, 336
  motor rehabilitation, 347
  optic neuritis, 339, 340
  pharmaceutical treatment, 347
  phenotype-specific RS fMRI patterns, 344
  sensorimotor network, 337, 338
  spinal cord RS FC, 341, 342
  structural substrates, 346
Musicogenic epilepsy, 203
Myoclonic astatic epilepsy (MAE), 184

N
Network breakdown modeling, 402
Network inhibition hypothesis, 202

Neuroanatomy and cortical landmarks
  anisotropic distortion, 5
  auditory cortex, 12
  coronal sections, 13
  insula
    sagittal sections, 9
    transverse sections, 10
  MPRage, 5
  sensorimotor cortex
    sagittal sections, 8, 9
    transverse sections, 6–8
  speech-associated frontal areas
    sagittal sections, 11–12
    transverse sections, 11
  speech-associated temporoparietal areas transverse sections, 12
  SPGR, 5
  visual cortex, 13
Neurodegeneration, 385
Neurodegenerative diseases, 385
Neurofibrillary tangle deposition, 364
Neuroimaging science, 433, 434
  ALE, 120–122
  preconditions and preliminaries, 119, 120
  Parkinson's disease
    functional connectivity assessed with resting-state fMRI, 419, 423
    motor control, functional MRI studies of, 423–425
    non-motor control, functional MRI studies of, 425–427
    preclinical compensation, 427, 428
  quantitative meta-analysis, 117–119
Neurologic deficits, 303
Neuronavigation, 304, 305
Nodal stress, 402
Non-fatigued (NF) MS, 345
Non-linear transformations, 99
Non-motor control, 425–427
Normalisation deformation model, 99
Nyquist ghost, 33

O

Occipital lobe seizures, 200
Optic neuritis (ON), 339, 340
Ordinary least squares (OLS) equation, 106
Oxygen extraction fraction (OEF), 225

P

Parahippocampal cortex, 359, 371, 372
Parenchymal vessels, 66, 67
Paresis, 277–279
Parkinson's disease (PD), 3, 41, 170
  clinical features and pathophysiology, 418
  neuroimaging, 418, 420–422
    functional connectivity assessed with resting-state fMRI, 419, 423
    motor control, functional MRI studies of, 423–425
    non-motor control, functional MRI studies of, 425–427
    preclinical compensation, 427, 428
Pattern separation, 363, 364
Perfusion-based MR techniques, 69–71
Perirhinal cortex, MTL, 358
  anterior border, 368, 369
  lateral border, 369
  posterior border, 369
  superolateral/medial border, 369
Periventricular nodular heterotopia (PVNH), 197
Photoparoxysmal response (PPR), 185, 208
Photosensitive epilepsy, 208
Picture Archiving and Communication System (PACS), 291
Positron emission tomography (PET), 52, 90, 117, 225, 226
Postcentral gyrus, 278
Posterior cingulate cortex (PCC), 288
Poststroke aphasia, 228
  language function, activation patterns *vs.* recovery of, 229, 230
  rTMS with activated imaging, 232–234
  treatment effect, 231, 232
Precentral gyrus, 271, 277–279
Presurgical planning, 287
  epilepsy, 297
  GSR, 295
  language system, 297, 298
  MLP, RSN mapping, 295, 296
  MRI and clinical protocols, 291, 292
  multiple studies, 296
  preprocessing, 293–295
  rsfMRI, processing methods for, 292
  somatomotor, 297
Primary motor cortex, somatotopic mapping, 274, 275, 277
Primary somatosensory cortex, somatotopic mapping, 277, 278
Principal component analysis (PCA), 57
Pseudo-continuous ASL (pCASL), 75
Psycho-physiological interactions (PPI), 328
PsycINFO, 119
PubMed, 119
Pulsed and (pseudo-)continuous ASL labeling methods, 75
Pulsed ASL (PASL), 75

Q

Quality control (QC), 291
Quantitative meta-analysis, 119
  basal ganglia, 122
  bilateral amygdala, 122
  deficient processing, 125
  depression, 124
  emotion processing, 124
  fusiform gyrus, 122
  posterior superior temporal sulcus, 122
  regional metabolic aberration, 126
  whole-brain renderings, 123

R

Radio frequency (RF), 29, 73
Random-effects (RFX) analyses, 113
Random field theory (RFT), 91, 102
Real-time fMRI, 138
Reference task, 136
Regional functional specialization, 322
Regional homogeneity (ReHo), 336
Regional structural specialization, 322, 323
Regional structure-function relationships, 324
Regions of interest (ROIs), 51
Relapsing-remitting (RR) MS, 337
Renormalized partial directed coherence (RPDC), 185
Repetitive transcranial magnetic stimulation (rTMS), 157, 232–234
Reporting strategy, 435
Resting state fMRI (rsfMRI), 281, 287
  auditory system and visual system, 51
  clinical uses of, 59–61
  covariance-based approaches, 48
  elastic abdominal belt traces, 48
  event-related designs, 47
  head motion causes artifacts, 50
  methodological issues, 336
  Midnight Scan Club, 53
  motion and respiratory signals, 50
  multiple sclerosis, 335
    between-network RS fMRI abnormalities, 342, 343
    cerebellar RS FC, 341
    clinical disability, ambulation and balance, 344
    cognitive impairment, depression and fatigue, 345, 346
    cognitive networks, 340
    cognitive rehabilitation, 347, 348
    deep gray matter RS FC, 340, 341
    diagnosis and differential diagnosis, 343, 344
    DMN, 338, 339
    graph analysis, large-scale network connectivity by, 343
    motor rehabilitation, 347
    optic neuritis, 339, 340
    pharmaceutical treatment, 347
    phenotype-specific RS fMRI patterns, 344
    sensorimotor network, 337, 338
    spinal cord RS FC, 341, 342
    structural substrates, 346
  MyConnectome scans, 53
  properties of, artifacts and variables of interest, 55, 56
  respiration and head motion, 50
  respiratory signals, 50
  ROIs, 51
  "seed map", 51
  sensorimotor network, 338
  signal denoising, 56–59
  simultaneous multi-slice sequences, 48
  spatial systems, 54
  "spring embedding" plots, 51
  task-free format, 48
  TMS, 53–55
  voxel signals, 50
  "winner-take-all" fashion, 53
Resting-state functional connectivity, 325–327, 341
Resting-state language network mapping, 245, 246
Resting state networks (RSN), 287, 289, 290, 337
Reverse inference, 126
ROI-based analysis, 144
Rolandic brain tumors
  primary motor cortex, somatotopic mapping of, 274, 275, 277
  primary somatosensory cortex, somatotopic mapping of, 277, 278
Rolandic neurosurgery, 265–267

S

Seed-based analysis, 387
Seed-based correlation (SBC) mapping, 292
Seed-based functional connectivity, 387
Seed-based technique, 340
Seizure-related hyperperfusion, 198
Sensorimotor cortex, 305
Sensorimotor network, 337, 338
Signal-to-noise ratio (SNR), 65, 74
Single-shot approaches, 79
Small-tipped microelectrode, 16
Small volume correction (SVC), 111
Somatomotor, 297, 298
Somatosensory fMRI, 272–274
Somatotopic mapping
  of primary motor cortex, 274, 276, 277
  of primary somatosensory cortex, 277, 278
Spatial independent component analysis (sICA), 292
Spatial normalisation, 98–100
Spatial resolution of fMRI
  BOLD technique, 65, 67–69
  hemodynamic response, 66, 67
  perfusion-based MR techniques, 69–71
  vascular structure, 66, 67
Spatial smoothing, 100, 102
Specific absorption rate (SAR), 30
Speech apraxia, 9
Speech-associated frontal areas, 11
Speech processing
  conceptual-semantic information, 219–220
  dual-stream model, 218
  monkey auditory cortex, 217
  posterior superior temporal regions, 221, 222
  sensory systems, 220–221
  STS, 219
Spinal cord RS FC, 341, 342
Spin-echo (SE) approaches, 80
Spin-echo BOLD, 35
SPM Software
  File Formats, 93
  installation, 91, 92
  interface, 92
  requirements, 91
Stack of Spirals (SoS), 80
Statistical parametric mapping (SPM)
  GLM, 90
  modelling and statistical inference
    contrasts, 109–110
    general linear model (*see* General linear model)
    population-level inference, 113, 114

topological inference, 110, 111
voxel by voxel hypothesis testing approach, 102
spatial transformations
coregistration, 94, 97, 98
data preparation, 95, 96
normalise function, 94
objective function, 94
optimisation algorithm, 94
realignment, 93, 95–97
rigid body transformation, 94
spatial normalisation, 98–100
spatial smoothing, 100, 102
SPM Software (*see* SPM Software)
Stimulation, DCS, 315, 316
Structural equation modeling (SEM), 127, 328
Structural Independent Component Analysis (sICA), 297
Subjective memory complaints (SMC), 396
Superior temporal gyrus (STG), 220, 228, 230
Superior temporal sulcus (STS), 217, 218
Supplementary motor area (SMA), 331, 423
Susceptibility-weighted images (SWI), 42
Sylvian fissure, 11–13

T

Tailoring temporal lobe resections, 246–248
Task-based functional connectivity, 326, 328
Tau burden, 398
Tau deposition, 401
Temporal lobe epilepsy (TLE), 180, 241
medial temporal lobe FMRI, 250
predicting naming outcome, 241–245
resting-state language network mapping, 245, 246
tailoring temporal lobe resections, 246–248
verbal memory outcome
language lateralization, 253–256
medial temporal lobe FMRI, memory outcome predictor, 248–250, 252
Temporal SNR (tSNR), 75
3D Gaussian probability distributions, 120
3D gradient and spin echo (GRASE), 80
Three-dimensional segmented echo-planar imaging (3D-EPI), 34, 82
3D SoS acquisition, 81
3D spin-echo readouts, 79
3D turbo spin echo (TSE), 80
Tissue perfusion, 73
Tonic seizures, 209–211
Tractography, 324
Transcranial magnetic stimulation (TMS), 53, 141, 149
adverse effects, 160
clinical and neuroscientific applications, 159
coil over placement, 160, 161
combine with fMRI, 161–162
human primary motor cortex, 158
offline combination of, 166–170
online TMS-fMRI approach
interleaved TMS-fMRI, 165–166
methodological issues, 163, 164
physical aspects of, 158–159
safety precautions, 160
time-varying electrical field, 157
Transentorhinal area, 370
Translational Imaging Platform (TIP), 291
Transneuronal spread model, 402
Trophic failure, 402
2D EPI, 82
2D turboFLASH (TFL), 75

U

Ultra-high field (UHF), 83, 84
Ultra-high-field fMRI
benefits, 29–30
BOLD-fMRI signals, 34
clinical applications
basal ganglia circuits, 41
basilar artery, 40
BCI technology, 37
cerebellum, 37
DTI, 41
finger-tapping task, 37, 40
functional mapping, 37
magnetic field strength, 39
PAG, 41
pre-surgical fMRI, 42
visually guided finger-tapping paradigm, 37
gradient-echo EPI sequences, 33
HSE BOLD signal, 33
limitations, 29–30
maximum physiological noise contribution, 35
memory-encoding task, 35
RF coils, 34
7-T fMRI, 30
SNR and BOLD signal, 31
thermal and physiological noise, 33
3D GRASE, 33
3D-EPI, 34
tissue-air boundaries, 32
Uncal sulcus, 367
Uncus, 365
Unified segmentation, 99

V

Velocity-selective arterial spin labeling (VSASL), 75
Verbal memory, 253
Verbal memory outcome, medial temporal lobe FMRI
language lateralization, 253–256
memory outcome predictor, 248–250, 252
Visual network, 339, 340
Visual word form area (VWFA), 142
Voxel-scaled brain, 120
Voxel-to-world mapping, 93

W

Wada memory test, 249
Wechsler Memory Scale, 253
Weighted least squares (WLS), 108
West syndrome, 186
Writing-induced seizures, 203

MIX
Papier aus verantwortungsvollen Quellen
Paper from responsible sources
FSC® C105338

If you have any concerns about our products,
you can contact us on
ProductSafety@springernature.com

In case Publisher is established outside the EU,
the EU authorized representative is:
Springer Nature Customer Service Center GmbH
Europaplatz 3, 69115 Heidelberg, Germany

Printed by Libri Plureos GmbH
in Hamburg, Germany